Ten Cate's

Oral Histology

Development, Structure, and Function

10th EDITION

Ten Cate's Oral Histology

Development, Structure, and Function

Antonio Nanci, PhD (McGill), PhD *Honoris causa* (University of Messina)
Professor and Canada Research Chair in Calcified Tissues, Biomaterials, and Structural Imaging
Department of Stomatology,
Faculty of Dental Medicine
Accredited with the Department of Biochemistry and Molecular Medicine,
Faculty of Medicine
Université de Montréal
Montréal, Quebec, Canada

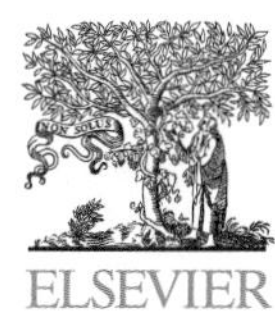

Elsevier
3251 Riverport Lane
St. Louis, Missouri 63043

TEN CATE'S ORAL HISTOLOGY: DEVELOPMENT, STRUCTURE, AND FUNCTION,
TENTH EDITION ISBN: 978-0-323-79895-2

Senior Content Strategist: Kelly Skelton
Senior Content Development Specialist: Sneha Kashyap
Publishing Services Manager: Deepthi Unni
Project Manager: Sindhuraj Thulasingam
Designer: Ryan Cook

Printed in India

Last digit is the print number: 9 8 7 6 5 4 3 2 1

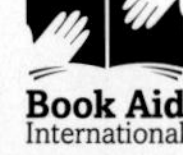

A particular thought goes to the ladies in my life—Irene, Kassandra, and Miriam—and charming little grandson "big boy" Émile.

Also, my heartfelt gratitude goes to my mentors—Feridoun Babaï (Université de Montréal), Hershey Warshawsky (McGill), and Harold C. Slavkin (University of Southern California)—who have shared with me their wisdom, enthusiasm, knowledge, and expertise that helped shape my career.

LIST OF CONTRIBUTORS

Florin Amzica, PhD
Associate Professor
Department of Stomatology,
Faculty of Dental Medicine
Department of Neurosciences,
Faculty of Medicine
Université de Montréal
Montreal, Quebec, Canada

James K. Hartsfield Jr., DMD, MS, MMSc, PhD
E. Preston Hicks Endowed Professor of Orthodontics and Oral Health Research
Department of Oral Health Science
University of Kentucky College of Dentistry
Lexington, Kentucky;
Volunteer Clinical Professor
Department of Orthodontics and Oral Facial Genetics
Indiana University School of Dentistry
Indianapolis, Indiana;
Adjunct Professor
Department of Oral Development and Behavioural Sciences
University of Western Australia Dental School
Perth, Western Australia, Australia;
Lecturer
Department of Developmental Biology
Harvard School of Dental Medicine
Boston, Massachusetts;
Adjunct Professor
Dental Medicine in Orthodontics
Touro College of Dental Medicine
Touro University
Hawthorne, New York

Jimmy K. Hu, PhD
Assistant Professor
School of Dentistry
University of California–Los Angeles
Los Angeles, California

Ophir Klein, MD, PhD
Adjunct Professor
Department of Craniofacial Biology
University of California–San Francisco
San Francisco, California;
Executive Director
Cedars-Sinai Guerin Children's
Los Angeles, California

Pierre Moffatt, PhD
Associate Professor
Shriners Hospitals for Children–Canada;
Faculty of Dental Medicine and Oral Health Sciences
McGill University
Montreal, Quebec, Canada

Antonio Nanci, PhD (McGill), PhD Honoris causa (University of Messina)
Professor and Canada Research Chair in Calcified Tissues, Biomaterials, and Structural Imaging
Department of Stomatology,
Faculty of Dental Medicine
Accredited with the Department of Biochemistry and Molecular Medicine,
Faculty of Medicine
Université de Montréal
Montréal, Quebec, Canada

Clarice Nishio, DDS, MSc, PhD, FRCD(C)
Associate Professor
Department of Oral Health,
Faculty of Dentistry
Université de Montréal
Montreal, Quebec, Canada

Ravi L. Rungta, PhD
Assistant Professor
Department of Stomatology,
Faculty of Dental Medicine
Department of Neurosciences,
Faculty of Medicine
Université de Montréal
Montreal, Quebec, Canada

Barry Sessle, MDS, PhD, DSc(hc)
Professor
Faculty of Dentistry and Department of Physiology,
Temerty Faculty of Medicine, and Centre for The Study of Pain
University of Toronto
Toronto, Ontario, Canada

Simon D. Tran, DMD, PhD
Professor
Faculty of Dental Medicine and Oral Health Sciences
McGill University
Montreal, Quebec, Canada

PREFACE

The first edition of *Oral Histology: Development, Structure, and Function* appeared in 1980 and was edited by A.R. Ten Cate. The textbook was subsequently renamed *Ten Cate's Oral Histology: Development, Structure, and Function* (6th edition) in 2003 in recognition of his contributions to oral histology and oral health. The present edition celebrates 44 years of a didactic style that remains fully relevant today and that has helped train multiple generations of oral health practitioners and researchers throughout the world.

The scope of this new edition remains to provide a solid treatise in oral histology with emphasis on structure–function relationships. Molecular concepts are integrated to help understand genes and mechanisms implicated in embryogenesis, development, cell function, and matrix events. The updates in information, in some cases, may appear subtle, and in others they are more significant. Boxed texts by key protagonists have been added to provide broader pictures, present novel concepts that may appear opposing and will likely continue to evolve, and discuss topics of clinical relevance.

Finally, I sincerely believe that, within the limits and purpose of an educational text, it is most important to keep an open mind.

Like previous editions, this 10th edition is intended to serve as a learning guide for students in a variety of disciplines. Although coverage is exhaustive, the text has been structured such that individual chapters and even selected sections can be used independently—in this regard, the digital edition will greatly facilitate the search and identification of information of specific interest. The focus continues to be on learning and understanding concepts rather than on memorization of detail, particularly numeric values. Thus dental hygienists, medical students, undergraduate and graduate dental students, and oral health researchers will find a degree of coverage suited for their respective needs.

Finally, a major objective is to sensitize students to the concept that, in addition to being pertinent to clinical practice, better understanding of the development and biology of oral tissues is expected to engender novel therapeutic approaches based on biologics that will likely be used by oral health practitioners in the foreseeable future. As progress is logically bound to occur in the coming years, the future practice of dentistry will inevitably undergo a shift from the traditional restorative approach to one more oriented toward the medical management of patients.

ACKNOWLEDGMENTS

The present edition builds on material from previous editions provided over the years by various contributors. I am most grateful to P. Mark Bartold, Paolo Bianco, Anne C. Dale, Jack G. Dale, Dale R. Eisenmann, Donald H. Enlow, Michael W. Finkelstein, Eric Freeman, Arthur R. Hand, Stéphane Roy, Paul T. Sharpe, Martha J. Somerman, Christopher A. Squier, Calvin D. Torneck, and S. William Whitson for their excellent past contributions. More recently, Shingo Kuroda, Matthieu Schmittbuhl, Eiji Tanaka, and Daniel Turgeon have also contributed.

Although every effort has been made to have a text free of factual and editorial errors, a few may still have managed to slip through, and for this I apologize. Timely identification of such slips is important, as the digital age now permits corrections to be carried on continuously through digital editions and, in some cases, in new batches of printed textbooks rather than having to wait for a new edition. Educators and students are most welcome to contact me should they find any inaccuracy or ambiguous text or want to share new perspectives.

The personnel who have over the years contributed to generating much of the illustration material deserve special thanks, as the quality of illustrations is ultimately a reflection of their personal talent. I thank Dainelys Guadarrama Bello and Katia J. Ponce for their general assistance with the assembly of text and figures. At Elsevier, I thank Kelly Skelton (Senior Content Strategist), Sneha Kashyap (Senior Content Development Specialist), and Sindhuraj Thulasingam (Project Manager) for their assistance and patience throughout preparation of this 10th edition.

Antonio Nanci

CONTENTS

1

Structure of the Oral Tissues: An Overview

Antonio Nanci

OUTLINE

This chapter presents an overview of the histology of the tooth and its supporting tissues (Fig. 1.1) and the salivary glands, bones of the jaw, and articulations between the jaws (temporomandibular joints [TMJs]) as a basis for subsequent detailed consideration.

THE TOOTH

Teeth constitute approximately 20% of the surface area of the mouth, the upper teeth significantly more than the lower teeth. Mastication is the function most associated with the human dentition, but teeth also are essential for proper speech. In the Animal Kingdom, teeth have important roles as weapons of attack and defense. Teeth must be hard and firmly attached to the bones of the jaws to fulfill most of these functions. In most submammalian vertebrates the teeth are fused directly to the jawbone. Although this construction provides a firm attachment, such teeth frequently are broken and lost during normal function. In these cases, many successional teeth form to compensate for tooth loss and to ensure continued function of the dentition.

The tooth proper consists of a hard, inert, acellular enamel formed by epithelial cells and supported by the less mineralized, more resilient, and vital hard connective tissue dentin, which is formed and supported by the dental pulp, a soft connective tissue (Fig. 1.2; see also Fig. 1.1). In mammals, teeth are attached to the jaw by tooth-supporting connective tissues consisting of cementum, periodontal ligament (PDL), and alveolar bone, which provide enough flexibility to withstand the forces of mastication. In human beings and most mammals, a limited succession of teeth still occurs, not to compensate for continual loss of teeth but to accommodate the growth of the face and jaws. The face and jaws of a human child are small and consequently can carry fewer teeth of smaller size. These smaller teeth constitute the deciduous or primary dentition. A large increase in the size of the jaws occurs with growth, necessitating not only more teeth but also larger ones. Because the size of teeth cannot increase after they are formed, the deciduous dentition becomes inadequate and must be replaced by a permanent or secondary dentition consisting of more and larger teeth.

Anatomically, the tooth consists of a crown and a root (see Figs 1.1 and 1.2); the junction between the two is the cervical margin. The term *clinical crown* denotes that part of the tooth that is visible in the oral cavity. Although teeth vary considerably in shape and size (e.g., an incisor compared with a molar), histologically they are similar.

Enamel

Enamel is an eccentric hard tissue because of its origin, its chemically distinct nature of the various noncollagenous matrix proteins expressed by ameloblasts, and its large mineral crystals. Enamel has evolved as an epithelial-derived protective covering for the crown of the teeth (see Figs. 1.1 and 1.2). The enamel is the most highly mineralized tissue in the body, consisting of more than 96% inorganic material in the form of apatite crystals and traces of organic material. The cells responsible for the formation of enamel (ameloblasts) cover the entire surface of the layer as it forms but are lost as the tooth emerges into the oral cavity. The loss of these cells renders enamel a nonvital and insensitive matrix that, when destroyed by any means (usually wear or caries), cannot be replaced or regenerated. To compensate for this inherent limitation, enamel has acquired a high degree of mineralization and a complex organization. These structural and compositional features allow enamel to withstand large masticatory forces and continual assaults by acids from food and bacterial sources. The apatite crystals within enamel pack together differentially to create a structure of enamel rods separated by interrod enamel (Fig. 1.3). Although enamel is a dead tissue in a strict biologic sense, it is permeable; ionic exchange can occur between the enamel and the environment of the oral cavity, in particular the saliva.

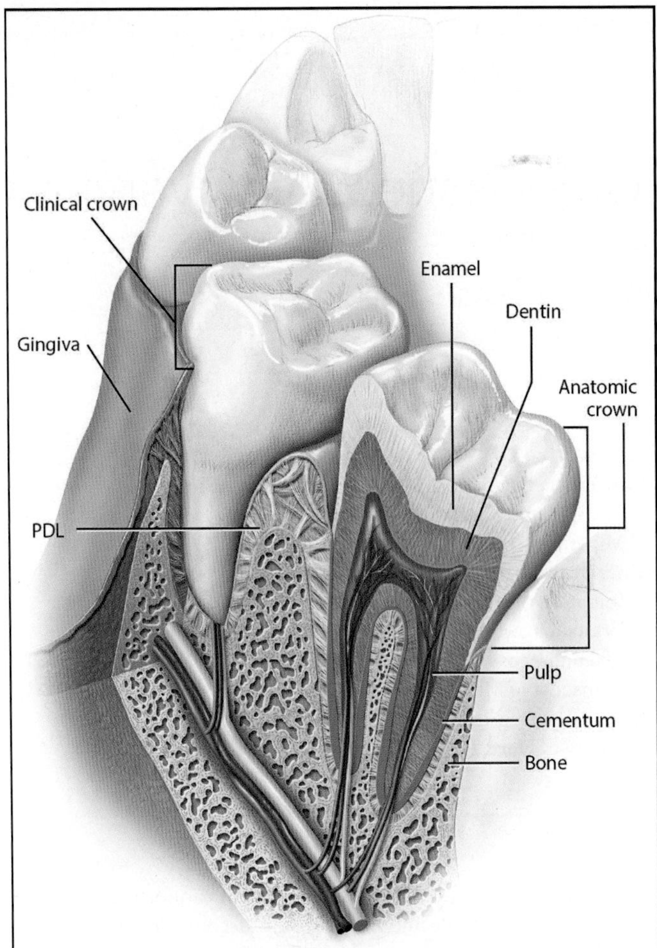

Fig. 1.1 The tooth and its supporting structure. *PDL*, Periodontal ligament.

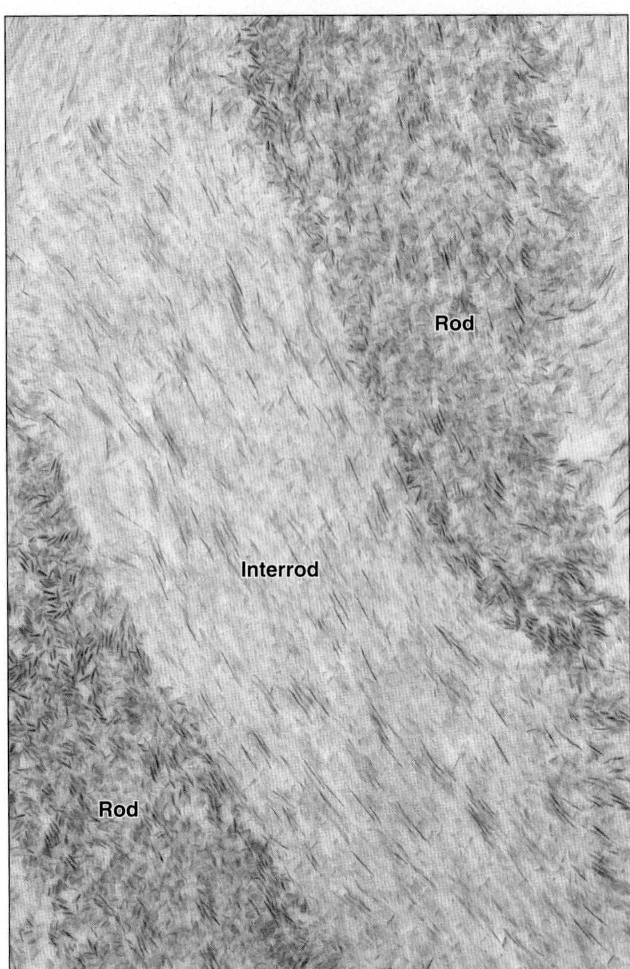

Fig. 1.3 Enamel. Electron micrograph showing that enamel consists of crystallites organized into rod and interrod enamel.

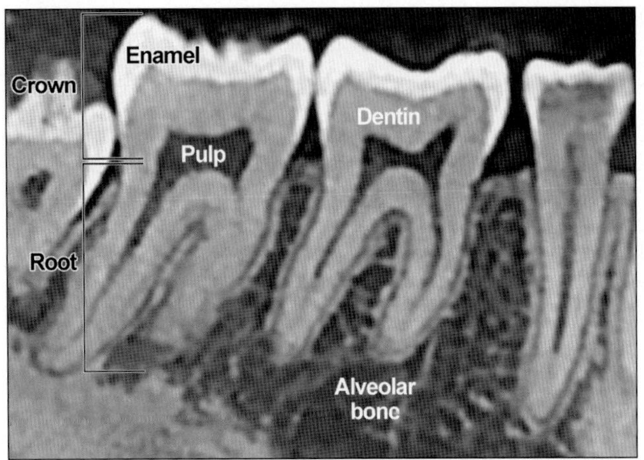

Fig. 1.2 Vertical cone beam computed tomography slice of mandibular molars and premolars. (Courtesy M. Schmittbuhl.)

Dentin

Because of its exceptionally high mineral content, enamel is a brittle tissue that cannot withstand the forces of mastication without fracture unless it has the support of a more resilient tissue, such as dentin. Dentin forms the bulk of the tooth, supports the enamel, and compensates for its brittleness.

Dentin is a mineralized, elastic, yellow-white, avascular tissue enclosing the central pulp chamber (Fig. 1.4; see also Figs. 1.1 and 1.2). The mineral is also apatite, and the organic component is mainly the fibrillar protein collagen. A characteristic feature of dentin is its permeation by closely packed tubules traversing its entire thickness and containing the cytoplasmic extensions of the cells that once formed it and later maintain it (see Fig. 1.4B). These cells are called *odontoblasts*; their cell bodies are aligned along the inner edge of the dentin, where they form the peripheral boundary of the dental pulp (see Fig. 1.4A). The very existence of odontoblasts makes dentin a vastly different tissue from enamel. Dentin is a sensitive tissue, and, more importantly, it is capable of repair because odontoblasts or cells in the pulp can be stimulated to deposit more dentin as the occasion demands.

Pulp

The central pulp chamber, enclosed by dentin, is filled with a soft connective tissue called *pulp* (see Fig. 1.4A). Dentin is a hard tissue; the pulp is soft (and is lost in dried teeth, leaving a clearly recognizable empty chamber). Despite distinctive histologic features, dentin and pulp are related embryologically and functionally and should be considered together. This unity is exemplified by the classic functions of pulp: It is (1) formative in that it produces the dentin that surrounds it; (2) nutritive in that it nourishes the avascular dentin; (3) protective in that it carries nerves that give dentin its sensitivity; and (4) reparative in that it is capable of producing new dentin when required.

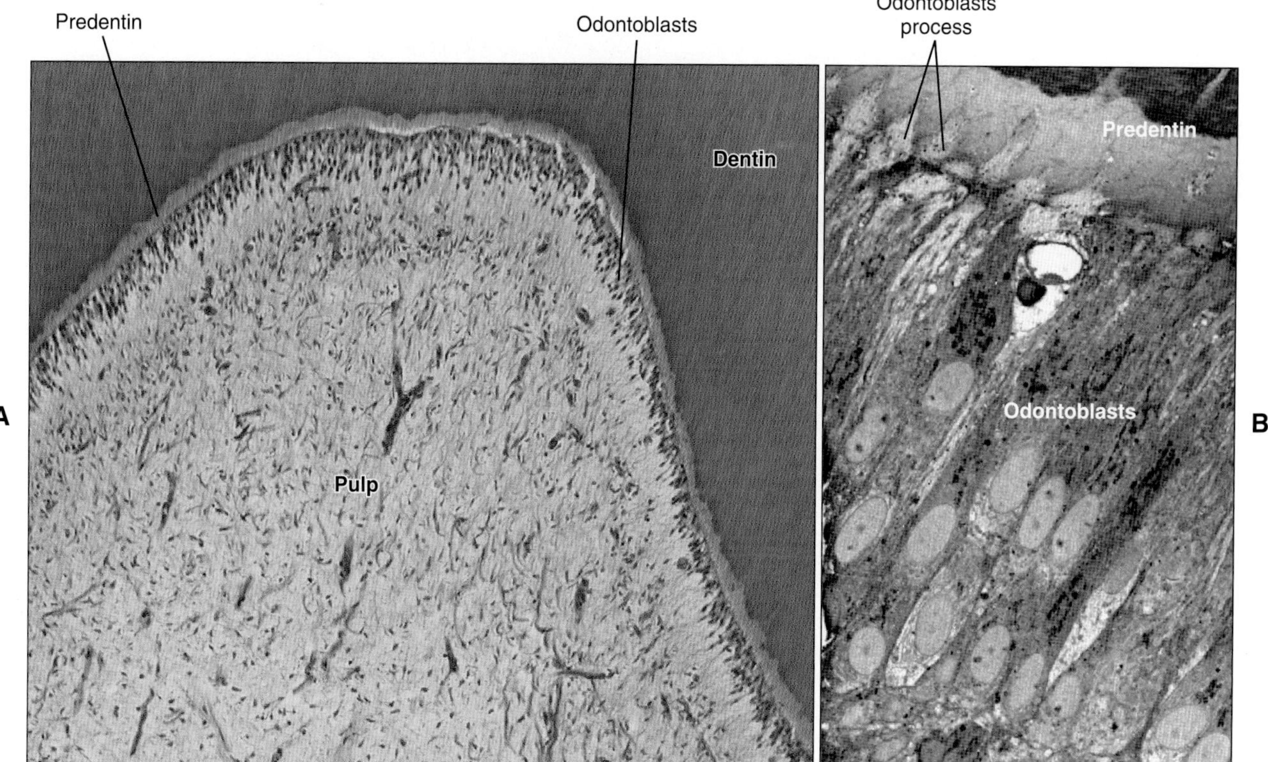

Fig. 1.4 Dentin and pulp. (A) The odontoblasts (cells that form dentin) line the pulp. (B) At higher magnification, these cells show processes extending into dentin.

In summary, the tooth proper consists of two hard tissues: the acellular enamel and the supporting dentin. The latter is a specialized connective tissue, the formative cells of which are in the pulp. These tissues bestow on teeth the properties of hardness and resilience. Their indestructibility also gives teeth special importance in paleontology and forensic science, for example, as a means of identification.

SUPPORTING TISSUES OF THE TOOTH

The tooth is attached to the jaw by a specialized supporting apparatus that consists of the alveolar bone, the PDL, and the cementum, all of which are protected by the gingiva (Fig. 1.5; also see Fig. 1.1).

Periodontal Ligament

The PDL is a highly specialized connective tissue situated between the tooth and the alveolar bone (see Fig. 1.5). The principal function of the PDL is to connect the tooth to the jaw, which it must do in such a way that the tooth will withstand the considerable forces of mastication. This requirement is met by the collagen fiber bundles that span the distance between the bone and the tooth and by ground substance between them. At one extremity the fibers of the PDL are embedded in bone; at the other extremity they are embedded in cementum. Each collagen fiber bundle is much like a spliced rope in which individual strands can be remodeled continually without the overall fiber losing its architecture and function. In this way the collagen fiber bundles can adapt to the stresses placed on them. The PDL has another important function, a sensory one. Tooth enamel is an inert tissue and therefore insensitive, yet the moment teeth come into contact with each other, we know it. Part of this sense of discrimination is provided by sensory receptors within the PDL.

Cementum

Cementum covers the roots of the teeth and is interlocked firmly with the dentin of the root (see Figs. 1.1, 1.2, and 1.5B). Cementum is a mineralized connective tissue similar to bone except that it is avascular; the mineral is also apatite, and the organic matrix contains collagen. The cells that form cementum are called *cementoblasts.*

The two main types of cementum are cellular and acellular. The cementum attached to the root dentin and covering the upper (cervical) portion of the root is acellular and thus is called *acellular (primary) cementum.* The lower (apical) portion of the root is covered by cellular (secondary) cementum. In this case, cementoblasts become trapped in lacunae within their own matrix, much like osteocytes occupy lacunae in bone; these entrapped cells are now called *cementocytes.* Acellular cementum anchors PDL fiber bundles to the tooth; cellular cementum has an adaptive role. Bone, the PDL, and cementum together form a functional unit of special importance when orthodontic tooth movement is undertaken.

ORAL MUCOSA

The oral cavity is lined by a mucous membrane that consists of two layers: an epithelium and subjacent connective tissue (the lamina propria) (Fig. 1.6). Although its major functions are lining and protecting, the mucosa also is modified to serve as an exceptionally mobile tissue that permits free movement of the lip and cheek muscles. In other locations it serves as the organ of taste.

Histologically, the oral mucosa can be classified into three types: (1) masticatory, (2) lining, and (3) specialized. The masticatory mucosa covers the gingiva and hard palate. The masticatory mucosa is bound down tightly by the lamina propria to the underlying bone (see Fig. 1.6B),

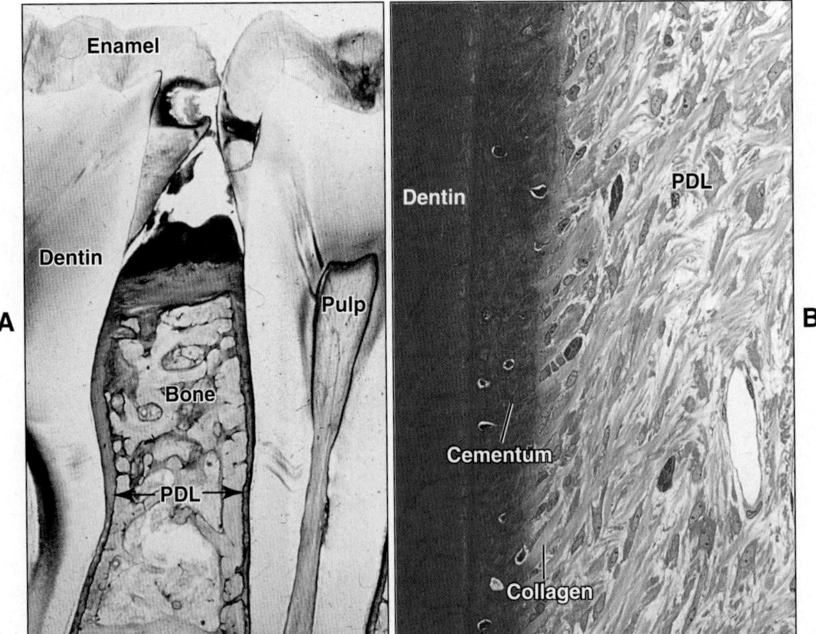

Fig. 1.5 Histologic sections of the periodontal ligament *(PDL)*. (A) Supporting apparatus of the tooth in longitudinal section. (B) At higher magnification, note the fibrocellular nature of the PDL.

and the covering epithelium is keratinized to withstand the constant pounding of food during mastication. The lining mucosa, by contrast, must be as flexible as possible to perform its function of protection. The epithelium is not keratinized; the lamina propria is structured for mobility and is not tightly bound to underlying structures (see Fig. 1.6C). The dorsal surface of the tongue is covered by a specialized mucosa consisting of a highly extensible masticatory mucosa containing papillae and taste buds.

A unique feature of the oral mucosa is that the teeth perforate it. This anatomic feature has profound implications in the initiation of periodontal disease. The teeth are the only structures that perforate epithelium anywhere in the body. Nails and hair are epithelial appendages around which epithelial continuity is always maintained. This perforation by teeth means that a sealing junction must be established between the gum and the tooth.

The mucosa immediately surrounding an erupted tooth is the gingiva. In functional terms the gingiva consists of two parts: (1) the part facing the oral cavity, which is masticatory mucosa, and (2) the part facing the tooth, which is involved in attaching the gingiva to the tooth and forms part of the periodontium. The junction of the oral mucosa and the tooth is permeable, and thus antigens can pass easily through it and initiate inflammation in gum tissue (marginal gingivitis).

SALIVARY GLANDS

Saliva is a complex fluid that, in health, almost continually bathes the parts of the tooth exposed within the oral cavity. Consequently, saliva represents the immediate environment of the tooth. Saliva is produced by three paired sets of major salivary glands (parotid, submandibular, and sublingual) and by the many minor salivary glands scattered throughout the oral cavity. A precise account of the composition of saliva is difficult because not only are the secretions of each of the major and minor salivary glands different, but their volume may vary at any given time. In recognition of this variability, the term *mixed saliva* has been used to describe the fluid of the oral cavity. Regardless of its precise composition, saliva has several functions. Saliva moistens the mouth, facilitates speech, lubricates food, and helps with taste by acting as a solvent for food molecules. Saliva also contains a digestive enzyme (amylase). Saliva not only dilutes noxious material mistakenly taken into the mouth, it also cleanses the mouth. Furthermore, it contains antibodies and antimicrobial substances, and by virtue of its buffering capacity plays an important role in maintaining the pH of the oral cavity.

The basic histologic structure of the major salivary glands is similar. A salivary gland may be likened to a bunch of grapes. Each so-called grape is the acinus (terminal secretory unit), which is a mass of secretory cells surrounding a central space. The spaces of the acini open into ducts running through the gland that are called successively the *intercalated, striated,* and *excretory ducts* (Fig. 1.7), analogous to the stalks and stems of a bunch of grapes. These ducts are more than passive conduits, however; their lining cells have a function in determining the final composition of saliva.

The ducts and acini constitute the parenchyma of the gland, the whole of which is invested by a connective tissue stroma carrying blood vessels and nerves. This connective tissue supports each individual acinus and divides the gland into a series of lobes or lobules, finally encapsulating it (Fig. 1.8).

BONES OF THE JAW

As stated, teeth are attached to bone by the PDL (see Figs 1.1 and 1.5A). This bone, the alveolar bone, constitutes the alveolar process, which is in continuity with the basal bone of the jaws. The alveolar process forms in relation to teeth. When teeth are lost, the alveolar process is gradually lost as well, creating the characteristic facial profile of the edentulous person whose chin and nose approximate because of a reduction in facial height. Although the histologic structure of the alveolar process is essentially the same as that of the basal bone, practically it is necessary to distinguish between the two. The position of teeth and supporting tissues, which include the alveolar process, can be modified easily by orthodontic therapy. However, modification of

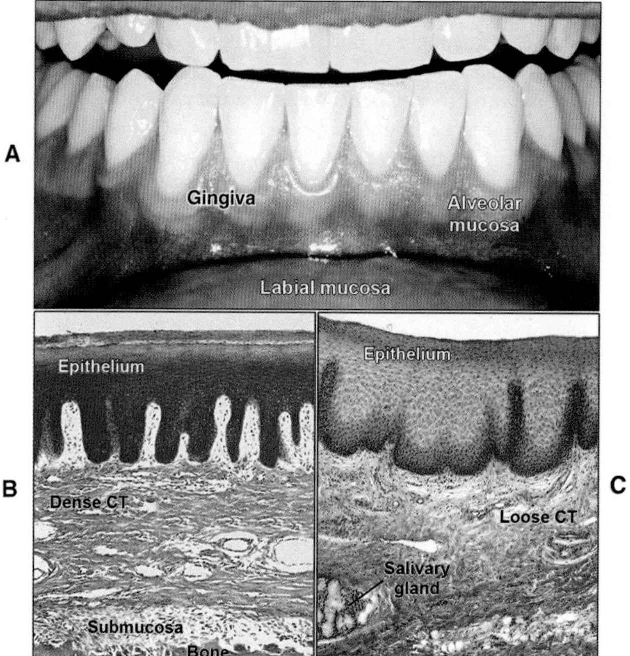

Fig. 1.6 Oral mucosa. (A) Note the difference between tightly bound mucosa of the gingiva (gum) and mobile mucosa of the labial sulcus (alveolar mucosa). (B) In histologic sections, the gingival epithelium is seen to be supported by dense connective tissue *(CT),* whereas the epithelium of the lip (C) is supported by a much looser connective tissue.

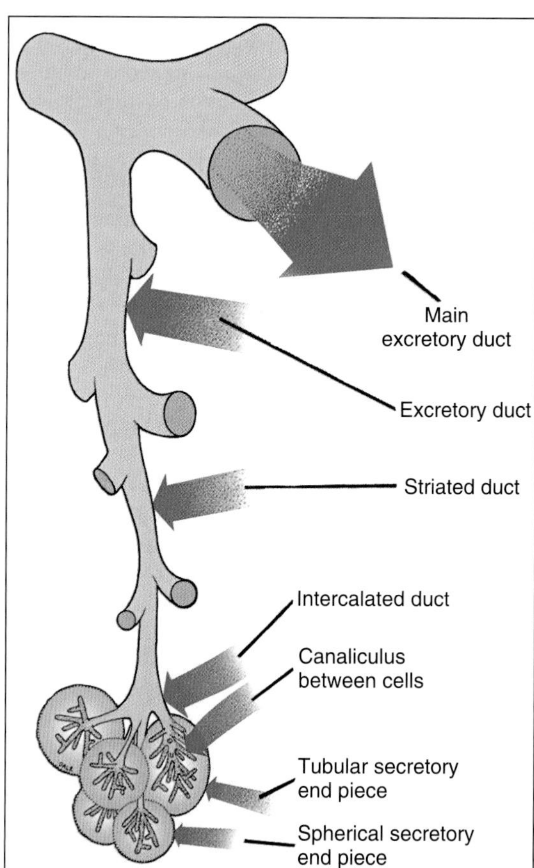

Fig. 1.7 Diagrammatic illustration of the ductal system of a salivary gland.

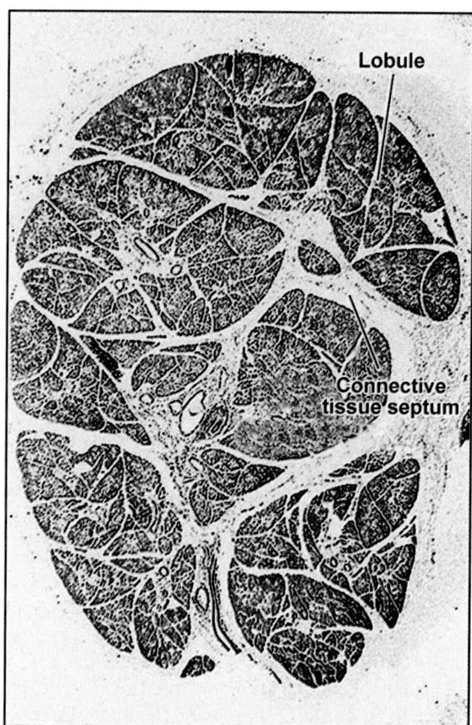

Fig. 1.8 Low-power photomicrograph of a salivary gland showing its lobular organization.

the position of the basal bone is usually much more difficult; this can be achieved only by influencing its growth. The way these bones grow is thus important in determining the position of the jaws and teeth.

TEMPOROMANDIBULAR JOINT

The relationship between the bones of the upper and lower jaws is maintained by the articulation of the condylar process of the mandible with the glenoid fossa of the temporal bone. This articulation, the TMJ, is a synovial joint with special features that permit the complex movements associated with mastication. The specialization of the TMJ is reflected in its histologic appearance (Fig. 1.9). The TMJ cavity is formed by a fibrous capsule lined with a synovial membrane and is separated into two compartments by an extension of the capsule to form a specialized movable disk. The articular surfaces of the bone are covered not by hyaline cartilage but by a fibrous layer that is a continuation of the periosteum covering the individual bones. A simplified way to understand the function of the TMJ is to consider it as a joint with the articular disk being a movable articular surface.

HARD TISSUE FORMATION

The hard tissues of the body—bone, cementum, dentin, and enamel—are associated with the functioning tooth. Because the practice of dentistry involves manipulation of these tissues, a detailed knowledge of them is obligatory (and each is discussed separately in later chapters). The purposes of this section are (1) to explain that a number of common features are associated with hard tissue formation, even though the final products are structurally distinct; (2) to indicate that the functional role of a number of these features is still not fully understood; and (3) to describe the common mechanism of hard tissue breakdown.

Three (i.e., bone, cementum, and dentin) of the four hard tissues in the body have many similarities in their composition and formation. They are specialized connective tissues, and collagen (principally type

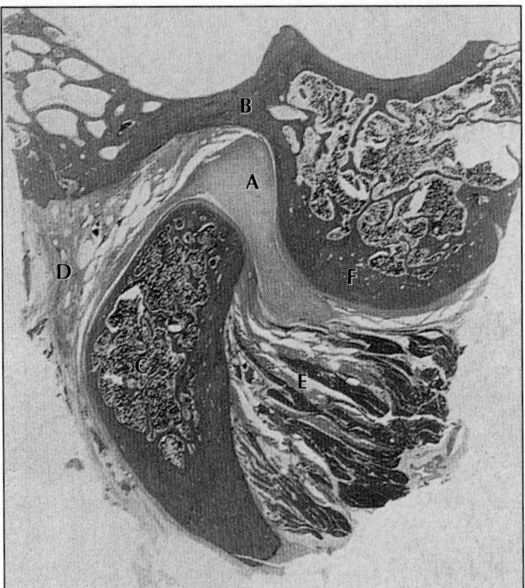

Fig. 1.9 Sagittal section through the temporomandibular joint. The disc (dividing the joint cavity into upper and lower compartments) is apparent. *A*, Intraarticular disc; *B*, mandibular (glenoid) fossa; *C*, condyle of mandible; *D*, capsule; *E*, lateral pterygoid muscle; *F*, articular eminence. (From Berkovitz BKB, et al.: *Oral anatomy, histology, and embryology*, ed 3, London, 2002, Mosby.)

I) plays a large role in determining their structure. Although enamel is not a connective tissue, and no collagen is involved in its makeup, its formation still follows many of the principles involved in the formation of hard connective tissue. Hard tissue formation may be summarized as the production by cells of an organic matrix capable of accommodating mineral. This rather simple concept, however, embraces complex events. How mineralization takes place is presented later.

The Organic Matrix in Hard Tissues

A hallmark of calcified tissues is the various matrix proteins that attract and organize calcium and phosphate ions into a structured mineral phase based on carbonated apatite. The formative blast cells of calcified tissues produce the organic matrix constituents that interact with the mineral phase. These cells specialize in protein synthesis and secretion, and they exhibit a polarized organization for vectorial secretion and appositional deposition of matrix proteins.

Of great interest is the fact that the proteins involved in these hard tissues, with one exception (enamel), are similar, comprising a predominant supporting meshwork of type I collagen with various added noncollagenous proteins functioning primarily as modulators of mineralization. Table 1.1 provides a comparative analysis of the characteristics of the various calcified tissues. This basic similarity of constituents is consistent with the general role of collagen-based hard tissues in providing rigid structural support and protection of soft tissues in vertebrates. Enamel has evolved to function specifically as an abrasion-resistant, protective coating that relies on its uniquely large mineral crystals for function. The organic matrix of enamel consists essentially of noncollagenous proteins that have no scaffolding role. However, enamel is not the only calcified tissue without collagen. Mineralization of cementum situated along the cervical margin of the tooth occurs within a matrix composed largely of noncollagenous matrix proteins also found in bone. In invertebrates, the shell of mollusks consists of laminae of calcium carbonate separated by a thin layer of organic material (acidic macromolecules, etc.).

Mineral

The inorganic component of mineralized tissues consists of hydroxyapatite, represented as $Ca_{10}(PO_4)_6(OH)_2$ and which has undergone substitutions with other ions. This formula indicates only the atomic content of a conceptual entity known as the *unit cell*, which is the least number of calcium, phosphate, and hydroxyl ions able to establish stable relationships. The unit cell of biologic apatite is hexagonal; when stacked together, these cells form the lattice of a crystal. The number of repetitions of this arrangement produces crystals of various sizes. Generally, the crystals are described as needlelike or platelike and, in the case of enamel, as long, thin ribbons. An unstable amorphous calcium phosphate phase may precede the formation of crystals.

Each apatite crystal has three compartments: the crystal interior, the crystal surface, and a layer of water called the *hydration shell*, all of which are available for the exchange of ions. Thus magnesium and sodium can substitute in the calcium position, fluoride and chloride in the hydroxyl position, and carbonate in the hydroxyl and phosphate positions. Fluoride substitution decreases the solubility of the crystals, whereas carbonate increases it. Magnesium inhibits crystal growth. The apatite crystal can retain its structural configuration while accommodating these substitutions.

In summary, biologic apatite is built on a definite ionic lattice pattern that permits considerable variation in its composition through substitution, exchange, and adsorption of ions. This pattern of ionic variability reflects the immediate environment of the crystal and is used clinically to modify the structure of crystals by exposing them to a fluoride-rich environment.

MINERALIZATION

Over the past few years there has been a shift in the perception of biologic mineralization, from a physiologic process highly dependent on sustained active promotion to one relying more on rate-limiting activities, including release from inhibition of mineralization (Box 1.1). Essentially, when calcium phosphate deposition is initiated, the crux is then to control spontaneous precipitation from tissue fluids supersaturated in calcium and phosphate ions and to limit it to well-defined sites. Formative cells achieve this by creating microenvironments that facilitate mineral ion handling and by secreting proteins that stabilize calcium and phosphate ions in body fluids and/or control their deposition onto a receptive extracellular matrix. Genome sequencing and gene mapping have shown that several of these proteins are located on the same chromosome and that there is synteny across several species.

Collectively, these proteins are referred to as the secretory calcium-binding phosphoprotein gene cluster that comprises (1) salivary proteins, (2) some enamel matrix proteins, and (3) bone/cementum/dentin matrix proteins. These proteins derive from the duplication and diversification of a common ancestral gene during evolution, with an enamel-related gene as an early intermediate in the process.

Initiation of Mineralization

Two mechanisms have been proposed for initiating mineralization of hard connective tissue. The first involves a structure called the *matrix vesicle* (Fig. 1.10), and the second is *heterogeneous nucleation*.

Matrix vesicles, first reported in 1967, have had an interesting history since their discovery, initially questioned as an artifact of tissue preparation. They are found in initial dentin, cementum, bone, and cartilage but not tooth enamel. Their abundance varies, and their detectability can be physiologically modulated (hypocalcemia); thus they appear to represent a *bona fide* entity but their exact role is questioned.

TABLE 1.1 Comparative Relationship Between Vertebrate Hard Tissues

	Enamel	Dentin	Fibrillar Cementum	Bone
Major Matrix Proteins				
Types	Amelogenin (several isoforms)	Collagen (type I) (+ type III, traces of V, VI)	Collagen (type I) (+ type III, XII, traces of V, VI, XIV)	Collagen (type I) (+ type III, traces of V, XII, XIV)
Conformation	Globular supramolecular aggregates; ribbons?	Random fibrils	Fibrils • Bundles (AEFC) • Sheets (CIFC)	Fibrils as random • Random (woven) • Sheets (lamellar)
Other Matrix Proteins				
	Nonamelogenins	Noncollagenous	Noncollagenous	Noncollagenous
Types	1. Ameloblastin	1. Dentin sialophosphoprotein as transcript • Dentin glycoprotein • Dentin phosphoprotein • Dentin sialoprotein	1. Bone sialoprotein	1. Bone sialoprotein
	2. Enamelin 3. Sulfated protein	2. Dentin matrix protein 1 3. Bone sialoprotein 4. Osteopontin 5. Osteocalcin 6. Osteonectin 7. Matrix extracellular phosphoglycoprotein	2. Osteopontin 3. Osteocalcin 4. Osteonectin 5. Dentin matrix protein 1 6. Dentin sialoprotein	2. Osteopontin 3. Osteocalcin 4. Osteonectin 5. Bone acidic glycoprotein-75 6. Dentin matrix protein 1 7. Dentin sialophosphoprotein as transcript 8. Matrix extracellular phosphoglycoprotein
Status of matrix proteins	Degraded along with amelogenins	Remain in matrix; also some present in peritubular dentin	Remain in matrix, but some may be degraded; also present in resting lines	Remain in matrix, but some may be degraded; also present in resting and reversal lines
Proteoglycans				
	Controversial	SLRP	SLRP	SLRP
Matrix Proteinases				
	1. MMP-20 (enamelysin) 2. KLK-4	Collagen-processing enzymes and others needed to degrade matrix	Collagen-processing enzymes and others needed to degrade matrix	Collagen-processing enzymes and others needed to degrade matrix
Mineral				
	Hydroxyapatite >90% ribbons (R) expand (mature crystallites can be millimeters in length)	Hydroxyapatite 67% Uniform small plates	Hydroxyapatite 45%–50% Uniform small plates	Hydroxyapatite 50%–60% Uniform small plates
Location of mineral	Between amelogenin nanospheres; related to ribbons?	Inside, at periphery, and between type I collagen fibril	Inside, at periphery, and between type I collagen fibril	Inside, at periphery, and between type I collagen fibril
Nucleated from	Controversial—Amelogenins? Nonamelogenins? Dentin?	Matrix vesicles then moving mineralization front, although additional mechanisms are most likely involved	Matrix vesicles then moving mineralization front, although additional mechanisms are most likely involved	Matrix vesicles then moving mineralization front, although additional mechanisms are most likely involved (See Boxes 1.1 and 1.2)
Prematrix				
	None present; crystallites abut plasma membrane of ameloblasts	Always present	Always present; usually very thin	Present only during formative phase

Continued

TABLE 1.1 Comparative Relationship Between Vertebrate Hard Tissues—cont'd

	Enamel	Dentin	Fibrillar Cementum	Bone
Growth Type				
	Appositional	Appositional	Appositional	Appositional
Cells				
Formative	Ameloblasts very tall and thin; multiple morphologies	Odontoblasts tall with long cytoplasmic processes	Cementoblasts short	Osteoblasts short
Microenvironment	Putatively sealed by secretory and ruffle-ended ameloblasts; leaky relative to smooth-ended ameloblasts	Incomplete, leaky junctions; cells act as limiting membrane	Cells widely spaced	No junctions at the level of the cell body; cells act as limiting membrane
Lifespan of formative cells	Limited to time until crown erupts	For life of tooth with gradual loss as pulp chamber occludes	Probably for life of tooth	Limited; associated with appositional growth phase
Maintenance	None	Odontoblast process	Cementocytes	Osteocytes
Lifespan of maintenance cells	NA	For life of tooth, with gradual loss as pulp chamber occludes	Limited by overall thickness of the layer	Long until area of bone undergoes turnover
Degradative	None per se; cells secrete proteinases	Odontoclasts	Odontoclasts/cementoclasts	Osteoclasts (limited lifespan)

Dentin, fibrillar cementum, and bone are collagen-based tissues. Enamel is outside rather than inside the body. Enamel, dentin, and cementum are not vascularized, and they do not turn over. Enamel, dentin, and primary cementum are acellular, but dentin contains the large, arborizing processes of odontoblasts embedded in the matrix.

AEFC, Acellular extrinsic fiber cementum; *CIFC*, cellular intrinsic fiber cementum; *KLK-4*, kallikrein-4; *MMP*, metalloproteinase; *NA*, not applicable; *SLRP*, small leucine-rich proteoglycans (biglycan, decorin).

From Nanci A, Smith CE: Matrix-mediated mineralization in enamel and the collagen-based hard tissues. In Goldberg M, Boskey A, Robinson C, editors: *Chemistry and biology of mineralized tissues*, Rosemont, IL, 1999, American Academy of Orthopedic Surgeons.

BOX 1.1 The Stenciling Principle of Extracellular Matrix Mineralization

The stenciling principle pertains to multilevel regulation of biologic mineralization within an extracellular matrix, as occurs in bones and teeth.[1] It describes a double-negative process whereby inhibition of inhibitors (i.e., release from inhibition at specific sites [stenciling]) activates/promotes mineralization, whereas the default condition of inhibition alone (without release) prevents mineralization elsewhere in soft connective tissues. It acts across multiple levels from the macroscale (skeleton/dentition vs. soft connective tissues) to the mesoscale (e.g., entheses and the tooth attachment complex where the soft periodontal ligament is situated between mineralized tooth cementum and mineralized alveolar bone), and to the microscale (mineral tessellation). It refers to inhibition of mineralization by both small molecules and proteins and then second level inhibition of these inhibitors by enzymes that degrade the inhibitors to permit and carefully regulate mineralization. The stenciling principle for extracellular matrix mineralization derives from the original pivotal paradigm for negative regulation discovered by Francois Jacob and Jacques Monod in the 1950s and published in 1961. Their paradigm at that time of the double-negative "repressing a repressor" to induce an activation effect—originally explaining genetic regulation of enzyme expression in bacteria—continues today and explains many processes in developmental biology, cancer biology, and even ecology.

The stenciling principle that promotes mineralization of extracellular matrices is best exemplified by two well-documented (mostly in bone, but also to some degree in tooth dentin) enzyme and inhibitor substrate relationships. The first inhibition-of-an-inhibitor relationship exists as an enzyme-substrate pair consisting of the enzyme tissue-nonspecific alkaline phosphatase (TNAP, TNSALP, ALPL), which degrades the inhibitory substrate small biomolecule pyrophosphate (PP_i). The second inhibition-of-an-inhibitor relationship exists as an enzyme-substrate pair consisting of the enzyme phosphate-regulating endopeptidase homolog X-linked (PHEX), which degrades the inhibitory protein osteopontin (OPN). It is thought that these enzyme-substrate pairs may act sequentially in the order given earlier, with the former providing for initial release from inhibition of mineralization and the latter providing for subsequent finer regulatory control over mineralization of the extracellular matrix. It is expected that other as yet unknown inhibitor-inhibitor pairs exist, and there indeed may be some tissue specificity to other pairs.

To achieve mineralization, the stenciling principle has at its core the notion that cell- and tissue-specific expression of the inhibitor-degrading enzymes occurs by differentiated resident cells at sites of skeletal and dental extracellular matrix production. In the presence of local inhibitory extracellular PP_i and OPN, in concert with appropriate levels of circulating (systemic) calcium and phosphorus mineral ions required for mineralization, gene expression patterns encoding for enzyme production/activity locally stencil early mineralization patterns and trajectories into the extracellular matrix. Mineralization initiates through degradation of inhibitory PP_i by TNAP, then continues through degradation of inhibitory OPN by PHEX. Given the ubiquity of inhibitory PP_i in most, if not all, tissue fluids, it can be considered that this widespread small biomolecule generally inhibits mineralization everywhere as a default pathway of inhibition except for skeletal and dental sites that will be released from this inhibition (stenciled) by PP_i-degrading TNAP. Thus the cells expressing TNAP are osteoblasts and osteocytes in bone, and odontoblasts, cementoblasts, and cementocytes in teeth. Once triggered in the extracellular matrix, mineralization trajectories are further stenciled (regulated) and propagated by OPN-degrading PHEX. Among connective tissue

BOX 1.1 The Stenciling Principle of Extracellular Matrix Mineralization—cont'd

cells, inhibitory OPN is produced most abundantly by bone and tooth cells as a major noncollagenous protein of their respective extracellular matrices, and thus its removal (degradation) is required for release from OPN inhibition such that continued bulk mineralization of extracellular matrix occurs. As part of the PHEX-OPN mineral-stenciling axis, but acting at a very fine scale, is the regulation of mineralization that occurs at the extensive cell-matrix interface found along the lacuno-canalicular network in which osteocytes and their cell processes reside.

In bone, the stenciling principle connects to the patterning of mineralization at the micrometer scale by describing how mineral propagation from small mineralization foci located in the collagenous osteoid subsequently forms a repeating, space-filling structural motif for the mineral, termed *crossfibrillar mineral tessellation.* The pattern first appears at the mineralization front and extends into the bone across its lamellar structure. The microscale mineral formations have been called *tesselles* (French, "tiles"), and they geometrically approximate irregular prolate ellipsoids. Although the tesselles are closely packed, they remain discrete with no complete fusion against their adjacent, abutting tesselle neighbors.

Deviations From the Stenciling Principle Cause Mineralization Defects in Skeletal and Dental Diseases

Hypomineralization of bones and teeth and defective and incomplete bone tessellation structure can be seen in certain single-gene mutation (monogenic) mineralization diseases (osteomalacias/odontomalacias). Consistent with the notions of the stenciling principle, this subset of the skeletal dysplasias manifests as bones and teeth that are soft (hypomineralized) and deformed because of defective mineralization originating from the enzyme mutations. This is caused, in part (there is also renal phosphate wasting in the hypophosphatemias), by an abnormal, unbalanced enzyme-substrate relationship stemming from an inactivating mutation in the enzyme gene that leads to decreased enzyme activity and causes mineralization-inhibiting substrate to accumulate in the extracellular matrix. For two cases of osteomalacia/odontomalacia, the gene for TNAP enzyme is mutated in the case of hypophosphatasia, and the gene for PHEX is mutated in the case of X-linked hypophosphatemia (XLH). Reduced or absent ability of the enzyme to remove its respective mineralization-inhibiting substrate from the extracellular matrix results in local accumulation of the inhibitor, and in the case of XLH, altered systemic mineral ion homeostatic controls, both of which ultimately reduce bone and tooth mineralization to compromise skeletal and dental structure and function. Particularly well-documented for XLH, mutations in the PHEX gene result in increased inhibitory OPN in the extracellular matrix, which prevents nascent mineral tesselles from enlarging such that they do not properly abut against one another and fail to pack into a three-dimensional tessellation pattern that would ensure appropriate stiffness (Box 1.1 Fig. 1). This results in debilitating, incomplete mineral tessellation at the microscale that clinically renders bones deformable under loading.

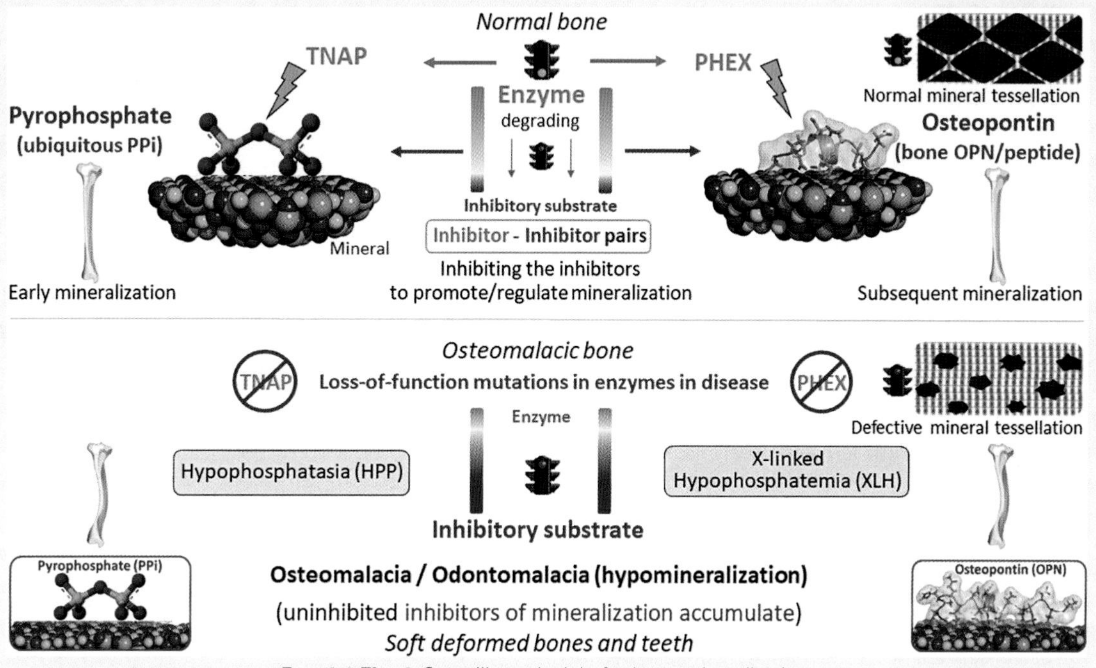

Box 1.1 Fig. 1 Stenciling principle for bone mineralization.

Marc D. McKee, *PhD*
Professor,
Faculty of Dental Medicine and Oral Health Sciences,
Department of Anatomy and Cell Biology,
Faculty of Medicine and Health Sciences,
McGill University,
Montreal, Quebec, Canada

Natalie Reznikov, *PhD, DMD*
Assistant Professor,
Department of Bioengineering,
Faculty of Engineering,
McGill University,
Montreal, Quebec, Canada

[1] From Buss DJ, et al.: Mineral tessellation in bone and the stenciling principle for extracellular matrix mineralization, *J Struct Biol* 214(1):107823, 2022. https://doi.org/10.1016/j.jsb.2021.107823.

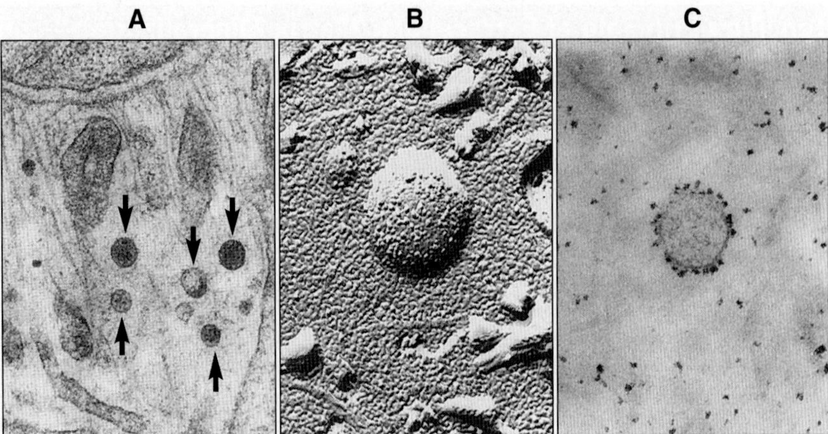

Fig. 1.10 (A) Matrix vesicles *(arrows)* as seen with an electron microscope. (B) Freeze fracture of the vesicle, showing many intramembranous particles thought to represent enzymes. (C) Histochemical demonstration of calcium-adenosine triphosphatase activity on the surface of the vesicle. (From Sasaki T, Garant PR: Structure and organization of odontoblasts, *Anat Rec* 22:235–249, 1996.)

A widely accepted view is that the matrix vesicle is a small, membrane-bound structure that buds off from the cell to form an independent unit within the first-formed organic matrix of hard tissues during initial mineralization. They provide a microenvironment in which proposed mechanisms for initial mineralization exist. Thus it contains alkaline phosphatase, calcium-adenosine triphosphatase, metalloproteinases, proteoglycans, and anionic phospholipids, which can bind calcium and inorganic phosphate and thereby form calcium–inorganic phosphate phospholipid complexes. The first morphologic evidence of a crystallite is seen within this vesicle. These membrane-bound extracellular vesicles have received much attention in the past few years for the biomolecules they contain, including nucleic acids, their ability to affect both physiologic and pathologic cell behavior, and their diagnostic and therapeutic potential.

In the second mechanism, during the formation of collagen-based calcified tissues, deposition of apatite crystals is catalyzed by charged amino acid side chains that line hole zones and channels of molecular assemblages of collagen fibrils (Figs. 1.11 and 1.12). These residues are thought to bind calcium and phosphate ions from solution and bring these ions into proximity so that they may interact to form initial prenucleation clusters and calcium phosphate nuclei inside and on the surface of fibrils. Osteocalcin has also been found at both sites, suggesting it could participate in nucleation and stabilization of mineral ions or phases. Altogether, this event leads to nucleation and the growth of crystals aligned inside collagen or disposed in random arrangements outside fibrils. This process is schematically represented in Fig. 1.13. Eventually, intrafibrillar and extrafibrillar collagen spaces are entirely mineralized, although extrafibrillar volume may vary with species, tissue, and speed of formation of the mineralizing matrix.

The role of type I collagen to mediate vertebrate mineral deposition may thus be modified to include contributions from certain noncollagenous proteins and possibly other molecules. More detailed discussion of the role of collagen in mineralization is presented by Landis et al. (see Recommended Reading). Neither of the two abovementioned mechanisms is involved in the mineralization of enamel; matrix vesicles are absent, and enamel contains no collagen. Initiation of enamel mineralization is believed to be achieved by crystal growth from the already mineralized dentin, by matrix proteins secreted by the ameloblasts, or by both processes.

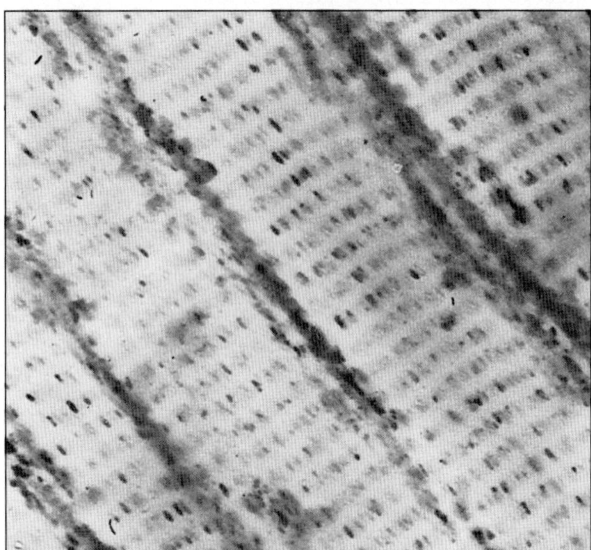

Fig. 1.11 Electron micrograph showing the disposition of crystals in collagen fiber bundles. The gaps in the collagen fibrils are where mineral has been deposited. (From Nylen MU, et al.: Mineralization of turkey leg tendon. II. Collagen-mineral relations revealed by electron and x-ray microscopy. In Sognnaes RF, editor: *Calcification in biological systems* [pub no 64], Washington, DC, 1960, American Association for the Advancement of Science, pp 129–142.)

Crystal Growth

When an apatite crystal has been initiated, its initial growth is rapid but then slows. Several factors influence crystal growth and composition, but especially important is the immediate environment of the growing crystal. For example, noncollagenous proteins can bind selectively to different surfaces of the crystal, preventing further growth and thereby determining the final size of the crystal. The accumulation of inorganic pyrophosphoric acid (pyrophosphate [PP_i]) at the crystal surface also blocks further growth.

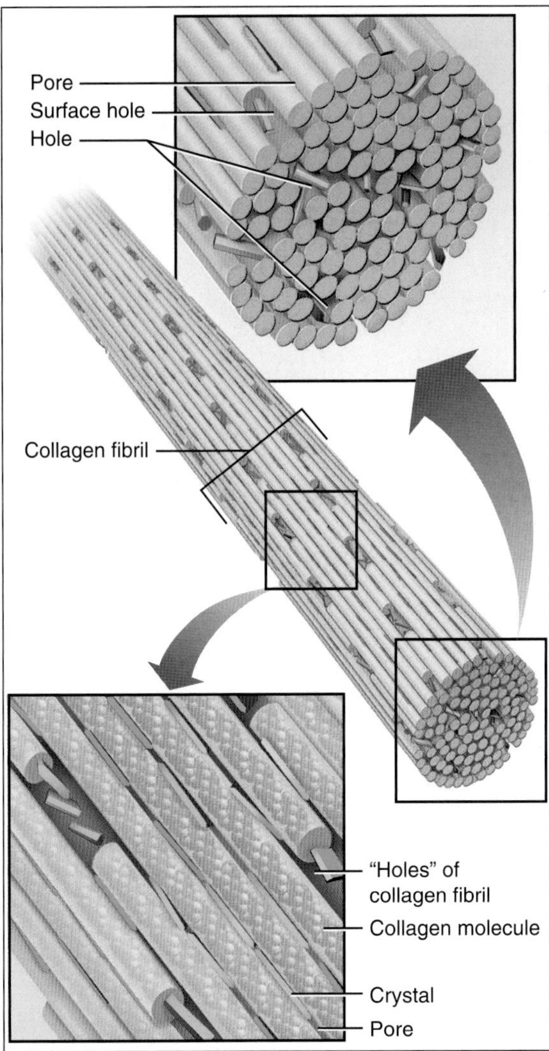

Fig. 1.12 Schematic illustration of the localization of mineral within the collagen fibril. (Redrawn from Glimcher MJ: On the form and function of bone: from molecules to organ. Wolffs law revisited, 1981. In Veis A, editor: *The chemistry and biology of mineralized connective tissues*, Amsterdam, 1981, Elsevier, pp 616–673.)

Alkaline Phosphatase

Alkaline phosphatase activity is always associated with the production of a mineralized tissue, and the implicated isozymes are part of the mammalian alkaline phosphatase gene family. Because the major isozyme is found in several other tissues, the isozyme is referred to as *tissue-nonspecific alkaline phosphatase.* In all cases, alkaline phosphatase exhibits a similar pattern of distribution and is involved with the blood vessels and cell membrane of hard tissue–forming cells. In hard connective tissues, alkaline phosphatase also is found in the organic matrix, associated with matrix vesicles (when present) and occurring freely within the matrix.

Although the enzyme alkaline phosphatase has a clearcut function, its role in mineralization is not yet fully defined. A precise description of this role is complicated by at least two factors. First, the term *alkaline phosphatase* is nonspecific, describing enzymes that have the capacity to cleave phosphate groups from substrates to provide phosphate ions at mineralization sites, most efficiently at an alkaline pH. Second, the enzyme may have more than one distinct function in mineralization.

The extracellular activity of alkaline phosphatase at mineralization sites occurs where continuing crystal growth is taking place. At these sites the enzyme is believed to have the function of cleaving PP_i. Hydroxyapatite crystals in contact with serum or tissue fluids are prevented from growing larger because PP_i ions are deposited on their surfaces, inhibiting further growth. Alkaline phosphatase activity breaks down PP_i, thereby permitting crystal growth to proceed.

The stenciling principle describes cell- and tissue-specific enzyme expression and activity to create at least two nested circuits of inhibition of inhibitors (or release from inhibition) for extracellular matrix mineralization—one that first permits mineralization and a second that sculpts in more detail hydroxyapatite crystal growth patterns. Together these act to ensure that mineralization in the skeleton and dentition occurs in the right locations and to the right extent. Both circuits arise from resident cell activity that also includes extracellular release of mineralization inhibitors (see Box 1.1).

Transport of Mineral Ions to Mineralization Sites

Although the subject has been studied extensively, the mechanism(s) whereby large amounts of phosphate and calcium are delivered to calcification sites is still not fully resolved. Mineral ions can reach a mineralization front by movement through or between cells. Tissue fluid is supersaturated in these ions, and it is possible that fluid simply needs to percolate between cells to reach the organic matrix where local factors then would permit mineralization. A priori, this mechanism is more likely to occur between cells, such as osteoblasts and odontoblasts, that have no complete tight junctions and where serum proteins, such as albumin, can be found in the osteoid and predentin matrix they produce. This also applies to cementoblasts that frequently are separated from each other by PDL fibers entering cementum. Several facts, however, complicate such a simple explanation. For example, hormones influence the movement of calcium in and out of bone. Thus it has been proposed that osteoblasts and odontoblasts form a sort of limiting membrane that would regulate ion influx into their respectable tissues.

The situation would seem more straightforward for enamel, where tight junctions between secretory stage ameloblasts restrict the passage of calcium. It has been concluded that during the secretory phase of enamel formation, some calcium likely passes between cells but that the majority of calcium entry into enamel occurs through a transcellular route. The situation is different during the maturation stage.

The possibility of transcellular transport is dictated by a particular circumstance: The cytosolic free calcium ion concentration cannot exceed 10^{-6} mol/L because a greater concentration would cause calcium to inhibit critical cellular functions leading to cell death. Two mechanisms have been proposed that permit transcellular transport of calcium without exceeding this critical threshold concentration. The first suggests that, as calcium enters the cell through specific calcium channels, it is sequestered by calcium-binding proteins that, in turn, are transported through the cell to the site of release. The second suggests that a continuous and constant flow of calcium ions occurs across the cell without the concentration ever exceeding 10^{-6} mol/L. Finally, intracellular compartments (e.g., endoplasmic reticulum and mitochondria) also play a role in calcium handling. Calcium has been localized to these structures not only in hard tissue–forming cells but

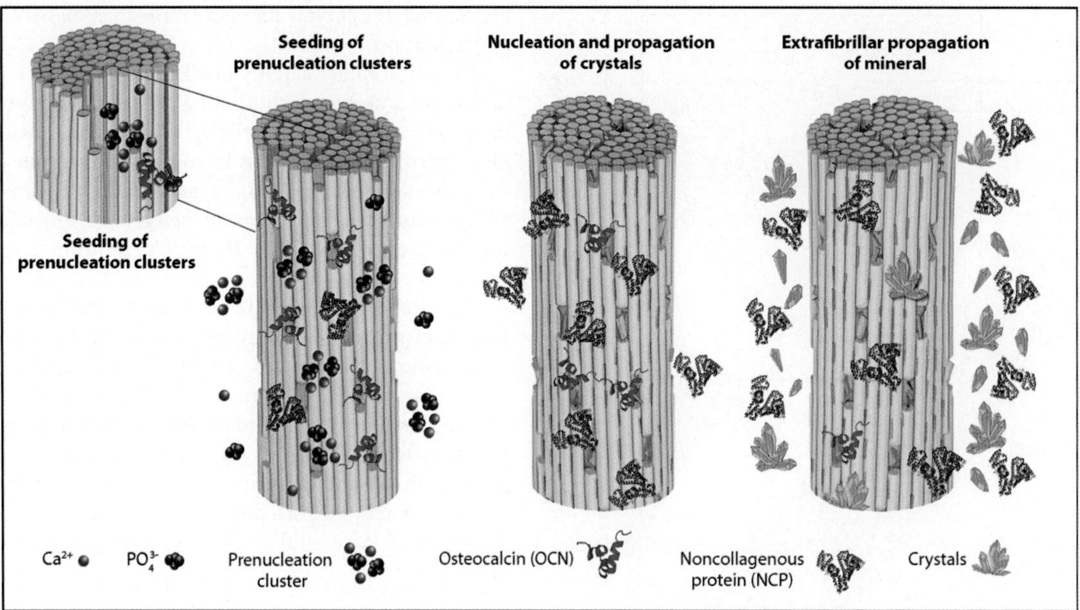

Fig. 1.13 Diagrammatic representation of intrafibrillar and extrafibrillar mineralization of collagen.

also in most other cells, and it is believed that the sequestration of calcium to these organelles is a safety device to control the calcium concentration of the cytosol.

Recent data from cryogenically preserved embryonal chicken bone (Box 1.2) have further shown the presence of numerous intracellular vesicles containing mineral precursors in osteocytes as well as in osteoblasts and preosteocytes. A series of nanochannels associated with the osteocyte lacunar system, has also been put in evidence for the passive transport of mineral precursor to the site of mineralization. The generalized presence and functionality of these nanochannels in other species, however, remain to be demonstrated.

HARD TISSUE DEGRADATION

Bone is remodeling constantly by an orchestrated interplay between removal of old bone and its replacement by new bone. Formative and destructive phases result from the activity of cells derived from two separate lineages. The osteoblasts, originating from mesenchyme in the case of long bones, are responsible for bone formation, whereas osteoclasts, originating from the blood (monocyte/macrophage lineage), destroy focal areas of bone as part of normal maintenance. Enamel under ameloblasts undergoes removal of matrix proteins by a process of extracellular enzymatic processing similar to that in the resorption lacuna under osteoclasts. The exact extent of the degradation of its organic matrix constituents and the exact manner by which their fragments leave the site of resorption are still not fully defined; in bone, transcytosis is involved (see Chapter 6). Such tissues as cementum and dentin do not normally undergo turnover, but all hard tissues of the tooth can be resorbed under certain normal eruptive conditions (e.g., deciduous teeth) and under certain pathologic conditions, including excessive physical forces and inflammation. The cells involved in their resorption have similar characteristics to osteoclasts but generally are referred to as *odontoclasts* (see Chapter 10).

SUMMARY OF HARD TISSUE FORMATION

Formative cells situated close to a good blood supply, producing an organic matrix capable of accepting mineral (apatite). These cells thus have the cytologic features of cells that actively synthesize and secrete protein. Mineralization in the connective hard tissues entails an initial nucleation mechanism involving a cell-derived matrix vesicle and the control of spontaneous mineral precipitation from supersaturated tissue fluids. After initial nucleation, further mineralization is achieved in relation to the collagen fiber and spread of mineral within and between fibers. In enamel, mineralization initiates either in relation to preexisting apatite crystals of dentin or enamel matrix proteins. Alkaline phosphatase is associated with mineralization, but its role is still not fully understood. The breakdown of hard tissue involves the macrophage system, which produces a characteristic multinucleated giant cell, the osteoclast. To break down hard tissue, this cell attaches to mineralized tissue and creates a sealed environment that is first acidified to demineralize the hard tissue. After exposure to the acidic environment, the organic matrix is broken down by proteolytic enzymes. In enamel, the challenge is to maintain a relatively neutral pH environment that will prevent mineral dissolution and allow optimal activity of the enzymes that break down the organic matrix components.

BOX 1.2 Mineralization Logistics During Bone Formation

During the formation and development of skeletal tissues, large amounts of calcium ions need to be transported from the bloodstream to the sites of mineralization. These ions must overcome huge distances and be moved through extracellular and intracellular compartments where calcium is highly regulated and cannot exceed millimolar and micromolar concentrations, respectively. Indeed, cells must maintain a very low calcium concentration in their cytosol that is crucial for their intracellular signaling functions. Yet, calcium concentration eventually reaches molar concentrations in the fully mineralized tissue. Thus the transportation of mineralization precursors in growing bone represents a major challenge.

New data acquired in the femur of the fast-growing chick embryo by focused ion beam with scanning electron microscopy (FIB-SEM) under cryogenic condition in the femur of the fast-growing chick embryo have shed some light on the understanding of how vertebrates overcome this major logistic problem.[1] The three-dimensional visualization of large volumes at high resolution and in a close-to-native state has revealed the presence of numerous intracellular vesicles containing mineral precursors (Box 1.2 Fig. 1) in osteocytes as well as in osteoblasts/preosteocytes. Based on the quantification of the volume of the different structures from the segmented data (see Box 1.2 Fig. 1C), an intracellular density of 0.037 vesicles per μmμ^3 on average can be estimated, and the mineral precursors found inside these vesicles occupy less than 10% of the volume.

Based on these FIB-SEM data and on the osteocytic lacunar density established using microCT, one can attempt to interpret the process of biomineralization in forming bone in a dynamic manner. To provide the calcium needed to mineralize the amount of bone tissue synthesized during 1 day, the available intracellular vesicles need to be transported at a velocity of 0.27 μm/s. Such a high velocity, similar to one of molecular motors involved in vesicle transport, suggests that the vesicles containing mineral precursors are trafficked through the cellular network by active cellular processes. In addition, an interconnected network of nanochannel of approximately 40 nm in diameter and in relation with the canaliculi was imaged. These nanochannels could facilitate the passive transport of the mineral precursor over the last 1 or 2 μm to the site of mineralization after being externalized by the cells; however, no extracellular vesicles were observed in the cryo-FIB/SEM experiments.

Although the presence of intracellular vesicles containing mineral precursors has been observed in various animal models,[2–6] our quantitative 3D study proposes an alternative calcium transport mechanism that requires revisiting the prominent existing theory on bone mineralization, the Matrix Vesicle-Mediated Mineralization, at least in chick embryos. Initially formulated by Anderson[7] and Bonucci,[8] this model suggests that chondrocytes/osteoblasts release small vesicles into the extracellular matrix, initiating the nucleation and growth of hydroxyapatite crystals for tissue mineralization. These vesicles have also been observed in initial dentin and cementum but not in tooth enamel. In addition, they are readily apparent among the abundant mineralization foci present in the osteoid seam of trabecular bone in a rat model of hypocalcemia, suggesting that they can be physiologically modulated.[9] Irrespective of the fact that no vesicles have been observed in the extracellular matrix in this study, matrix vesicles are characterized by a small diameter (20 to 200 nm) and a relatively lower occurrence,[10] prompting concerns about their ability to meet the essential mineralization demands for chick embryo development.

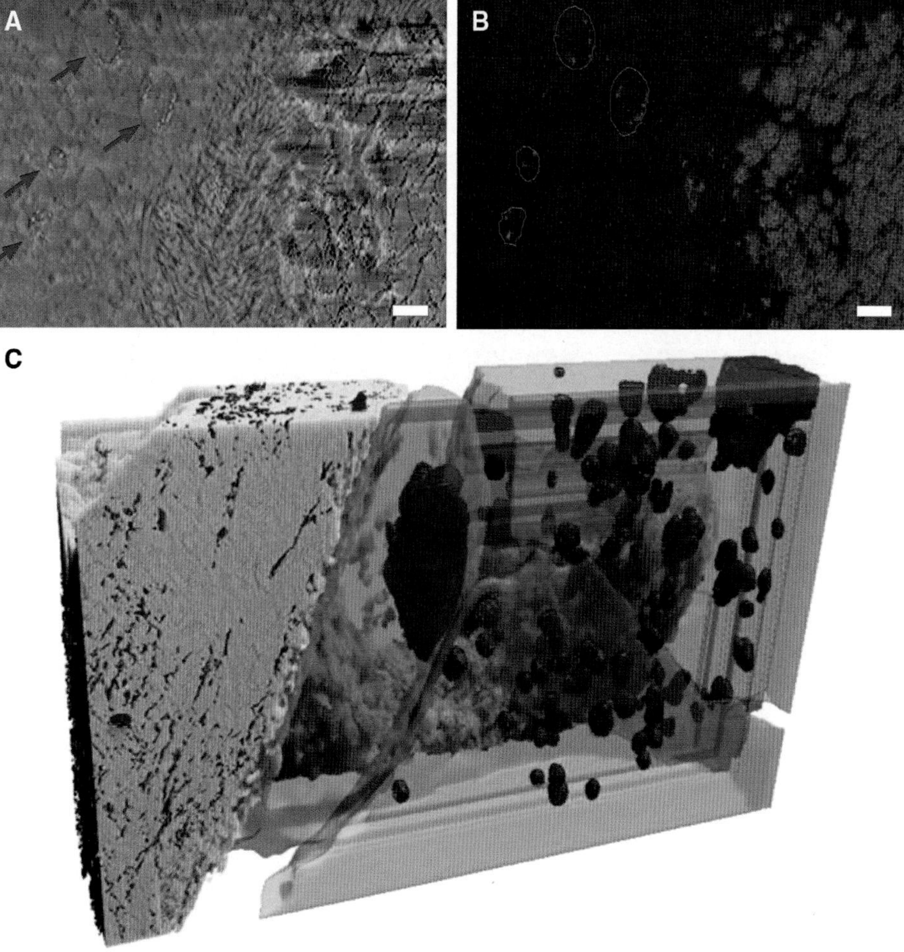

Box 1.2 Fig. 1 Scanning electron microscope images acquired in cryomode of (A) mixed in-lens/secondary electron detector *(arrows)* showing the presence of intracellular vesicles *(arrows)*. Mineral precursors are found inside some of the vesicles and appear brighter in the corresponding backscattered electron detector image *(contour of the vesicle is shown in red)* (scale bar: 1 μm). (C) Perspective rendering of three-dimensional segmented data showing the different structural features: Numerous vesicles containing mineral precursors *(red)* are found inside the cells *(light blue)*. Nuclei are shown in purple. Canaliculi *(dark blue)* penetrate the mineralized bone matrix *(light yellow)*, the latter being also composed of an extensive network of nanochannels *(green)*.

(Continued)

BOX 1.2 Mineralization Logistics During Bone Formation—cont'd

However, the density of matrix vesicles has not been firmly established, making a direct comparison precarious. It remains conceivable, though, that both mechanisms—intracellular and matrix vesicles—may act simultaneously in different regions of the long chick bone.

Hence this study revisited the embryonal bone mineralization from the viewpoint of calcium transportation. The new proposed model (Box 1.2 Fig. 2), based on experimental and conceptual data, suggests that bone mineralization is enabled by different transport mechanisms in which calcium ions first transit in the vasculature, probably regulated by the action of calcium-binding proteins. Active transport of calcium-loaded vesicles within the osteocytic cellular network is then at play, allowing mineral ions to be trafficked over long distance (tens of micrometers). Finally, diffusion through a nanochannel network could be the way to bridge the last micrometers. Many open questions remain, such as the specific mechanism by which calcium ions are packaged into intracellular vesicles and then released from them into the matrix. Moreover, the observations have been made in embryonal chicken skeleton, and it cannot be excluded that different skeletal materials use different strategies in the mineralization process.

References

1. Raguin E, et al.: Logistics of bone mineralization in the chick embryo studied by 3D cryo FIB-SEM imaging, *bioRxiv* 2:527853, 2023.
2. Mahamid J, et al.: Amorphous calcium phosphate is a major component of the forming fin bones of zebrafish: indications for an amorphous precursor phase, *Proc Natl Acad Sci U S A* 105:12748–12753, 2008.
3. Mahamid J, et al.: Bone mineralization proceeds through intracellular calcium phosphate loaded vesicles: a cryo-electron microscopy study, *J Struct Biol* 174(3):527–535, 2011.
4. Akiva A, et al.: On the pathway of mineral deposition in larval zebrafish caudal fin bone, *Bone* 75:192–200, 2015.
5. Kerschnitzki M, et al.: Bone mineralization pathways during the rapid growth of embryonic chicken long bones, *J Struct Biol* 195(1):82–92, 2016.
6. Kerschnitzki M, et al.: Transport of membrane-bound mineral particles in blood vessels during chicken embryonic bone development, *Bone* 83:65–72, 2016.
7. Anderson HC: Vesicles associated with calcification in the matrix of epiphyseal cartilage, *J Cell Biol* 41(1):59–72, 1969.
8. Bonucci E: Fine structure of early cartilage calcification, *J Ultrastruct Res* 20(1):3350, 1967.
9. Mocetti P, et al.: A histomorphometric, structural, and immunocytochemical study of the effects of diet-induced hypocalcemia on bone in growing rats, *J Histochem Cytochem* 48(8):1059–1077, 2000.
10. Golub EE: Role of matrix vesicles in biomineralization, *Biochim Biophys Acta* 1790(12):1592–1598, 2009.

Emeline Raguin, *PhD*
Group leader,
Department of Biomaterials,
Max Planck Institute of Colloids and Interfaces,
Potsdam, Germany

Richard Weinkamer, *PhD*
Group leader,
Department of Biomaterials,
Max Planck Institute of Colloids and Interfaces,
Potsdam, Germany

Peter Fratzl, *PhD*
Professor,
Department of Biomaterials,
Max Planck Institute of Colloids and Interfaces,
Potsdam, Germany

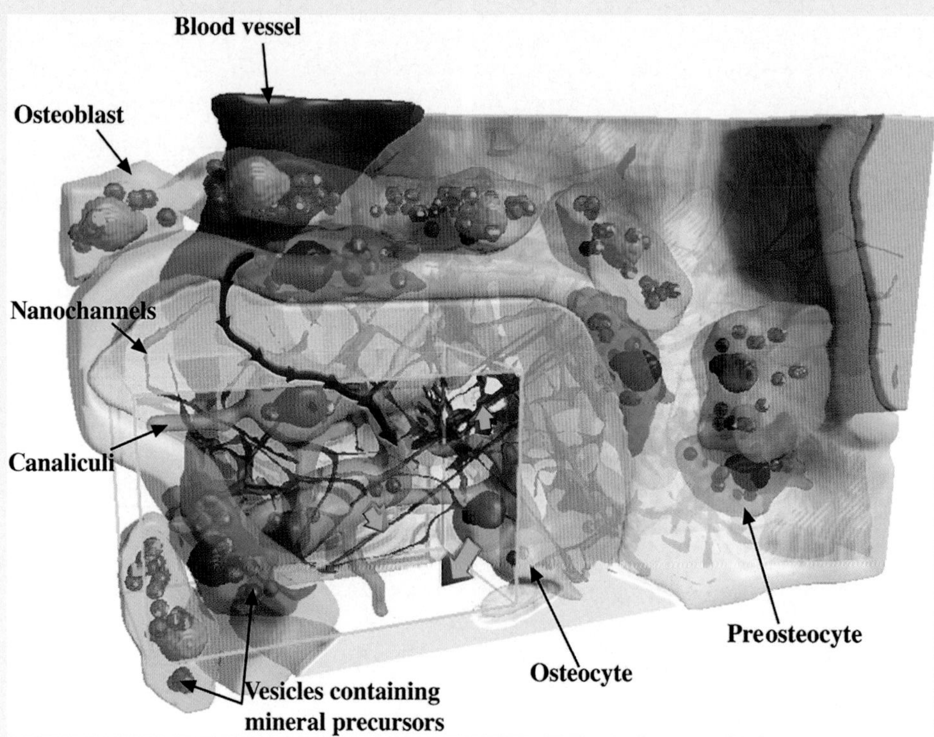

Box 1.2 Fig. 2 Schematic representation of the new model of calcium transportation during mineralization of a forming bone showing the active transportation of vesicles containing mineral precursors *(red arrows)* that subsequently shed their content into the matrix. This mineral content is then passively transported by diffusion through the nanochannels network to finally reach the sites of mineralization.

RECOMMENDED READING

Landis WJ, editor, et al.: *Current concepts of the mineralization of type I collagen in vertebrate tissues*, 1st ed., United Kingdom, 2021, Taylor & Francis Group.

2

General Embryology

Antonio Nanci

OUTLINE

This chapter provides basic general embryology information needed to explain the development of the head, particularly the structures in and around the mouth. It supplies a background for understanding (1) origins of the tissues associated with facial and dental development and (2) the cause of many congenital defects that manifest in these tissues.

GERM CELL FORMATION AND FERTILIZATION

The human somatic (body) cell contains 46 chromosomes, 46 being the diploid number for the cell. Two of these are sex chromosomes; the remaining are autosomes. Each chromosome is paired so that every cell has 22 homologous sets of paired autosomes, with one sex chromosome derived from the mother and one from the father. The sex chromosomes, designated X and Y, are paired as XX in the female and XY in the male.

Fertilization is the fusion of male and female germ cells (the spermatozoa and ova, collectively called *gametes*) to form a zygote, which commences the formation of a new individual. Germ cells are required to have half as many chromosomes (the haploid number) so that, on fertilization, the original complement of 46 chromosomes will be reestablished in the new somatic cell. The process that produces germ cells with half the number of chromosomes of the somatic cell is called *meiosis.* Mitosis describes the division of somatic cells.

Before mitotic cell division begins, DNA is first replicated during the synthetic phase of the cell cycle so that the amount of DNA is doubled to a value known as tetraploid (four times the amount of DNA found in the germ cell). During mitosis the chromosomes containing this tetraploid amount of DNA are split and distributed equally between the two resulting cells; thus both daughter cells have a diploid DNA quantity and chromosome number, which duplicates the parent cell exactly.

Meiosis, by contrast, involves two sets of cell divisions occurring in quick succession. Before the first division, DNA is replicated to the tetraploid value (as in mitosis). In the first division the number of chromosomes is halved, and each daughter cell contains a diploid amount of DNA. The second division involves the splitting and separation of the chromosomes, resulting in four cells; thus the final composition of each cell is haploid with respect to its DNA value and its chromosome number.

Meiosis is discussed in this textbook because the process occasionally malfunctions by producing zygotes with an abnormal number of chromosomes and individuals with congenital defects that sometimes affect the mouth and teeth. For example, an abnormal number of chromosomes can result from the failure to separate a homologous chromosome pair during meiosis so that the daughter cells contain 24 or 22 chromosomes. If, on fertilization, a gamete containing 24 chromosomes fuses with a normal gamete (containing 23 chromosomes), the resulting zygote will possess 47 chromosomes; one homologous pair has a third component. Thus the cells are trisomic for a given pair of chromosomes. If one member of the homologous chromosome pair is missing, a rare condition known as *monosomy* prevails. The best-known example of trisomy is Down syndrome (trisomy 21). Among features of Down syndrome are facial clefts, a shortened palate, a protruding and fissured tongue, and delayed eruption of teeth.

Approximately 10% of all human malformations are caused by an alteration in a single gene. Such alterations are transmitted in several ways, of which two are of special importance. First, if the malformation results from autosomal dominant inheritance, the affected gene generally is inherited from only one parent. The trait usually appears in every generation and can be transmitted by the affected parent to statistically half of the children. Examples of autosomal dominant conditions include achondroplasia, cleidocranial dysostosis, osteogenesis imperfecta, and dentinogenesis imperfecta; the latter two conditions result in abnormal formation of the dental hard tissues. Dentinogenesis imperfecta (Fig. 2.1) arises from a mutation in the dentin sialophosphoprotein gene. Second, when the malformation is a result of autosomal recessive inheritance, the abnormal gene can express itself only when it is received from both parents. Examples include chondroectodermal dysplasia, some cases of microcephaly, and cystic fibrosis.

All of these conditions are examples of abnormalities in the genetic makeup or genotype of the individual and are classified as genetic defects. The expression of the genotype is affected by the environment in which the embryo develops, and the outcome of development is termed the *phenotype.* Adverse factors in the environment can result in excessive deviation from a functional and accepted norm; the outcome is described as a congenital defect. Teratology is the study of such developmental defects.

PRENATAL DEVELOPMENT

Prenatal development is divided into three successive phases (Fig. 2.2). The first two, when combined, constitute the embryonic stage, and the third is the fetal stage. The forming individual is described as an embryo or fetus depending on its developmental stage.

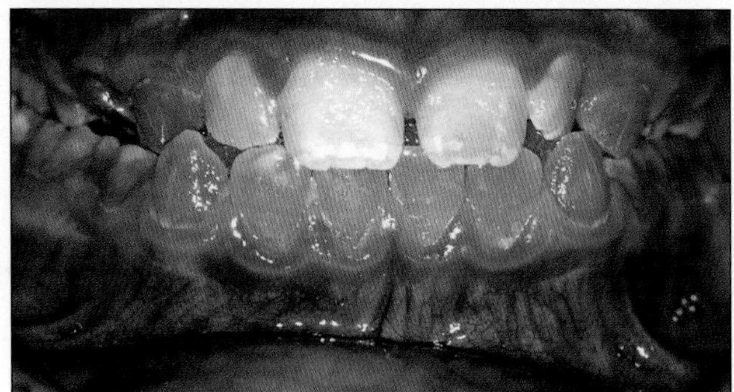

Fig. 2.1 Intraoral view of the dentition of a child with dentinogenesis imperfecta, an autosomal dominant genetic defect. (Courtesy A. Kauzman.)

The first phase begins at fertilization and spans the first 4 weeks or so of development. This phase involves largely cellular proliferation and migration, with some differentiation of cell populations. Few congenital defects result from this period of development because, if the perturbation is severe, the embryo is lost.

The second phase spans the next 4 weeks of development and is characterized largely by the differentiation of all major external and internal structures *(morphogenesis)*. The second phase is a particularly vulnerable period for the embryo because it involves many intricate embryologic processes; during this period, many recognized congenital defects develop.

From the end of the second phase to term, further development is largely a matter of growth and maturation, and the embryo now is called a fetus.

INDUCTION, COMPETENCE, AND DIFFERENTIATION

Patterning is key in development from the initial axial (head-to-tail) specification of the embryo through its segmentation. It is a spatial and temporal event that implicates the classical processes of induction, competence, and differentiation. These concepts also apply to the

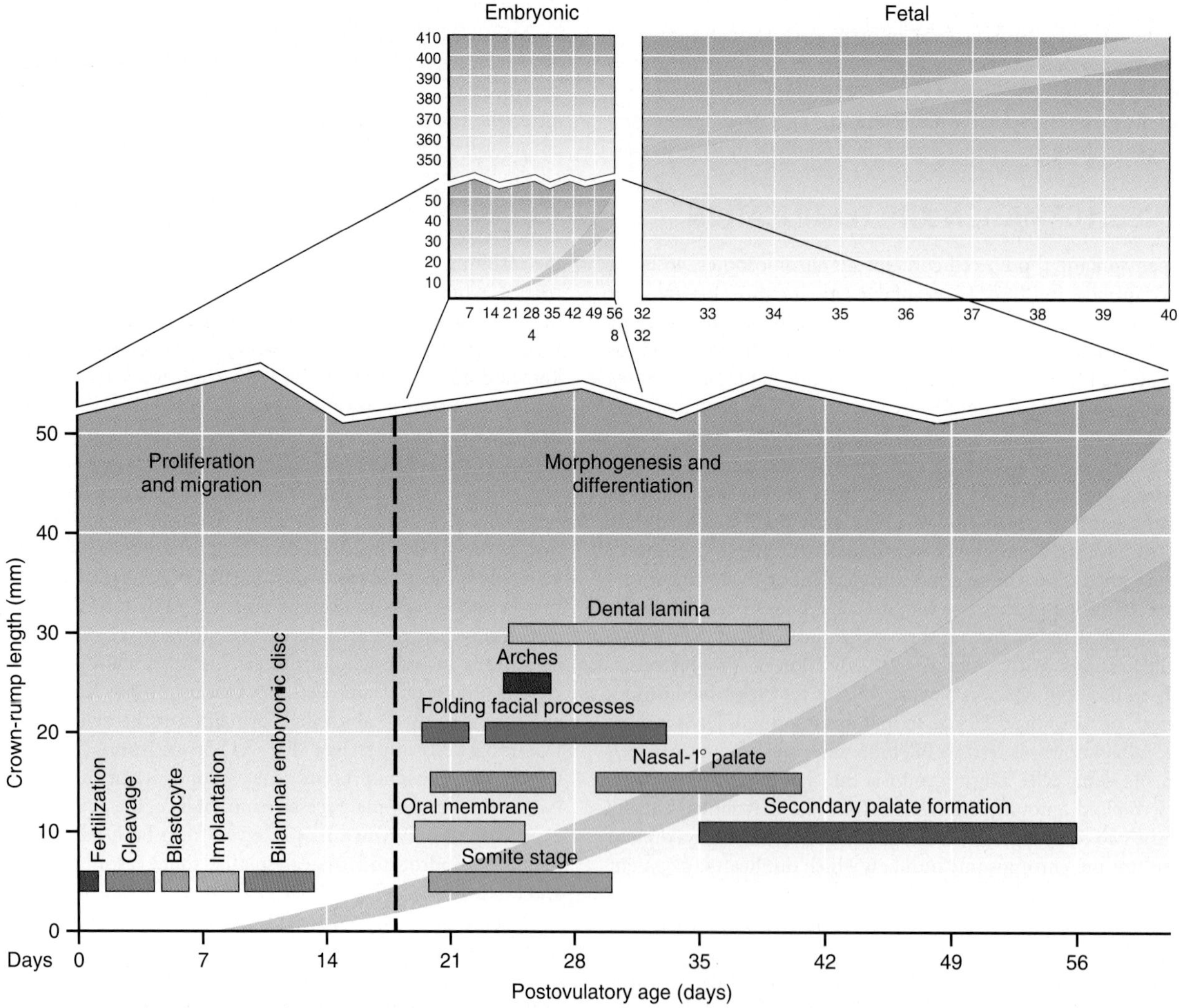

Fig. 2.2 Sequences of prenatal development. The upper diagram shows the distinction between embryonic and fetal stages. The lower part of the embryonic diagram is expanded in the bottom diagram, which distinguishes the stages of proliferation and migration and morphogenesis and differentiation. The timing of key events also is indicated. (From Waterman RE, Meller SM: Congenital craniofacial abnormalities. In Shaw JH, et al., editors: *Textbook of oral biology*, Philadelphia, 1978, WB Saunders Co, pp. 863–896.)

development of the tooth and its supporting tissues, as exemplified by regional development of incisors, canines, premolars, and molars.

Every cell of an individual stems from the zygote. Clearly, they have differentiated somehow into populations that have assumed particular functions, shapes, and rates of turnover. The process that initiates differentiation is induction; an inducer is the agent that provides cells with the signal to enter this process. Furthermore, each compartment of cells must be competent to respond to the induction process. Windows of competence of varying duration exist for different populations of cells.

Homeobox genes and growth factors play crucial roles in development. All homeobox genes contain a similar region of 180 nucleotide base pairs (the homeobox) and function by producing proteins (transcription factors) that bind to the DNA of other downstream genes, thereby regulating their expression. By knocking out such genes or by switching them on, it has been shown that they play a fundamental role in patterning. Furthermore, combinations of differing homeobox genes provide codes or sets of assembly rules to regulate development; one such code is involved in dental development (see Chapter 5).

Homeobox genes act in concert with other groups of regulatory molecules (i.e., growth factors and retinoic acids). Growth factors are polypeptides that belong to a number of families. For them to have an effect, cells must express cell-surface receptors to bind them. When bound by the receptors, there is transfer of information across the plasma membrane and activation of cytoplasmic signaling pathways to cause alteration in the gene expression. Thus a growth factor is an inductive agent, and the appropriate expression of cell-surface receptors bestows competency on a cell. A growth factor produced by one cell and acting on another is described as *paracrine regulation,* whereas the process of a cell that recaptures its own product is known as *autocrine regulation* (Fig. 2.3). The extensive and diverse effects of a relatively few growth factors during embryogenesis can be achieved by cells expressing combinations of cell-surface receptors requiring simultaneous capture of different growth factors to respond in a given way (Fig. 2.4). Such combinations represent another example of a developmental code. By contrast, the retinoic acid family freely enters a cell to form a complex with intracellular receptors, which eventually affects gene expression. Growth factors and retinoids regulate the expression of homeobox genes, which, in turn, regulate the expression of growth factors, an example of the role of regulatory loops in development.

FORMATION OF THE THREE-LAYERED EMBRYO

After fertilization, mammalian development involves a phase of rapid proliferation and migration of cells with little or no differentiation. This proliferative phase lasts until three germ layers have formed.

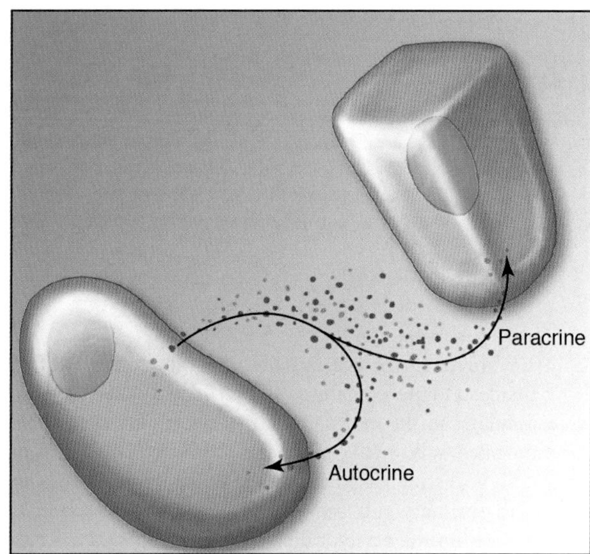

Fig. 2.3 Autocrine and paracrine regulation. On the left, the cell captures its own cytokine (autocrine); on the right, the cytokine is captured by a nearby target cell (paracrine).

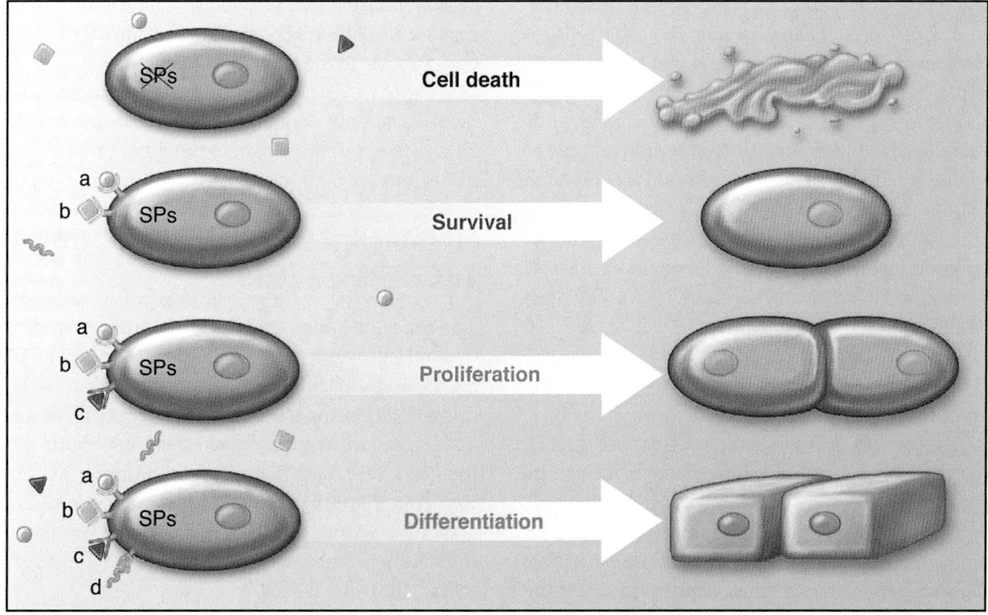

Fig. 2.4 Modulation of the expression of cell-surface receptors *(colored membrane-bound forms)* results in the binding of different combinations of growth factors *(a-d, colored geometric forms)* that influence cellular outcome. When binding occurs, there is transfer of information across the plasma membrane and activation of cytoplasmic signaling pathways *(SPs)* to cause alteration in gene expression. In the absence of receptors, binding with grown factors cannot take place, and cell death occurs.

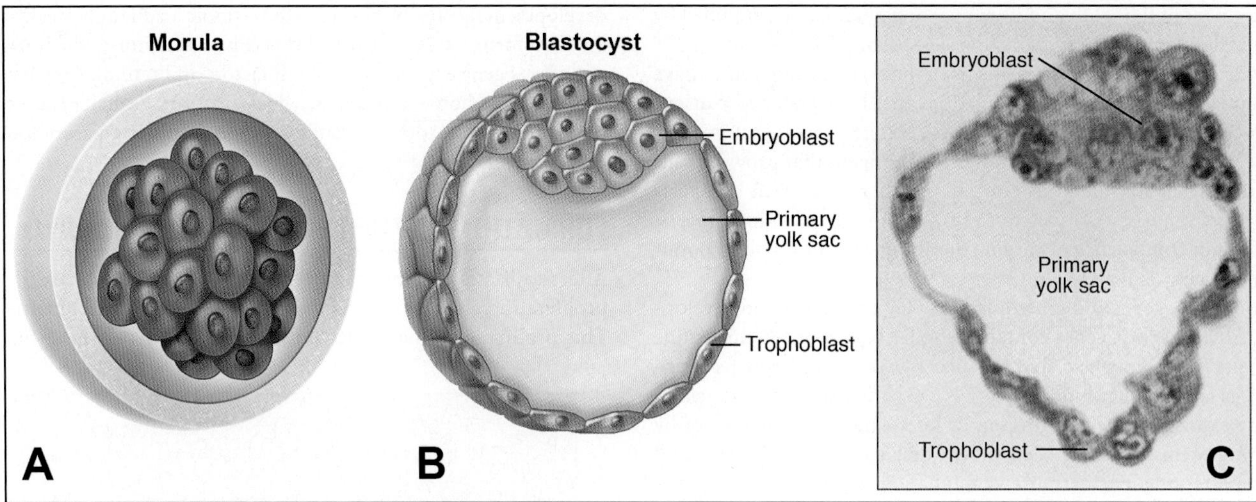

Fig. 2.5 Drawing of the transformation of the (A) morula into a (B) blastocyst. (C) Colorized histologic section illustrates the differentiation at this time of the blastocyst into trophoblast cells that line the cavity of the primary yolk sac and are involved in maintenance of the embryo and of embryoblast cells that form a small cluster within the cavity that are involved in the development of the embryo. Adapted from Hertig AT, et al.: *Contrib Embryol* 35:199–220, 1954, Used with permission from Carnegie Institution for Science.

In summary, the fertilized egg initially undergoes a series of rapid divisions that lead to the formation of a ball of cells called the *morula.* Fluid accumulates in the morula, and its cells realign themselves to form a fluid-filled hollow ball, called the *blastocyst.* Two cell populations now can be distinguished within the blastocyst: (1) those lining the cavity (the primary yolk sac), called *trophoblast cells;* and (2) a small cluster within the cavity, called the *inner cell mass* or *embryoblast* (Fig. 2.5). The embryoblast cells form the embryo proper, whereas the trophoblast cells are associated with implantation of the embryo and formation of the placenta (they are not described further here).

At about day 8 of gestation, the cells of the embryoblast differentiate into a two-layered disk called the *bilaminar germ disk.* The cells on the dorsal aspect, the ectodermal layer, are columnar and reorganize to form the amniotic cavity. Those on the ventral aspect, the endodermal layer, are cuboidal and form the roof of a second cavity (the secondary yolk sac), which develops from the migration of peripheral cells of the extraembryonic endodermal layer. This configuration is completed after 2 weeks of development (Fig. 2.6). During this time the axis of the embryo is established and is represented by a slight enlargement of the ectodermal and endodermal cells at the head (cephalic or rostral) end of the embryo in a region known as the *prochordal* (or *prechordal*) plate where ectoderm and endoderm are in contact (Fig. 2.7A; see also Fig. 2.6A).

During the third week of development, the embryo enters the period of gastrulation during which the germ layers forming the bilaminar embryonic disk are converted to a trilaminar disk (see Fig. 2.7). As previously described, the floor of the amniotic cavity is formed by ectoderm, and, within it, a structure called the *primitive streak* develops along the midline by cellular convergence (see Fig. 2.7A). This structure is a narrow groove with slightly bulging areas on each side. The rostral end of the streak finishes in a small depression called the *primitive node,* or *pit.* Cells of the ectodermal layer migrate through the streak and between the ectoderm and endoderm. The cells that pass through the streak change shape and migrate away from the streak in lateral and cephalic directions. The cells from the cephalic regions form the notochord process, which pushes forward in the midline as far as the prochordal plate. Through canalization of this process, the notochord is formed to support the primitive embryo.

Elsewhere alongside the primitive streak, cells of the ectodermal layer divide and migrate toward the streak where they invaginate and spread laterally between the ectoderm and endoderm. These cells, sometimes called the *mesoblast,* infiltrate and push away the extraembryonic endodermal cells of the hypoblast, except for the prochordal plate, to form the true embryonic endoderm. They also pack the space between the newly formed embryonic endoderm and the ectoderm to form a third layer of cells called the *mesoderm* (see Fig. 2.7B–D). In addition to spreading laterally, cells spread progressively forward, passing on each side of the notochord and prochordal plate. The cells that accumulate anterior to the prochordal plate because of this migration give rise to the cardiac plate, the structure in which the heart forms (see Fig. 2.7A). As a result of these cell migrations, the notochord and mesoderm now separate the ectoderm from the endoderm (see Fig. 2.7C), except in the region of the prochordal plate and in a similar area of fusion at the tail (caudal) end of the embryo called the *cecal plate.*

FORMATION OF THE NEURAL TUBE AND FATE OF THE GERM LAYERS

The series of events leading to the formation of the three-layered, or triploblastic, embryo during the first 3 weeks of development now has been sketched. These initial events involve cell proliferation and migration. During the next 3 to 4 weeks of development, major tissues and organs differentiate from the triploblastic embryo; these include the head, face, and tissues contributing to development of the teeth. Key events are the differentiation of the nervous system and neural crest tissues from the ectoderm, the differentiation of mesoderm, and the folding of the embryo in two planes along the rostrocaudal (head-to-tail) and lateral axes.

The nervous system develops as a thickening within the ectodermal layer at the rostral end of the embryo. This thickening constitutes the neural plate, which rapidly forms raised margins (neural folds). These folds, in turn, encompass and delineate a deepening midline depression—the neural groove (Fig. 2.8). The neural folds eventually fuse so

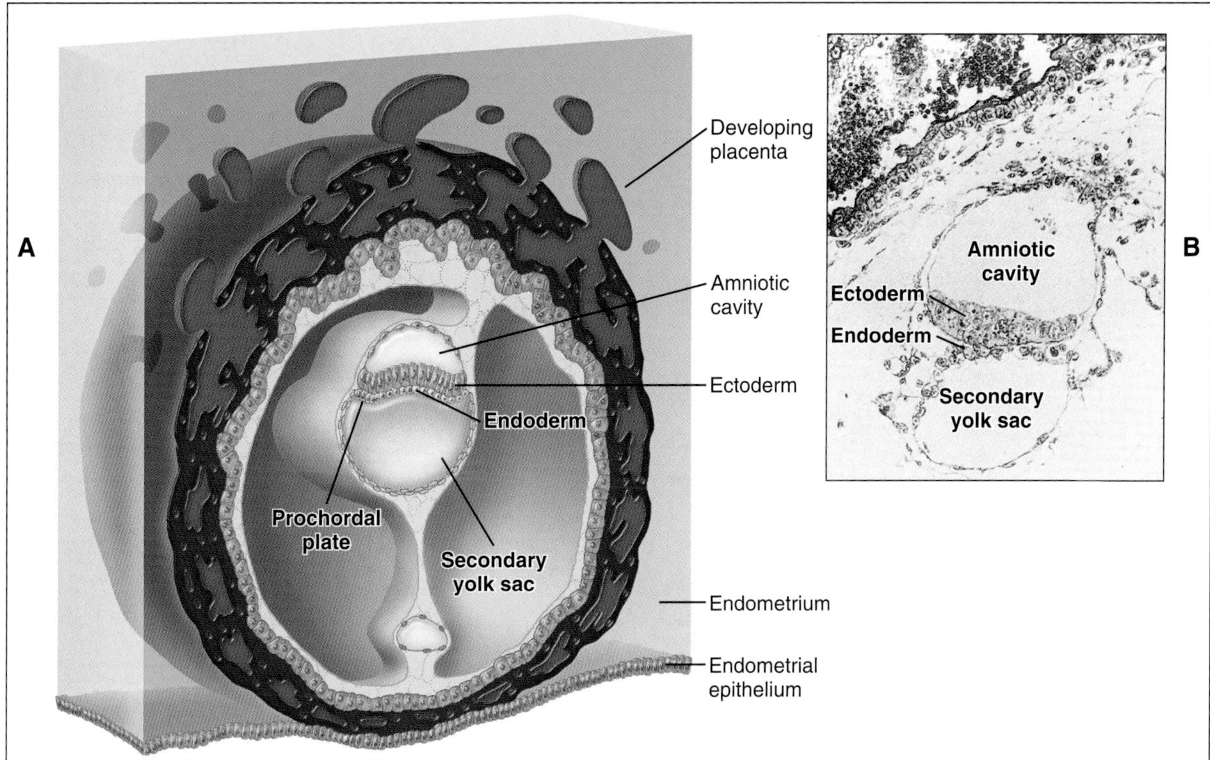

Fig. 2.6 (A) Schematic representation and (B) histologic section of a human blastocyst at 13 days of gestation. An amniotic cavity has formed within the ectodermal layer. Proliferation of endodermal cells forms a secondary yolk sac. The bilaminar embryo is well established. (B, From Brewer JI: A human embryo in the bilaminar blastodisc stage [the Edwards-Jones-Brewer ovum], *Contrib Embryol Carnegie Instn* 27:85–93, 1938.)

that a neural tube separates from the ectoderm to form the floor of the amniotic cavity with mesoderm intervening.

As the neural tube forms, changes occur in the mesoderm adjacent to the tube and the notochord. The mesoderm first thickens on each side of the midline to form paraxial mesoderm. Along the trunk of the embryo, this paraxial mesoderm breaks into segmented blocks called *somites*. Each somite has three components: (1) the sclerotome, which eventually contributes to two adjacent vertebrae and their disks; (2) the myotome, which gives origin to a segmented mass of muscle; and (3) the dermatome, which gives rise to the connective tissue of the skin overlying the somite. In the head region, the mesoderm only partially segments to form a series of numbered somitomeres, which contribute in part to the head musculature. At the periphery of the paraxial mesoderm, the mesoderm remains as a thin layer (intermediate mesoderm), which becomes the urogenital system. Further laterally the mesoderm thickens again to form the lateral plate mesoderm, which gives rise to (1) the connective tissue associated with muscle and viscera; (2) the serous membranes of the pleura, pericardium, and peritoneum; (3) the blood and lymphatic cells; (4) the cardiovascular and lymphatic systems; and (5) the spleen and adrenal cortex.

A different series of events takes place in the head region. First, the neural tube undergoes massive expansion to form the forebrain, midbrain, and hindbrain. The hindbrain exhibits segmentation by forming a series of eight bulges, known as *rhombomeres,* which play an important role in the development of the head (see Chapter 3).

Folding of the Embryo

A crucial developmental event is the folding of the embryo in two planes along the rostrocaudal axis and along the lateral axis (Fig. 2.9). The head fold is critical to the formation of a primitive stomatodeum or oral cavity; ectoderm comes through this fold to line the primitive stomatodeum, with the stomatodeum separated from the gut by the buccopharyngeal membrane (Fig. 2.10).

Fig. 2.11 illustrates how the lateral folding of the embryo determines this disposition of mesoderm. As another result, the ectoderm of the floor of the amniotic cavity encapsulates the embryo and forms the surface epithelium. The paraxial mesoderm remains adjacent to the neural tube and notochord. The lateral plate mesoderm cavitates to form a space (coelom), and the mesoderm bounding the cavity lines the body wall and gut. Intermediate mesoderm is relocated to a position on the dorsal wall of the coelom. The endoderm forms the gut. Fig. 2.12 indicates the final disposition of the mesoderm and the derivatives of the ectoderm, endoderm, and cranial neural crest.

The Neural Crest

As the neural tube forms during neurulation, a group of cells along the dorsal-lateral margins of the closing neural folds become distinct from the neuroectoderm. These so-called *neural crest cells (NCCs)* receive inductive signals to undergo an epithelial-mesenchymal transition (EMT), a process whereby their cell adhesive properties and cytoskeletal organization change, allowing them to delaminate and migrate extensively away from the neural tube to multiple locations in the embryo, where they give rise to a myriad of cell types throughout the body (Figs. 2.13 and 2.14; see also Fig. 2.12). NCCs exhibit the exceptional capacity of stem and progenitor cells, and advances in the NCC field continue to uncover the genes, proteins, and regulatory networks that endow them with such capacity (Box 2.1). Pathway signaling molecules belonging to the bone morphogenetic proteins, Wnt (wingless homologue in vertebrates), fibroblast growth factor and secreted by the surrounding nonneural ectoderm and underlying mesoderm, play a critical role in inducing the NCC cascade. At the molecular level, NCC competence is indicated by the expression

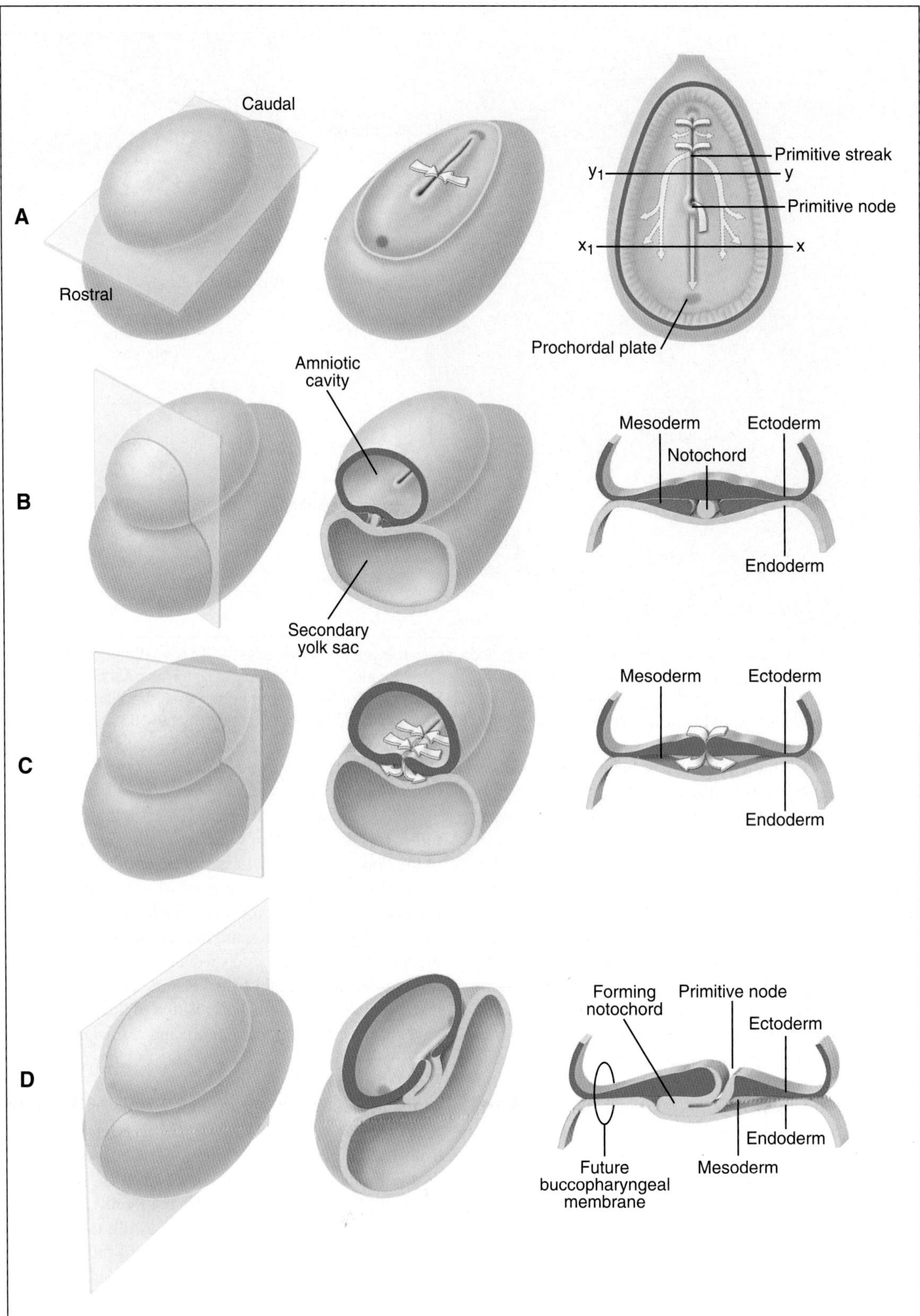

Fig. 2.7 Gastrulation conversion of the bilaminar embryo into a trilaminar embryo. *(Left column)* The plane of section for the middle and right columns. *(Middle column)* A three-dimensional view. *(Right column)* A two-dimensional representation. (A) The floor of the amniotic cavity, formed by the ectodermal layer of the bilaminar embryo. Ectodermal cells converge toward the midline to form the primitive streak, a narrow groove terminating in a circular depression called the *primitive node*. Ectodermal cells then migrate through the streak and between the ectodermal and endodermal layers in lateral and cephalic directions *(arrows)*. A notochord process extends forward from the primitive node. (B) A transverse section through x-x_1, showing the notochord flanked by mesoderm. (C) A section through y-y_1. (D) Notochord pushing rostrally as seen in longitudinal section.

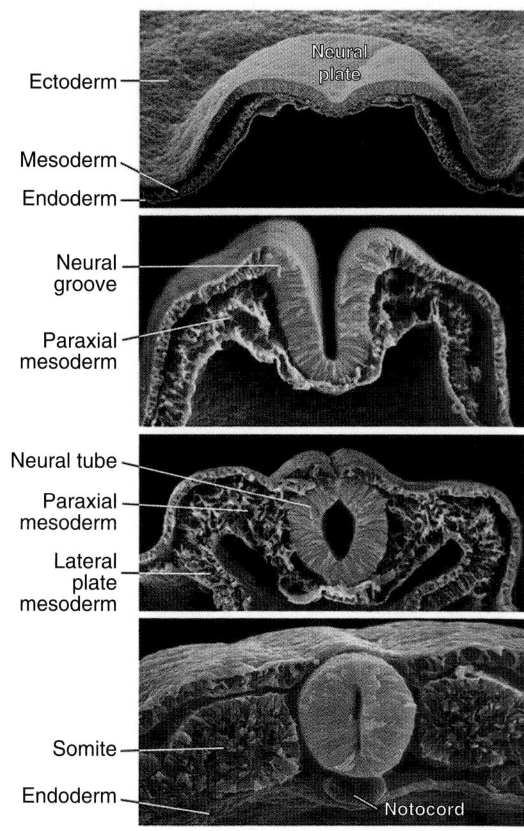

Fig. 2.8 Scanning electron micrograph views of formation and closure of the neural fold elevations. (Courtesy G. Schoenwolf.)

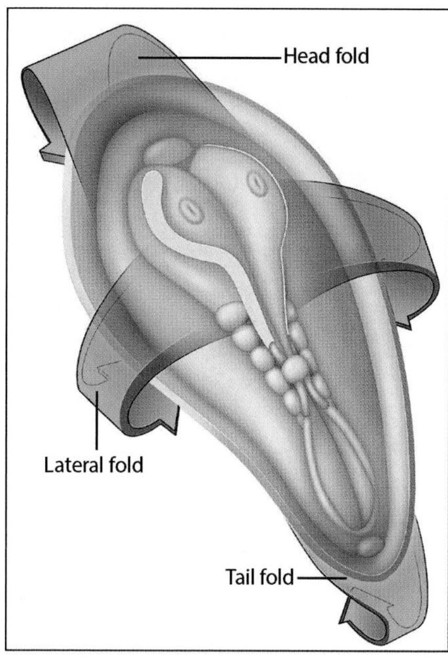

Fig. 2.9 Embryo at 21 days of gestation, before folding. The arrows indicate where folding occurs.

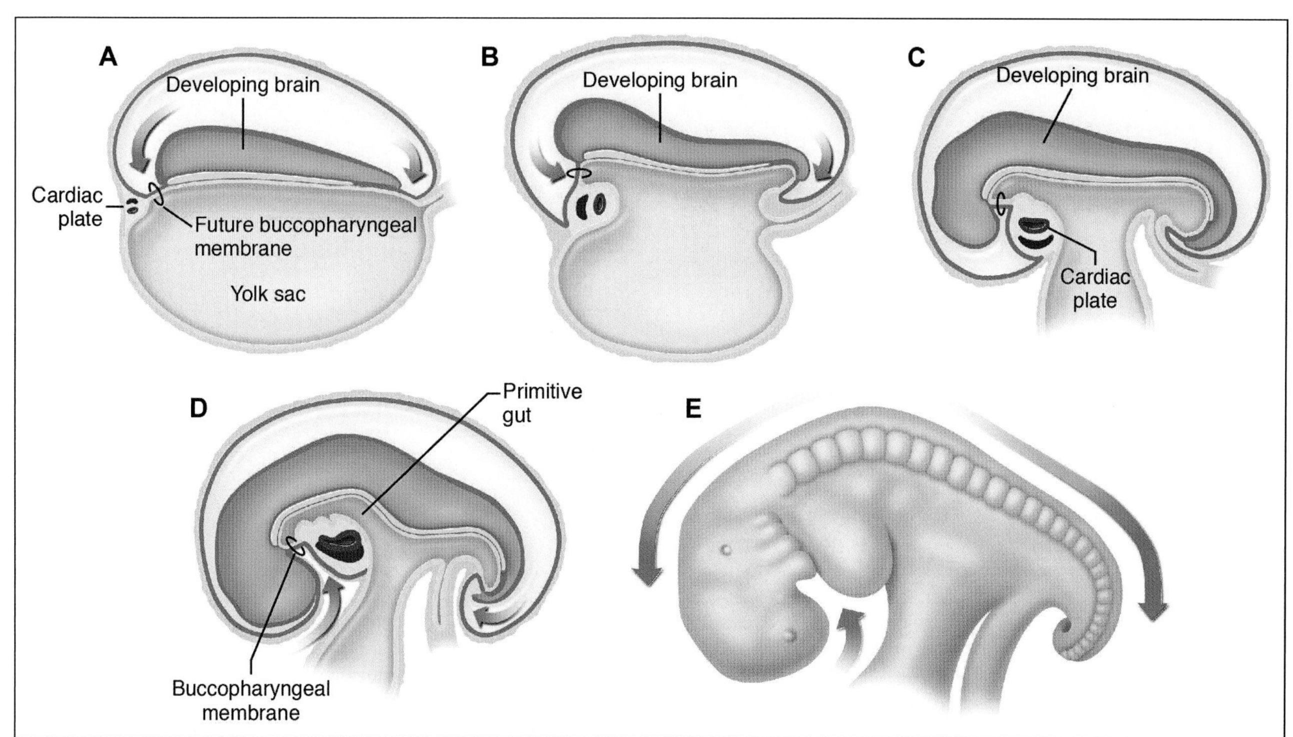

Fig. 2.10 Sagittal sections of embryos illustrate the effects of the caudocephalic foldings. (A) Where folding begins; (B) the onset of folding at 24 days of gestation. (C, D) Days 26 and 28, respectively, show how the head fold establishes the primitive stomatodeum, or oral cavity *(arrow),* bounded by the developing brain and cardiac plate. It is separated from the foregut by the buccopharyngeal membrane. (E) The embryo at completion of folding.

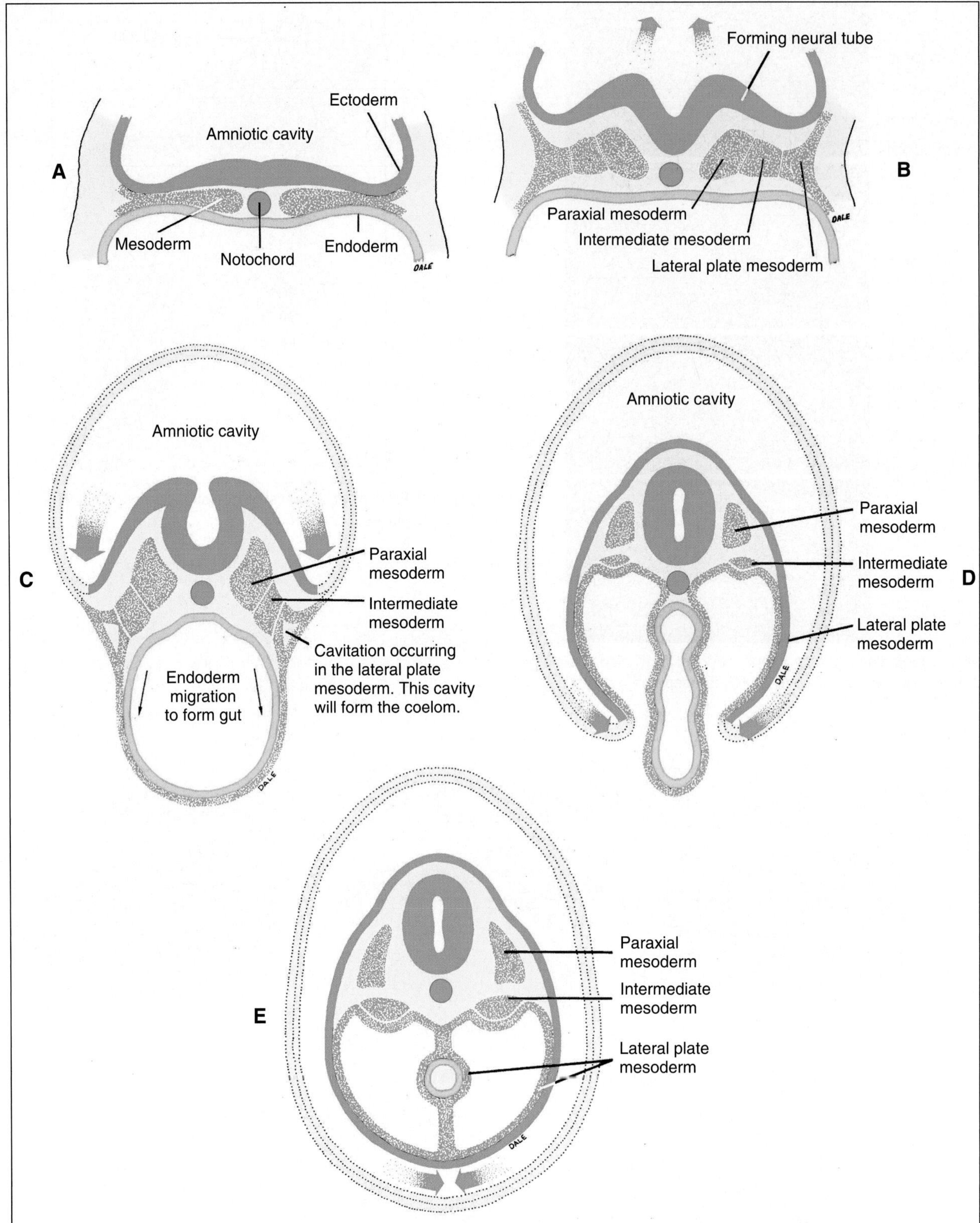

Fig. 2.11 Cross-sectional profiles. (A) The mesoderm, situated between the ectoderm and endoderm in the trilaminar disk. (B) Differentiation of the mesoderm into three masses: the paraxial, intermediate, and lateral plate mesoderm. (C–E) With lateral folding of the embryo, the amniotic cavity encompasses the embryo, and the ectoderm, constituting its floor, forms the surface epithelium. Paraxial mesoderm remains adjacent to the neural tube. Intermediate mesoderm is relocated and forms urogenital tissue. Lateral plate mesoderm cavitates, forming the coelom and its lining the serous membranes of the gut and abdominal cavity.

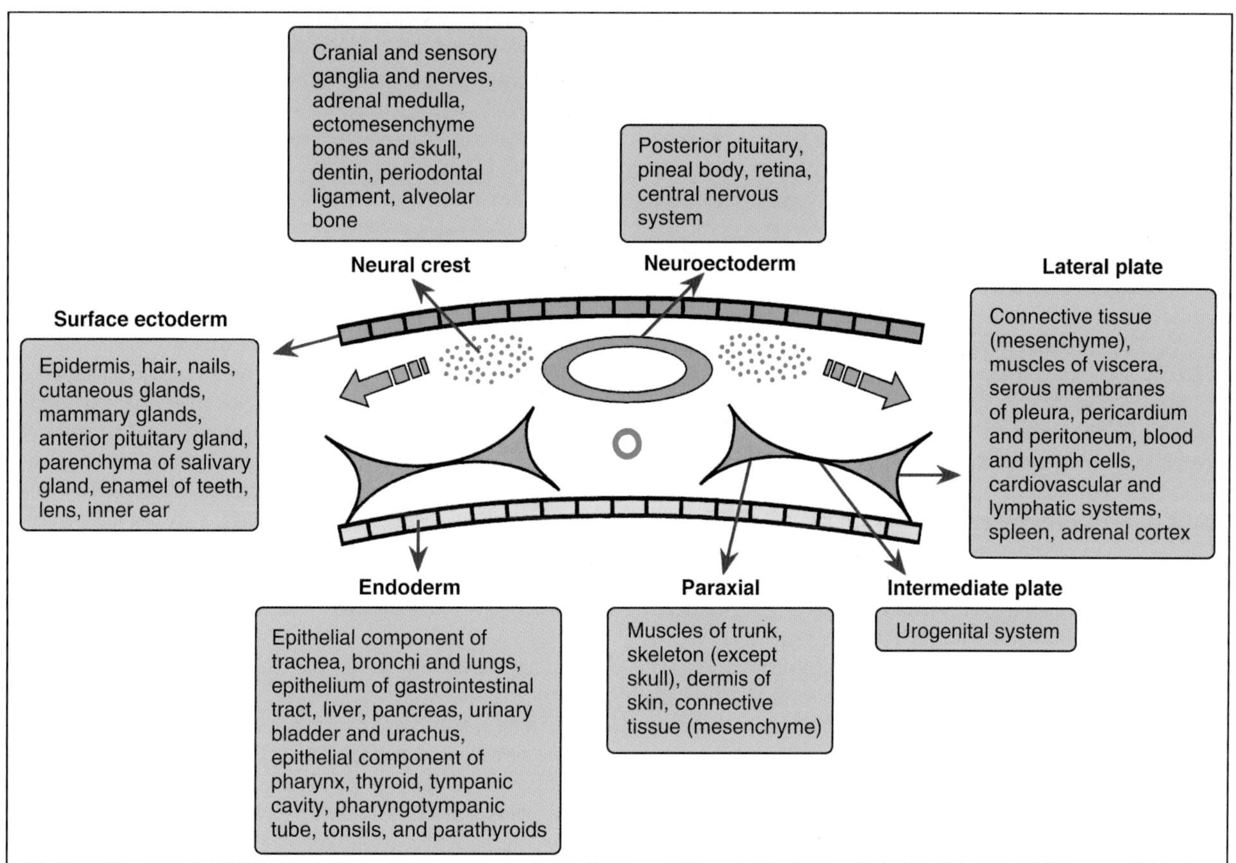

Fig. 2.12 Derivatives of the germ layers and cranial neural crest.

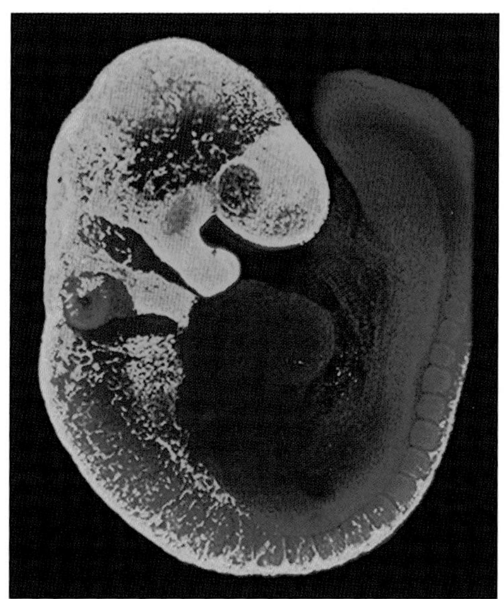

Fig. 2.13 Migration of neural crest cells throughout the embryo traced in a knock-in Pax3-GFP *(green)* transgenic mouse model. (Courtesy A. Barlow and P. Trainor, Stowers Institute for Medical Research.)

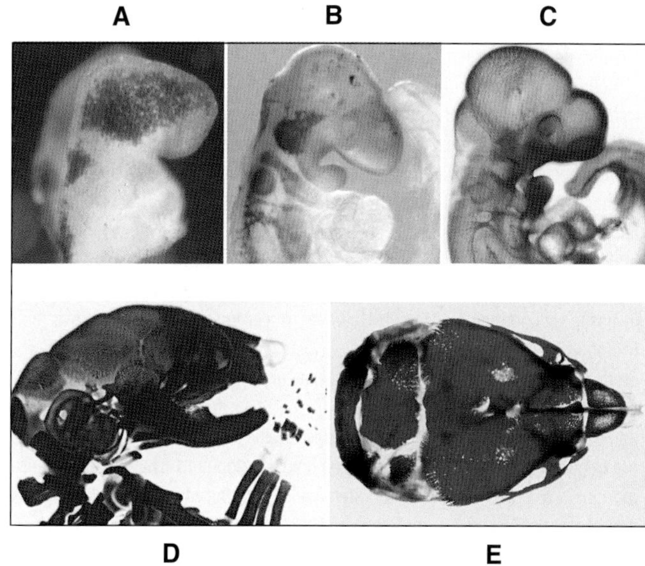

Fig. 2.14 Migration and differentiation of cranial neural crest cells (NCCs). (A) Migrating NCC. (B, C) Neuronal differentiation of NCC. (D) Skeletal differentiation of NCC. (E) Neurocranium (bone, *red;* cartilage, *blue*). (From Trainor P: Specification of neural crest cell formation and migration in mouse embryos, *Semin Cell Dev Biol* 16(6):683–693, 2005.)

BOX 2.1 Neural Crest Cells and Their Application in Regenerative Medicine

Neural crest cells (NCCs) comprise a migratory stem and progenitor cell population that forms during the third to fourth weeks of human embryonic development. Derived from the ectoderm during the period of neurulation, NCCs are essential both for embryo development and throughout adult life. NCCs are formed along almost the entire length of the embryo and can be subdivided into distinct axial populations: cranial, cardiac, trunk, and sacral. Cranial NCCs give rise to the precursors of most of the cranial cartilage, bone and connective tissue of the craniofacial skeleton, the meninges surrounding the brain, and odontoblasts of the teeth. Cranial and trunk NCCs generate neurons and glia within the peripheral and enteric nervous systems, and they differentiate into melanoblasts (pigment cells of the skin). Cardiac NCCs generate smooth muscle cells of the cardiovascular system and form the septum of the heart. Vagal and sacral NCCs give rise to neurons and glia in the gastrointestinal tract. Trunk NCCs also differentiate into hormone-secreting cells of the adrenal gland. In fact, there is barely a tissue or organ throughout the human body that does not receive a contribution from NCCs.

NCCs are considered a vertebrate-specific cell type that has played a central role in the evolution of novel morphologic structures and their variation and adaptation; however, the evolutionary origins of NCCs remain an enigma. One hypothesis suggests that NCCs may have initially emerged in tunicates. Advances in the NCC field continue to uncover the genes, proteins, and regulatory networks that endow NCCs with their stem and progenitor cell–like properties and astonishing array of lineage descendant cell fates. Much of the focus on NCCs therefore currently revolves around their contributions to congenital disorders and diseases, which are collectively termed *neurocristopathies.* This includes disorders of craniofacial development such as cleft palate and craniosynostosis; anomalies of cardiac development, including persistent truncus arteriosus; malformation of gastrointestinal development as occurs in Hirschsprung disease; and cancers such as neuroblastoma and melanoma, which affect the peripheral nervous system and skin, respectively. Understanding the genetic etiology and cell and tissue pathogenesis of individual neurocristopathies offers the potential for developing reparative, regenerative, or preventive therapies for treating neurocristopathies.

Stem cell transplantations have been touted as a therapeutic strategy in the treatment of neurocristopathy disorders and diseases. Although embryonic stem cells were once considered ideal for this purpose because of their extraordinary pluripotency, their derivation is still ethically controversial, and the potential for host rejection remains high. In contrast, adult stem cells are available from numerous tissue sources and can be derived from an affected individual without ethical concern or fear of transplant rejection. The identification of multipotent NCC progenitors in adults has therefore facilitated their therapeutic application in tissue engineering and repair. However, in contrast to stem cells, less than 5% of NCCs exhibit true multipotency. Most NCCs exhibit a limited capacity for producing identical daughter cells, and they are typically unipotent or bipotent, with their fate determined by a combination or intrinsic and extrinsic genetic and environmental cues. Furthermore, despite their persistence in adults, NCCs are generated only transiently during embryo development. Therefore NCCs are more akin to progenitor cells than stem cells, with the true stem cell being the neural stem cell in the neuroepithelium from which NCCs are derived. Nonetheless, studies of NCC contribution to the sciatic nerve in rats revealed that pure populations of NCCs can be isolated through flow cytometry and (more important) that these isolated NCCs retain the capacity to form neurons and glia after transplantation into host avian embryos. Similar populations of NCCs also persist in the gut, epidermis dental pulp, heart, bone marrow, cornea, hard palate, and oral mucosa of adult organisms, providing multiple accessible sources of cells for replacement therapy.

The developmental potential of neural crest stem and progenitor cells may, however, decrease with age. Whereas mouse embryo–derived gut neural crest progenitor cells migrate great distances away from a transplantation site in avian embryos and differentiate into neurons, adult gut–derived neural crest progenitor cells only engraft structures in the proximity of their site of transplantation. Nonetheless, gut-derived neural crest progenitor cells transplanted into the aganglionic gut of a rat model of the Hirschsprung disease engrafted and differentiated into neurons. Furthermore, NCCs isolated from fetal human gut tissue remained viable, engrafted, and established functional connections after transplantation into the bowel of immunodeficient mice.

NCCs derived from the epidermis of the skin also appear to hold considerable therapeutic promise. Not only are they readily accessible for isolation, but the hair follicle contains a mixed population of epidermal, keratinocyte, and melanocyte stem cells, each of which exhibits a high degree of plasticity. Within the hair follicle is a multilayered region of the outer root sheath called the *bulge.* The bulge is where new hair growth occurs and, interestingly, the inner layers are derived from NCCs. Neural crest–derived cells, harvested from the bulge region, can undergo self-renewal, indicating these cells are stem cells. Furthermore, these cells are multipotent, and under differentiation conditions they produce colonies of neurons, smooth muscle cells, rare Schwann cells, melanocytes, and even chondrocytes. These cells have therefore been called *epidermal neural crest stem cells,* and the bulge in which they are found represents their niche.

Recently, neural crest–derived cells isolated from hair follicles were shown to repair sciatic nerve function in vivo in mice. Isolated stem cells from the hair follicle were used in transplants to treat two different injured nerves, the sciatic and tibial nerve. After transplantation, the follicle stem cells incorporated into the nerve, precipitating the recovery of proper nerve function. Functional studies of the gastrocnemius revealed consistent contractions upon stimulation. Furthermore, tibial nerve function was recovered in mice that received a follicle stem cell transplant, as demonstrated by normal walking ability. In contrast, control mice with a severed sciatic nerve but without transplantation displayed no muscle contraction upon stimulation. Taken together, these results determined that transplantation of follicular neural crest stem cells promotes regenerative axonal growth, resulting in the recovery of peripheral nerve function. Consistent with this model, the neuroprotective properties and therapeutic potential of epidermis-derived neural crest stem cells were also demonstrated in the rescue of long-term potentiation and cognitive disability in a rat model of vascular dementia. These experiments elegantly demonstrate the potential of follicle stem cells (of which epidermal neural crest stem cells are a component) as a potential source of cells to be used in stem cell therapies.

Tooth-derived NCCs, such as those from the dental pulp, are also a promising cell source for regeneration because, similar to the epidermis, they are easy to isolate, maintain in culture, and manipulate. Furthermore, their application in peripheral nerve injuries in animal models has revealed their regeneration capacity through glial differentiation and neuroprotection function.

In addition to autologous transplantation without immune rejection, the isolation of adult neural crest progenitor cells, or their induced pluripotent stem cell (iPSC) derivation from patients affected with a neurocristopathy, provides a powerful platform for modeling disease and informing its pathogenesis, as well as drug screening for therapeutics. For example, enteric NCC progenitors derived from human iPSC can migrate, engraft, and differentiate into neurons, rescuing disease-related mortality in mice with Hirschsprung disease. This raises the possibility of generating neural crest progenitor cells via iPSC or isolating them directly from the ganglionic region of the gut of a patient with Hirschsprung disease and then transplanting these cells into the aganglionic region of the same individual. This type of approach may provide a treatment option for Hirschsprung disease and, similarly, familial dysautonomia, a neurodegenerative disorder of the peripheral nervous system that is characterized by autonomic dysfunction without incurring problems with histocompatibility and immunosuppression, which are typical of transplantation surgery.

BOX 2.1 Neural Crest Cells and Their Application in Regenerative Medicine—cont'd

In other studies, human iPSC–derived NCCs were shown to be capable of producing erythropoietin such that when transplanted subcutaneously into anemic mice, they induce erythropoiesis, illustrating their potential clinical use in treating renal and nonrenal anemia. Furthermore, transplanted human iPSC–derived NCCs can rapidly restore corneal thickness and clarity in a rabbit model of corneal endothelial regeneration in rabbits. Lastly, human iPSC–derived NCCs can be differentiated into brain pericyte–like cells that have the molecular and functional characteristics of pericytes.

Human iPSC–derived NCCs exhibit low immunogenicity, which is encouraging for their use in cellular therapy. However, there is still much to learn because not all endogenous NCCs that can be derived from adult tissues or human iPSC are equivalent. This is born out in tests of their capacity in craniofacial regeneration, which revealed the importance of NCC origin for optimal success and surgical outcomes.

Conclusions

Although NCCs are a discrete population, generated only transiently in the embryo, numerous populations of neural crest stem and progenitor cells have been isolated from embryonic and adult tissues. Neural crest–derived stem cells are extremely useful for disease modeling, for drug screening, and in stem cell therapy. They are easily accessible, are relatively easy to maintain in culture, and provide an autologous source of tissue for replacement therapies, thereby bypassing immunorejection. These approaches, when used in combination with advances in genome engineering, make it possible to isolate neural crest progenitor cells from an affected individual, correct a genetic defect in those cells, then transplant those cells back into the same individual, possibly preventing or correcting the disorder. As proof of principle, a similar type of combinatorial stem cell and gene editing approach has recently been successful in the treatment of sickle cell anemia. The application of modern genomic and proteomic techniques, including single-cell RNA sequencing, assay for transposase-accessible chromatin sequencing, identification of posttranslational modifications of proteins, and protein-protein interaction networks will continue to deepen our understanding of the regulation of NCC development and their capacity for tissue-specific regeneration.

Paul A. Trainor, *BSc, PhD*
Investigator
Stowers Institute for Medical Research
Kansas City, Missouri, United States
Professor
The Graduate School of the Stowers Institute for Medical Research
Kansas City, Missouri, United States
Professor
Department of Cell Biology and Physiology
University of Kansas School of Medicine
Kansas City, Missouri, United States

Recommended Reading

Gandhi S, Bronner ME: Seq your destiny: neural crest cell fate determination in the genomic era, *Ann Rev Genet* 55:349–376, 2021.

Le Dourain NM, Kalchein C, editors: *the neural crest*, Cambridge, England, 1999, Cambridge University Press.

Okuno H, Okano H: Modelling human congenital disorders with neural crest cell developmental defects using patient-derived induced pluripotent stem cells, *Regen Ther* 18:275–280, 2021.

Saint-Jeannet JP, editor: *Advances in experimental medicine and biology*, New York, 2006, Landes Bioscience.

Trainor PA, editor: *Neural crest cells: evolution, development and disease*, New York, 2014, Elsevier.

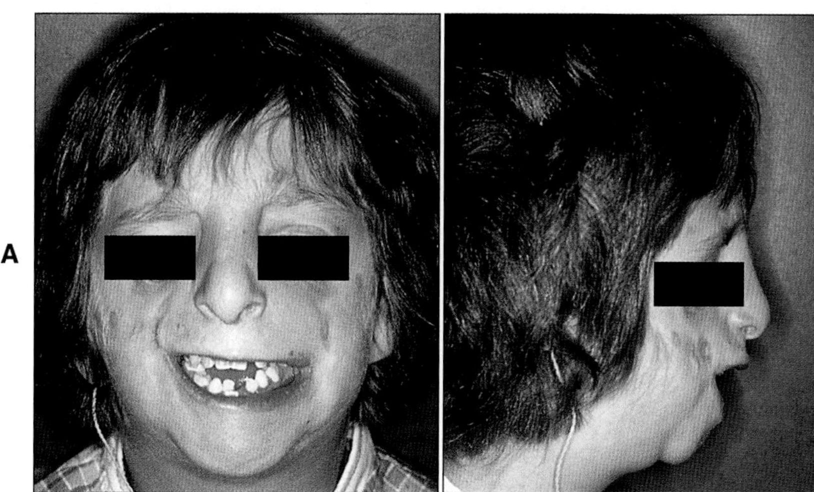

Fig. 2.15 (A, B) A child with mandibulofacial dysostosis (Treacher Collins syndrome). The underdevelopment results from a failure of the neural crest cells to migrate to the facial region. (Photograph courtesy Dr. L.B. Kaban.)

of members of the Snail (Snail and Slug) zinc-finger transcription factor family, who, as master regulators of EMT, repress the expression of the cell adhesion molecule E-cadherin in concert with upregulation of N-cadherin as part of the cadherin switch.

NCCs are formed along almost the entire length of the embryo and can be subdivided into distinct axial populations: cranial, cardiac, trunk, and sacral. Cranial NCCs play a particularly important role in head and facial development. In addition to contributing to formation of the cranial sensory ganglia, cranial NCCs also differentiate to form most of the connective tissue of the head. Embryonic connective tissue elsewhere is derived from mesoderm, known as *mesenchyme*, whereas in the head it is known as *ectomesenchyme*, reflecting its origin from neuroectoderm. Proper migration of NCCs is essential for the development of the craniofacial skeleton and the teeth, and many craniofacial anomalies are therefore considered disorders of NCC development, termed *neurocristopathies*. In Treacher Collins syndrome (Fig. 2.15), for example, full facial development does not occur because of the insufficient generation, proliferation, and survival of NCCs in the facial region. With respect to the teeth, all the tissues (except enamel and perhaps some cementum) and their supporting apparatus are derived directly from NCCs, and their depletion prevents proper dental development.

RECOMMENDED READING

Cordero DR, et al.: Cranial neural crest cells on the move: their roles in craniofacial development, *Am J Med Genet A* 155:270, 2011.

Dash S, Trainor PA: The development, patterning and evolution of neural crest cell differentiation into cartilage and bone (Special Issue *"Imaging and Computational Methods in Musculoskeletal Biology"*), *Bone* 137:115409, 2020.

Minoux M, Rijli FM: Molecular mechanism of cranial neural crest cell migration and patterning in craniofacial development, *Development* 137:2605, 2010.

Moore KL, et al.: *The developing human: clinically orientated embryology*, ed 8, Philadelphia, 2008, Saunders.

Munoz WA, Trainor PA: Neural crest cell evolution: how and when did a neural crest cell become a neural crest cell. In Trainor PA, editor: *Neural crest and placodes,* New York, 2015, Elsevier, pp 3–26. Current topics in developmental biology, vol. 111.

Sadler TW, editor: *Langman's essential medical embryology*, vol 1, Baltimore, 2005, Lippincott Williams & Wilkins.

3

Embryology of the Head, Face, and Oral Cavity

Antonio Nanci

OUTLINE

Knowledge of the evolutionary development of the skull, face, and jaws is helpful in understanding the complex events involved in cephalogenesis (formation of the head). Early chordates have a fairly simple anatomic plan with (1) a notochord for support, (2) a simple nervous system and sense organs, (3) segmented muscle blocks, and (4) at the beginning of the pharynx in its lateral wall, a series of branchial arches supported by cartilage associated with clefts to permit gaseous exchange. The first vertebrates evolved from this simple plan and were jawless (agnathia). Cartilaginous blocks (occipital and parachordal) evolved to support the notochord in the head region, along with cartilaginous capsules (nasal, optic, otic) to protect the sense organs. These cartilages collectively form the neurocranium. The branchial arches, as mentioned, are supported by a series of cartilaginous rods originally numbered 0, 1, 2, and so on that constitute the viscerocranium. The first cartilage (cartilage 0) of the branchial arches migrated to the neurocranium to provide additional support as the trabecular cartilage. Because of this, the actual second arch cartilage became the first arch cartilage (Fig. 3.1A and B). The neurocranium and viscerocranium together form the chondrocranium.

From this simple model, vertebrates came to possess jaws (gnathostomata) through modification of the jointed first arch cartilage, with the upper element, the palatopterygo-quadrate bar, becoming the upper jaw and the lower element and Meckel's cartilage becoming the lower jaw (see Fig. 3.1C). The fibrous connection between the two formed the jaw joint. In addition to jaws, vertebrate evolution also brought about massive expansion of the head region and associated larger neural and sensory elements. For protection, dermal bones developed as additional bony skeletal elements to form the vault of the skull and the facial skeleton, which included bony jaws and teeth. This cephalic expansion demanded a source of new connective tissue, the neuroectoderm (see Chapter 2) from which neural crest cells (NCCs) migrate and differentiate into ectomesenchyme. Fig. 3.2 shows a comparison between the cranial components of the primitive vertebrate skull and the cranial skeleton of a human fetus.

NEURAL CREST CELLS AND HEAD FORMATION

The folding of the three-layered embryo has been described, and the rostral or head fold is important at this point. As discussed in Chapter 2, the neural tube is produced by the formation and fusion of the neural folds, which sink beneath surface ectoderm (see Fig. 2.8). The anterior portion of this neural tube expands greatly as the forebrain, midbrain, and hindbrain form (Fig. 3.3), and the part associated with the hindbrain develops a series of eight bulges, the rhombomeres (Fig. 3.4). Lateral to the neural tube is the paraxial mesoderm, which partially segments rostrally to form somatomeres and fully segments caudally to form somites, the first in the series being the occipital somites (see Fig. 3.3).

NCCs from the midbrain and the first two rhombomeres transform and migrate as two streams to supply additional embryonic connective tissue needed for craniofacial development (see Fig. 3.4). The first stream provides much of the ectomesenchyme associated with the face, whereas the second stream is targeted to the first arch where they contribute to formation of the jaws. NCC subpopulations, depending on their anteroposterior location along the neural tube, are subject to a complex temporal and spatial set of signaling events. A plethora of molecules are used as cues to guide them to their destination within restricted areas of the head. Their eventual differentiation is also tightly controlled through reciprocal signaling with neighboring ectodermal cells. The various intracellular signaling events and cross talk between cells eventually culminate to elicit various cellular responses, including proliferation, migration, differentiation, and survival or apoptosis.

NCCs from rhombomere 3 and beyond migrate into arches that will give rise to pharyngeal structures. Because homeobox transcription factor genes are not expressed anterior to rhombomere 3, a different set of coded patterning genes has been adapted for development of cephalic structures (Fig. 3.5). This new set of transcription factor genes, reflecting the later development of the head in evolutionary terms, includes orthodenticle homeobox 2 (Otx2), muscle segment homeobox (Msx), the distal-less homeobox (Dlx), and the

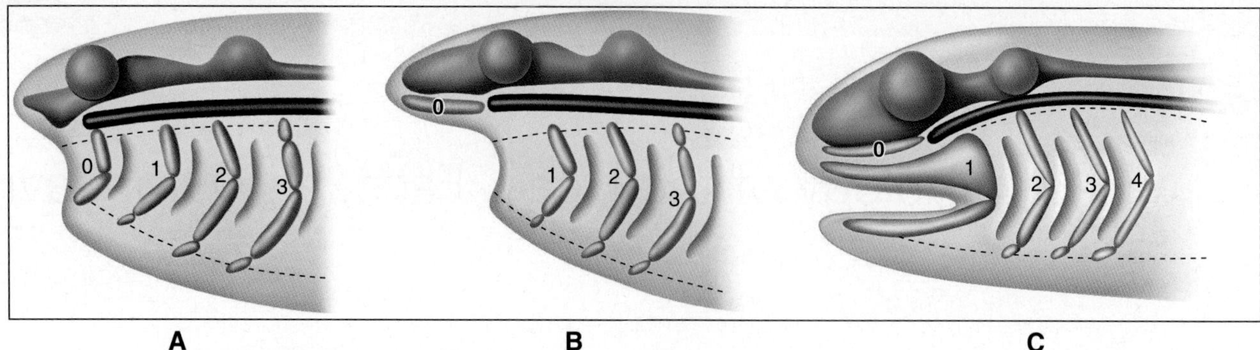

Fig. 3.1 (A, B) The viscerocranium and the movement of arch 0 to the neurocranium. (C) The jaws developed from the first branchial arch cartilage of the viscerocranium. (Redrawn from Osborn JW, editor: *Dental anatomy and embryology,* vol 2, Oxford, UK, 1981, Blackwell Scientific.)

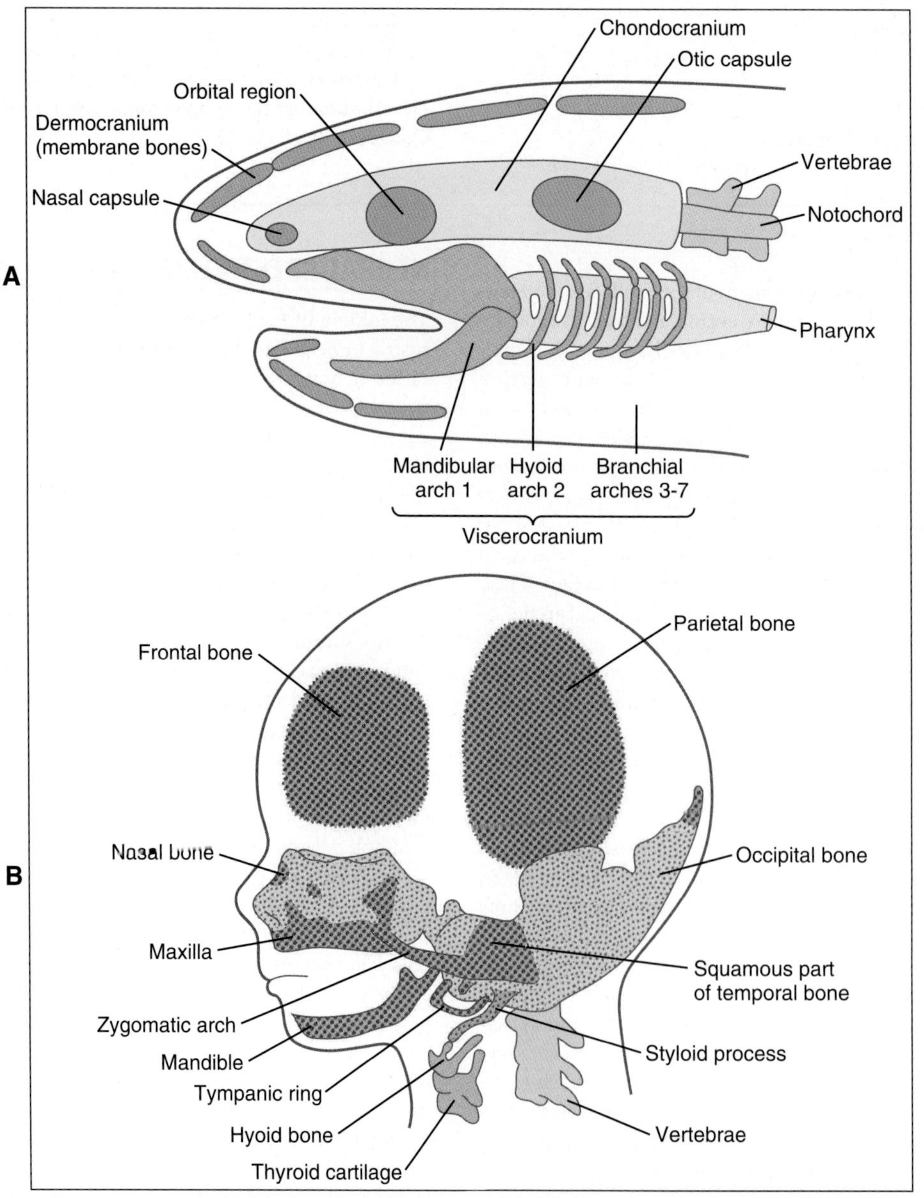

Fig. 3.2 The major components of (A) the primitive vertebrate cranial skeleton and (B) a human fetal head. (B) Bones of the cranial vault and face are formed by intramembranous ossification *(coarse stippling),* whereas bones of the cranial base form by endochondral ossification *(fine stippling).* (From Carlson BM: *Human embryology and developmental biology,* Philadelphia, PA, 2004, Mosby.)

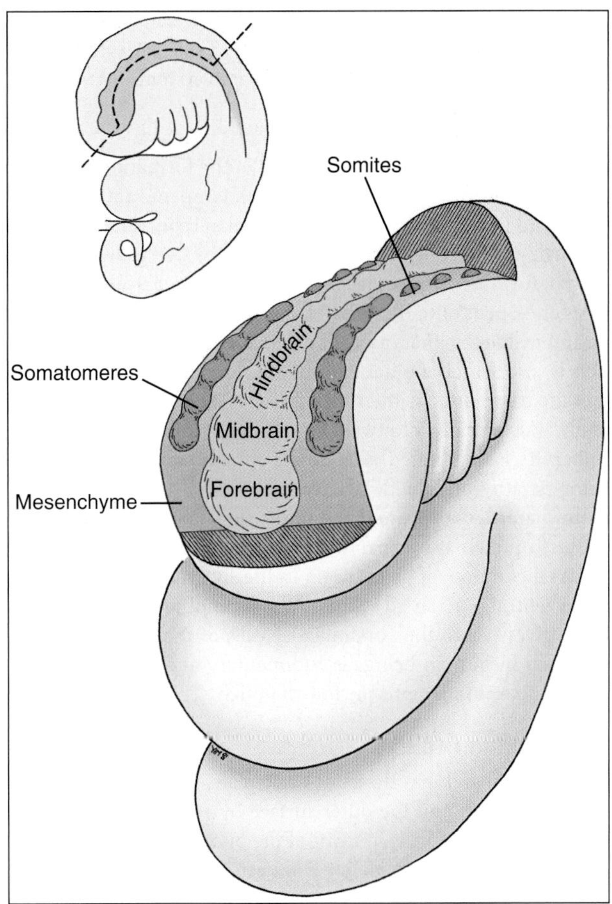

Fig. 3.3 The building blocks for cephalogenesis.

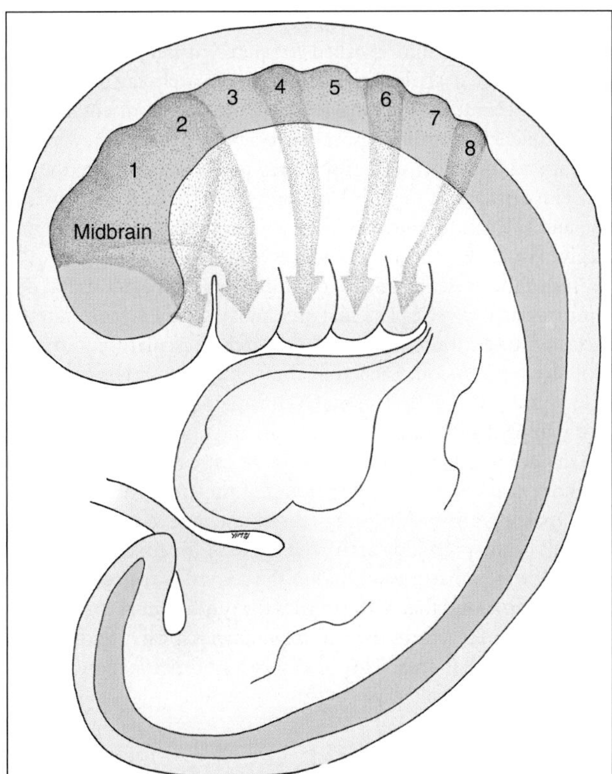

Fig. 3.4 The source and pattern of neural crest migration to the developing face and branchial arch system. The midbrain and rhombomeres 1 and 2 contribute to the face and first branchial arch.

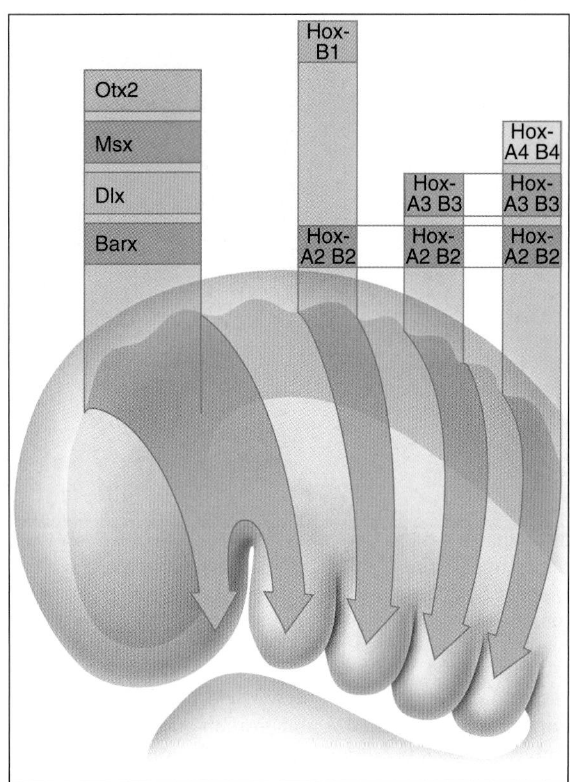

Fig. 3.5 Migrating neural crest cells express the same *homeobox* (*Hox*) genes as their precursors in the rhombomeres from which they derive. Note that Hox genes are not expressed anterior to rhombomere 3. A new set of patterning genes (*Otx2, Msx, Dlx, Barx*) has evolved to bring about development of cephalic structures so that a Hox code also is transferred to the branchial arches and developing face.

BarH-like homeobox (*Barx*). Homeobox genes also are implicated in dental development, and their effects are discussed in Chapter 5.

Some NCC populations require instructions from their local microenvironment. The resulting cross talk involves common signaling pathways, such as sonic hedgehog (*Shh*), fibroblast growth factor (*Fgf*), and bone morphogenetic proteins (*Bmp*). Enzymes that modify chromatin architecture regulating the accessibility of transcription factors to DNA also participate in craniofacial patterning. Environmental factors that transmit repulsive and/or attractive signals are also instrumental in specifying the segregation and fate of NCCs in their migration to branchial arches. Several secreted ligands and their membrane-bound receptors provide repulsive cues, especially in the NCC-free regions of mesenchyme adjacent to rhombomeres 3 and 5. Among others, important players in this process are the membrane-anchored receptors v-erb-b2 avian erythroblastic leukemia viral oncogene homolog 4 (*Erbb4*), ephrin and neurolipin along with their respective soluble ligands, neuregulins, ephrins, and semaphorins. On the other hand, directional guidance (attraction) of NCCs into their respective arches is provided by another elaborate set of species-specific molecules, such as Twist, T-box 1 (Tbx1), stromal cell–derived factor 1/chemokine cxc motif receptor 4 (Sdf1b/Cxcr4a), neuropilin 1/vascular endothelial growth factor (Npn1/Vegf), and Fgf receptor 1 (Fgfr1).

The species-specific patterning of the head and face, especially the shape and size of the beak and muzzle, has been suggested to depend on the canonical (β-catenin–dependent) Wnt signaling pathway that seems to be an upstream modulator of critical effector molecules, such as Fgf8, Bmp2, and Shh, present in the frontonasal ectodermal zone (FEZ) center. This center is another major determinant of

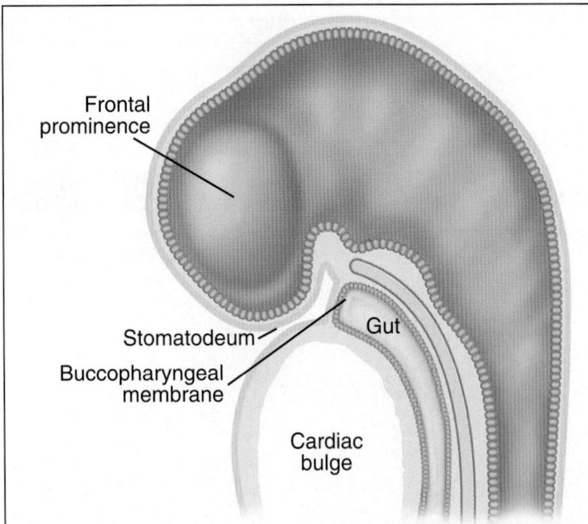

Fig. 3.6 Sagittal section through a 4-week-old embryo showing the stomatodeum delimited by the frontal prominence above and the developing cardiac bulge below. The buccopharyngeal membrane separates the stomatodeum from the primitive gut.

species-specific patterning and outgrowth of the upper face. Variation in the organization, relative size, and position of the FEZ, together with other molecules such as calmodulin, are partly responsible for the very different shapes encountered in nature.

Although understanding of molecular analyses has made significant progress, the cell biologic activities resulting from various molecular cascades are still being clarified. Planar polarity genes are attracting much attention not only because of their role in regulating cell polarity and morphogenesis, but also because of their implication in positioning cellular structures and coordinating activities, such as cell intercalation. One such structure is the cilium, which is found on the surface of most vertebrate cells and acts as a mechanical/chemical sensor. Ciliary dysfunction is present in some syndromes, such as facial-digital syndrome and Bardet-Biedl syndrome, which exhibit facial changes, as well as cleft palate and micrognathia. Experimentally, it has been shown that a neural crest–targeted mutation of the *kif3* gene, encoding for a kinesin-like protein implicated in ciliogenesis and intraflagellar transport, affects polarized growth and cell shape, resulting in shortened mandibles and defects in development of the cranial base.

BRANCHIAL (PHARYNGEAL) ARCHES AND THE PRIMITIVE MOUTH

When the stomatodeum first forms, it is delimited rostrally by the frontal prominence and caudally by the developing cardiac bulge (Figs. 3.6 and 3.7A). The buccopharyngeal membrane, a bilaminar structure consisting of apposed ectoderm and endoderm, separates the stomatodeum from the foregut (see Fig. 3.6), but this soon breaks down so that the stomatodeum communicates directly with the foregut (Fig. 3.8). Laterally the stomatodeum becomes limited by the first pair of pharyngeal or branchial arches (see Fig. 3.8; see also Fig. 3.7A). The branchial arches form in the pharyngeal wall as a proliferation of mesoderm infiltrated by migrating NCCs. Six cylindric thickenings thus form; however, the fifth and sixth are transient structures in humans. They expand from the lateral wall of the pharynx and approach their anatomic counterparts, expanding from the opposite side. In doing so, the arches progressively separate the primitive stomatodeum from the developing heart. The arches are seen clearly as bulges on the lateral aspect of the embryo and are separated externally by small clefts called *branchial grooves.* On the inner aspect of the pharyngeal wall are corresponding small depressions called *pharyngeal pouches* that separate each of the branchial arches internally. Table 3.1 summarizes the derivatives of the branchial (pharyngeal) arch system.

Fate of Grooves and Pouches

The first groove and pouch are involved in the formation of the external auditory meatus, tympanic membrane, tympanic antrum, mastoid antrum, and pharyngotympanic or eustachian tube. The second, third, and fourth grooves normally are obliterated by overgrowth of the second arch, forming a transitory cervical sinus (Fig. 3.9) that sometimes persists and opens onto the side of the neck (branchial fistula) or on the neck and inside the pharynx (pharyngocutaneous fistula). The second pouch is also largely obliterated by the development of the palatine tonsil; a part persists as the tonsillar fossa. The third pouch expands dorsally and ventrally into two compartments, and its connection with the pharynx is obliterated. The dorsal component gives origin to the inferior parathyroid gland, whereas the ventral component, with its anatomic counterpart from the opposite side, forms the thymus gland. The fourth pouch also expands into dorsal and ventral components. The dorsal component gives origin to the superior parathyroid gland, and the ventral portion gives rise to the ultimobranchial body, which, in turn, gives rise to the parafollicular cells of the thyroid gland. The fifth pouch in human beings is rudimentary and thus disappears or becomes incorporated into the fourth pouch.

Anatomy of an Arch

Every branchial arch has the same basic plan. The inner aspect is covered by endoderm and the outer surface by ectoderm, except for the first arch because it forms in front of the buccopharyngeal membrane and therefore derives completely from ectodermally covered surfaces. The central core consists of mesenchyme derived from lateral plate mesoderm invaded by NCCs, referred to as *ectomesenchyme.* This neural-derived mesenchyme condenses to form a bar of cartilage, the arch cartilage (Fig. 3.9). The cartilage of the first arch is called *Meckel's cartilage,* and the second is called *Reichert's cartilage,* after the anatomists who first described them. The other arch cartilages are not named. The contribution of Meckel's cartilage is discussed subsequently. Reichert's cartilage gives rise to a bony process, the stylohyoid ligament and the upper part of the body and lesser horns of the hyoid bone. The cartilage of the third arch gives rise to the lower part of the body, and the greater horns of the hyoid bone and that of the fourth arch give rise to the cartilages of the larynx.

Some of the mesenchyme surrounding this cartilaginous bar develops into striated muscle. The first arch musculature gives origin to the muscles of mastication and the second arch musculature to the muscles of facial expression. Each arch also contains an artery and a nerve (Fig. 3.9 and Table 3.2). The nerve consists of two components, one motor (supplying the muscle of the arch) and one sensory. The sensory nerve divides into two branches: a posttrematic branch, supplying the epithelium that covers the anterior half of the arch, and a pretrematic branch, passing forward to supply the epithelium that covers the posterior half of the preceding arch. The nerve of the first arch is the fifth cranial (or trigeminal) nerve, that of the second is the seventh cranial (or facial) nerve, and that of the third is the ninth cranial (or glossopharyngeal) nerve. Structures derived from any arch carry with them the nerve supply of that arch. Thus the muscles of mastication are innervated by the trigeminal nerve.

Fusion of Processes

The first, second, and third branchial arches play an important role in the development of the face, mouth, and tongue. Classically, the formation of the face is described in terms of the formation and fusion of several processes or prominences (Fig. 3.10). In some

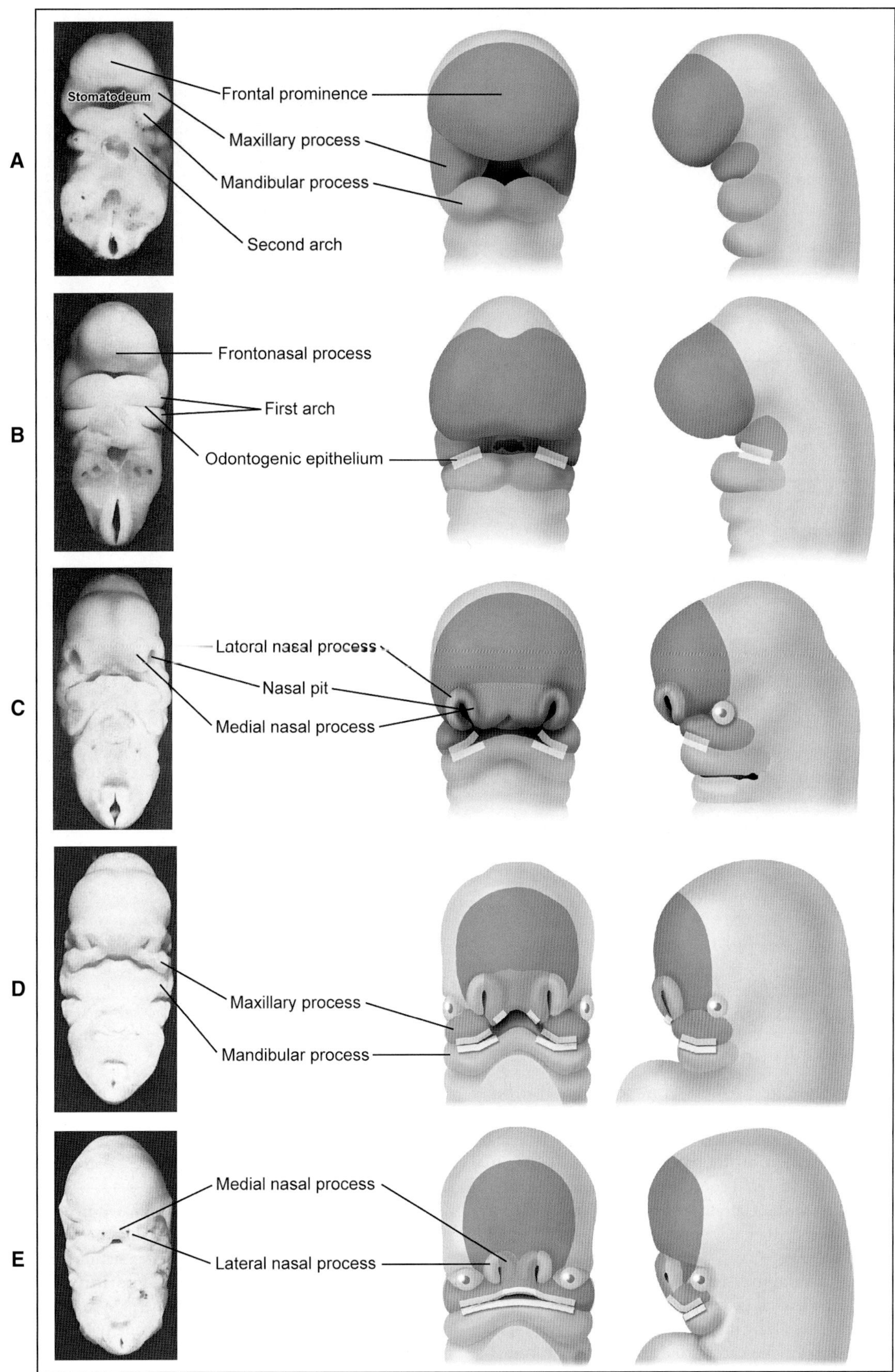

Fig. 3.7 Summary of human facial development from about weeks 4 through 6 of development. Left-column photographs show actual embryos; the middle and right columns are diagrammatic representations of frontal and lateral views, respectively. (A) Boundaries of the stomatodeum in a 26-day-old embryo. The stomatodeum is limited cranially by the frontal prominence, laterally by the newly formed maxillary process (derived from the first arch), and ventrally by the mandibular process (also derived from the first arch). (B) A 27-day-old embryo. The nasal placode is about to develop, and odontogenic epithelium can be identified in the regions delimited by the white bars. The beginning elements for facial development and the boundaries of the stomatodeum are apparent. (C) A 34-day-old embryo. The nasal pits have formed, thereby delineating the lateral and medial nasal processes. (D) A 36-day-old embryo shows the fusion of various facial processes that are completed by 38 days of gestation (E). (Redrawn from Nery EB, et al.: Timing and topography of early human tooth development, *Arch Oral Biol* 15:1315, 1970. Photographs courtesy H. Nishimura.)

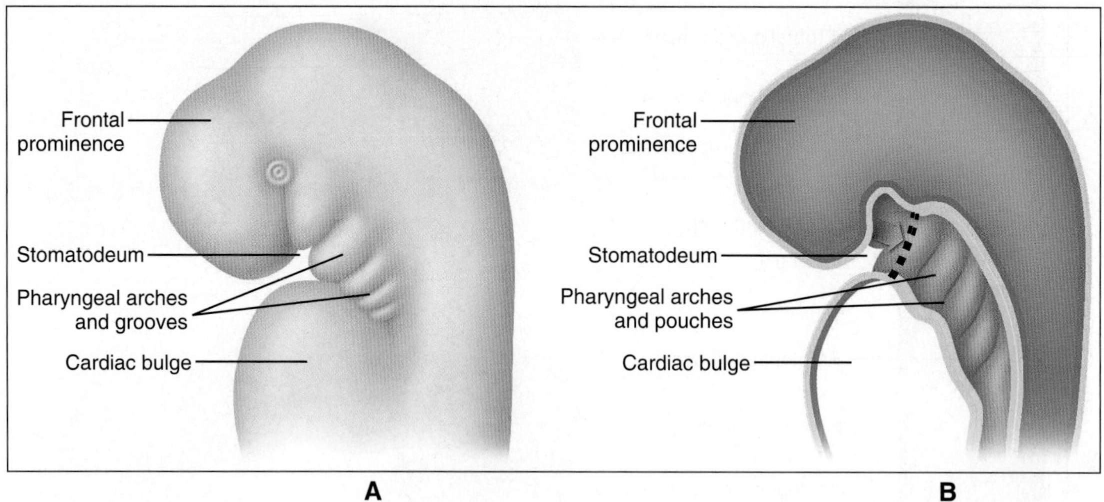

Fig. 3.8 (A) Development of pharyngeal arches and the grooves between them in a 35-day-old embryo. (B) Midline section showing reflection of the arches on the pharyngeal wall and the pharyngeal pouches separating them. The dotted line *(arrow)* represents the site where the buccopharyngeal membrane was.

TABLE 3.1 Derivatives of the Branchial (Pharyngeal) Arch System

	Arch	Groove	Pouch
First	1. Mandible and maxilla 2. Meckel's cartilage: a. Incus and malleus of inner ear b. Sphenomalleolar ligament c. Sphenomandibular ligament	External auditory meatus	Tympanic membrane Tympanic cavity Mastoid antrum Eustachian tube
Second	1. Reichert's cartilage: a. Styloid process of temporal bone b. Stylohyoid ligament c. Lesser horns of the hyoid bone d. Upper part of the body of the hyoid bone	Obliterated by the down-growth of the second arch	Largely obliterated Contributes to tonsil
Third	1. Lower part of the body of the hyoid bone 2. Greater horns of the hyoid bone		Inferior parathyroid gland Thymus
Fourth	Cartilages of the larynx		Superior parathyroid gland Ultimobranchial body
Fifth	Transient	Transient	Transient
Sixth	Transient	Transient	Transient

instances, these processes are swellings of mesenchyme that cause furrows between apparent processes so that the ostensible fusion of processes involves the elimination of a furrow. Only in certain instances, such as the union of the palatal processes, does actual fusion occur (Fig. 3.11). To avoid confusion, the conventional term *process* (rather than the more accurate terms *swelling* or *prominence*) is used to describe the further development of the face and oral cavity.

To recapitulate, the primitive stomatodeum is, at first, bounded above (rostrally) by the frontal prominence, below (caudally) by the developing heart, and laterally by the first branchial arch. With spread of the arches midventrally, the cardiac bulge is distanced from the stomatodeum, and the floor of the mouth is now formed by the epithelium covering the mesenchyme of the first, second, and third branchial arches.

At about day 24 of gestation, the first branchial arch establishes another process, the maxillary process, so that the stomatodeum is limited cranially by the frontal prominence covering the rapidly expanding forebrain, laterally by the newly formed maxillary process, and ventrally by the first arch (now called the *mandibular process*) (see Fig. 3.7B).

FORMATION OF THE FACE

Early development of the face is dominated by the proliferation and migration of ectomesenchyme involved in the formation of the primitive nasal cavities. At about day 28 of gestation, localized thickenings develop within the ectoderm of the frontal prominence, just above the opening of the stomatodeum. These thickenings are the olfactory placodes. Rapid proliferation of the underlying mesenchyme around the placodes bulges the frontal eminence forward and produces a horseshoe-shaped ridge that converts the olfactory placode into the nasal pit (see Fig. 3.7C). The lateral arm of the horseshoe is called the *lateral nasal process*, and the medial arm is called the *medial nasal process*. The region of the frontal prominence where these changes occur and the nose will develop is referred to as the *frontonasal process (region)*. The medial nasal processes of both sides, together with the frontonasal process, give rise to the middle portion of the nose.

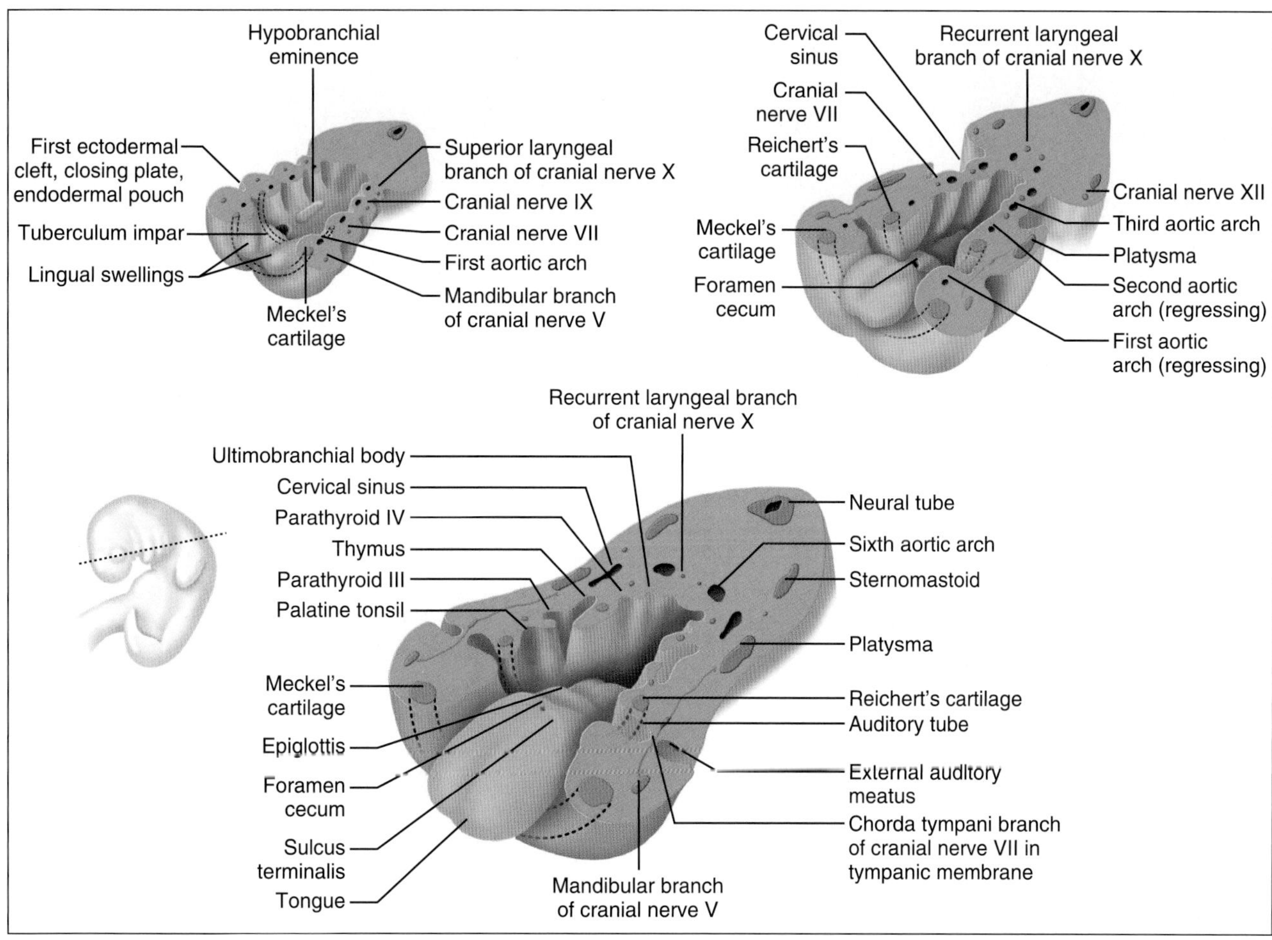

Fig. 3.9 Progressive stages in development of pharyngeal arches and their derivatives during the second month in utero. (Redrawn from Shaw JH, et al.: *Textbook of oral biology,* Philadelphia, PA, 1978, Saunders.)

TABLE 3.2 Innervation and Vascularization of Pharyngeal Arches

Arch	Blood Vessel	Nerve
First	First aortic arch	Mandibular (and maxillary) division of the trigeminal nerve (cranial nerve V)
Second	Second aortic arch	Facial (VII)
Third	Third aortic arch	Glossopharyngeal (IX)
Fourth	Fourth aortic arch	Vagus (X)

The maxillary process grows medially and approaches the lateral and medial nasal processes but remains separated from them by distinct grooves, the nasolacrimal groove and the bucconasal groove (Fig. 3.12). As the process continues to grow, the medial nasal process is displaced toward the midline, where it merges with its anatomic counterpart from the opposite side. In this way the middle portion of the upper lip or philtrum is formed. The merging of the two medial nasal processes also results in the formation of that part of the maxilla carrying the incisor teeth and the primary palate. Fusion occurring between the forward extent of the maxillary process and the lateral aspect of the medial nasal process will obliterate the bucconasal groove and result in the formation of the lateral aspects of the upper lip. The lower lip is formed by merging of the two streams of ectomesenchyme of the mandibular processes. The parts of the face resulting from these developmental steps are illustrated in Fig. 3.13.

An unusual type of fusion occurs between the maxillary process and the lateral nasal process. As with most other processes associated with facial development, the maxillary and lateral nasal processes initially are separated by a deep groove (see Fig. 3.12). The epithelium in the floor of this groove forms a solid cord that separates from the surface and becomes surrounded by mesenchyme. This detached epithelial cord eventually canalizes to form the nasolacrimal duct.

The face develops between days 24 and 28 of gestation. Already at this early time, some of the epithelium covering the facial processes will start assuming odontogenic, or tooth-forming, capacity (see Fig. 3.7). In the region of the future upper and lower jaws, the epithelium will proliferate and thicken to form U-shaped primary epithelial bands along which teeth will develop.

FORMATION OF THE SECONDARY PALATE

Initially there is a common oronasal cavity bounded anteriorly by the primary palate and occupied mainly by the developing tongue. Only after the development of the secondary palate is distinction between the oral and nasal cavities possible. The palate proper develops from primary and secondary components.

The formation of the primary palate from the frontonasal and medial nasal processes has been described already. The formation of the secondary palate commences between 7 and 8 weeks of gestation and completes around the third month of gestation. Three outgrowths appear in the oral cavity; the nasal septum grows downward from the frontonasal process along the midline, and two palatine shelves or

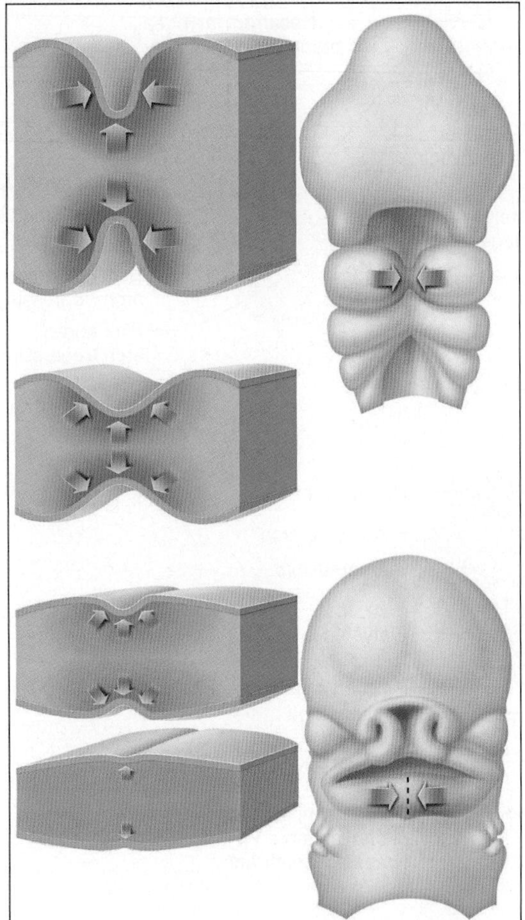

Fig. 3.10 Fusion of facial processes involves elimination of furrows between them. The arrows indicate the general direction of the fusion events (compare with Fig. 3.11).

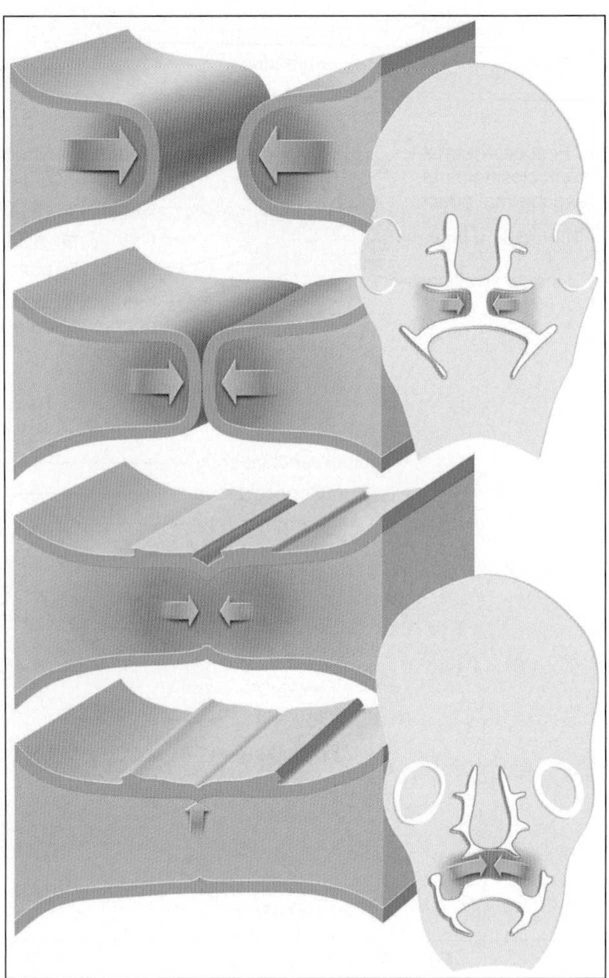

Fig. 3.11 During palate formation there is fusion of palatal processes involving the breakdown of surface epithelium.

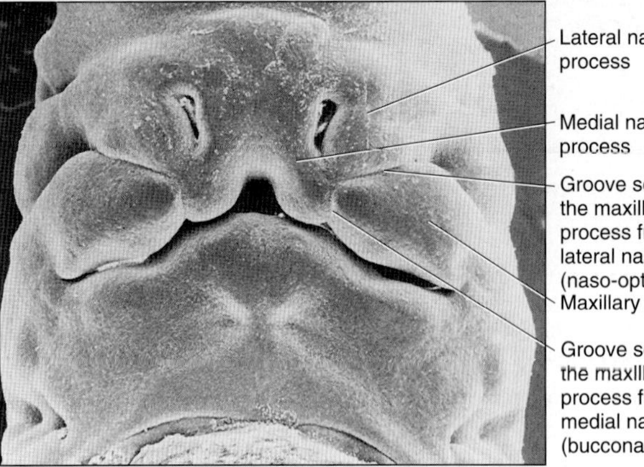

Fig. 3.12 Scanning electron micrograph of a human embryo at around 6 weeks of development. (Courtesy K.K. Sulik.)

processes, one from each side, extend from the maxillary processes toward the midline (Figs. 3.14 and 3.15). The shelves are directed first downward on each side of the tongue. After 7 weeks of development, the tongue is withdrawn from between the shelves, which now elevate and fuse with each other above the tongue and with the primary palate. The septum and the two shelves converge and fuse along the midline, thus separating the primitive oral cavity into nasal and oral cavities. The closure of the secondary palate proceeds gradually from the primary palate in a posterior direction. A factor contributing to closure of the secondary palate is displacement of the tongue from between the palatine shelves by the growth pattern of the head.

Between 7 and 8 weeks of gestation the tongue and mandible in the embryo are small relative to the upper facial complex, and the lower lip is positioned behind the upper one (Fig. 3.16A). The head is folded onto the developing thoracic region, and the tongue occupies an elevated position between the palatine shelves (see Figs. 3.14D and 3.16A).

By 9 weeks of gestation, the upper facial complex has lifted away from the thorax and thus permits the tongue and lower jaw to grow forward (more anterior), and the tongue is now situated below the palatine shelves (see Fig. 3.16B).

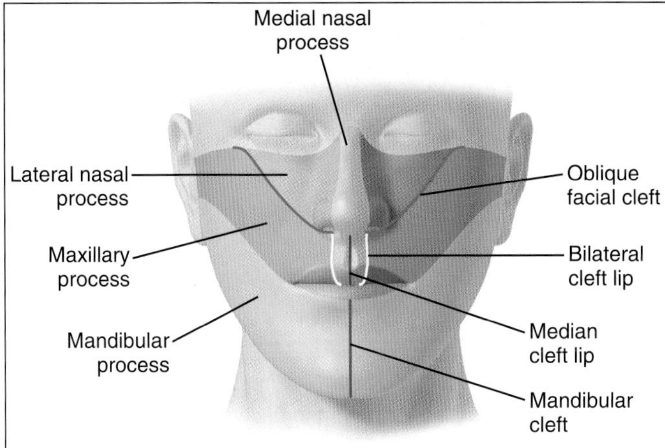

Fig. 3.13 Schematic representation of the origin of different parts of the face. The solid lines indicate sites of potential malformations resulting from lack of fusion between facial processes.

For fusion of the palatine shelves to occur, elimination of the epithelial covering of the shelves is necessary. As the two palatine shelves meet, adhesion of the epithelia occurs so that the epithelium of one shelf becomes indistinguishable from that of the other and a midline epithelial seam that consists of two layers of basal epithelial cells forms. This midline seam must be removed to permit ectomesenchymal continuity between the fused processes. As palatal growth proceeds, the seam first thins down and then breaks up into discrete islands of epithelial cells (Fig. 3.17). The basal lamina surrounding these cells then is lost, and the epithelial cells lose their epithelial characteristics and assume fibroblast-like features. In other words, epithelial cells transform into mesenchymal cells—that is, they undergo an epitheliomesenchymal transformation (transition). This is a fundamental embryonic process that also is implicated in the invasive behavior of epithelial neoplastic cells. During craniofacial development, such a transformation is a prerequisite for NCC migration (see Chapter 2) and may be implicated in cementoblast differentiation (see Chapter 9).

FORMATION OF THE TONGUE

The tongue begins to develop at about 4 weeks of gestation. The pharyngeal arches meet in the midline beneath the primitive mouth. Local proliferation of the mesenchyme then gives rise to a number of swellings in the floor of the mouth (Fig. 3.18, see also Fig. 3.9). First, a

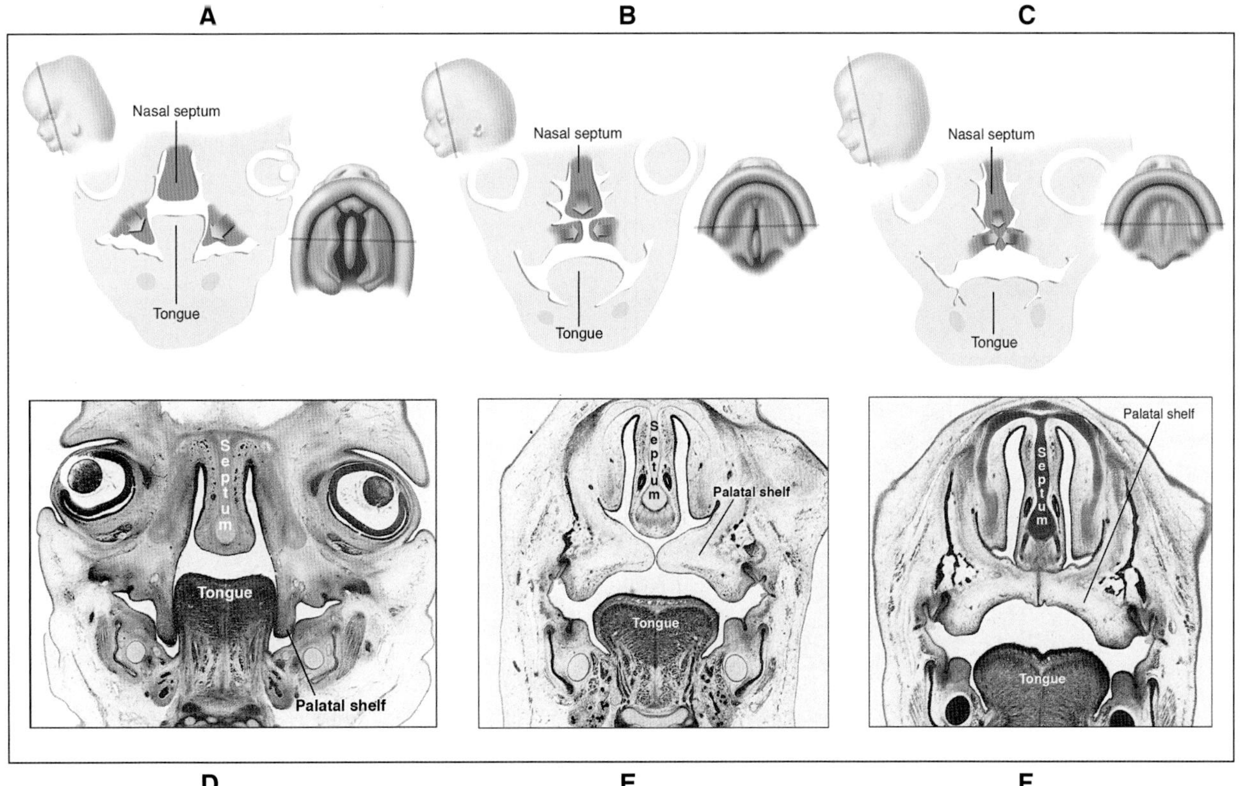

Fig. 3.14 Formation of the secondary palate. (A) At 7 weeks of development, the palatine shelves are forming from the maxillary processes and are directed downward on each side of the developing tongue. (B) At 8 weeks, the tongue has been depressed, and the palatine shelves are elevated but not fused. (C) Fusion of the shelves and the nasal septum is completed. Formation of the secondary palate. Coronal sections through human embryos at approximately (D) 7 weeks, (E) 8 weeks, and (F) 9 weeks of development. The initial disposition of palatine shelves on each side of the tongue is shown in (D), their elevation coincident with depression of the tongue in (E), and their final fusion with each other and with the nasal septum in (F). (Redrawn from Diewert VM: A morphometric analysis of craniofacial growth and changes in spatial relations during secondary palatal development in human embryos and fetuses, *Am J Anat* 167:495, 1983.)

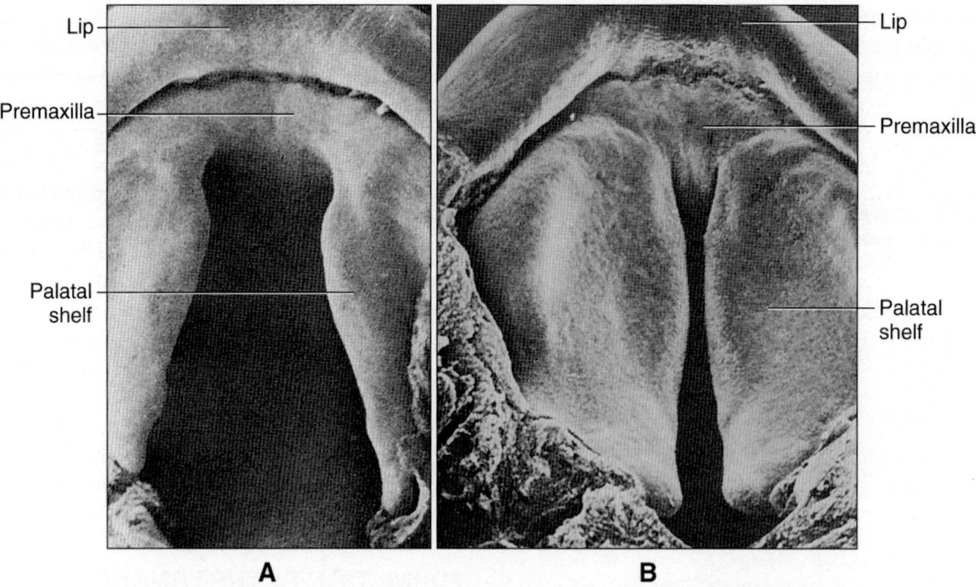

Fig. 3.15 Palatine shelves in (A) 7-week-old and (B) 8-week-old human embryos seen from the underside. (From Waterman RE, Meller SM: Alterations in the epithelial surface of human palatal shelves prior to and during fusion: a scanning electron microscopic study, *Anat Rec* 180:111, 1974.)

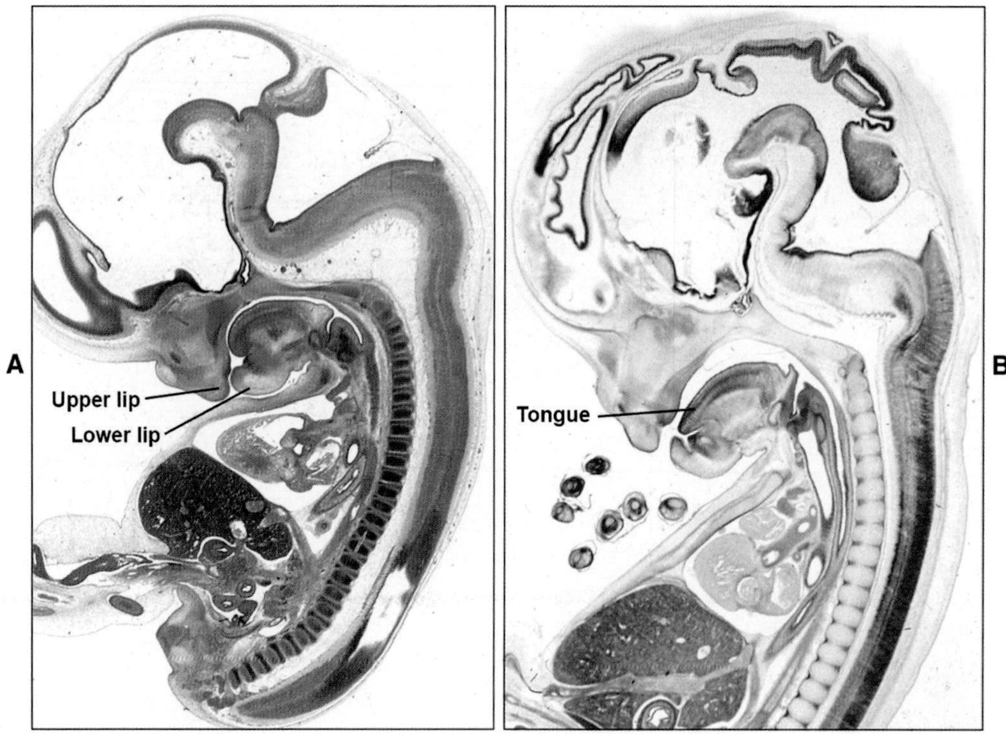

Fig. 3.16 Sagittal sections through human embryos. (A) At 7 weeks of development, the folded head has the upper lip in front of the lower lip with the tongue elevated. (B) By 9 weeks of development, the head is raised so that the tongue not only is lowered but also has grown forward. (From Diewert V: Contribution of differential growth of cartilages to changes in craniofacial morphology. In Dixon AD, Sarnat BG, editors: *Factors and mechanisms influencing bone growth,* New York, NY, 1982, Alan R. Liss.)

swelling (the tuberculum impar) arises in the midline in the mandibular process and is flanked by two other bulges, the lingual swellings. These lateral lingual swellings quickly enlarge and merge with each other and the tuberculum impar to form a large mass from which the mucous membrane of the anterior two-thirds of the tongue is formed. The root of the tongue arises from a large midline swelling developed from the mesenchyme of the second, third, and fourth arches. This swelling consists of a copula (associated with the second arch) and a large hypobranchial eminence (associated with the third and fourth arches). As the tongue develops, the hypobranchial eminence overgrows the copula, which disappears. The posterior part of the fourth arch marks the development of the epiglottis.

The tongue separates from the floor of the mouth by a downgrowth of ectoderm around its periphery, which subsequently degenerates to form the lingual sulcus and gives the tongue mobility. The muscles of the tongue have a different origin; they arise from the occipital somites, which have migrated forward into the tongue area, carrying with them their nerve supply, the twelfth cranial (hypoglossal) nerve.

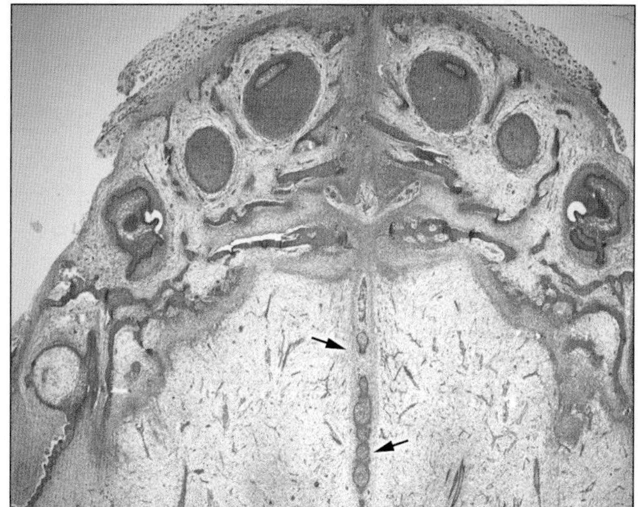

Fig. 3.17 Ventrodorsal histologic section of the forming maxilla from a human embryo passing through the developing teeth and fusing palatal shelves. Remnants of the surface epithelium of the shelves *(arrows)* are visible along the line of fusion. (Courtesy M. Seccani Galassi.)

This unusual development of the tongue explains its innervation. Because the mucosa of the anterior two-thirds of the tongue is derived from the first arch, it is supplied by the nerve of that arch, the fifth cranial (trigeminal) nerve, whereas the mucosa of the posterior third of the tongue, derived from the third arch, is supplied by the ninth cranial (glossopharyngeal) nerve. As previously indicated, the motor supply to the muscles of the tongue is the twelfth cranial nerve.

The development of the tongue and palate and the formation of the oral cavity are diagrammed in Fig. 3.19, which illustrates midline sagittal sections through the developing embryo at progressively advancing stages of gestation.

DEVELOPMENT OF THE SKULL

The skull can be divided into three components: (1) the cranial vault, (2) the cranial base, and (3) the face (Fig. 3.20). Membranous bone formed directly in mesenchyme with no cartilaginous precursor forms the cranial vault and face (Fig. 3.21; see also Fig. 3.2) while the cranial base undergoes endochondral ossification (see Fig. 3.2). Some of these membrane-formed bones may develop secondary cartilages to provide rapid growth. Intramembranous and endochondral ossification are discussed in Chapter 6.

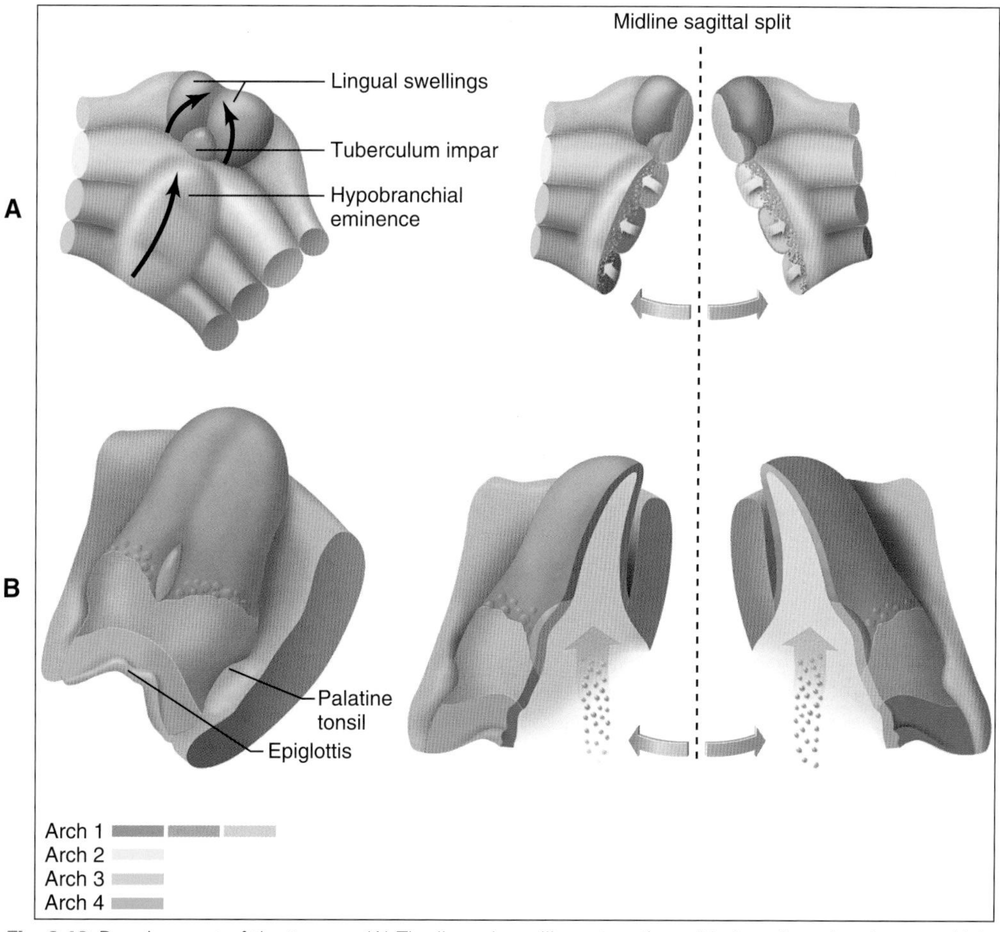

Fig. 3.18 Development of the tongue. (A) The lingual swellings, together with the tuberculum impar, which arise from the first arch, will form the anterior two-thirds of the tongue. The hypobranchial eminence overgrows the second arch. (B) Final disposition of the tongue and the relative contributions of the first to fourth arch. The arrow depicts the route of incoming occipital myotomes that form the tongue muscle.

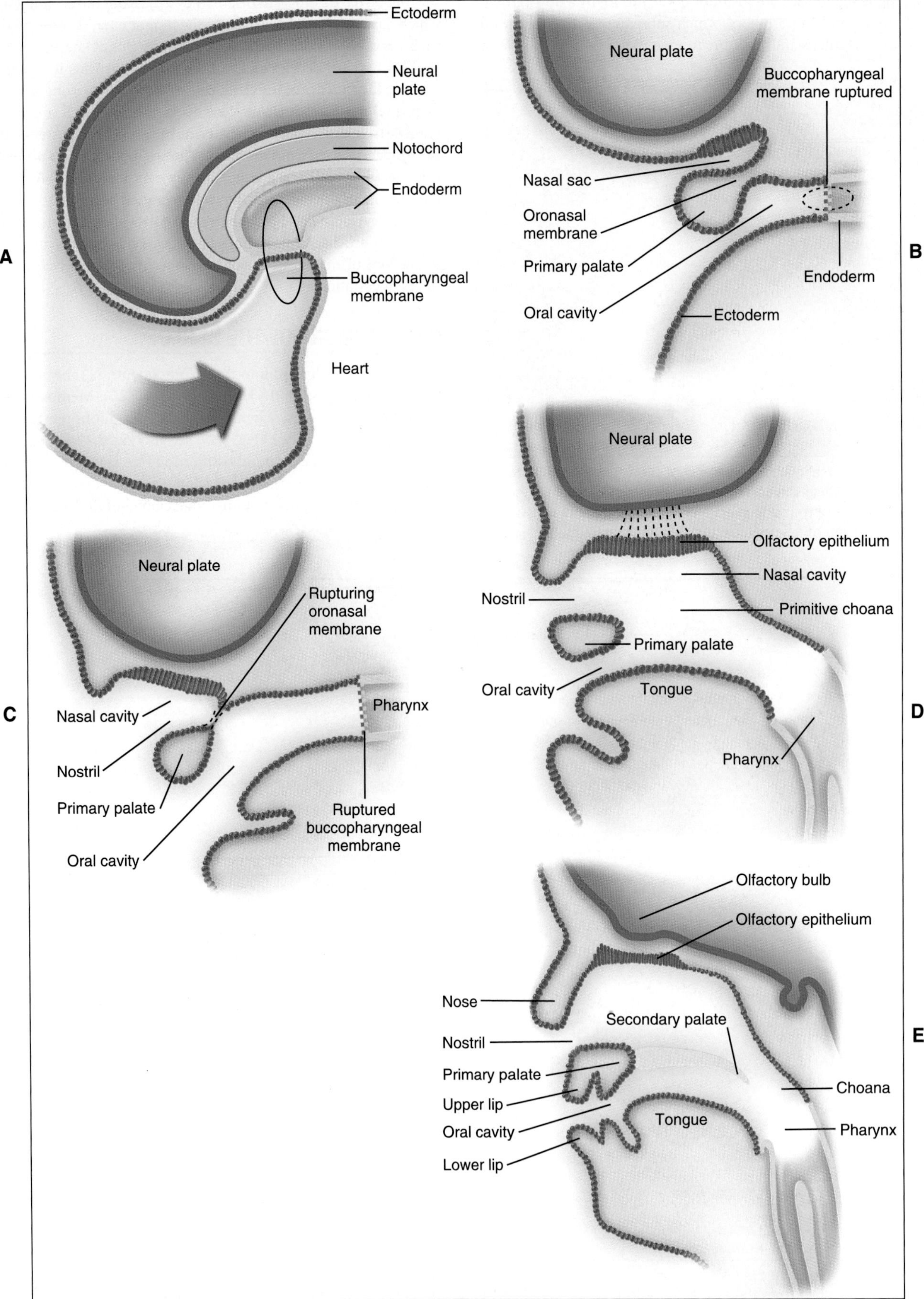

Fig. 3.19 Summary of the development of the oral cavity as seen in midsagittal section. (A) Head fold and formation of the stomatodeum, or oral cavity. (B) Formation of the nasal pit and primary palate. (C) Establishment of the continuity between the presumptive nasal and oral cavities. (D, E) Final anatomy of the nasal and oral cavities established by development of the secondary palate.

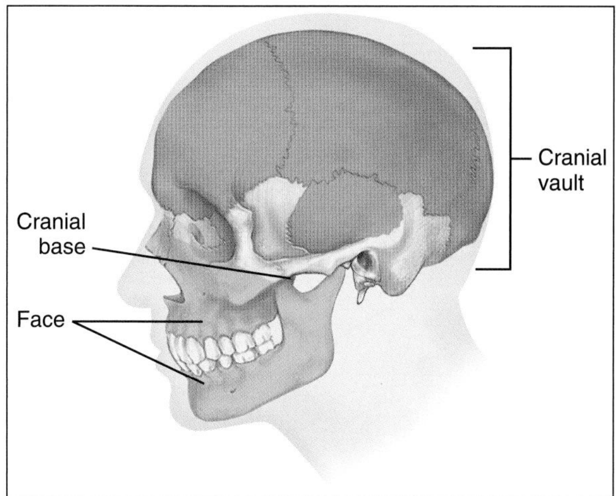

Fig. 3.20 Subdivisions of the skull.

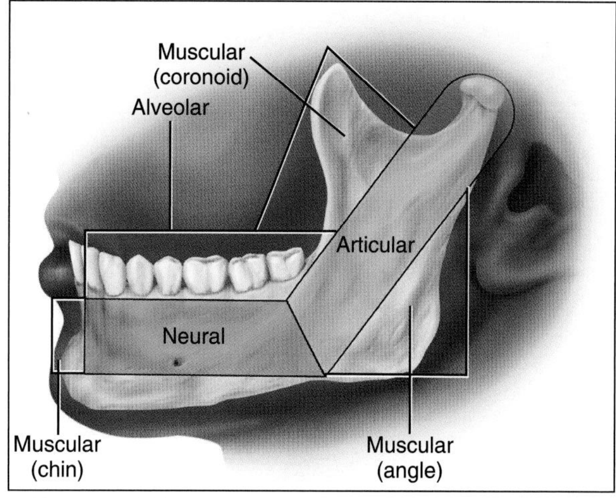

Fig. 3.22 Differing developmental blocks for the mandible.

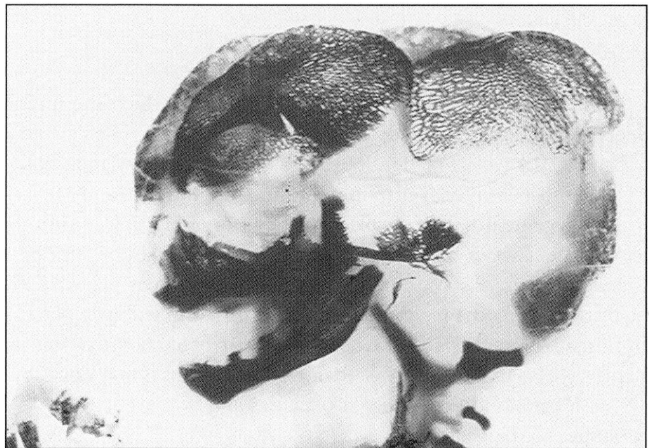

Fig. 3.21 A 14-week-old cleared human embryo in which the mineralized bone has been stained with alizarin red. (Courtesy V.M. Diewert. Photographed from the University of Washington collection.)

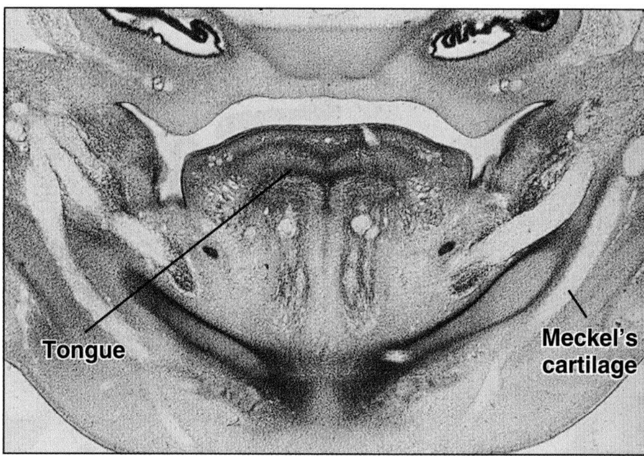

Fig. 3.23 Slightly oblique coronal section of an embryo demonstrating nearly the extent of Meckel's cartilage. (From Diewert VM: A morphometric analysis of craniofacial growth and changes in spatial relations during secondary palatal development in human embryos and fetuses, *Am J Anat* 167:495, 1983.)

For skull development, standard texts on embryology should be consulted. This text considers in detail only the development of the jaws.

DEVELOPMENT OF THE MANDIBLE AND MAXILLA

The mandible and the maxilla form the tissues of the first branchial arch, the mandible forming within the mandibular process and the maxilla within the maxillary process.

Mandible

As discussed later, the mandible is a membranous bone developed in relation to the nerve of the first arch and almost entirely independent of Meckel's cartilage. The mandible has neural, alveolar, and muscular elements (Fig. 3.22), and its growth is assisted by the development of secondary cartilages.

The cartilage of the first arch, Meckel's cartilage, forms the lower jaw in primitive vertebrates. In humans, Meckel's cartilage has a close positional relationship to the developing mandible. At 6 weeks of development, this cartilage extends as a solid hyaline cartilaginous rod surrounded by a fibrocellular capsule from the developing ear region (otic capsule) to the midline of the fused mandibular processes (Fig. 3.23). The two cartilages of each side do not meet at the midline but are separated by a thin band of mesenchyme. The mandibular branch of the trigeminal nerve (the nerve of the first arch) has a close relationship to Meckel's cartilage, beginning two-thirds of the way along the length of the cartilage. At this point the mandibular nerve divides into lingual and inferior alveolar branches, which run along the medial and lateral aspects of the cartilage, respectively (Fig. 3.24). The inferior alveolar nerve further divides into incisor and mental branches more anteriorly.

On the lateral aspect of Meckel's cartilage, during the sixth week of embryonic development, a condensation of mesenchyme occurs in the angle formed by the division of the inferior alveolar nerve and its incisor and mental branches (see Fig. 3.24). At 7 weeks of development, intramembranous ossification begins in this condensation, forming the first bone of the mandible. From this center of ossification, bone formation spreads rapidly anteriorly to the midline and posteriorly toward the point where the mandibular nerve divides into its lingual and inferior alveolar branches. Anteriorly, this spread of new bone formation occurs along the lateral aspect of Meckel's cartilage, forming a trough that consists of lateral and medial plates that unite beneath the incisor nerve (Fig. 3.25). This trough of bone extends to the midline, where it comes into approximation with a similar trough formed in the adjoining mandibular process. The two separate centers of ossification remain separated at the mandibular symphysis until shortly after birth. The trough soon is converted into a canal as bone forms over the nerve, joining the lateral and medial plates.

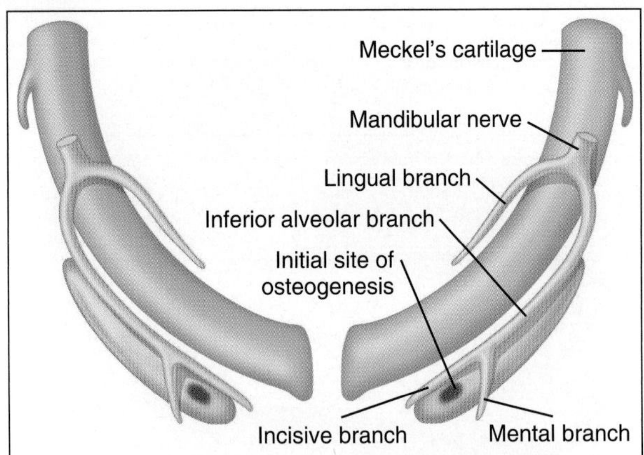

Fig. 3.24 Site of initial osteogenesis related to mandible formation. Bone formation extends from this anteriorly and posteriorly along Meckel's cartilage.

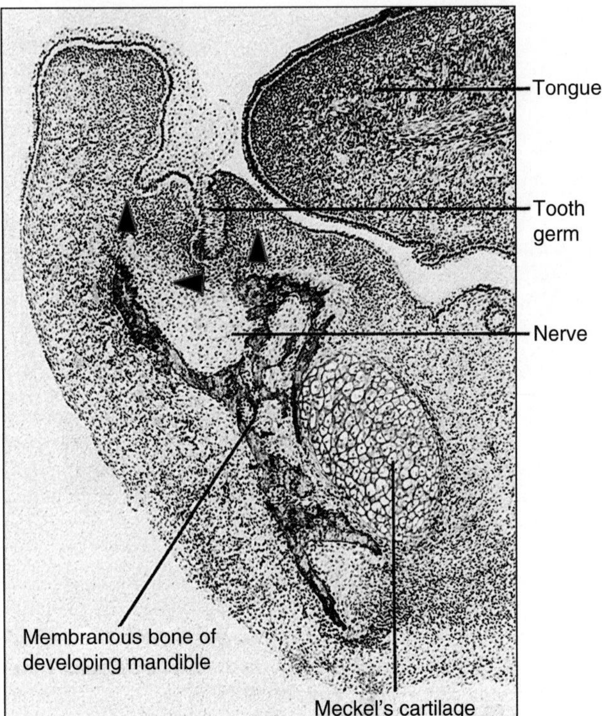

Fig. 3.25 Photomicrograph of a coronal section through an embryo showing the general pattern of intramembranous bone deposition associated with formation of the mandible. The relationship among nerve, cartilage, and tooth germ is evident. Arrowheads indicate the future directions of bone growth to form the neural canal and lateral and medial alveolar plates. Compare this with the development of the maxilla (see Fig. 3.28).

Similarly, there is a backward extension of ossification along the lateral aspect of Meckel's cartilage to the point where the mandibular nerve divides into the inferior alveolar and lingual nerves. From this point where the nerve divides to the midline, medial and lateral alveolar plates of bone develop in relation to the forming tooth germs subdividing the trough of bone. Thus the teeth come to occupy individual compartments, which finally are enclosed by growth of bone over the tooth germ. In this way the body of the mandible essentially is formed.

The ramus of the mandible develops by a rapid spread of ossification posteriorly into the mesenchyme of the first arch, turning away from Meckel's cartilage (Fig. 3.26). This point of divergence is marked by the lingula in the adult mandible, the point at which the inferior alveolar nerve enters the body of the mandible.

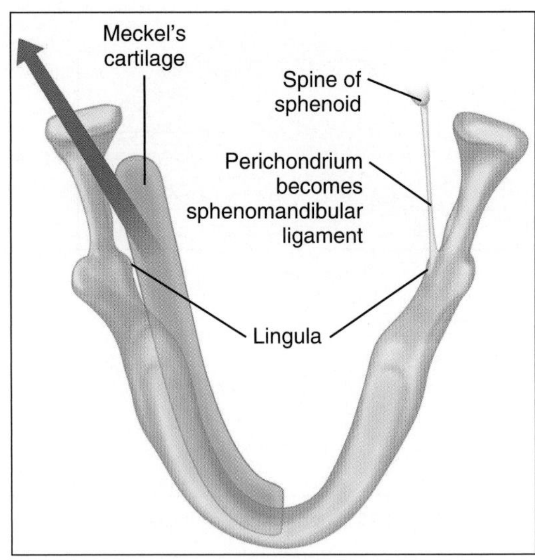

Fig. 3.26 Spread of mandibular ossification away from Meckel's cartilage at the lingula.

Thus by 10 weeks of development, the rudimentary mandible is formed almost entirely by intramembranous ossification, and Meckel's cartilage degenerates to make place for new bone (Fig. 3.27). Although Meckel's cartilage is widely believed not to be directly implicated in ossification, there is some emerging evidence that it may play an active role by delimiting the region where bone formation will take place. In addition, new notions on the osteogenic capacity of chondrocytes (see Chapter 6) also make it possible that in some regions it may contribute to bone formation in the space it occupies and that eventually fills in with bone (see Fig. 3.27B).

Meckel's cartilage has the following fate (see Table 3.1): Its most posterior extremity forms the incus and malleus of the inner ear and the sphenomalleolar ligament. From the sphenoid to the division of the mandibular nerve into its alveolar and lingual branches, the cartilage is lost totally, but its fibrocellular capsule persists as the sphenomandibular ligament (see Fig. 3.26). From the lingula forward to the division of the alveolar nerve into its incisor and mental branches, Meckel's cartilage degenerates. Forward from this point to the midline, some evidence exists that the cartilage might make a small contribution to the mandible by means of endochondral ossification.

The further growth of the mandible until birth is influenced strongly by the appearance of three secondary (growth) cartilages and the development of muscular attachments. These secondary cartilages include (1) the condylar cartilage, which is most important; (2) the coronoid cartilage; and (3) the symphyseal cartilage. These cartilages are referred to as *secondary cartilage* to distinguish them from the primary Meckel's cartilage. They have a different histologic structure from the primary cartilages in that their cells are larger, and less intercellular matrix is formed.

The condylar cartilage appears at 12 weeks of development and rapidly forms a cone- or carrot-shaped mass that occupies most of the developing ramus. This mass of cartilage is converted quickly to bone by endochondral ossification (see Chapter 6) so that at 20 weeks of development only a thin layer of cartilage remains in the condylar head. This remnant of cartilage persists until the end of the second decade of life, providing a mechanism for growth of the mandible, in the same way as the epiphyseal cartilage does in the limbs.

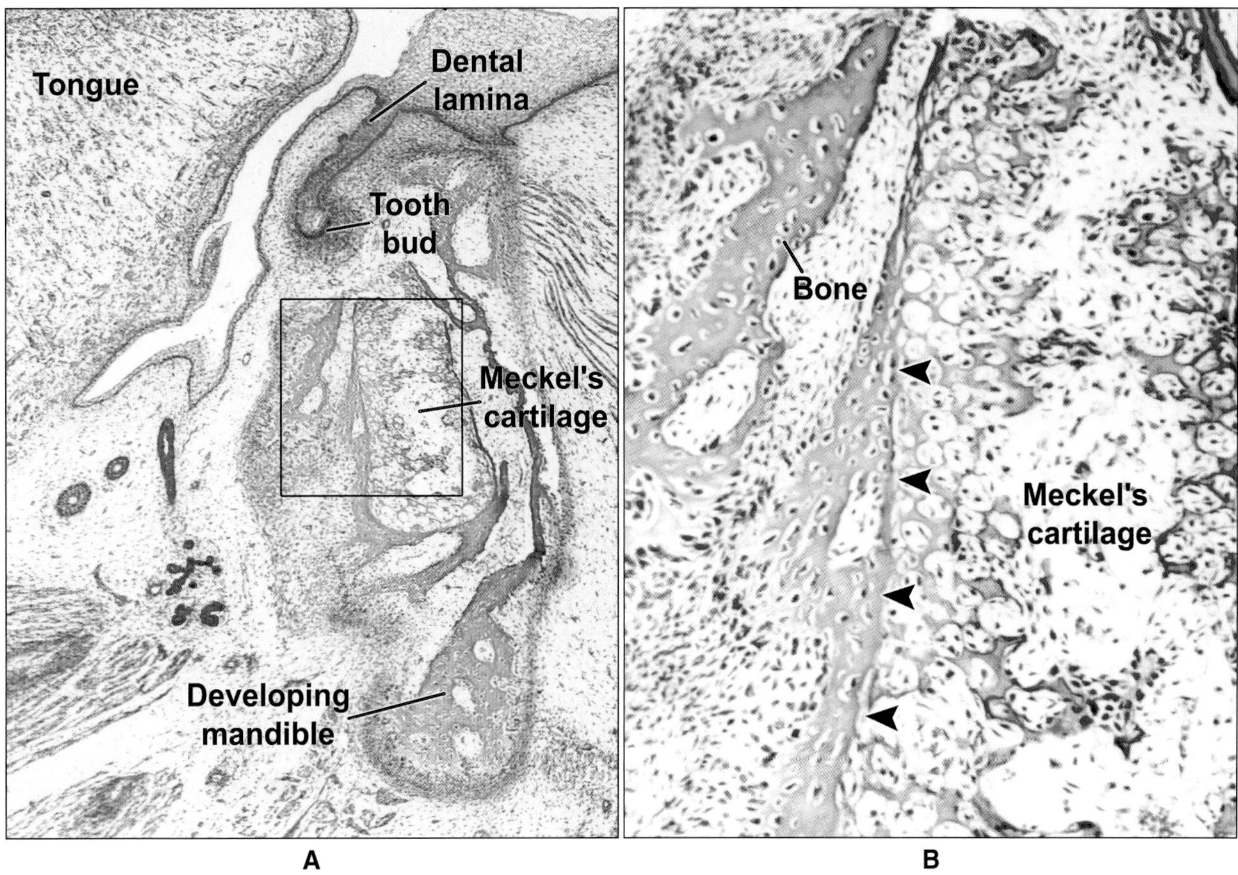

Fig. 3.27 (A) Photomicrograph of a sagittal section through the developing mandible of an embryo showing how bone forms around the outer aspect of Meckel's cartilage. As the cartilage is degraded, the space previously occupied by cartilage becomes filled with new bone. (B) Higher magnification view of the boxed area in (A). Somewhat reminiscent to what takes place when the bony collar forms at the primary ossification center of the cartilage analogue of long bones (see Chapter 6), some bone appears to form on the surface of Meckel's cartilage.

The coronoid cartilage appears at about 4 months of development, surmounting the anterior border and top of the coronoid process. Coronoid cartilage is a transient growth cartilage and disappears long before birth.

The symphyseal cartilages, two in number, appear in the connective tissue between the two ends of Meckel's cartilage but are independent of it. They are obliterated within the first year after birth. Small islands of cartilage also may appear as variable and transient structures in the developing alveolar processes.

Maxilla

The maxilla also develops from a center of ossification in the mesenchyme of the maxillary process of the first arch. No arch cartilage or primary cartilage exists in the maxillary process, but the center of ossification is associated closely with the cartilage of the nasal capsule. As in the mandible, the center of ossification appears in the angle between the divisions of a nerve (i.e., where the anterosuperior dental nerve is given off from the inferior orbital nerve). From this center, bone formation spreads posteriorly below the orbit toward the developing zygoma and anteriorly toward the future incisor region (Fig. 3.28). Ossification also spreads superiorly to form the frontal process. As a result of this pattern of bone deposition, a bony trough forms for the infraorbital nerve. From this trough a downward extension of bone forms the lateral alveolar plate for the maxillary tooth germs. Ossification also spreads into the palatine process to form the hard palate. The medial alveolar plate develops from the junction of the palatal process and the main body of the forming maxilla. This plate, together with its lateral counterpart, forms a trough of bone around the maxillary tooth germs, which eventually become enclosed in bony crypts in the same way as described for the mandible.

A secondary cartilage also contributes to the development of the maxilla. A zygomatic, or malar, cartilage appears in the developing zygomatic process and for a short time adds considerably to the development of the maxilla.

At birth the frontal process of the maxilla is well marked, but the body of the bone consists of little more than the alveolar process containing the tooth germs and small though distinguishable zygomatic and palatal processes. The body of the maxilla is relatively small because the maxillary sinus has not developed. This sinus forms during week 16 as a shallow groove on the nasal aspect of the developing maxilla. At birth the sinus is still a rudimentary structure about the size of a small pea.

Interestingly, even though both mandibular and maxillary primordia originate from similar NCCs and possess similar molecular features, they develop into very different structural entities. In the first branchial arch, a gradient of gene expression involving the Dlx family of transcription factors (1–6), the so-called intraarch Dlx code, promotes coordinated gene expression along the dorsoventral axis that regulates jaw patterning. Distinct sets of Dlx family members are important for determining the identity of the mandible (Dlx1/2/5/6) versus the

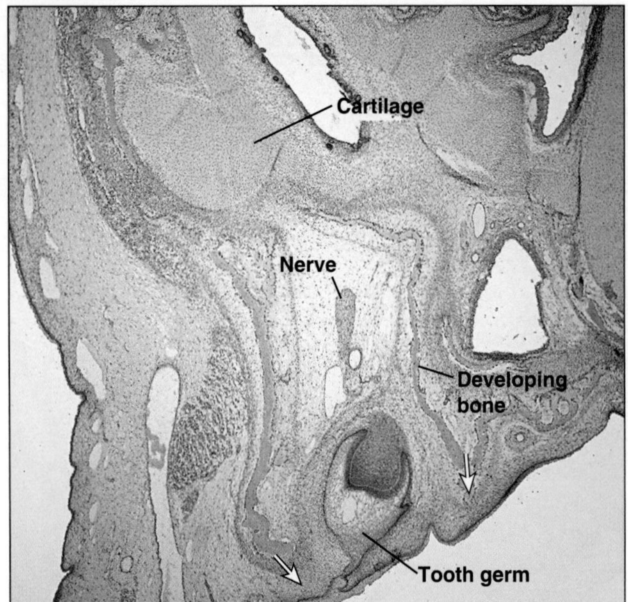

Fig. 3.28 Coronal section through an embryo showing the general pattern of intramembranous bone deposition associated with formation of the maxilla. The relationship between cartilage, nerve, and tooth germ is evident. Arrows indicate the future directions of bone growth to form the lateral and medial alveolar plates. Compare this with the developing mandible in Fig. 3.25. (Courtesy B. Kablar.)

maxilla (Dlx1/2). A dramatic demonstration of the importance of the selective set of Dlx molecules in jaw specification is observed in mice lacking both Dlx5 and 6 genes. Lack of Dlx5/6 causes a reversal of the mandible into a maxilla, generating an animal with two mirror-image upper jaws. Dlx5/6 activate expression of other downstream transcription factors (Dlx3/4, heart- and neural crest derivatives–expressed 1 and 2[Hand1/2], Alx3/4, Pitx1, gastrulation brain homeobox 2 [Gbx2], bone morphogenic protein 7 [Bmp7]) important for mandibular development processes and repress others (pou domain class 3, transcription factor 3 [Pou3f3], forkhead box l2 [Foxl2], Iroquois homeobox protein 5 [Irx5]) that are themselves important for maxillary processes and under control of Dlx1/2. Thus Dlx family members are critical for determining the identity of the mandible versus the maxilla. Another level of complexity is brought about by local environmental signaling cross talk that directly or indirectly modulates the transcriptional Dlx program. One such regulator is endothelin, a secreted molecule produced mostly by the ectoderm that signals through the endothelin receptor Ednra in NCCs and promotes, possibly through mads box transcription enhancer factor 2 polypeptide c (Mef2C), Dlx5/6 expression. Targeted ablation of the endothelin pathway in mice causes duplication of maxillary processes, whereas ectopic expression induces duplication of the mandibular processes. Other signaling events coming from the endoderm (Vegf and Shh) or the ectoderm (Fgf, Bmp, wingless-type MMTV integration site family [Wnt]) also promote dorsoventral guidance by modulating many different cellular processes such as migration, survival, apoptosis, and/or differentiation.

Common Features of Jaw Development

This account of jaw development shows that, in their development, the mandible and maxilla have much in common. Both begin from a single center of membranous ossification related to a nerve, both form a neural element related to the nerve, and both develop an alveolar element related to the developing teeth. Finally, both develop secondary cartilages to assist in their growth.

DEVELOPMENT OF THE TEMPOROMANDIBULAR JOINT

The temporomandibular joint is an articulation between two bones initially formed from membranous centers of ossification. Before the condylar cartilage forms, a broad band of undifferentiated mesenchyme exists between the developing ramus of the mandible and the developing squamous tympanic bone. With formation of the condylar cartilage, this band is reduced rapidly in width and is converted into a dense strip of mesenchyme. The mesenchyme immediately adjacent to this strip breaks down to form the joint cavity, and the strip becomes the articular disk of the joint.

CONGENITAL DEFECTS

The complicated changes that occur during embryogenesis between weeks 4 and 8 of development have been described. They lead to, among other things, the formation of the face, mouth, and tongue and their associated structures. After 8 weeks, development is essentially a matter of growth. Embryogenesis is a complicated and delicately balanced process; malfunctions produce congenital defects. The genetic basis of some of these defects has been discussed previously.

Environmental factors, including teratogens (agents causing congenital defects), also must be considered. The types of environmental factors affecting the embryo can be classified into five groups: (1) infectious agents, (2) x-ray radiation, (3) drugs, (4) hormones, and (5) nutritional deficiencies. The classic example of an infectious agent causing a congenital defect is the rubella virus, which induces German measles. Among the widespread malformations that result from this infection of the mother are cleft palate and deformities of the teeth. The teratogenic effect of x-ray radiation is well understood, and many defects, including cleft palate, can result from the irradiation of pregnant women. In addition to affecting the embryo directly, x-ray radiation also may affect the germ cells of the fetus, causing genetic mutations that lead to congenital malformations in succeeding generations. Cortisone injected into mice and rabbits causes a high percentage of cleft palates in the offspring. The same is also true for nutritional deficiencies, especially vitamin deficiencies. Although vitamin deficiencies have been shown to be teratogenic in experimental animals, this effect has not been demonstrated in human beings.

The timing of environmental factors can be critical. If a teratogen exerts its effect during the first 4 weeks of life when the embryo is developing rapidly, the teratogen usually damages so many cells that death of the embryo occurs. However, if only a few cells are damaged, normal proliferation is great enough that minor damage is eliminated readily. Probably, many teratogenic agents acting in this first phase of development are not appreciated because the embryo dies and is miscarried. During the next stage of development, between 4 and 8 weeks of gestation when histodifferentiation and organ differentiation are taking place, teratogenic agents are most likely to produce malformation. The subsequent growth phase is not as susceptible to teratogenic agents.

Not surprisingly, therefore, most teratogenic agents leading to facial and dental malformations exert their effects during the period of morphogenesis and histodifferentiation within the embryo. These malformations include the various types of clefts, which can be understood readily from knowledge of embryology (Figs. 3.29 and 3.30): the oblique facial cleft (results from lack of fusion between the maxillary process and lateral nasal process), the median cleft lip (results from lack of fusion between the two medial nasal processes), bilateral cleft lip (results from lack of fusion between the maxillary process and median nasal process), microstomia (an excessive merging of the mandibular and maxillary processes), the converse or macrostomia (results from failure of the

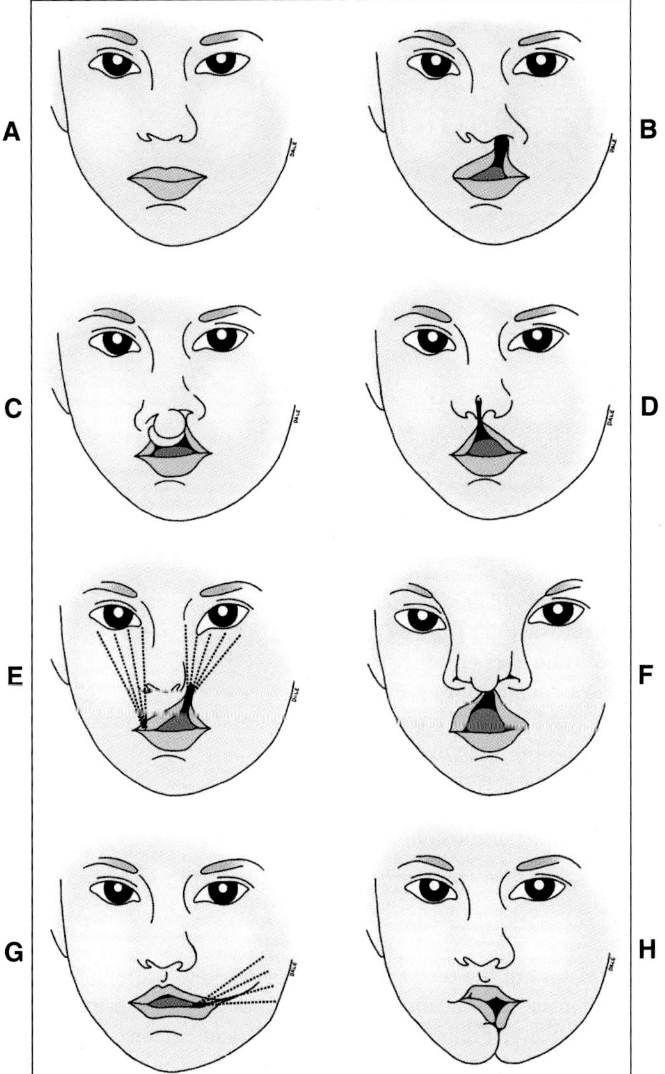

Fig. 3.29 Types of facial clefts. (A) Normal fusion. (B) Unilateral cleft lip. (C) Bilateral cleft lip. (D) Median cleft lip. (E) Oblique facial cleft. (F) Median cleft (frontonasal dysplasia). (G) Lateral facial cleft. (H) Mandibular cleft.

maxillary and mandibular processes to fuse), and the rare mandibular cleft, which, in minor form, involves only the lower lip (results from failure of the first branchial arches to fuse or malformation of the symphysis).

Often when clefts of the lip and anterior maxilla occur, the distortion of facial development prevents the palatine shelves from making contact when they swing into the horizontal position; thus clefts of the primary palate often are accompanied by clefts of the secondary (hard and soft) palate. When clefts of the palate occur with no corresponding

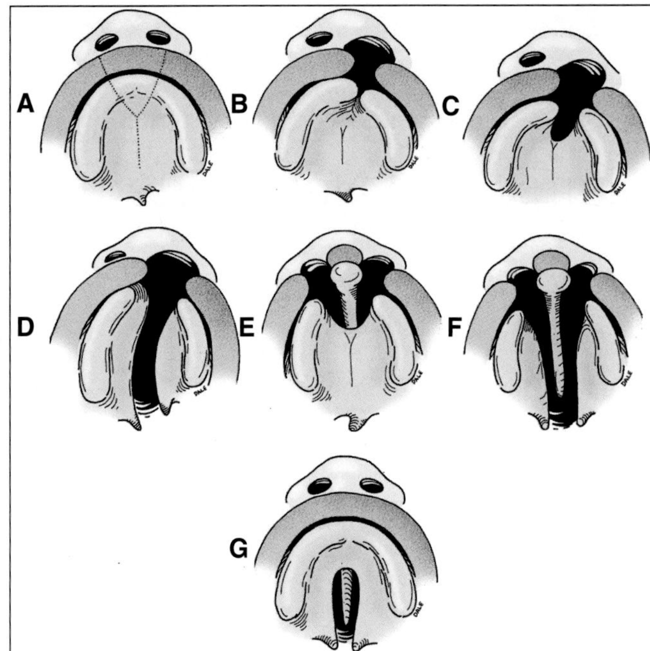

Fig. 3.30 Palatal clefts seen from a ventral view. (A) Normal fusion. (B) Cleft of lip and alveolus. (C) Cleft of lip and primary palate. (D) Unilateral cleft lip and palate. (E) Bilateral cleft lip and primary palate. (F) Bilateral cleft lip and palate. (G) Cleft palate only.

facial cleft, the cause is different (see Fig. 3.30G). Such palatal clefts may result from (1) failure of the shelves and septum to contact each other because of a lack of growth or because of a disturbance in the mechanism of shelf elevation, (2) failure of the shelves and septum to fuse after contact has been made because the epithelium covering the shelves does not break down or is not resorbed, (3) rupture after fusion of the shelves, or (4) defective merging and consolidation of the mesenchyme of the shelves. The extent of clefting reflects the time when the processes involved in closure of the secondary palate have been affected. Full clefting results from interference at the start of closure and partial clefting later as the process proceeds posteriorly.

RECOMMENDED READING

Creuzet S, et al.: Patterning the neural crest derivatives during development of the vertebrate head: insights from avian studies, *J Anat* 207:447, 2005.

Gitton Y, et al.: Evolving maps in craniofacial development, *Semin Cell Dev Biol* 21:301–308, 2010.

Liu B, et al.: Molecular control of facial morphology, *Semin Cell Dev Biol* 21:309–313, 2010.

Moore KL, Persaud TV: *The developing human: clinically orientated embryology*, ed 8, Philadelphia, PA, 2007, Saunders.

Sadler TW, editor: Langman's essential medical embryology, vol 1, Baltimore, MD, 2005, Lippincott Williams & Wilkins.

Szabo-Rogers HL, et al.: New directions in craniofacial morphogenesis, *Dev Biol* 341:84–94, 2010.

4

Basic Concepts on the Cell, Extracellular Matrix, and Neural Elements

Antonio Nanci, Florin Amzica, and Ravi L. Rungta

OUTLINE

The various cells, tissues, and organs that compose the oral cavity and related structures are complex entities that exhibit developmental characteristics. However, they have several structural and functional features in common with other cells and tissues in various parts of the body. This chapter focuses on the cell membrane, cytoskeleton, and cellular junctions because they are critical to the understanding of cellular biology in general. It also elaborates on the fibroblast and the extracellular matrix it forms because this cell type is implicated in several oral tissues. The basic physiology of the nervous system is also considered here as it is fundamental for understanding pain, mastication, sensation in the mouth, taste, and salivary gland function. The roles of specific oral tissue cells in their formation, growth, maintenance, and function are described fully in following chapters.

THE CELL MEMBRANE

To understand the functioning of cells and communication mechanisms between them, one needs to understand the structure and properties of the cell membrane. In addition to delimiting and maintaining integrity of the cell, this specialized envelope is involved in various processes, such as cell adhesion to extracellular matrices, cell signaling, cellular junctions and intercellular communication, ion movement, and release and uptake of proteins. It also interacts with the cytoskeleton.

In 1972 Singer and Nicholson proposed that the cell membrane is a mosaic supramolecular structure consisting of a bilayer of phospholipids interweaved with cholesterol and proteins (Fig. 4.1). Phospholipids are amphipathic molecules with a hydrophilic head containing a phosphate group and a hydrophobic tail containing two fatty acid chains (see Fig. 4.1A). The hydrophobic tails of the phospholipids are directed toward the center of the bilayer, and the hydrophilic heads are in contact with the intracellular or extracellular fluids. This phospholipid bilayer exhibits fluidic properties and confers flexibility to the membrane. The cholesterol molecules between phospholipids (see Fig. 4.1B) oppose excessive fluidity and ensure some stability to the membrane.

Proteins are distributed within the lipid bilayer of the membrane in a mosaic pattern. There are two types of membrane proteins: integral (or intrinsic) and peripheral (or extrinsic). The former are incorporated into the phospholipid bilayer and have both polar and nonpolar domains. The nonpolar regions of the integral proteins contact those of the phospholipids, whereas the polar parts of the proteins are in contact with the aqueous phase of intracellular or extracellular fluids and contain openings that constitute the pores or channels. Extrinsic proteins are located on one side of the membrane, with their polar domain in contact with the hydrophilic head group of the phospholipids or with the polar groupings of intrinsic proteins. Their attachment to the membrane is much looser than that of integral proteins, and they accomplish structural functions or act as receptors, pumps, or enzymes. Of particular importance, proteins on the internal face of the cell membrane act as anchoring points for cytoskeletal proteins to control the cell shape and strengthen the cell. Finally, on the external face of the cell membrane, there can be polysaccharides attached either to proteins (glycoproteins) or to lipids (glycolipids) that act as receptors or mediators to immunologic reactions.

Aside from their limiting function, cell membranes also display to some extent an important physiologic property—they are permeable. That is, they selectively allow molecules to cross them by a variety of mechanisms. Nonpolar molecules such as gasses (e.g., oxygen,

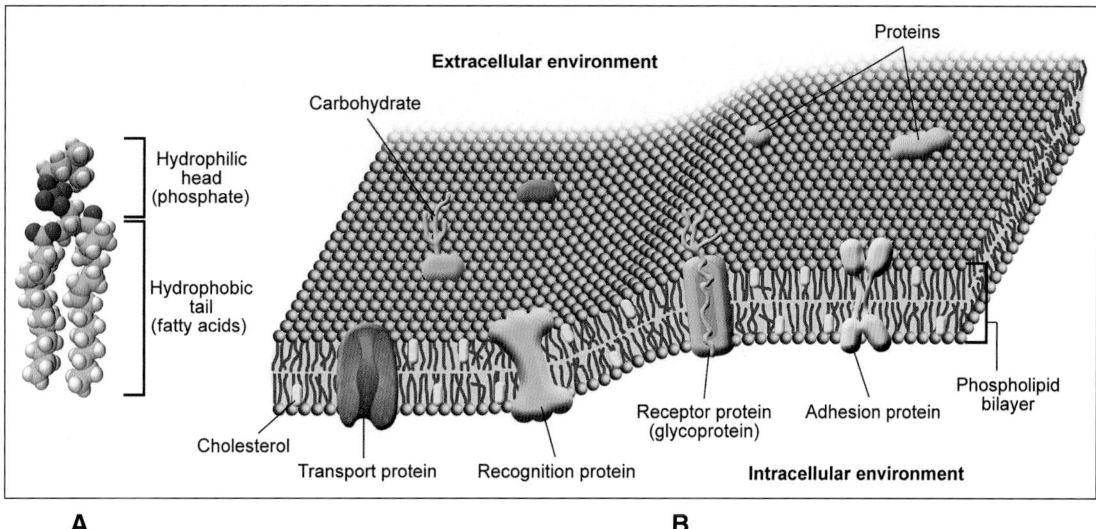

Fig. 4.1 Schematic representation of the structure of the cell membrane. (A) Phospholipid constituting the building block of cellular membranes. (B) Distribution of phospholipids in a bilayer membrane, as well as localization of various molecules within this structure. (Courtesy A. Paz Ramos.)

carbon dioxide, nitrogen) cross the cell membrane by simple diffusion according to their concentration gradient because they are liposoluble in the membrane. Ions, on the contrary, are polar particles and cannot easily diffuse through the phospholipidic bilayer. They will, however, cross the membrane through channels, as a function of their respective concentration and electric gradients, provided their size allows the physical passage through the channel pore. In general, when evaluating the propensity of a given ion to cross a membrane, one should consider the size of the hydrated ion. For instance, monovalent ions cross easier than multivalent ions, and potassium crosses easier than sodium because its hydrated complex is smaller (~0.4 nm in diameter) than that of sodium (~0.5 nm). Water itself easily crosses the cellular membranes because of the very small diameter of its molecule (~0.3 nm) and because the membrane is endowed with specific water channels. The aquaporins that constitute these channels were discovered by Peter Agre in 1992 for which he received the Nobel Prize in 2003. The channels allow very fast transition of water molecules from one side of the membrane to the other.

Permeability to large organic molecules depends essentially on their liposolubility. However, their passage through the hydrophilic poles of the phospholipidic bilayer may encounter some difficulties and reduce their passage, despite their liposolubility. Other large molecules, such as glucose, amino acids, and proteins, are too polar and too large to cross the cell membrane by simple diffusion. Some of them proceed by active transport and/or facilitated diffusion (glucose, amino acids), whereas others (proteins) proceed by endocytosis and exocytosis.

CYTOSKELETON

Cells possess a cytoskeleton that provides a structural framework, facilitates intracellular transport, supports cell junctions, transmits signals about cell contact and adhesion, and permits motility. The three structural elements of the cytoskeleton are microfilaments, intermediate filaments, and microtubules. All are dynamic structures assembled from protein subunits and disassembled as cellular activities and external influences on the cell change.

Microfilaments are 6 to 8 nm in diameter and consist of globular actin molecules polymerized into long filaments (Fig. 4.2). Microfilaments form tracks for the movement of myosin and serve as intracellular muscles for the maintenance of cell shape, movement, and contractility. Microfilament networks, along with actin-binding and actin-bundling proteins, are found in association with adhesive cell junctions; as a web beneath cell membranes, especially the apical membrane; and as the structural core of microvilli, filopodia, and lamellipodia. Actin interacts with the other two components of the cytoskeleton.

Intermediate filaments are approximately 10 nm in diameter and have a diverse protein composition. They are not contractile but are important in the maintenance of cell shape and contact between adjacent cells and the extracellular matrix. In cells of mesenchymal origin, such as fibroblasts and osteoblasts, intermediate filaments are polymers of the protein vimentin (Fig. 4.3). In epithelial cells, intermediate filaments consist of cytokeratins. The filaments form bundles, called *tonofilaments,* which anchor onto desmosomes (see Fig. 4.3B). Cytokeratins are a multigene family of proteins that occur as linked acidic and basic pairs with differing combinations in different types of epithelia. Their expression patterns have been used to determine the relationship between cell types and as an indication of the origin of various tumors.

Microtubules are tubular or cylindric structures with an average diameter of 25 nm (Fig. 4.4). Microtubules are composed of the protein tubulin arranged in rings stacked end to end, making up the tubules. Microtubules provide internal support for the cell; are the basis of motility for certain organelles, such as cilia; act as guide paths and part of the motor mechanism for the movement of secretory vesicles and other organelles; and serve to position and organize certain organelles within the cell.

INTERCELLULAR JUNCTIONS

Specialized areas of the plasma membrane form contacts and junctions between cells and with the extracellular matrix. When cells come into contact with one another, and sometimes with the extracellular matrix, specialized junctions may form at specific sites on the contacting cell membranes. These specialized junctions may be classified into the following categories:

1. Tight junctions (zonula occludens)
2. Adhesive junctions

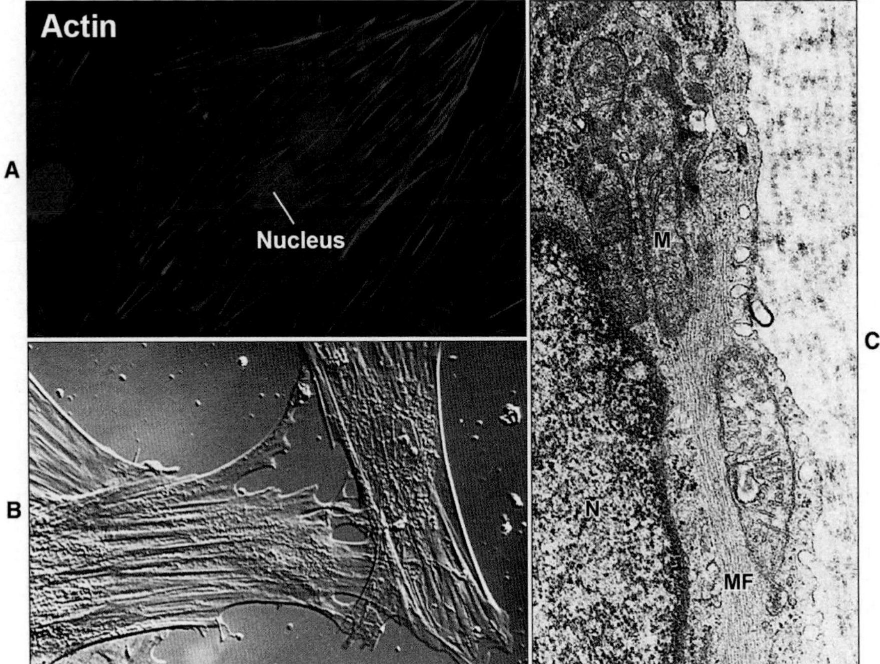

Fig. 4.2 Microfilaments *(MFs).* (A) Cultured osteogenic cells labeled with fluorescent rhodamine-phalloidin for actin, the main protein constituting MFs (nuclei are stained using 4,6-diamino-2-phenylindole [DAPI] and appear blue). (B) Nomarski differential interference contrast image of MF bundles appearing as elongated raised lines in the cytoplasm of cultured fibroblasts. (C) Electron micrograph of MFs in the cytoplasm of a fibroblast. *M,* Mitochondria; *N,* nucleus. (Courtesy Jane Aubin.)

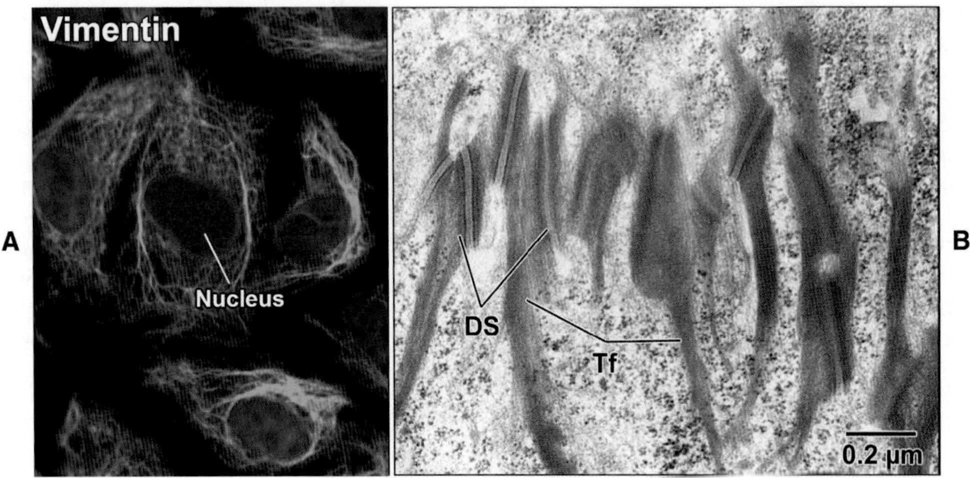

Fig. 4.3 (A) Intermediate filaments consisting of vimentin polymers in Saos osteogenic cells revealed by green immunofluorescence. The filaments radiate outward from the perinuclear region (nuclei are stained using 4,6-diamino-2-phenylindole and appear blue). (B) Electron micrographs of intermediate filaments consisting of cytokeratins in epithelial cells; these form discrete bundles called *tonofilaments (Tf)* that insert into the desmosomal plaques *(DS)* or distribute around the periphery of a cell. (A, Courtesy K. Patel.)

   a. Cell-to-cell
      i. Zonula adherens
      ii. Macula adherens (desmosome)
   b. Cell-to-matrix
      i. Focal adhesions
      ii. Hemidesmosomes
3. Communicating (gap) junctions

The term *zonula* describes a junction that completely encircles the cell; macula indicates a junction that is more circumscribed in extent (e.g., patchlike). Junctions may occur in certain combinations. A junctional complex present between cells of a simple or pseudostratified epithelium usually consists of a tight junction, a zonula adherens, and desmosomes (Fig. 4.5). On the molecular level, intercellular junctions typically consist of three components: a transmembrane adhesive protein, a cytoplasmic adapter protein, and a cytoskeletal filament. These three components differ depending on the type of junction.

In occluding (tight) junctions (Fig. 4.6A; see also Fig. 4.5), the opposing cell membranes are held in close contact by the presence of transmembrane adhesive proteins arranged in anastomosing strands that encircle the cell. The intercellular space essentially is obliterated

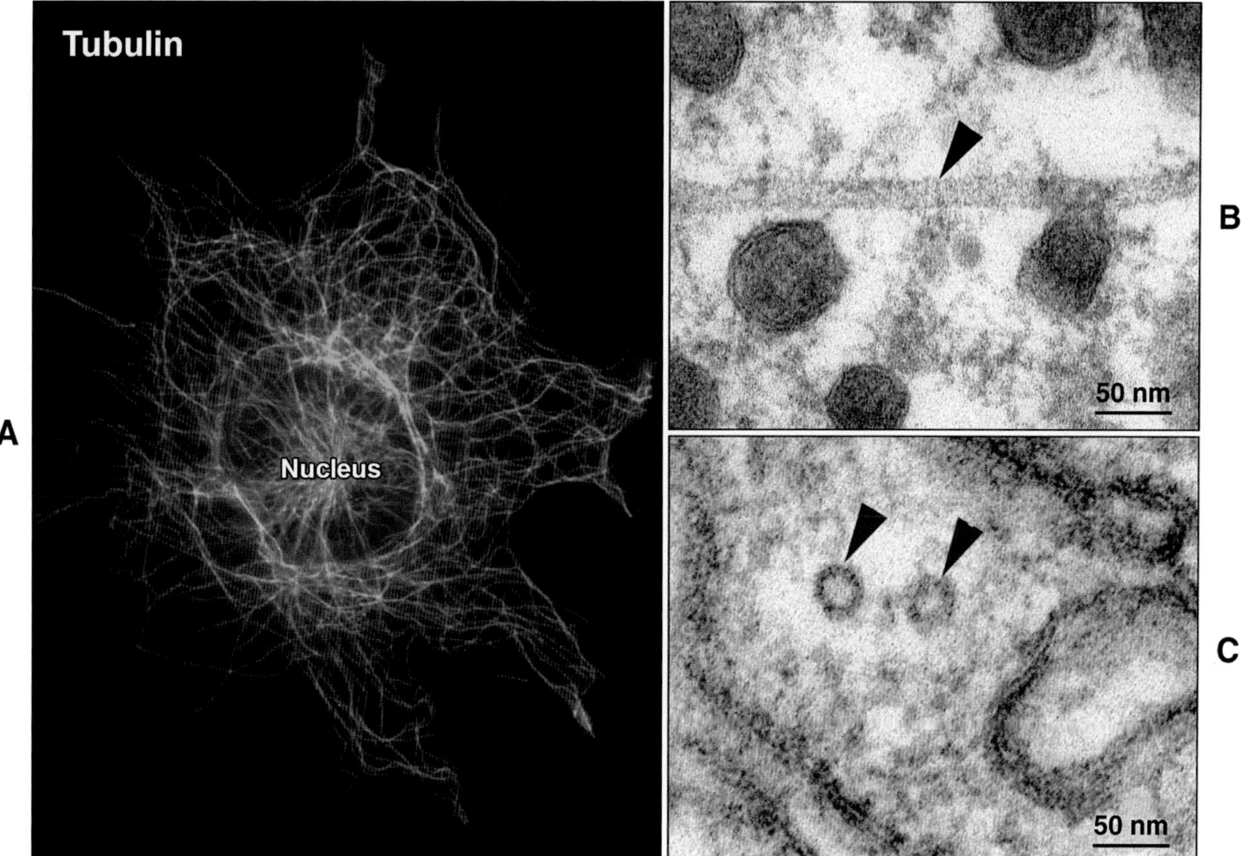

Fig. 4.4 Microtubules. (A) Fluorescent micrograph of cultured osteogenic cells labeled with an antibody to tubulin *(green)*, the main protein of microtubules (nuclei are stained using 4,6-diamino-2-phenylindole and appear blue). Electron micrographs of longitudinally oriented (B) cross-sectioned (C) microtubules *(arrowheads)*. (A, Courtesy D. Guadarrama Bello.)

at the tight junction. The transmembrane adhesive proteins, which include occludin, members of the claudin family, and (in some tissues) junctional adhesion molecule, interact homotypically with the same proteins on the adjacent cell. Several cytoplasmic proteins associate with the intracellular portions of the transmembrane proteins; these include cell polarity–related proteins, vesicular transport–related proteins, kinases, transcription factors, and a tumor suppressor protein. In addition, some of the cytoplasmic proteins of the tight junctions bind to actin filaments. Tight junctions control the passage of material through the intercellular spaces (e.g., from the interstitium to the lumen of a gland). They also have an important role as a so-called fence to define and maintain the two major domains of the cell membrane, the apical and basolateral surfaces. The tightness of the junction to water and ions (especially cations) is related to the specific claudin(s) present and is correlated with the number of strands of transmembrane proteins. For example, tight junctions joining salivary gland secretory cells have only two or three junctional strands and are relatively permeable to water, whereas those joining salivary gland striated duct cells may have six to nine strands and are relatively impermeable to water.

Adhesive junctions hold cells together or anchor cells to the extracellular matrix. In contrast to tight junctions, the intercellular space in cell-cell adhesive junctions is maintained at approximately 20 nm. Adhesive junctions also are important in cellular signaling. Their cytoplasmic components may interact with the cytoskeleton, triggering changes in cell shape or motility, or with certain tumor suppressor molecules, or they may act as nuclear transcription factors or coactivators. In some instances, the loss of cell-cell or cell-matrix contact may lead to apoptosis (programmed cell death), whereas in others, loss of contact may lead to loss of cell polarity and differentiation or unregulated cell proliferation. In cell-cell adhesive junctions the principal transmembrane proteins are members of the cadherin family. Cadherins are calcium ion–dependent proteins that interact homotypically with cadherins on the adjacent cell. The cytoplasmic adapter proteins are members of the catenin family. Catenins interact with the cytoplasmic domain of the transmembrane cadherin molecule, with the cytoskeleton, and with a number of other proteins, including kinases, and tumor suppressor molecules that are associated with adhesive junctions. In the zonula adherens (see Figs. 4.5 and 4.6B), the cadherin family member is E-cadherin, α- and β-catenin are the cytoplasmic adapters, and actin filaments are the cytoskeletal component. The catenins and actin filaments are concentrated on the cytoplasmic side of the cell membrane at the zonula adherens to form a dense web that is continuous with the terminal web of actin at the apical (and sometimes the basal) end of the cells. Another transmembrane adhesive protein present in the adherens junction is nectin, a member of the immunoglobulin superfamily. Nectin has an important role during junction formation, establishing the initial adhesion site and recruiting E-cadherin and other proteins to the junction. Other cytoplasmic proteins associated with the zonula adherens include p120 catenin, a signaling molecule associated with E-cadherin that is important in stabilizing the junction; afadin, which links nectin to the actin cytoskeleton; vinculin and α-actinin, which are actin-binding proteins; and ponsin, which links afadin and vinculin (see Fig. 4.6B).

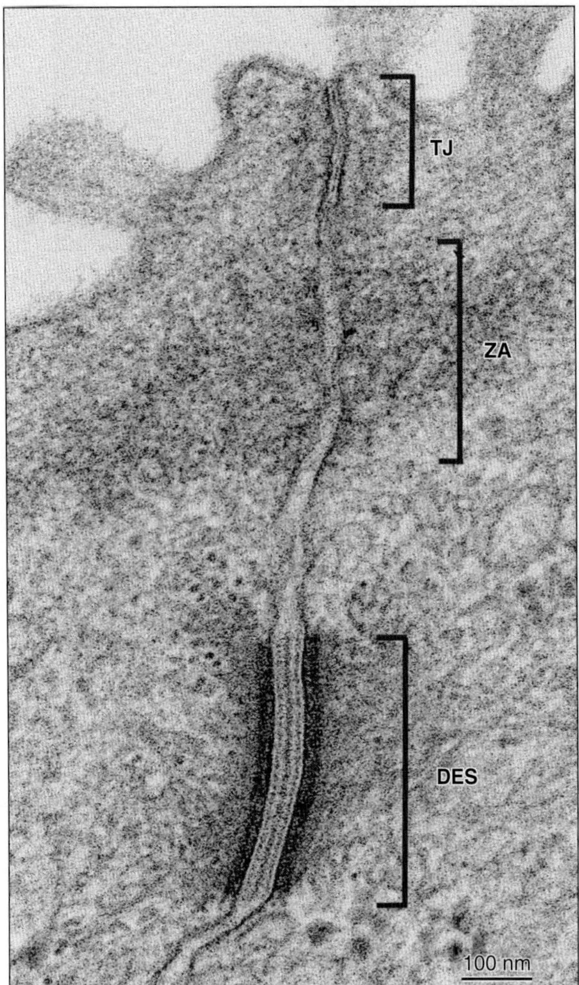

Fig. 4.5 Electron micrograph of a junctional complex between epithelial cells of a salivary gland. In the tight junction (*TJ*, zonula occludens), located at the boundary of the apical and lateral cell membranes, the intercellular space is obliterated. In the adherens junction (zonula adherens [*ZA*], the cell membranes are separated by ~20 nm, and a dense mat of microfilaments is present in the cytoplasm. In the desmosome (*DES*), the cell membranes are parallel and separated by ~25 nm, and a central dense line is present in the intercellular space. Intermediate filaments insert into dense plaques on the cytoplasmic surface of the desmosome.

In the desmosome (see Figs. 4.5 and 4.6C), the cadherins are desmoglein and desmocollin. The interaction of these transmembrane proteins with those from the adjacent cell results in a dense line in the middle of the intercellular space at the desmosome. The catenins are desmoplakin, plakoglobin, and plakophilin, which form an electron-dense plaque on the cytoplasmic side of the desmosome. This plaque serves as an attachment site for the cytoskeletal components, which, in the case of the desmosome, are intermediate filaments.

Cell-matrix junctions have a structural organization similar to that of cell-cell adhesive junctions. Focal adhesions link the actin-rich cytoskeleton of cells with the extracellular matrix to mediate cell adhesion and migration, mechanosensing, and intracellular signaling events (Fig. 4.7). The formation of focal adhesions is a highly complex process that requires the assembly of multiple cellular proteins, including vinculin, talin, paxillin, tensin, zyxin, focal adhesion kinase, and α-actinin. The transmembrane component is a member of the integrin family of adhesion molecules. Integrins are heterodimers of different

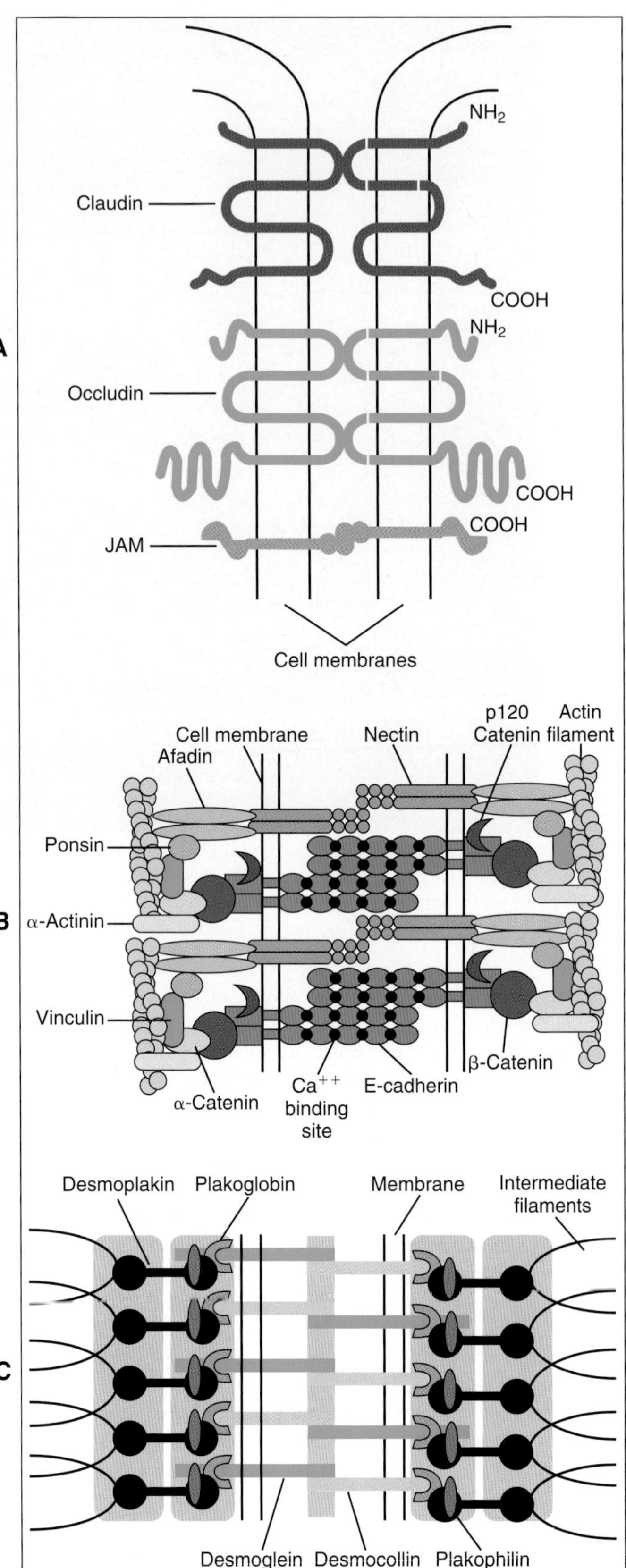

Fig. 4.6 Diagrams showing molecular structures of intercellular junctions. (A) Tight junction. (B) Adhering junction. (C) Desmosome. *JAM*, Junctional adhesion molecule. (Courtesy A.R. Hand.)

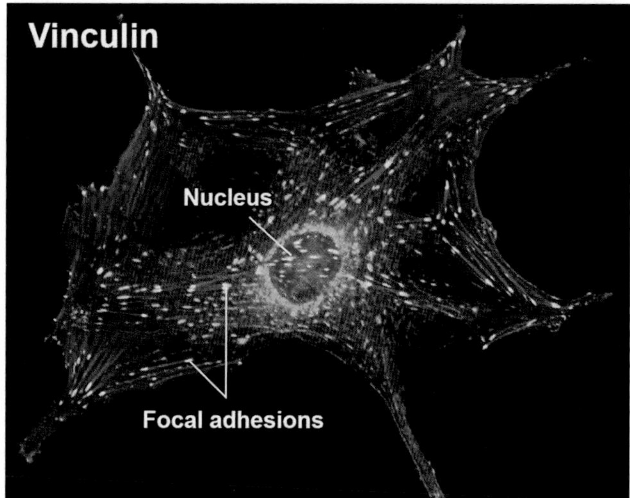

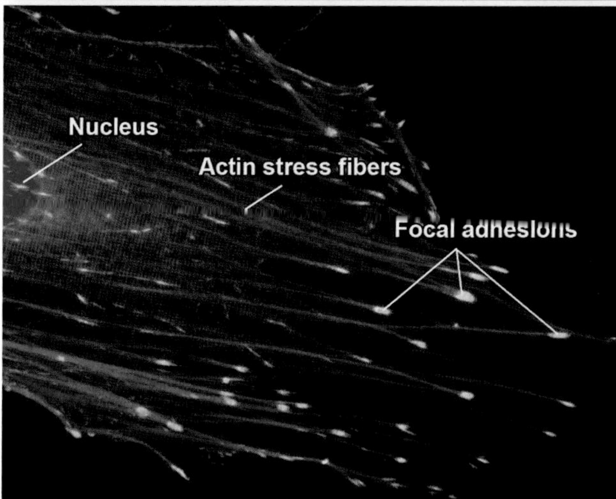

Fig. 4.7 Visualization of focal adhesions in an osteogenic cell by immunofluorescence detection of vinculin *(green)*, an abundant protein in focal adhesions. These localize at the cell periphery and are associated with the extremity of actin stress fibers, here stained in red using rhodamine-phalloidin (nuclei are stained using 4,6-diamino-2-phenylindole and appear blue). (Courtesy D. Guadarrama Bello.)

alpha and beta subunits that occur in different combinations with specificity for various extracellular matrix molecules. The cytoplasmic adapter proteins, which include the actin-binding proteins α-actinin, vinculin, and talin, link the transmembrane integrins to the actin cytoskeleton. Binding of the integrin to collagen, laminin, fibronectin, and other extracellular matrix proteins results in recruitment and remodeling of the actin cytoskeleton. Ligand binding by integrins also leads to the recruitment and activation of various intracellular signaling molecules, including guanine nucleotide–binding proteins and several protein kinases. Mature focal adhesions are larger and lead to stronger interactions between the cytoskeleton and substrate.

Hemidesmosomes link the cell to the basal lamina and, through additional extracellular molecules, to the rest of the extracellular matrix. The transmembrane adhesive molecules present in hemidesmosomes (Fig. 4.8) are the integrin $\alpha_6\beta_4$, which binds specifically to the basal lamina glycoprotein laminin, and collagen XVII (also identified as BP180). Like in the desmosome, the cytoplasmic adapter proteins (bullous pemphigoid antigen 230 [BP230] and plectin) form a dense plaque on the cytoplasmic surface of the hemidesmosome, which functions as an attachment site for intermediate filaments.

Gap junctions are plaquelike regions of the cell membrane where the intercellular space narrows to 2 to 3 nm and transmembrane proteins of the connexin family form aqueous channels between the cytoplasm of adjacent cells (Fig. 4.9). These proteins have specific tissue and cellular distributions and confer differing permeability properties to the gap junctions. Six connexin molecules form a connexon, which has a central channel approximately 2 nm in diameter (see Fig. 4.9D). The connexons in one cell pair with connexons in the adjacent cell to create a patent channel. Small molecules, such as ions and signaling molecules, can move readily from one cell to another. Gap junctions electrically couple cells and allow for a coordinated response to a stimulus by the cells that are interconnected.

Cell-cell and cell-matrix junctions have important roles in the differentiation, development, and function of normal cells, tissues, and organs. However, the functions of these junctions may be altered or disrupted by genetic abnormalities of junctional or cytoskeletal proteins by autoimmune diseases in which circulating antibodies to junctional proteins are present or by modifications of the ionic environment (e.g., pH). Mutations of connexin genes have been identified as the bases for certain types of deafness, congenital cataracts, a demyelinating disease (Charcot-Marie-Tooth), and oculodentodigital dysplasia (a disease that exhibits craniofacial abnormalities, syndactyly, conductive hearing loss, and hair and nail abnormalities). Several types of epidermolysis bullosa (a blistering skin disorder) are caused by mutations of the genes for various desmosomal, hemidesmosomal, and intermediate filament proteins. In addition, some forms of the disease are caused by mutations of the genes for extracellular matrix proteins involved in cell-matrix adhesion. Pemphigus vulgaris and pemphigus foliaceus (blistering diseases of the oral mucosa and skin, respectively) are caused by autoantibodies to desmoglein-3 and -1, the cadherin in desmosomes. Another debilitating skin disease, bullous pemphigoid, results from the presence of autoantibodies to the hemidesmosomal components collagen XVII (BP180) and BP230.

EPITHELIUM–CONNECTIVE TISSUE INTERFACE

All epithelia are separated from the underlying connective tissue by a layer of extracellular matrix organized as a thin sheet immediately adjacent to the epithelial cells. This is the basal lamina (also known as *basement membrane* in light microscopy), which is a product of the epithelium and connective tissue. The basal lamina, along with hemidesmosomes, attaches the epithelium to the underlying connective tissue, functions as a filter to control the passage of molecules between the epithelium and connective tissue, and acts as a barrier to cell migration. The basal lamina also has important signaling functions that are essential for epithelial differentiation and the development and maintenance of cell polarity.

The basal lamina has an overall thickness of 50 to 100 nm and consists of two structural components: the lamina lucida, adjacent to the basal cell membrane, and the lamina densa, between the lamina lucida and the connective tissue (Fig. 4.10). In epithelia there is a third layer, the lamina fibroreticularis, closely associated with the lamina densa. The main constituents of the basal lamina are type IV collagen, which forms a chicken-wire type of network; the adhesive glycoprotein laminin; and a heparan sulfate proteoglycan. Fibronectin, an adhesive glycoprotein, type III collagen (reticular fibers), type VII collagen (anchoring fibrils), and other types of collagen all made by fibroblasts are present in the lamina fibroreticularis and help maintain the attachment of the basal lamina to the underlying connective tissue. There also exists a special, atypical basal lamina between the ameloblasts and maturing enamel (see Chapter 7) and between the gingiva and tooth surface (see Chapter 12).

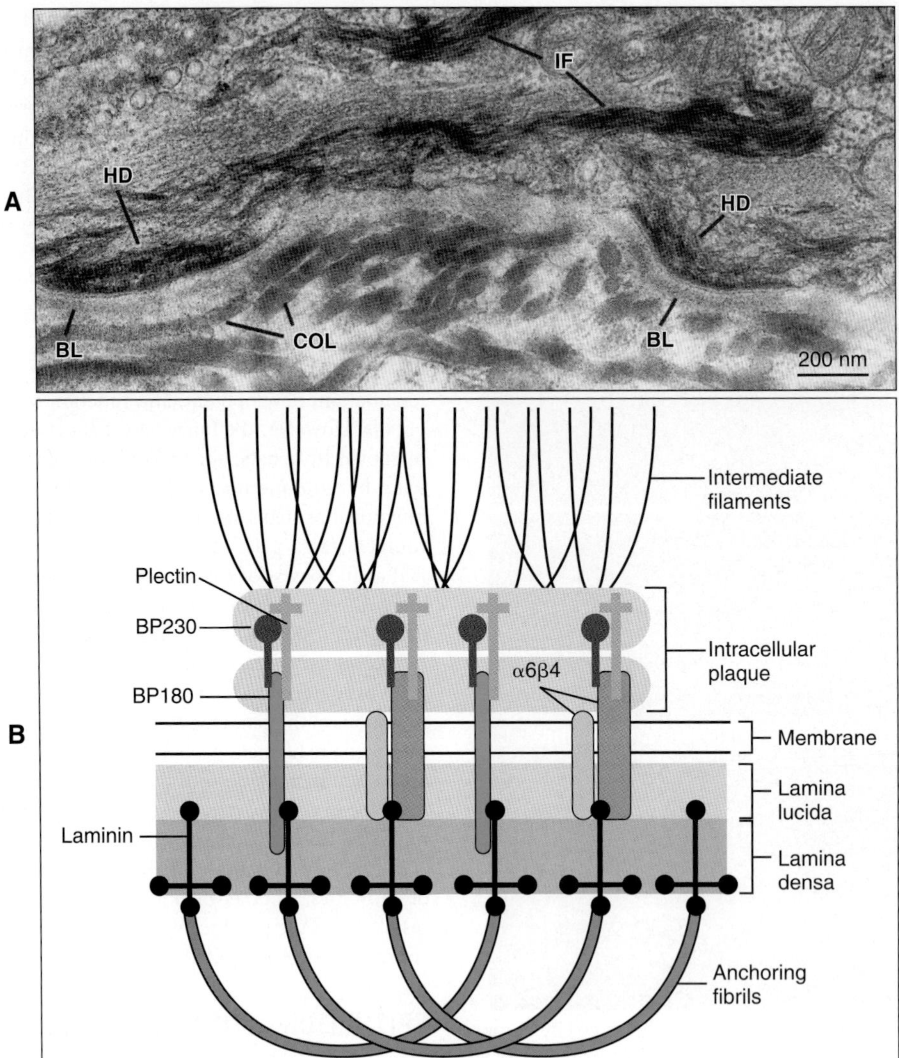

Fig. 4.8 (A) Electron micrograph of hemidesmosomes *(HD)* of a basal epithelial cell from a rat salivary gland excretory duct. (B) Diagram of a hemidesmosome. *BL,* Basal lamina; *COL,* collagen fibrils; *IF,* intermediate filaments.

FIBROBLASTS

Fibroblasts are the most abundant cells of soft connective tissues and play central roles in the normal physiologic function of the gingiva, the periodontal ligament, the dental pulp, bone marrow spaces, the fibrous periosteum covering alveolar bone, the stroma of salivary glands, and the mucosal connective tissues of the oral cavity. Fibroblasts synthesize and secrete the fibrous elements of extracellular matrices and interfibrillar molecules that contribute to the structure and function of connective tissues. The importance of this unique cell in oral biology is highlighted in Box 4.1.

Cellular Organization

Fibroblasts are anchorage-dependent cells that are tightly associated with fibrillar collagen and are often oriented along their axes to large bundles of collagen fibers, a phenomenon that is commonly seen in the principal fibers of the gingiva and periodontal ligament (Figs. 4.11 and 4.12). The resting fibroblast is an elongated cell with little cytoplasm and a dark-staining, flattened nucleus containing condensed chromatin, indicative of low levels of transcriptional activity (see Fig. 4.11). Active fibroblasts have an oval-shaped, pale-staining nucleus and a greater amount of cytoplasm (see Fig. 4.11). The degree of synthetic and secretory capacity of fibroblasts is evidenced by the amount of rough endoplasmic reticulum, secretory granules, and mitochondria and the extent of the Golgi complex in their cytoplasm (see Fig. 4.12).

Contraction and Motility

Fibroblasts exhibit motility and contractility, which are important during connective tissue formation and remodeling and during wound repair. The actin cytoskeleton of fibroblasts allows them to move through the ground substance. In certain tissues, fibroblasts have significant contractile properties called *myofibroblasts.*

Junctions

In most connective tissues, fibroblasts are separated from one another by the extracellular matrix components; therefore intercellular junctions are not present. Exceptions are embryonic tissue in which gap junctions are common and the periodontal ligament in which fibroblasts commonly exhibit cell-cell contacts of the adherens type. Fibroblasts also form specialized focal contacts with components of the extracellular matrix known as a *fibronexus* (Fig. 4.13).

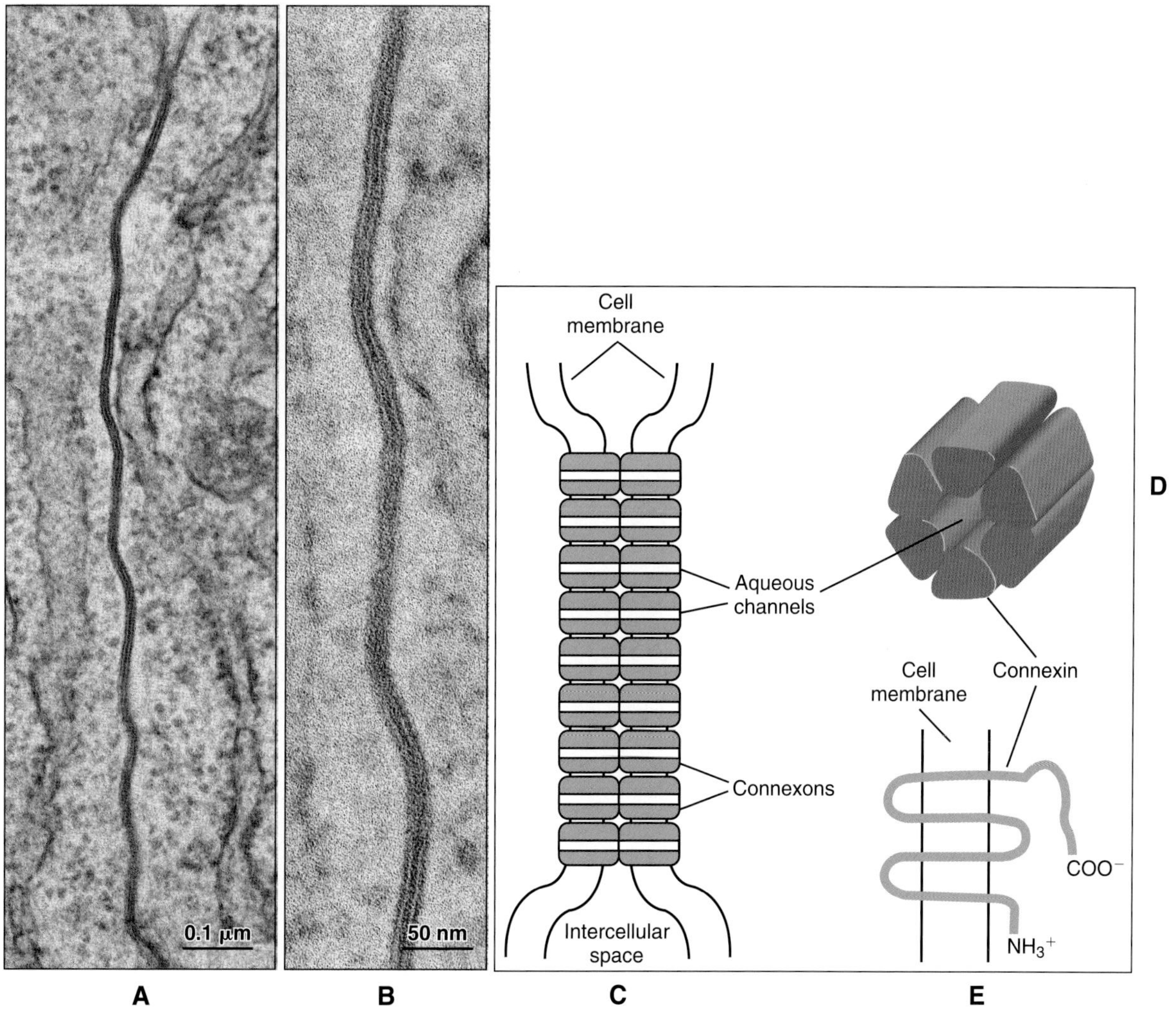

Fig. 4.9 (A, B) Electron micrographs of a gap junction. The adjacent cell membranes are separated by 2 to 3 nm. Indistinct regions in the junction result from the varying orientation of the membranes in the section. (C–E) Diagrams of gap junction structure. (C) View corresponding to thin-section electron micrographs. (D) A single connexon consists of six connexin molecules. (E) A connexin molecule has four transmembrane domains, and the N- and C-terminal domains are located in the cytoplasm. (C–E, Courtesy A.R. Hand.)

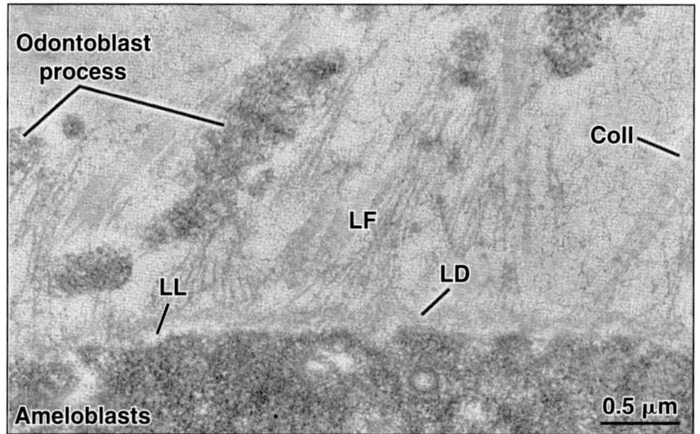

Fig. 4.10 Electron micrograph illustrating the three components—the lamina lucida *(LL)*, lamina densa *(LD)*, and lamina fibroreticularis *(LF)*—forming the basal lamina associated with epithelial cells, here interposed between differentiating ameloblasts and odontoblasts. *Coll,* Collagen fibrils.

Heterogeneity

Although fibroblasts of different tissues have similar appearances, which have historically been distinguishable mainly as active or quiescent, there is considerable heterogeneity within fibroblast populations. This heterogeneity is manifested as differences in their synthetic products, rates of synthesis and turnover, response to regulatory molecules, proliferation rates, among other critical factors. For example, it has been estimated that collagen in the periodontal ligament has a turnover rate approximately eight times that of collagen in the skin and about two times that of gingival collagen. More recent work using single-cell sequencing of mRNA expression repertoires of fibroblasts from lung and skin has shown thousands of different fibroblast subtypes based on their mRNA expression repertoire.

Aging

Fibroblasts originate from mesenchymal cells. When differentiated, they can replicate by mitosis. An inverse correlation has been found between the age of a donor and the number of divisions that cultured fibroblasts can undergo before they become senescent. The exact cause of this replicative senescence is unknown. Fibroblasts from long-lived species can

BOX 4.1 The Fibroblast: An Extracellular Matrix Cell With Key Functions in Oral Biology

Origin of Fibroblasts

Debate over the general origins of fibroblasts began with 19th-century pathologist Virchow, who favored the idea of local division of undifferentiated mesenchymal cells. In the 1920s Maximow suggested a hematogenous origin after observing a rapid accumulation of cells in tissue culture without obvious increase of local mitotic activity. Experiments by Russell Ross and colleagues at the University of Washington clarified this issue with a rat parabiotic model in which the identity of labeled cells was established using electron microscopy and radioautography. These data demonstrated that fibroblasts taking up tritiated thymidine after wounding are not bloodborne and that proliferation is associated with local division of cells closely associated with blood vessels. A follow-up in vitro study of human bone marrow fibroblasts added further support to the idea of separate origins for fibroblasts and macrophages. Since these early experiments, sophisticated molecular methods using bar codes to mark fibroblast lineages have shown that multiple subtypes of fibroblasts differentiate from local precursors and from bone marrow–derived, bloodborne precursors (e.g., fibrocytes). It now seems that much of the structural complexity of connective tissues that are exhibited in specialized oral tissues, such as periodontal ligament, arises from the existence and specific functions of these fibroblast subtypes.

In the context of tissue development, fibroblasts in the periodontal ligament originate embryologically from the dental follicle. Early electron microscopy examination of developing mouse tooth germs demonstrated that cell division is confined to paravascular cells. The cells of the investing layer around the developing periodontal ligament exhibit the ultrastructural characteristics of undifferentiated fibroblasts, suggesting that these cells are not yet specialized and have yet to become oriented toward synthesis of the extracellular matrix proteins that characterize the fibroblasts of the gingiva and the periodontal ligament. These cells, then, are likely to act as a reservoir of progenitor cells, that, go on to form the connective tissues of the gingiva and the periodontal ligament.

Fibroblasts in the Gingiva and Periodontal Ligament

The fibroblasts of gingival and periodontal ligament connective tissues maintain the integrity of the dentogingival junction and the attachment of the tooth root to the bone, in part, by mediating collagen turnover and by preserving collagen fiber attachments to the root surface.

The dentogingival junction comprises epithelial and soft connective tissues, which collectively provide a continuously adapting sealing system around the neck of the tooth. This sealing system is critical for preventing bacterial invasion and maintaining adaptation of the gingiva to the tooth root, while loss of the normal regulation of this sealing system can lead to destruction of the underlying periodontal attachments to the alveolar bone. Throughout the lifetime of mammals, the size, structure, and anatomic configuration of the healthy dentogingival junction remain remarkably stable. Gingival fibroblasts mediate the synthesis and remodeling of gingival fiber attachments that insert into the root surfaces of teeth. The bulk of the gingival connective tissues comprises type I collagen, secreted by fibroblasts. Because collagen is turned over rapidly in periodontal tissues, deviations of the balance between synthesis and degradation can lead to loss of tissue form, net collagen loss, and, ultimately, tooth loss.

The periodontal ligament is critical for the development of the periodontium, regulation of tooth eruption, dissipation of masticatory forces, orthodontic tooth movement, and provision of proprioception for controlling mastication. The periodontal ligament is exposed to a range of mechanical forces that are physiologic (mastication, speech) and pathophysiologic (orthodontic or parafunctional behaviors that serve no direct physiologic function). Successful treatment outcomes of a wide variety of dental procedures rely on the integrity of the periodontal ligament and its fibroblast populations. Oral parafunctional occlusal habits, such as bruxism (a disorder characterized by grinding and clenching of teeth), exert supraphysiologic forces to the teeth, which lead to periodontal ligament destruction, loss of fiber attachment to teeth secondary to force-induced cell death, and eventual tooth loss.

It has been known for many years that the functions of the periodontal ligament include proprioception, tooth support, and attachment; these latter functions are provided by the principal collagen fibers of the periodontal ligament, which undergo rapid turnover in health and are dependent on the activities of fibroblasts in these tissues. Homeostasis of the periodontal ligament structure and contiguous periodontal tissues is maintained by the fibroblasts. Although there is rapid collagen turnover in the periodontal ligament, the turnover of cells is very slow. Under normal conditions of function, these cells are actively engaged in protein metabolism for periodontal ligament homeostasis rather than in proliferation.

Extracellular Matrix Structure and Function

The collagen matrix of gingival and periodontal connective tissues is organized into bundles of fibers, which constitute the supraalveolar fiber apparatus in gingiva and the principal collagen fibers of the periodontal ligament. In gingiva, collagen is organized into highly ordered arrays of transseptal, circular, dentogingival, gingival-periosteal, and dentoperiosteal fibers. These fibers prevent rotation, maintain tooth linkages during mesial drift, and are critically important in providing the biologic seal of the gingiva to the roots of the teeth. In the periodontal ligament, fibroblasts contribute to the synthesis and remodeling of collagen fibers and interfibrillar ground substance that is critical for maintaining tooth support in the alveolar bone. Tractional forces generated by contractile machinery in gingival and periodontal ligament fibroblasts are important for creating tension in the collagen matrix; these forces ensure that the gingiva is tightly bound to the tooth roots and the alveolar bone.

Role of the Extracellular Matrix in Tissue Physiology

The extracellular matrix, which was once believed only to provide physical structural support for cell adhesion and migration, is now recognized as serving a critical role in the form and function of all oral tissues. The extracellular matrix provides mechanical cues that influence decisions regarding the form, function, fate of cells, and, in particular, the fibroblasts of soft connective tissues. In connective tissues, direct transfer of forces to cells may involve cell-to-cell and/or cell-to-matrix contacts. Periodontal ligament fibroblasts perceive and transmit mechanical force through elements of the extracellular matrix, such as collagen, which support and transmit mechanical loads. Transmembrane adhesion molecules, such as integrins, are the main cellular components that mediate the sensing and regulation of extracellular matrix mechanics. Integrins act as matrix receptors and connect the matrix to the cytoskeleton. Furthermore, integrins functionally integrate cell adhesion and cell-signaling processes and transfer forces from the extracellular matrix to the cytoskeleton. The cytoskeleton, in turn, can transmit cellular forces and contributes to information processing of mechanically derived signals. The cytoskeleton of fibroblasts comprises three different polymer systems: actin microfilaments, vimentin intermediate filaments, and tubulin-based microtubules. Notably, the actin-based cytoskeleton is critically important for the determination of cell shape, cell migration, remodeling of the extracellular matrix, and, in force-loaded tissues such as the periodontal ligament, maintenance of cell survival in the face of potentially lethal applied mechanical forces. The fibroblasts of the periodontal ligament and gingiva exhibit specialized arrays of cross-linked actin filaments in the submembrane cortex that protect them against mechanical force–induced death. One of the important proteins that mediates protection against force-induced cell death is filamin A, an actin–cross-linking protein that stabilizes the cell cortex and helps regulate the adhesive activities of integrins.

The integrity and function of the extracellular matrix is pivotal to its mechanobiologic function, which is tightly maintained by the fibroblasts that reside in these tissues. The rate of extracellular matrix turnover is positively related with mechanical loading: Increasing force levels associated with mastication and bruxism tend to increase both the production and removal of extracellular matrix structural elements. Collagen (type I) is the most abundant structural extracellular matrix

BOX 4.1 The Fibroblast, an Extracellular Matrix Cell With Key Functions in Oral Biology—cont'd

protein of mammalian connective tissues and in all oral tissues. Collagen provides the necessary foundational support for the periodontal ligament to withstand the mechanical loads delivered to teeth as a result of masticatory and parafunctional activities. The high rate of collagen turnover that is exhibited by fibroblasts in the gingiva and periodontal ligament is an intrinsic characteristic that maintains normal cellular architecture and function of the periodontium.

Remodeling of the Extracellular Matrix in Connective Tissues

In health, the synthesis and remodeling of collagen by fibroblasts enable dynamic attachment of the gingiva and the periodontal ligament to the tooth root. Physiologic remodeling of collagen occurs largely by internalization and degradation of collagen in acidic, membrane-bound vacuolar compartments (i.e., phagolysosomes). In high-prevalence inflammatory lesions of the gingiva such as gingivitis, matrix metalloproteinases remodel collagens and affect gingival tissue architecture and function, possibly enabling maintenance of gingival attachment to tooth roots.

Intracellular collagen degradation, which is mediated by phagocytosis by fibroblasts, is required for physiologic matrix remodeling and wound healing. During collagen phagocytosis, fibroblasts adhere to collagen, followed by partial digestion of collagen fibril extracellularly; shorter segments are then internalized and digested intracellularly by lysosomal cathepsins (B, L, K). In tissues with rapid matrix remodeling (e.g., involuting uterus, periodontium) and in healing wounds, collagen turnover is directly related to the volume density of collagen fibrils in phagosomes within fibroblasts, indicating that phagocytosis is critical for collagen turnover. Although much is known about the mechanisms that control the matrix metalloproteinase pathway, the regulation of fibroblast collagen phagocytosis is not well understood. Although Ca^{2+}, collagen structure, lectins, cytokines, the urokinase plasminogen activator receptor–associated protein, and integrins can modulate phagocytosis by fibroblasts in vitro, the regulation of collagen degradation by phagocytosis in vivo is poorly understood.

Collagen receptor–dependent phagocytosis uniquely engages markedly different cortical structures and membrane protrusions than phagocytosis that is initiated by complement or immunoglobulin receptors. In contrast to phagocytic cells such as macrophages in which cells first extend processes and then bind their targets, the initial rate-limiting step in collagen phagocytosis by fibroblasts is cell adhesion to collagen, which is controlled by beta 1-integrin activation. Electron microscopic analysis of gingival fibroblast–mediated remodeling of collagen in vivo shows that after adhesion to collagen, actin-rich pseudopods are formed that pull and reshape collagen fibrils. In vitro studies have indicated that these critical steps in collagen phagocytosis are dependent on nonmuscle myosins and actin filaments. Thus the actin cytoskeleton, in concert with attachment to integrins (which is mediated by actin-binding proteins), provides a dynamic system that enables fibroblasts to interact dynamically and reciprocally with extracellular matrix polymers such as collagen and underscores the importance of the actin cytoskeleton in controlling collagen remodeling.

Christopher A. McCulloch
Matrix Dynamics Group
Faculty of Dentistry
University of Toronto
Toronto, Canada

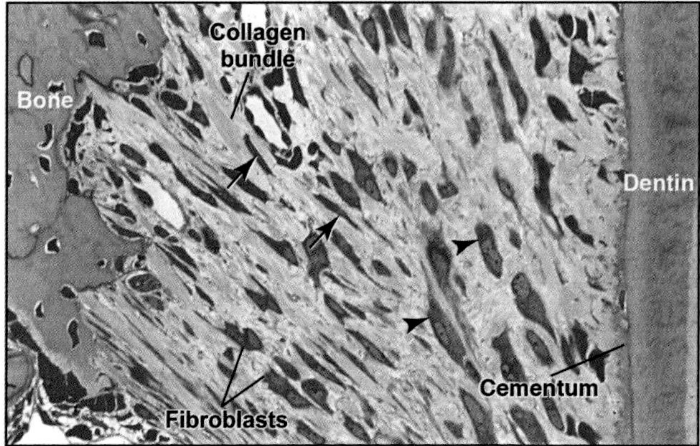

Fig. 4.11 Light microscope image. Inactive fibroblasts *(arrows)* can be identified by their relationship to collagen bundles; their dark-staining, usually elongated nuclei; and their sparse cytoplasm. Active fibroblasts *(arrowheads)* have larger, less densely stained nuclei and clearly visible cytoplasm.

divide more times than fibroblasts from short-lived species, suggesting a genetic component. Some have demonstrated a relationship between the gradual loss of telomere DNA at the ends of the chromosomes that occurs during each mitotic cycle and the onset of senescence. Other studies suggest that the accumulation of oxidative damage to DNA and proteins also contributes to senescence. Fibroblasts that become senescent remain viable but exhibit changes in metabolism and gene expression that suggest an aging phenotype (e.g., a decrease in the production of extracellular matrix proteins and an increase in the production of degradative enzymes). Altogether these changes result in many of the signs associated with human aging (e.g., skin fragility, loss of elasticity, and decreased capacity for wound healing).

SECRETORY PRODUCTS OF FIBROBLASTS

Fibroblasts can synthesize and secrete a variety of extracellular molecules. These include the components of the fibrous elements of the extracellular matrix, the components of the amorphous ground substance, and a number of biologically active molecules (e.g., proteinases, cytokines, and growth factors).

Collagens

The collagen superfamily contains at least 27 types of collagens that, together, constitute the most abundant proteins found in the body (Table 4.1). All collagens are composed of three polypeptide alpha chains coiled around each other to form the typical collagen triple-helix configuration. Common features include the presence of the amino acid glycine in every third position (Gly-X-Y repeating sequence), of hydroxyproline and hydroxylysine, and of noncollagenous domains and a high proportion of proline residues. Variations among the collagens include differences in the assembly of the basic polypeptide chains, lengths of the triple helix, interruptions in the helix, and terminations of the helical domains.

Mesenchymal cells and their derivatives (fibroblasts, chondrocytes, osteoblasts, odontoblasts, and cementoblasts) are the major producers of collagens. Other cell types (such as epithelial, endothelial, muscle, and Schwann cells) also synthesize collagens, although on a more limited basis in terms of amount and variety of collagen types.

The collagen superfamily is subdivided into nine subfamilies largely based on their supramolecular assemblies (see Table 4.1):

1. Fibrillar collagens (types I, II, III, V, XI, XXIV, XXVII): These collagens aggregate in a highly organized manner in the extracellular compartment to form fibrils with a typical 64-nm banding pattern. Type I collagen is the most abundant in most connective collagen

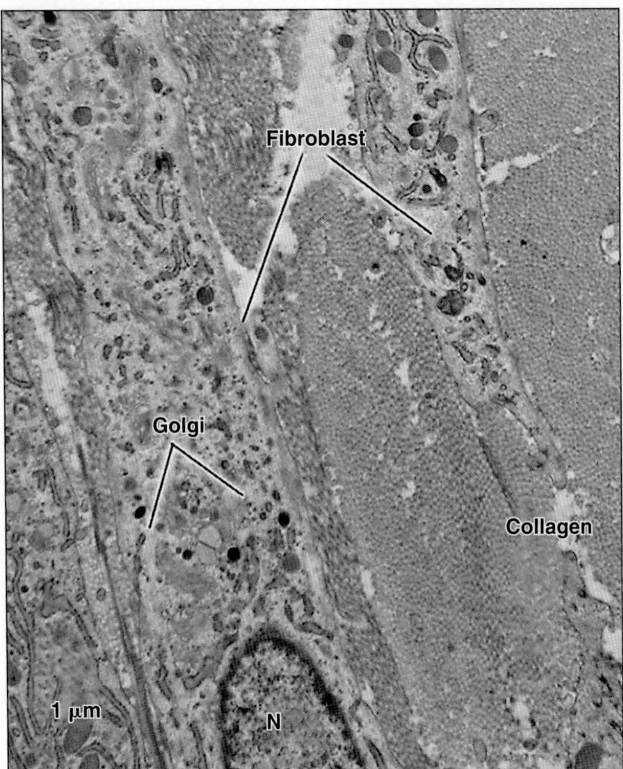

Fig. 4.12 In electron micrographs, fibroblasts typically lie adjacent to collagen fibrils and have elongated cell bodies. The quantity and density of heterochromatin in nuclei *(N)* is indicative of their activity; active fibroblasts have less heterochromatin, and it is less condensed. Protein synthetic organelles are more abundant in active fibroblasts, and the Golgi complex, in particular, is more extensive in these cells.

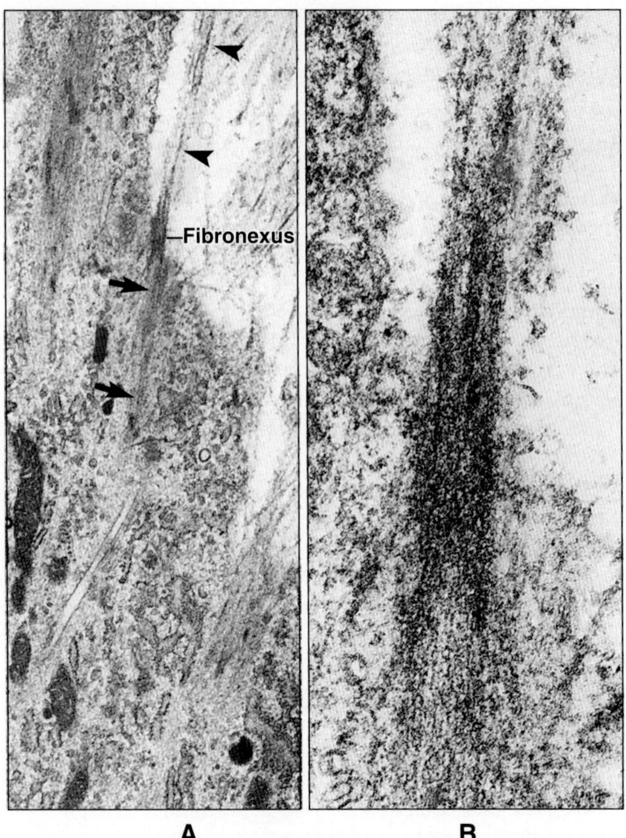

Fig. 4.13 (A, B) Electron micrographs illustrating a fibronexus in a periodontal ligament fibroblast. Intracellular filaments of actin *(arrows)* are linked to extracellular filaments of fibronectin *(arrowheads)* via transmembrane integrin receptors. (From Garant PR, et al.: Attachment of periodontal ligament fibroblasts to the extracellular matrix in the squirrel monkey, *J Periodontal Res* 17:70–79, 1982.)

tissues. Collagen fibrils often are composed of more than one type of collagen. For example, type I collagen fibrils often contain small amounts of types III, V, and XII. Type V collagen is believed to regulate fibril diameter.

2. Basal lamina collagen (type IV): Collagen type IV is similar in size to type I collagen but does not assemble as fibrils. It contains frequent nonhelical sequences and aggregates in a sheetlike, chicken-wire configuration. Type IV collagen is a major component of the basal lamina and is a product of epithelial cells.
3. Fibril-associated collagens with interrupted triple helices (FACIT): Collagens IX, XII, XIV, XVI, XIX, XX, XXI, and XXII consist of chains that have different lengths and contain a variety of noncollagenous domains. They exhibit several interruptions in the triple helix and are found in various locations in different tissues. Several of the FACIT collagens associate with fibrillar collagens and other extracellular matrix components. Of these, type XIX collagen is found in basal laminae and appears to be important for skeletal muscle cell differentiation.
4. Network-forming collagens: Type VIII collagen assembles into a hexagonal lattice, which is believed to impart compressive strength while providing an open, porous meshwork. Type X collagen has a similar size and structure and is largely restricted to the hypertrophic zone of the epiphyseal cartilage growth plate.
5. Anchoring-fibril collagen: Collagen VII has unusually large nonhelical ends making up two-thirds of the size of the molecule. The C-terminal ends associate to form dimers that subsequently are assembled into the anchoring fibrils that extend from the basal lamina into the underlying connective tissue.
6. Microfibril-forming collagen: Type VI collagen, which has large N- and C-terminal globular domains that associate in an end-to-end fashion, forms beaded filaments. Type VI collagen is present in most connective tissues. This collagen has binding properties for cells, proteoglycans, and type I collagen and may serve as a bridge between the cells and the matrix.
7. Transmembrane collagen types XIII, XVII, XXIII, and XXV: These collagens are transmembrane proteins with extracellular collagenous domains and a C-terminal noncollagenous domain that functions in cell adhesion. Type XVII collagen is found in hemidesmosomes of basal epidermal cells and attaches the cells to the basal lamina. Type XIII collagen is present in focal adhesion sites of fibroblasts and at cell-matrix interfaces in some epithelia, muscle, and nerves. Type XIII collagen also is present in the cell-cell adhesive specializations. These collagens may interact with other cell surface or extracellular matrix molecules to alter cell behavior.
8. Multiplexin (endostatin-forming) collagens: Type XVIII collagen is a component of basal laminae of epithelial and endothelial cells and is believed to stabilize structures of the basal lamina. Type XVIII collagen has multiple interruptions in the central helical domain and a large, unique C-terminal nonhelical domain. This C-terminal domain can be cleaved by extracellular proteases to form endostatin, a potent inhibitor of endothelial cell migration and angiogenesis. In the brain, endostatin may be deposited in the amyloid plaques of Álzheimer's disease. Type XV collagen has a similar structure and a wider distribution, including the papillary

TABLE 4.1 **The Collagens**

Type	Gene Name	Chains	Supramolecular Assembly	Characteristic Features	Tissue Distribution	Major Function
Fibril-Forming Collagens						
I	COL1A1, COL1A2	$[\alpha1(I)]_3$, $[\alpha1(I)]_2\alpha2(I)$	Fibrils 300 nm	Most abundant collagen	Abundant in skin, bone, dentin, cementum, tendons, ligaments, and most connective tissue	Provides tensile strength to connective tissue
II	COL2A1	$[\alpha1(II)]_3$	Fibrils 300 nm	Forms heterofibrils with Col IX and XI	Cartilage, vitreous humor, intervertebral disk	Provides tensile strength to connective tissue
III	COL3A1	$[\alpha1(III)]_3$	Fibrils 300 nm	Abundant in elastic tissues	Embryonic connective tissue, pulp, skin, blood vessels, lymphoid tissue (reticular fibers)	Provides tensile strength to connective tissue
V	COL5A1, COL5A2, COL5A3	$[\alpha1(V)]_2\alpha2(V)$	Fibrils 390 nm	Forms core of type I fibrils Binds to DNA, heparan sulfate, thrombospondin, heparin, and insulin	Basal laminae, blood vessels, ligaments, skin, dentin, periodontal tissues	Provides tensile strength
		$\alpha1(V)\alpha2(V)\alpha3(V)$			Placenta	
		$[\alpha1(V)]_3$			Present in tumor cells	
XI	COL11A1, COL11A2	$\alpha1(XI)\alpha2(XI)\alpha3(XI)$	Fibrils	Forms core of type II fibrils	Cartilage, vitreous humor, placenta	Provides tensile strength, controlling lateral growth of type II fibrils
XXIV	COL24A1	$[\alpha1(XXIV)]_3$	Fibrils	Displays structural features unique to invertebrate fibrillar collagens	Bone, cornea	Regulation of type I fibrillogenesis
XXVII	COL27A1	$[\alpha1(XXVII)]_3$	Fibrils	Presence of triple-helix imperfections	Cartilage, eye, ear, lungs	Possible association with type II fibrils
Microfibril-Forming Collagens						
VI	COL6A1, COL6A2, COL6A3, COL6A4,	$\alpha1(VI)\alpha2(VI)\alpha3(VI)$	Beaded filaments 150 nm	Highly disulfide cross-linked	Ligament, skin, cartilage, placenta	Bridging between cells and matrix
	COL6A5 (also known as COL29A1) COL6A6				Skin, lung, small intestine, colon, testis	
Transmembrane Collagens						
XIII	COL13A1	$[\alpha1(XIII)]_3$	Linear	Single transmembrane domain and a large, mainly collagenous ectodomain	Epidermis, hair follicle, cell surfaces, focal adhesions, intercalated disks	Cell-matrix, cell-cell adhesion
XVII	COL17A1	$[\alpha1(XVII)]_3$	Linear		Hemidesmosomes	Cell attachment to matrix
XXIII	COL23A1	$[\alpha1(XXIII)]_3$	Linear	Single-pass hydrophobic transmembrane domain	Heart, retina, metastatic tumor cells	Cell-matrix interaction
XXV	COL25A1	$[\alpha1(XXV)]_3$	Linear	Extracellular domain deposited in β-amyloid plaques	Neurons	Neuron adhesion
Multiplexin (Endostatin-Forming Collagens)						
XV	COL15A1	$[\alpha1(XV)]_3$	Linear	Contains antiangiogenic factor	Epithelial and endothelial basement membranes, internal organs (adrenal gland, pancreas, kidney)	Stabilizes skeletal muscle cells
XVIII	COL18A1	$[\alpha1(XVIII)]_3$		Contains antiangiogenic factor	Epithelial and endothelial basement membranes, liver, lung, kidney	Eye development; anchors vitreal collagen fibrils, determination of the retinal structure and the closure of the neural tube

Continued

TABLE 4.1 **The Collagens—cont'd**

Type	Gene Name	Chains	Supramolecular Assembly	Characteristic Features	Tissue Distribution	Major Function
Fibril-Associated Collagens With Interrupted Triple Helices (FACIT)						
IX	COL9A1, COL9A2, COL9A3	$\alpha1(IX)\alpha2(IX)\alpha3(IX)$	200 nm	Interacts with glycosaminoglycans in cartilage	Cartilage, vitreous humor	Attaches functional groups to surface of type II fibrils
XII	COL12A1	$[\alpha1(XII)]_3$			Widespread in many connective tissues (type I–containing tissues); enriched in periodontal ligament fibroblasts	Modulates fibril interactions
XIV	COL14A1	$[\alpha1(XIV)]_3$		Associated with type I	Widespread in many connective tissues	Modulates fibril interactions
XVI	COL16A1	$[\alpha1(XVI)]_3$		Numerous interruptions in the triple helix may make this molecule elastic or flexible	Endothelial, perineural, muscle, some epithelial basal laminae, cartilage, placenta	Associates with heterotypic II/IX/XI fibrils and fibrillin-1 filaments
XIX	COL19A1	$[\alpha1(XIX)]_3$			Endothelial, perineural, muscle, and some epithelial basal laminae	Muscle differentiation
XX	COL20A1	$[\alpha1(XX)]_3$			Corneal epithelium, skin, cartilage, tendon, heart, muscle, kidney, pancreas, spleen, testis, ovary, subthalamic nucleus	Associates with fibrils
XXI	COL21A1	$[\alpha1(XXI)]_3$			Widespread in developing connective tissues, abundant in vascular walls	Maintains extracellular matrix integrity
XXII	COL22A1	$[\alpha1(XXII)]_3$			Tissue junctions: myotendinous junction, articular cartilage—synovial fluid, hair follicle—dermis	Cell adhesion ligand
Meshwork-Forming Collagens						
IV	COL4A1, COL4A2, COL4A3, COL4A4, COL4A5, COL4A6	$[\alpha1(IV)]_2\alpha2(IV)$	Sheetlike network 390 nm	Interactions with type IV, perlecan, laminin, nidogen, integrin	Basal laminae	Structural network of basal laminae together with laminins, proteoglycans, and entactin/nidogen
VIII	COL8A1, COL8A2	$[\alpha1(VIII)]_2\alpha2(VIII)$	Hexagonal network 130 nm		Fibroblast gr Cornea (Descemet membrane), endothelium	Tissue support, porous meshwork
X	COL10A1	$[\alpha1(X)]_3$	Hexagonal network 150 nm		Hypertrophic zone of cartilage growth plate	Calcium binding
Anchoring-Fibril Collagen						
VII	COL7A1	$[\alpha1(VII)]_3$	450 nm	Forms bundles made of dimers anchorod in anchoring plaques and basal laminae	Epithelium (skin, mucosa)	Strengthens epithelial–connective tissue junction
Other Collagen[a]						
XXVI	COL26A1	$[\alpha1(XXVI)]_3$	Unknown	Disulfide bonds that form the trimer are made in an N-terminal noncollagenous domain	Developing and adult testis and ovary	Unknown
XXVIII	COL28A1				Dorsal root ganglia, peripheral nerves, adult sciatic nerves	

[a]A number of proteins containing helical collagenous domains have also been described.

dermis. However, its C-terminal endostatin-like domain (restin) has less potent antiangiogenic activity than that of type XVIII collagen. Both collagens have glycosaminoglycan side chains and can be classified as proteoglycans. The C-terminal domain of type IV collagen also inhibits endothelial cell migration and angiogenesis.

9. Other collagens: There are other collagens and proteins containing helical collagenous domains that cannot be classified into the other categories. Type XXVI is found in the extracellular matrix of the testis and ovary; however, its function and association with other collagens or matrix proteins have not been established. The structure of type XXVIII has some similarities with type IV, but the triple helical domain is longer than that of type IV. Type XXVIII is predominantly expressed in the basement membranes around Schwann cells of the peripheral nervous system (PNS) and dorsal root ganglia. There is also a highly heterogeneous group of proteins that contain helical collagenous domains but have not been clearly defined as collagens.

Collagen Synthesis and Assembly

Production of type I collagen by fibroblasts, odontoblasts, and osteoblasts is essentially the same. As a secretory protein, fibrous collagen is synthesized as a proprotein (procollagen) (Fig. 4.14). mRNA directs the assembly of specific amino acids into polypeptide chains on ribosomes associated with the rough endoplasmic reticulum. These initial pro alpha polypeptide chains are about one and a half times longer than those in the final collagen molecule because they have N- and C-terminal extensions that are important for assembly of the triple-helical molecule. As the chains are synthesized, they are translocated into the cisternae of the rough endoplasmic reticulum, where some posttranslational modifications occur. The first modification is hydroxylation of many of the proline and lysine residues in the chain, which permits hydrogen bonding with the adjacent chains as the triple helix is assembled. The vitamin C–dependent enzymes prolyl hydroxylase and lysyl hydroxylase are required for this step. In vitamin C deficiency, fewer collagen molecules are formed, and they are less stable. Tissues with a high collagen content and a high rate of turnover of collagen, such as the periodontal ligament, are affected severely; one of the early symptoms of vitamin C deficiency (scurvy) is loosening of the teeth. Through the action of galactosyltransferase in the rough endoplasmic reticulum, some of the hydroxylysine residues are glycosylated by addition of galactose.

Proper alignment of the chains in a triple helix is achieved by disulfide bonding at the C-terminal extension, a process catalyzed by the enzyme protein disulfide isomerase. The three chains then twist around themselves to weave the helix. The assembled helix is transported through the Golgi complex, where glycosylation is completed by the addition of glucose to the O-linked galactose residues. Molecular chaperones, including Hsp47, Bip, and Grp94, are implicated in this translocation. Secretory granules containing the procollagen molecules are formed at the *trans* face of the Golgi complex and are released subsequently by exocytosis at the cell surface.

The formation of typical banded collagen fibrils occurs extracellularly (Fig. 4.15). The C-terminal extensions, and at least part of the N-terminal ones, are removed by the action of C- and N-proteinases as the molecules are about to be secreted and/or extracellularly soon after their release. The main C-proteinase is identical to bone morphogenetic protein 1. The shortened collagen molecules align as five-unit, quarter-staggered microfibrils, which then assemble in a parallel fashion, giving rise to a regular series of gaps or holes within the fibril (see Chapter 1). These gaps are the location of the initial deposits of mineral associated with the collagen fibrils in bone, dentin, and cellular cementum. After the fibrils are assembled, the remaining portions of the N-terminal extensions are removed by procollagen peptidase. The oxidation of some lysine and hydroxylysine residues by the extracellular enzyme lysyl oxidase, forming reactive aldehydes, results in intermolecular cross-links that further stabilize the fibrils. The newly deposited fibrils are of small diameter and length. As the tissues mature, the fibrils may increase in diameter (by as much as tenfold) and length to further strengthen the tissue.

Inherited Diseases Involving Collagens

Several mutations occur in collagen genes, resulting in a variety of different phenotypes depending on the affected collagen. Some of the more common mutations include osteogenesis imperfecta (brittle bone disease) caused by mutations of the type I collagen genes and often including dental abnormalities; several types of Ehlers-Danlos syndrome (hyperextensible skin, hypermobile joints, tissue fragility), resulting from mutations in the type I, III, or V collagen genes; Stickler syndrome caused by mutations in the type II or XI collagen genes and characterized by retinal detachments, cataracts, hearing loss, joint problems, cleft palate, and facial and dental abnormalities; Alport syndrome, nephrosis caused by defects of the basal lamina in the kidney glomerulus and sensorineural hearing loss because of mutations in certain type IV collagen genes; and different forms of epidermolysis bullosa, a separation of the epidermis and dermis caused by mutations of the type VII or XVII collagen genes. Other mutations in collagen genes causing less common diseases have been identified, and it is likely that additional mutations that cause or contribute to other human diseases will be discovered.

Elastin

Elastin is produced by fibroblasts and smooth muscle cells. Its formation follows a pathway similar to that described for collagen, with final assembly into sheets (laminae) or fibers occurring outside the cell (Figs. 4.16 and 4.17). The elastic properties of elastin result from numerous intermolecular cross-links between lysine groups formed by the enzyme lysyl oxidase and its highly hydrophobic nature. To form an elastic fiber, the glycoproteins fibrillin-1, fibrillin-2, and several microfibril-associated glycoproteins are secreted first and assembled into microfibrils. The microfibrils then provide a scaffold for the accumulation of elastin and assembly of elastic fibers (see Fig. 4.17). Immature elastic fibers consisting only of microfibrillar subunits are referred to as *oxytalan fibers.* As the fibers mature, the microfibrils are displaced peripherally, resulting in a core of elastin surrounded by a sleeve of microfibrils. During formation, the ratio of microfibrils to elastin is greater than in mature elastic fibers; these developing elastic fibers have been called *elaunin fibers.*

Mutations in the fibrillin-1 gene result in Marfan syndrome, the second most common inherited connective tissue disease.

Proteoglycans

The ground substance of the extracellular matrix appears amorphous in the microscope but contains a complex mixture of macromolecules with important function. These macromolecules require special stains to reveal; they interact with cells and the fibrous components of the matrix and are involved in adhesion and signaling events (see Fig. 4.16B). The ground substance also is highly hydrated, providing a mechanism for regulating tissue water content and the diffusion of nutrients, waste products, and other molecules. Fibroblasts synthesize two main classes of macromolecules making up the ground substance: proteoglycans and glycoproteins.

Proteoglycans are a large group of extracellular and cell surface–associated molecules that consist of a protein core to which glycosaminoglycan chains are attached (Fig. 4.18). Glycosaminoglycans are long

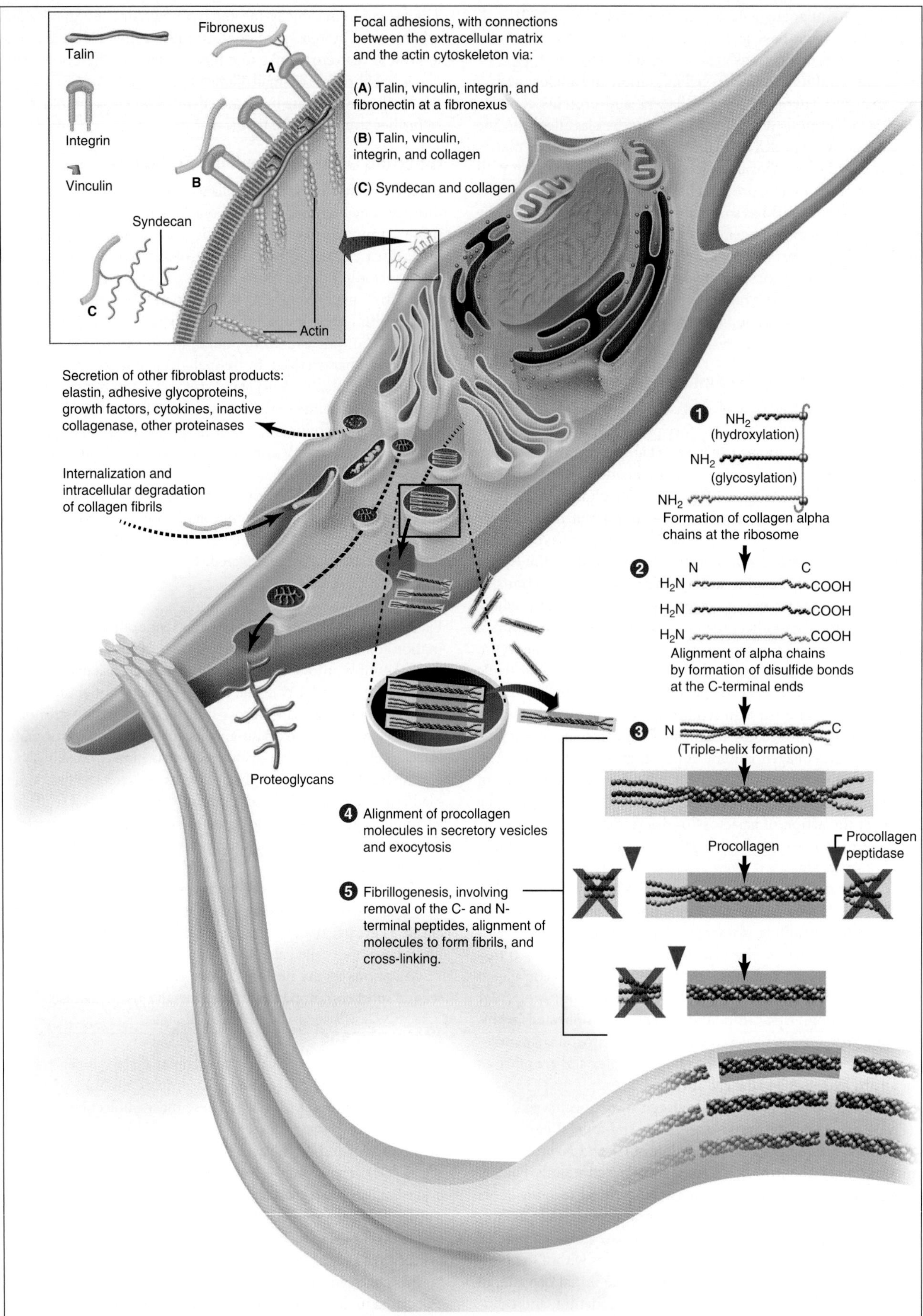

Fig. 4.14 Diagrammatic illustration of some of the structural and functional aspects of fibroblasts, and formation of collagen fibrils.

chains of repeating disaccharide units consisting of a hexosamine and uronic acid. Depending on the combination of hexosamine and uronic acid, several different glycosaminoglycans are recognized. The large number of carboxyl and sulfate groups in glycosaminoglycans makes them acidic (negatively charged). They readily bind various proteins and other molecules, and their hydrophilic nature allows them to bind large amounts of water.

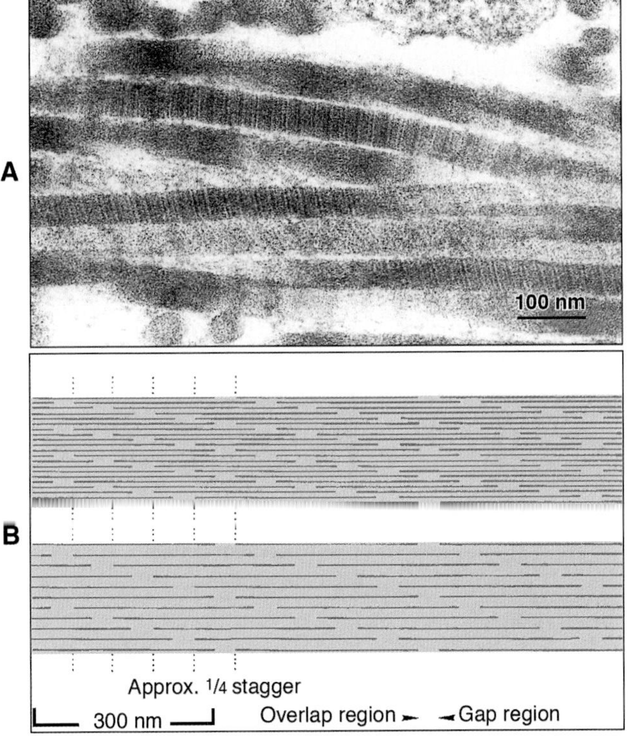

Fig. 4.15 (A) Transmission electron micrograph of collagen fibrils showing the typical banding pattern revealed by the differential binding of heavy metal stains used in such preparations. (B) Diagram illustrating the arrangement of collagen molecules in a banded collagen fibril.

Hyaluronic acid is a large glycosaminoglycan present in most connective tissues and is especially abundant in embryonic tissues and cartilage. With its bound water, hyaluronic acid forms a viscous hydrated gel. In cartilage, hyaluronic acid forms a large aggregate with 50 to 100 molecules of the proteoglycan monomer aggrecan. This aggregated proteoglycan, with its bound water, accounts for the resistance of cartilage to compressive forces. A similar aggregating proteoglycan, versican, is present in many connective tissues. Nonaggregating proteoglycans, typically containing one to a few glycosaminoglycan chains, include decorin, fibromodulin, perlecan, agrin, glypican, syndecan, and CD44. Decorin and fibromodulin bind to collagen and probably function in regulating the growth and/or diameter of collagen fibrils (Fig. 4.19). Perlecan and agrin are heparan sulfate proteoglycans of basal laminae and bind to several matrix glycoproteins. Perlecan is present in almost all basal laminae and in cartilage, whereas agrin is found in high concentrations in basal lamina at specific sites (e.g., neuromuscular junction, kidney glomerulus). Glypican is a lipid-anchored membrane proteoglycan, and syndecan and CD44 are transmembrane proteoglycans that bind cells to collagen, fibronectin, hyaluronic acid, and other matrix molecules.

An important property of cell surface and matrix proteoglycans is their ability to bind growth factors, cytokines, and other biologically active molecules. At the cell surface, membrane-associated proteoglycans, such as syndecan and glypican, are capable of binding members of the fibroblast growth factor and transforming growth factor β families, hepatocyte growth factor, and others and presenting them to their specific receptors on the surface of the same cell. In some cases, proteoglycans modulate the activity of the bound growth factor; in other cases, they are essential coreceptors for the growth factor. Through interactions of the cytoplasmic domain of its core protein with cytoskeletal elements, kinases, and other proteins, syndecan is involved in transmembrane signaling. In the extracellular matrix, growth factors bound to proteoglycans constitute a reservoir of active molecules that can exert their effects on nearby cells. In matrices that are remodeled

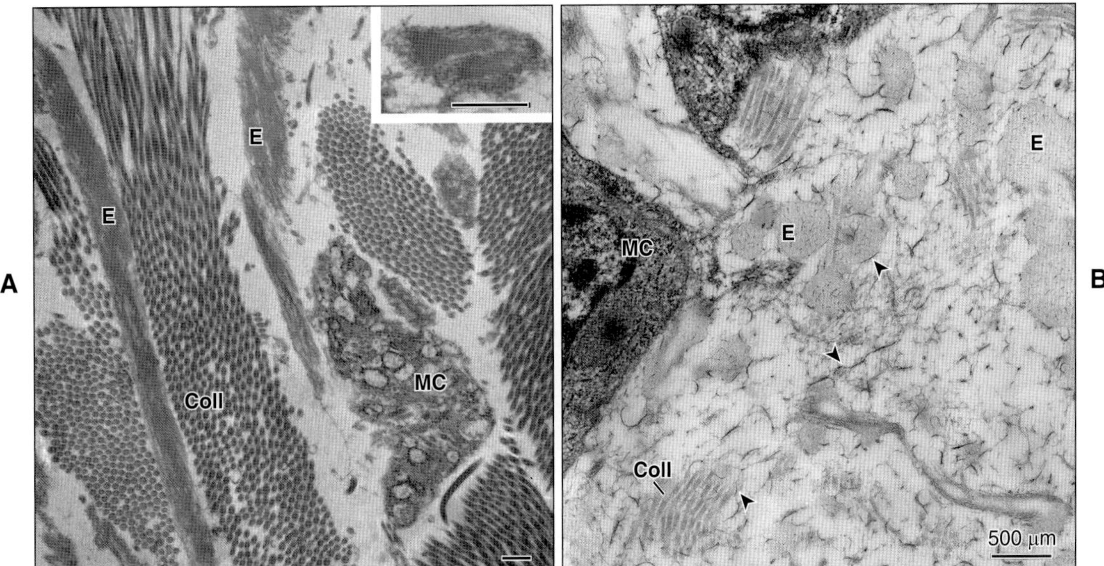

Fig. 4.16 (A) Electron micrograph showing the accumulation of elastin *(E)* among collagen fibers *(Coll)* in the skin dermis. (B) Micrograph from a preparation specially stained to reveal proteoglycans in the ground substance of an elastic connective tissue. These appear as fine filaments *(arrowheads)*, which interact with the elastin and collagen fibers. *MCs*, Mesenchymal cells. (Courtesy D. Quaglino.)

continually, such as that of bone, bound growth factors may be released during matrix turnover.

Glycoproteins

Several glycoproteins are found in the ground substance; a number of these have adhesive properties. One of their primary functions is to bind cells to extracellular matrix elements.

Fibronectin is a major extracellular matrix and plasma glycoprotein synthesized primarily by hepatocytes and fibroblasts. Fibronectin consists of two disulfide-linked polypeptide chains that have several structural domains capable of reacting with cell membrane receptors of the integrin family and other extracellular matrix components such as heparin, collagen, and fibrin. Through these interactions, fibronectin is involved in the cell attachment, migration, differentiation, and growth. As such, it plays an important role in embryonic development and wound healing.

Tenascin is a large molecule with a six-arm, star-shaped structure. Tenascin is synthesized at specific times and locations during embryogenesis and is present in adult connective tissues but with a more restricted distribution. Tenascin binds to fibronectin and to proteoglycans, particularly the cell surface proteoglycan syndecan. Tenascin blocks the binding capacity of syndecan, thereby allowing cells to move more freely. The migratory pathway for neural crest cells is forecast by the expression of tenascin along that pathway. Tenascin also is present in developing cartilage.

Thrombospondin is expressed in a number of tissues and is synthesized by several cell types. Thrombospondin has a trimeric or pentameric structure and functions at the cell surface and in the extracellular matrix to promote cell attachment, spreading, and migration. Thrombospondin also is important for the proper organization of collagen fibrils in the skin and cartilage.

Growth Factors and Cytokines

Fibroblasts, particularly those activated and responding to some type of stimulation, such as inflammation or mechanical forces, secrete a number of growth factors, cytokines, and inflammatory mediators (Box 4.2). These molecules, principally acting locally in a paracrine or autocrine fashion, have important roles in developmental processes, wound healing, and tissue remodeling.

Extracellular Matrix Degradation

In addition to their important function in the synthesis and assembly of the extracellular matrix, fibroblasts also participate in the remodeling of connective tissues through the degradation of collagen and other extracellular matrix molecules and their replacement by newly synthesized molecules. These processes are essential for certain aspects of normal embryonic development, tissue morphogenesis, and remodeling and occur during wound repair, inflammatory diseases, and tumor growth and metastasis. Two mechanisms for the degradation of collagen have been recognized: (1) the secretion by cells of enzymes that sequentially degrade collagen and other matrix molecules extracellularly, and (2) the selective ingestion of collagen fibrils by fibroblasts and their intracellular degradation.

The collagen triple helix is highly resistant to proteolytic attack. The matrix metalloproteinase (MMP) family is a large family of proteolytic

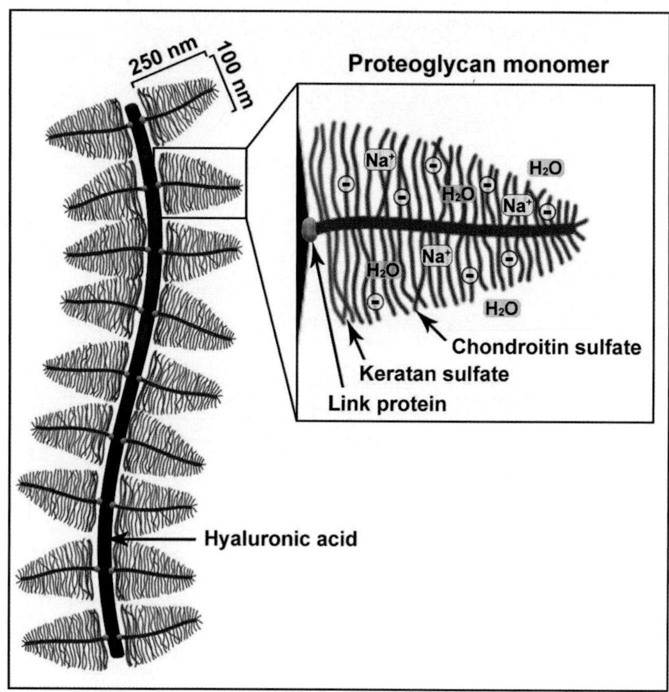

Fig. 4.18 Diagram of a proteoglycan aggregate. Aggregating proteoglycans are abundant in cartilage. Fibrous connective tissues contain similar aggregating proteoglycans and smaller nonaggregating proteoglycans. These smaller proteoglycans are similar in structure to the proteoglycan monomers shown in this figure; some may have only one or two glycosaminoglycan chains. (Courtesy A. Paz Ramos.)

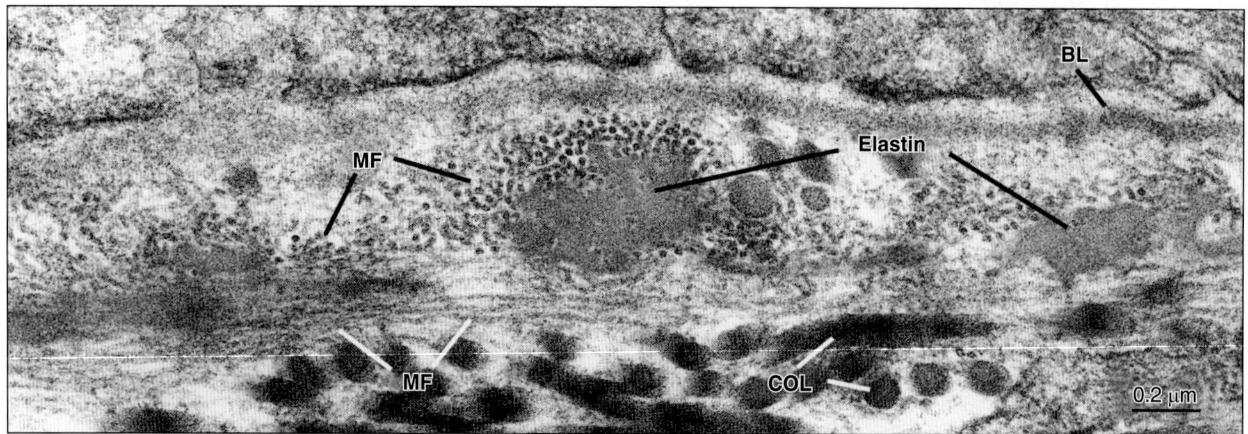

Fig. 4.17 Electron micrograph of elastic fibers adjacent to epithelial cells of a salivary gland excretory duct. Elastin has a dense, amorphous appearance; numerous longitudinal and cross-sectioned microfibrils *(MFs)* surround the elastin. *BL,* Basal lamina; *COLs,* collagen fibrils.

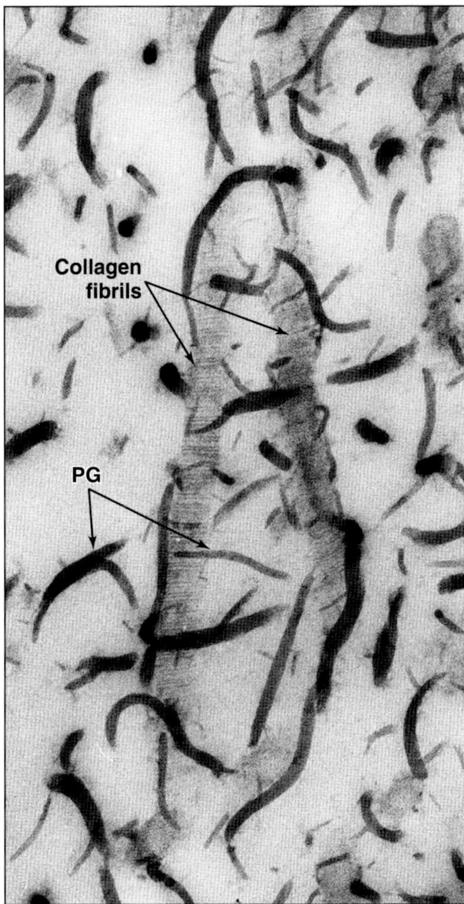

Fig. 4.19 Collagen fibrils in loose connective tissue surrounded and connected by small and large proteoglycans *(PGs).* The proteoglycans are stained densely because of special tissue preparation procedures. (From Erlinger R, et al.: Ultrastructural localisation of glycosaminoglycans in human gingival connective tissue using cupromeronic blue, *J Periodontal Res* 30:108–115, 1995.)

enzymes that includes collagenases (MMP-1, -8, and -13), gelatinases (MMP-2 and -9), metalloelastase (MMP-12), stromelysins (MMP-3, -10, and -11), and matrilysins (MMP-7 and -26). In addition to these secreted enzymes, several membrane-type (MT) MMPs (MT-MMPs) exist and have transmembrane domains and extracellular active sites. These enzymes are capable of degrading collagen and other matrix macromolecules into small peptides extracellularly (Fig. 4.20). The MMPs are synthesized and secreted by fibroblasts, inflammatory cells, and some epithelial and tumor cells. Extracellular degradation often occurs in inflammatory lesions or when large amounts of collagen must be degraded rapidly. Several mechanisms are used to regulate this process, which is necessary to prevent indiscriminate degradation of matrix components at other times. Some of the normal components of serum, such as α_2-macroglobulin, inhibit MMPs. The MMPs are secreted as inactive precursors (proenzymes) and must be cleaved proteolytically themselves to become active. MT-MMPs, which are activated intracellularly before insertion into the membrane, can activate certain MMPs such as gelatinase A (MMP-2) and collagenase 3 (MMP-13). Activated gelatinases, along with other extracellular proteinases, in turn can activate collagenases and other soluble MMPs. Finally, many cells secrete inhibitors of MMPs, called tissue inhibitors of metalloproteinases. Fibroblasts secrete the activators and the inhibitors of MMPs, which allow these cells to participate in regulating extracellular degradation.

BOX 4.2 Repertoire of Factors Produced by Fibroblasts

FGF2	Fibroblast growth factor-2
HGF	Hepatocyte growth factor
IGF1	Insulin-like growth factor-1
IL1	Interleukin-1
IL6	Interleukin-6
IL8	Interleukin-8
KGF	Keratinocyte growth factor
PGE2	Prostaglandin E_2
PDGF	Platelet-derived growth factor
TGF-β	Transforming growth factor β
TNF-α	Tumor necrosis factor α
VEGF	Vascular endothelial growth factor

Intracellular degradation is considered the most important mechanism for the physiologic turnover and remodeling of collagenous connective tissue (Fig. 4.21). This process involves recognition of the fibrils to be degraded, possibly through binding to fibroblast integrin receptors; partial digestion of the fibrils into smaller fragments, probably by gelatinase A (MMP-2); phagocytosis of the fragments; formation of a phagolysosome; and intracellular digestion of the collagen fragments within the acidic environment of the phagolysosome by lysosomal enzymes, particularly the cathepsins. Little is known about how these processes are regulated and carried out.

In summary, cells interact with and respond to their neighbors and to their environment in many ways. These interactions include the formation of specialized cell-cell and cell-matrix junctions and the synthesis and secretion of a variety of products to create and maintain the cellular environment. Cell-cell and cell-matrix junctions are involved in cell adhesion, organization of the cytoskeleton, intercellular and intracellular signaling, and development and maintenance of the differentiated state. The proteins, glycoproteins, and proteoglycans of the extracellular matrix function in cell-matrix adhesion and signaling; regulate diffusion of nutrients, waste products, and soluble signaling molecules; impart connective tissues with their characteristic properties of tensile and compressive strength and elasticity; and, in certain tissues, provide the appropriate conditions for the nucleation and growth of mineral crystals.

ORGANIZATION AND PHYSIOLOGY OF THE NERVOUS SYSTEM

The various tissues and their composing molecules need to be recognized and understood through their functional mission. For instance, dental pain starts with an aggression on peripheral tissue (e.g., bone, dentin, gum) but only fully develops after the inflammatory response has been translated by nerves into electric signals that are conveyed by specialized anatomic nerve pathways toward the brain, where it becomes a sensation of pain. Similarly, mastication becomes a movement only after specific brain structures have produced a command, which has a biochemical and biophysical substrate, and further relayed it through precise anatomic pathways toward the effector muscles. This section discusses basic neurophysiology notions important to understanding these mechanisms. The reader is invited to consult a dedicated neurophysiology textbook for a more detailed account.

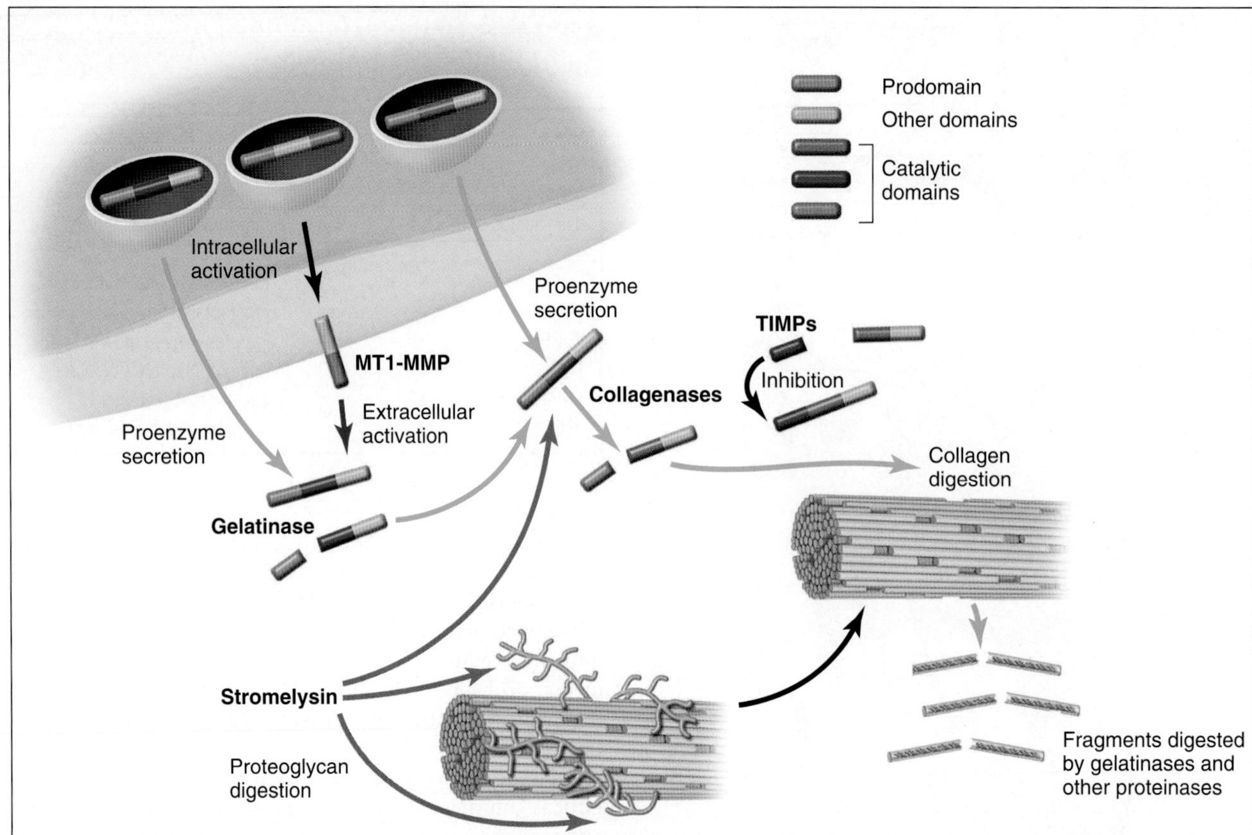

Fig. 4.20 Diagrammatic illustration of the sequence of events in the extracellular degradation of collagen fibrils. Fibroblasts, inflammatory cells, epithelial cells, and tumor cells produce soluble and/or membrane-type matrix metalloproteinases *(MMPs)*. The prodomain of membrane-type MMPs *(MT-MMPs)* is cleaved intracellularly by a furin like enzyme, and the active enzyme is inserted into the cell membrane. Soluble MMPs are secreted as inactive proenzymes. The prodomains of gelatinase A *(MMP-2)* and stromelysin 1 *(MMP-3)* are cleaved by MT1-MMP or other extracellular proteinases; the activated stromelysin and gelatinase then can activate collagenases (e.g., *MMP-1* and *MMP-13*). Stromelysin also digests proteoglycans and other matrix glycoproteins. The activated collagenases cleave the collagen molecules of the fibril into two smaller fragments, which may be further digested by gelatinases and other proteinases. MT1-MMP also can digest collagen fibrils and other extracellular matrix molecules. Collagenases and other MMPs are inhibited by tissue inhibitors of metalloproteinases *(TIMPs)*, which bind to the active site of the enzyme.

The Nervous System

The nervous system is the most complex system of the human body. Structurally it is divided into the central nervous system (CNS) and the PNS. The CNS comprises the brain and the spinal cord, both well protected by the bony structures of the skull and the spine. The PNS extends the nerve functions outside of the CNS by means of the nervous pathways (peripheral nerves and plexus) and the ganglion relay stations.

From a functional point of view, the nervous system has several divisions (Fig. 4.22): First, if one considers the principle of the reflex arc, the nervous system is made of (1) the afferent pathways (mainly internal or external sensors [e.g., pain terminals] and the bundles of sensory nerves [spinal and cranial nerves]), (2) the encephalon (made of the white matter [axons, mostly myelinated but also unmyelinated for certain pain pathways] and the grey matter, consisting of groups of cells organized in layers [e.g., the neocortex and hippocampus] or nuclei [e.g., the thalamus and basal ganglia]), and (3) the efferent pathways (mainly motor nerves [spinal, cranial, and autonomous] connecting to effecting organs [mostly muscles and glands] involved in necessary corrections in homeostatic processes).

According to the type of regulated activity, the nervous system is also subdivided into (1) the somatic nervous system, responsible for the voluntary and/or conscious muscle activity, and (2) the autonomous nervous system, involved in unconscious or automatic activities (e.g., digestion, blood circulation, and secretion).

Cells of the Nervous System

The essential building blocks of the nervous system are the neurons and the glia (Figs. 4.23 and 4.24). Both are critically involved in conveying information between cerebral structures. As discussed later, this function relies on their electrophysiologic properties. In addition, glial cells regulate the extracellular concentration of ions and mediate the nourishment of neurons. Further, glial and other nonneuronal cell types are important for maintaining the integrity of a complex vascular system, which is vital for supplying energy and removing metabolites.

The mammalian CNS develops from the neural plate, a thickened region of ectoderm on the dorsal aspect of the embryo, which gives rise to the neural fold, neural crest, and neural tube. Multipotential neural stem cells in these structures give rise to most of the neurons and glial cells of the CNS. As indicated in Box 2.1, neural crest cells generate the

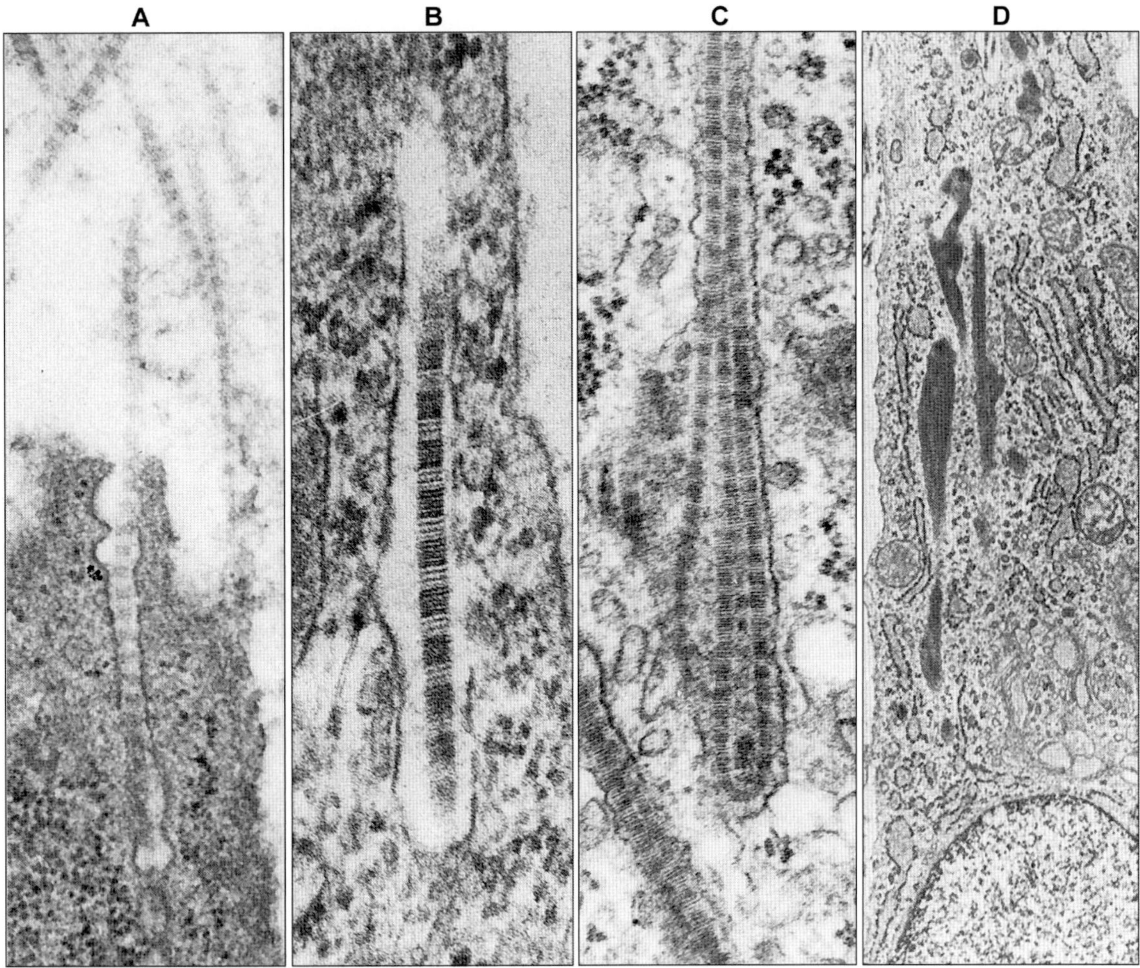

Fig. 4.21 Intracellular degradation of collagen by fibroblasts. (A) Ingestion of extracellular collagen fibrils. (B) Formation of phagosome. (C) Initial fusion of lysosomes with collagen-containing phagosome. (D) Advanced stages of intracellular collagen degradation in dense lysosomal structures. (B, From Ten Cate AR, et al.: The role of fibroblasts in the remodeling of periodontal ligament during physiologic tooth movement, *Am J Orthod* 69:155–168, 1976.)

neurons and glia associated with the peripheral and enteric nervous systems. Most neurons required by the brain are believed to be already present at birth, but there is now growing evidence that neurogenesis (the formation of neurons) continues throughout life. Evidence so far supports adult neurogenesis in the dentate gyrus of the hippocampus, subventricular zone, and olfactory bulb.

The neuron is the basic working unit of the brain; it transmits information to other nerve cells, muscle, and gland cells (see Figs 4.22–4.24). The Italian physician and Nobel laureate Camillo Golgi developed a silver impregnation method that stains neurons, which allowed him to visualize their path by light microscopy for the first time in 1873. There are three classes of neurons: (1) Sensory neurons carry information from sense organs (pain, proprioception, thermic information, etc.) to the brain, (2) motor neurons carry messages from the brain to the muscles and control voluntary muscle activity (e.g., speech, mastication), and (3) interneurons (local circuit cells), which are generally inhibitory, locally control the amount of excitation. Within each of these classes are hundreds of different types of neurons with distinct message-carrying abilities. The vast extent and variety of communicating pathways between these neurons underlie the complexity of human behavior.

Histologically, neurons (see Fig. 4.23) consist of three compartments: the dendritic arbor, the soma (or cell body), and the axon. Dendrites are multiple ramified processes that collect signals from other nervous cells to convey them to the soma. The soma contains the nucleus and various cytoplasmic organelles (mitochondria, endoplasmic reticulum, Golgi apparatus, and special filaments called *neurofibrils*). Functionally, the soma represents the compartment where information from the dendrites converges and is integrated. The axon is a relatively long extension that in some cases can almost reach 1 m in length. It is single at its point of origin from the soma (axon hillock) but often divides into multiple collaterals or terminals.

Many axons are covered with myelin, a layered sheath consisting of 70% to 85% lipids and 15% to 30% proteins, that insulates and protects them and accelerates transmission of electric signals along their length (see Fig. 8.62). Swellings (boutons) form at the axonal terminals or along the length of the axon (en passant) and are the site where one or several chemical messengers, the neurotransmitters, accumulate. The role of the axon is to transmit the information that has been processed at the somatic level to the terminal boutons and, from there, to the next neuron in the information chain.

Glial cells were discovered in 1856 by Rudolph Virchow and are by some estimates 10 times more numerous than neurons. They are specialized nervous cells that, in addition to their supportive, protective, and nutritional role, are important signaling partners for neurons. Morphologically they are characterized by a central body with abundant somatic extensions called *processes* (see Figs. 4.23 and 4.24).

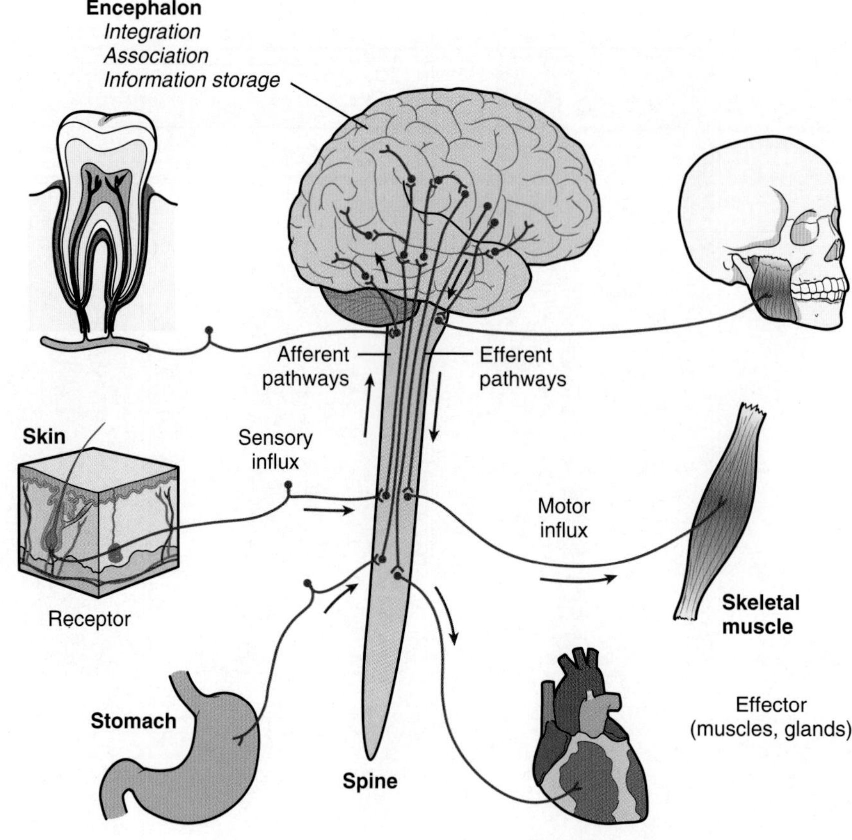

Fig. 4.22 Schematic organization of the nervous system and of the main communication pathways: afferent and efferent.

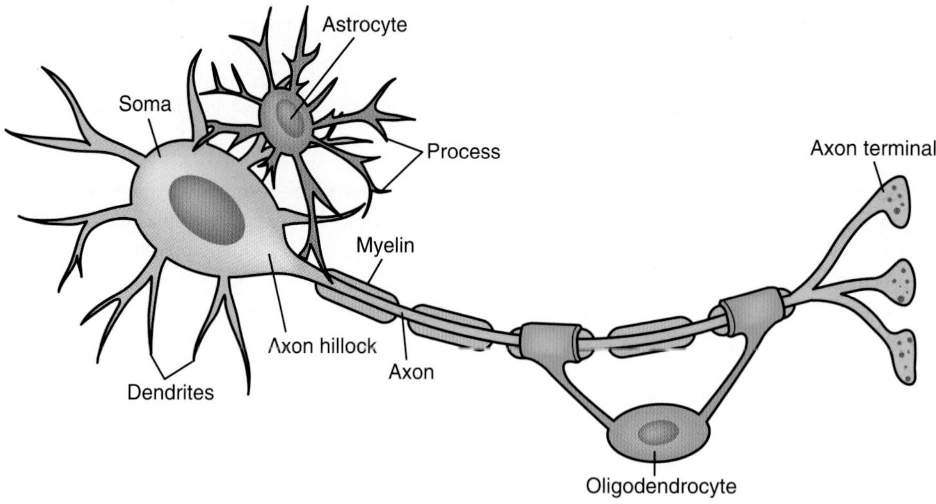

Fig. 4.23 Schematic representation of a neuron and its association with glial cells.

There are several types of glial cells, among which the best known are (1) astrocytes, with communication and homeostatic roles; (2) oligodendrocytes, which are called *Schwann cells* in the PNS that form the myelin sheath; and (3) microglia, which play a role in the immune protection of the nervous system.

THE NEUROVASCULAR UNIT

The brain is a hungry organ, which accounts for approximately 20% of the body's energy demands despite weighing only about 2% of the body weight. Importantly, as the brain largely lacks energy reserves, it relies on a constant source of oxygen and glucose supplied via the blood. The relationship between the vasculature and the brain is extremely important in maintaining proper cognitive function and a healthy brain, with vascular dysfunction as a major cause for neurologic disorders and neurodegenerative diseases such as Álzheimer's.

There exists a large amount of communication between the brain and its vasculature via specialized cells that form a neurovascular unit comprised of endothelial cells, mural cells (pericytes and vascular smooth muscle cells), and astrocytes (a type of glial cell; see Fig.

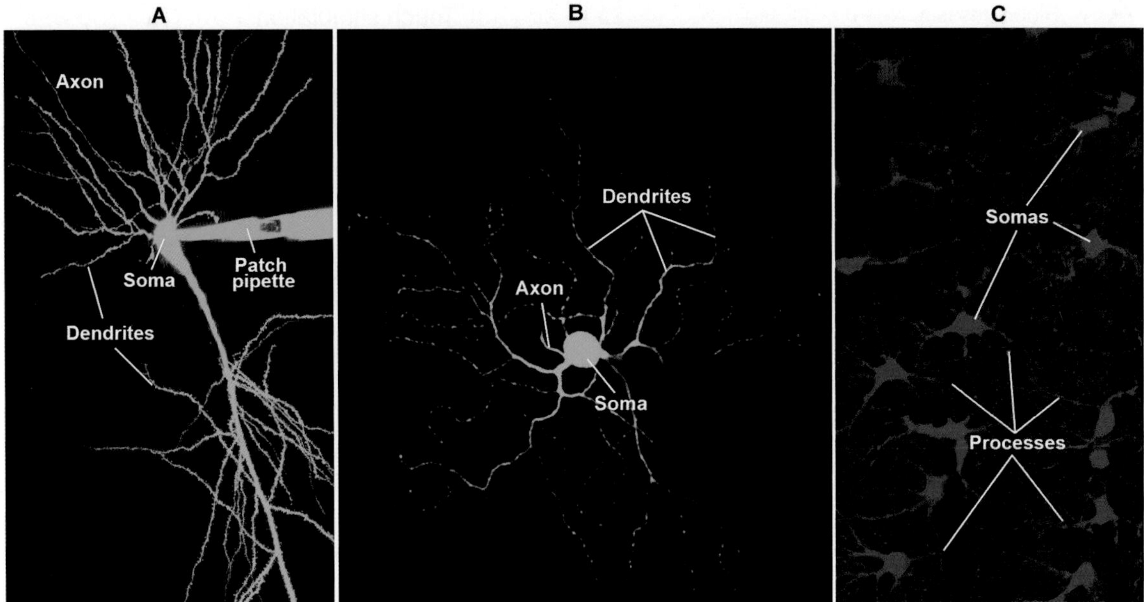

Fig. 4.24 Fluorescence preparations of a neuron from (A) the hippocampus (CA1 pyramidal neuron filled with a patch pipette) and (B) the retina. These two images illustrate well the wide range in neuronal shapes. (C) Astrocytes from the hippocampus with multiple somatic extensions, termed processes. (A, Courtesy D.A. MacVicar; B, from Morquette B, et al.: REDD2-mediated inhibition of mTOR promotes dendrite retraction induced by axonal injury, *Cell Death Differ* 22:612–625, 2015; C, courtesy B.A. MacVicar.)

4.24C). This neurovascular unit (Fig. 4.25) plays two fundamental roles in maintaining proper brain homeostasis: (1) maintaining the integrity of the blood-brain barrier and (2) regulating cerebral blood flow via the process of neurovascular coupling.

BLOOD-BRAIN BARRIER

The blood-brain barrier is a semipermeable border between the brain tissue and the blood, and is made up of endothelial cells; the barrier is critical for brain health because it protects the brain from toxins and pathogens. The endothelial cells are tightly overlapped and connected by tight-junctions (see earlier), which limit the passage of nonlipid-soluble substances from the blood into the brain. The endothelial cells are further covered by pericytes, which reside in the basement membrane, and astrocyte end-feet (specialized types of processes that enwrap the vasculature). The astrocytes and pericytes are critical components of the blood-brain barrier because they regulate its integrity via reciprocal signaling with the endothelial cells. Importantly, the expression of specific transporters on the endothelial cells selectively control the passage of specific molecules into the brain (e.g., the brain endothelium possesses an extremely high density of the glucose transporter [Glut1] to help meet the high energy requirements of the brain). In addition to diffusion and transport-mediated entry across the blood-brain barrier, nonpermeable macromolecules can gain entry to the brain via the process of transcytosis, in which they are endocytosed and transported in vesicles from the luminal to abluminal side of the endothelium.

NEUROVASCULAR COUPLING

Active neurons signal to blood vessels to cause vasodilation and increase the amount of local blood flow through neurovascular coupling. Many cellular pathways and vasoactive compounds exist for mediating vascular dilation, and this depends on the cell types that are activated. For example, both excitatory and inhibitory neurons can release vasoactive compounds, such as potassium, nitric oxide, and prostaglandins, which then act on either contractile pericytes or smooth muscle cells to dilate vessels. Astrocytes are also important regulators of vascular tone: Calcium variations at their end-feet can lead to either dilation or constriction of the adjacent blood vessel. Endothelial cells can also contribute to neurovascular coupling via voltage and calcium signals that propagate along the endothelial network via gap junctions. The final effector cells of neurovascular coupling are contractile mural cells, which express the contractile protein alpha smooth muscle actin, which undergo rearrangements between actin and myosin filaments leading to dilation. The increase in blood flow that results from neurovascular coupling results in more oxygen to the local tissue than is needed, and this mismatch is the basis for the blood oxygen level–dependent functional magnetic resonance imaging signal, which is a commonly utilized method for noninvasive brain activity mapping in humans.

Electrophysiologic Features of Nervous System Cells

The importance of physiology within medical sciences relates to the fact that disease, or anomalous behavior, is a deviation from the healthy state or from homeostasis. Thus physiology allows a better understanding of disease and more rational and efficient interventions. In this sense, understanding the electrophysiology of nervous cells is of fundamental importance because it provides a measurable feature to the functional aspect.

The membrane of neurons and glia is electrically polarized. At rest, the inside is negatively charged with respect to the outside. The voltage difference (resting membrane potential) is approximately −70 mV for neurons and −80 mV for glial cells. This voltage mainly results from a net flow of potassium ions toward the extracellular milieu. This concentration gradient is maintained by the Gibbs-Donnan equilibrium and by the activity of sodium-potassium adenosine triphosphate (ATP) pumps. The Gibbs-Donnan equilibrium describes a phenomenon occurring on both sides of a semipermeable membrane—here the cell membrane—leading to an uneven distribution of the ions across the membrane and its consequent polarization.

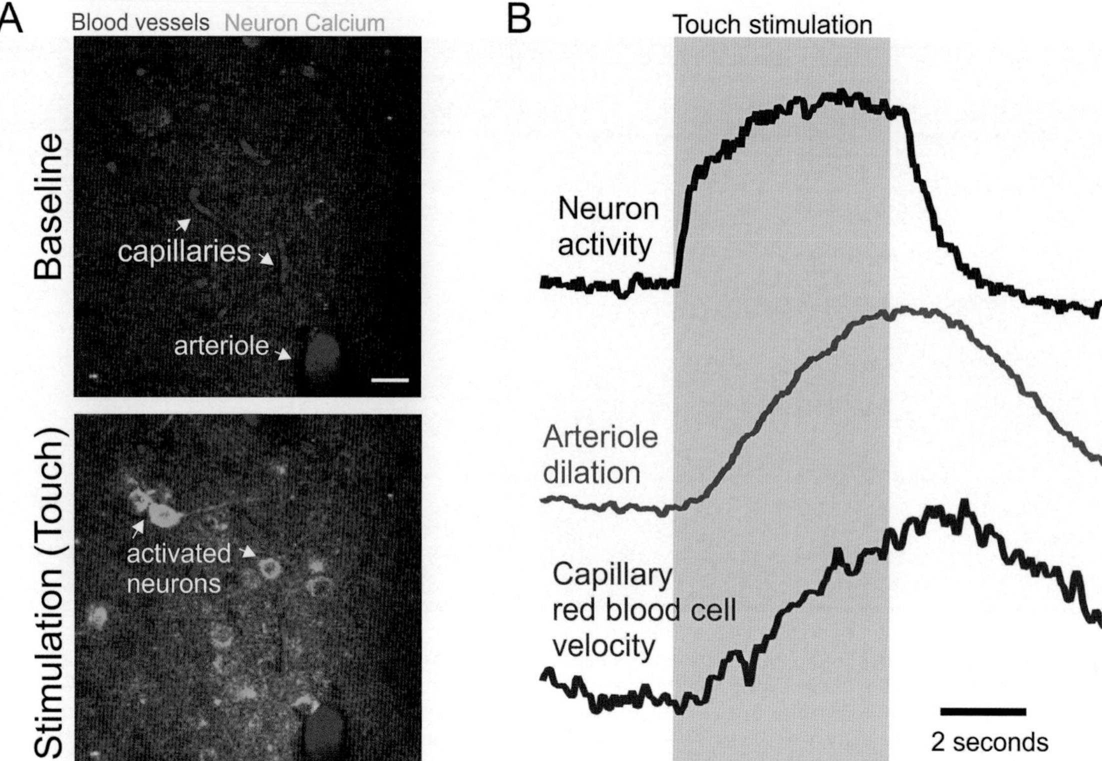

Fig. 4.25 Neurovascular coupling. Increased neuronal activity evokes a cascade of signaling events, which cause local blood flow to increase. (A) Images of blood vessels *(red)* and neurons *(green)* in the primary somatosensory cortex of the mouse. Following touch of the mouse whiskers, neurons surrounding the brain vasculature are activated (indicated by an increase in fluorescence). (B) Touch of the mouse whiskers leads to an increase in neuronal activity in primary somatosensory cortex *(top)*, followed by a local arteriole dilation that occurs with a delay *(middle)*, and an increase in the speed of red blood cells within the capillaries where most of the metabolic exchange occurs. (From Rungta RL, et al.: Diversity of neurovascular coupling dynamics along vascular arbors in layer II/III somatosensory cortex, *Commun Biol* 4:855, 2021.)

A transient decrease of the resting membrane potential (also termed *depolarization*) at a specific site of the cellular membrane, the axon hillock, may trigger an action potential. This initial depolarization may arise in the dendrites as a consequence of the activation of one or more membrane receptors or at any other place on the membrane after an electric stimulation. Once the initial depolarization crosses a voltage threshold at the axon hillock, the action potential is generated and propagates in the axon with a speed that varies between 0.7 and 100 m/s.

Once the action potential has reached the axonal terminals, it triggers the release of a chemical messenger (neurotransmitter), which further conveys the information across the synapse to the next cell, whose receptors respond specifically to the released neurotransmitter. This protocol is typical for the neuron-to-neuron communication. Recently it has been established that glial cells also use the synaptic structure to react to or to influence the neuronal activity. It is, however, important to keep in mind that glial cells are not endowed with the mechanism to generate action potentials (hence the absence of the axons) and that the glial release of neurotransmitters is subject to other mechanisms. In addition, glial cells are very sensitive to variations in the extracellular potassium concentrations and modulate their membrane potential in accordance. The glia-to-glia communication mainly relies on the presence of networks of gap junctions through which various ions or molecules may travel rapidly from cell to cell, following concentration gradients.

The physiology of cells of the nervous systems relies heavily on membrane permeability, and the basic aspects of this process described previously should be carefully studied to facilitate understanding of the following sections.

The Resting Membrane Potential

The Gibbs-Donnan equilibrium predicts that the cellular membranes are polarized and that a potential difference would be recorded across the membrane (negative inside the cell). This hypothesis was fully confirmed once electrodes could be inserted through the cellular membrane (intracellular recordings). This potential difference was termed membrane potential (V_m); it was additionally called resting V_m because initially it was seen in unstimulated neurons. However, it is now well established that nervous cells (both neurons and glia) in vivo almost never display a membrane potential with a fixed value; rather, they have a continuously changing polarization that is a function of the rich synaptic and ionic activities of the elements surrounding such a cell. Therefore the term resting is more or less adequate and is used here to distinguish it from the action potential.

There are two major factors that generate the resting membrane potential:

1. The unbalance between diffusible ions across the membrane because of its impermeability to intracellularly located proteins (as determined by the Gibbs-Donnan equilibrium). This unbalance is further maintained by the sodium-potassium pump.
2. The difference in membrane permeability for various ions (mainly potassium, sodium, and chloride, in this order). Because the permeability is significantly higher for potassium than for the other two, it is the outward leak of this ionic species that mainly determines the membrane potential.

Ions that may cross the cellular membrane are submitted to electrochemical gradients. When the concentration and electric gradients are equal and opposed, no net charge traffic exists; thus the ion flux is in equilibrium. The voltage potential where this occurs is called *Nernst potential,* after the German chemist who first described it. The equilibrium potential for various ionic species is given in Table 4.2. Obviously these are only informative values because the given concentrations are average values that vary (although not by much) continuously during the spontaneous activity of nervous cells.

An immediate consequence of the Nernst potentials is that, for any given membrane potential, at least two ionic species will compete to bring the membrane potential to their respective equilibrium potential. Assuming that in a neuron, at a given moment in time, its membrane potential is −60 mV, and provided that appropriate channels are open, chloride would enter the cell to bring its membrane potential to −89 mV, potassium would leave the cell (to bring it close to −97 mV), and sodium will rush into the neuron (to depolarize it toward +61 mV). A similar behavior is seen in glial cells, except for chloride: At a similar membrane potential, because of its equilibrium potential (see Table 4.2), opening of chloride channels in the glia drives this ion outside the cell (to reach −28 mV). Thus various ions have conflicting interests when it comes to crossing the cellular membrane.

The Action Potential

All living cells have a membrane potential. In addition, neurons (as well as muscular cells) are excitable—that is, when stimulated they may produce an action potential, which is a fast change of their membrane potential mediated by some specific proteins situated, with a critical density, in a precise location, the axon hillock. Glial cells, although they seem to possess the same proteins, albeit with an insufficient density, are not able to generate action potentials.

The action potential (Fig. 4.26) is made of several phases: the depolarization (*2,* in figure), the repolarization (*3*), and the afterhyperpolarization (*4*). These periods are preceded by a resting membrane potential (*1*) during which, if the polarization crosses a firing threshold of −57 mV, an action potential is generated. After the hyperpolarization there is a recovery period (*5*), during which the membrane potential is brought back to control values. During the depolarizing phase, the intracellular potential becomes positive with respect to the exterior and tends to the sodium equilibrium potential (+61 mV) because it is generated by a massive entrance of sodium into the neuron by both electric and concentration gradients.

During the repolarization phase (*3*), the intracellular polarity again becomes negative with respect to the outside and reaches the control resting value. This phenomenon is related to two factors: the inactivation of sodium channels that had favored the entrance of sodium during the previous phase, and the opening of potassium channels through which this ion will leave the cell. The following afterhyperpolarization (*4*) is more negative than the control level and aspires to reach −97 mV, suggesting that during this phase there is increased permeability for potassium. It results from the delayed closing of potassium channels that were open during the repolarization phase. Eventually, the membrane potential slowly returns to control values (*5*). During this phase, sodium-potassium pumps reestablish the ionic concentrations on both sides of the cellular membrane.

It is noteworthy that the action potential itself (phases 2 and 3) of excitatory neurons lasts approximately 1 ms. However, interneurons (inhibitory, local circuit cells) produce remarkably short action potentials (~0.5 ms), which allow them to sustain very high discharge rates. In contrast with the stability of this rule, the afterhyperpolarization and the recovery have variable durations (from a few milliseconds to tens of milliseconds) and are highly variable among different types of neurons.

The generation of an action potential critically depends on two types of protein channels. One allows the passage of sodium ions, the other of potassium. Both are voltage dependent; their functional configuration (open vs. closed or inactivated) depends on the polarization across the membrane in which they are embedded.

Although calcium does not play a direct role in the genesis of the neuronal action potential, it may modulate the excitability of a neuron. Calcium concentration is maintained at extremely low levels within the cytoplasm. In the extracellular space it tends to accumulate in front of voltage-gated sodium channels because, whenever they open, calcium is attracted by electric and concentration gradients toward the interior of the neuron. However, the high specificity of the sodium channels (and their small inner diameter) prevents calcium from crossing through them. Calcium ions accumulating in front of sodium channels will nevertheless constitute electric screens for sodium by repelling some of them. A possible absence (or lower concentration) of calcium in the extracellular space would render the neuronal membrane potential less negative (more depolarized, thus closer to the excitability threshold) and would lead to the production of more spontaneous action potentials.

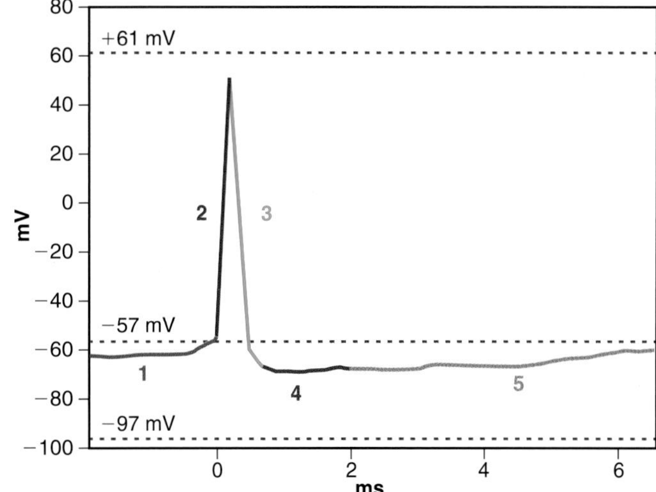

Fig. 4.26 Time course of an action potential with its phases: *(1)* resting membrane potential, *(2)* depolarization, *(3)* repolarization, *(4)* afterhyperpolarization, *(5)* recovery period.

TABLE 4.2 Equilibrium Potential for Various Ions

Cell Type	Ions	Ionic Concentration [mEq/L] (Extracellular/Intracellular)	Equilibrium Potential [mV]
Neurons	Na^+	145/14	+61
	K^+	4/157	-97
	Cl^-	116/4	-89
Glia	Cl^-	116/40	-28

The production of an action potential is associated with a period of refractoriness. This is a property of an excitable membrane not to respond to stimuli. The refractoriness of the action potential has two phases: a period of absolute refractoriness and one of relative refractoriness. The absolute refractory period roughly corresponds to the depolarizing and repolarizing phases (see *[2]* and *[3]* in Fig. 4.26) and means that whatever supplementary stimulus might be applied, no additional action potential can be triggered because either all voltage-gated sodium channels are already open or the same channels are inactivated and no stimulus can change that state. The absolute refractoriness confers on an action potential its all-or-none characteristic.

The relative refractory period follows the absolute refractory period and mainly corresponds to the afterhyperpolarization and recovery (see *[4]* and *[5]* in Fig. 4.26). During this time, another action potential can be triggered; however, because of the more hyperpolarized membrane potential, a stronger stimulus is required to bring the polarization of the membrane to the excitability threshold.

Propagation of the Action Potential

The axonal propagation of an action potential represents a particular case of spreading of intracellular signals through a neuron. It has, however, some peculiarities, especially because of the all-or-none feature of the action potential, and is of paramount importance in the transmission of information through the neuronal networks. As an example, in the case of pain transmission through the axons of sensory neurons, preventing the propagation of action potentials, thus of pain, is the main goal of local anesthesia (Box 4.3).

An action potential generated at the axon hillock of a neuron propagates toward the axonal terminals (called orthodromic propagation), where it triggers the synaptic function (see later discussion). Recently it has been proposed that an action potential generated at the axon hillock may also travel through the soma toward the dendrites (back-propagation). In addition, it has been known for a long time that action potentials could be generated, with appropriate stimulation, at any location of an axon, in which case the propagation of this action potential occurs in both directions (orthodromic and antidromic) (Fig. 4.27). Thus an action potential generated at one site in an axon will always propagate in one direction, distally from the initiating site, and will never propagate backward.

The example presented in Box 4.4 represents a case in which the axonal membranes are continuously coated with sodium and

BOX 4.3 Local Anesthesia

Axons of peripheral sensory neurons are grouped in bundles (e.g., in the trigeminal nerve) that convey, among others, pain stimuli. The purpose of local anesthesia is to block, somewhere on its anatomic pathway, the propagation of painful information toward the brain. Local anesthetics are amphipathic substances; some are esters and others are amides that readily cross the axonal membranes. Once the anesthetic molecules have reached the intracellular compartment, they couple to specific receptor sites within the sodium voltage-gated channel and inactivate its functioning, thus preventing the generation at that site of action potentials. In other terms, a region that has been inactivated by a local anesthetic blocks the propagation of action potentials beyond that zone and mutes the transmission of sensory (pain included) information. The end of the local anesthetic effect is produced either by local hydrolysis (esters) or by the washing out of the agent into the bloodstream and further metabolizing in the liver (amides).

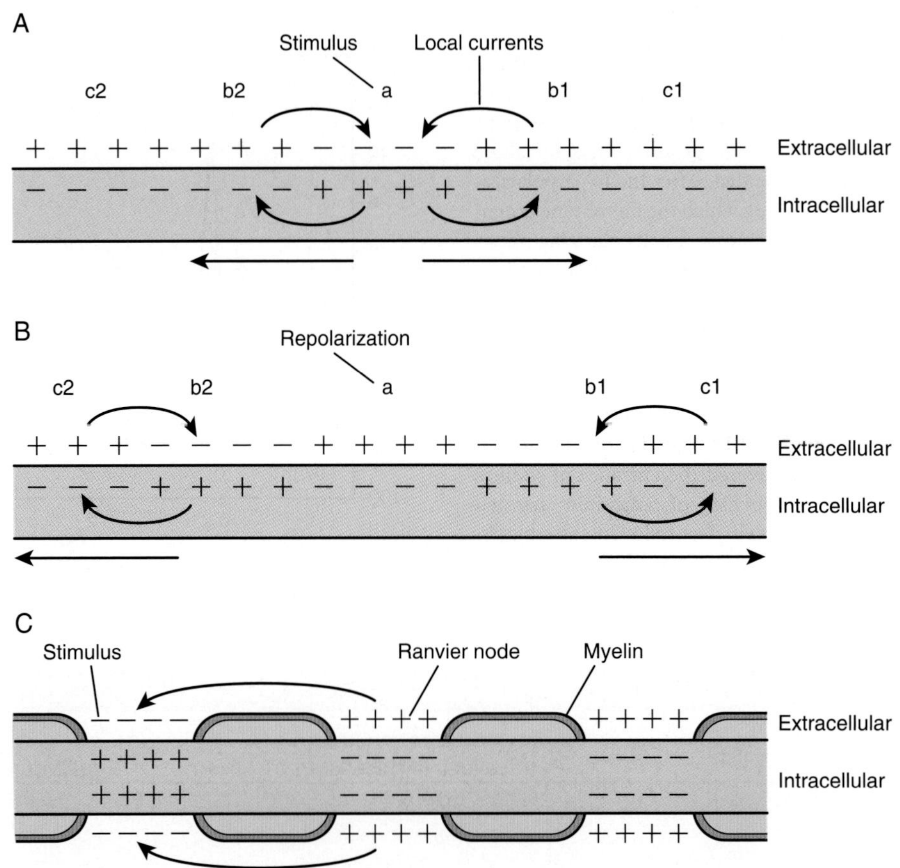

Fig. 4.27 (A) Generation of the action potential upon stimulation. (B) Propagation through a nonmyelinated axon. (C) Propagation through a myelinated axon.

potassium voltage-gated channels. These are axons through which action potentials propagate at relatively low speed and consume high amounts of ATP for the ionic rebalance. A much faster and economic propagation of action potentials is achieved through myelinated axons (see Fig. 4.27C), axons whose membrane is almost continuously coated with myelin. It is interrupted at regular intervals to expose the axonal membrane to the extracellular space. These sites are called nodes of Ranvier, where the membrane is endowed with sodium and potassium voltage-gated channels, thus constituting the sites where action potentials regenerate. Between Ranvier nodes action potentials propagate intracellularly through passive diffusion of ions, which is much faster than the near-to-near propagation in nonmyelinated axons. Moreover, an action potential unbalances ionic concentrations only at Ranvier nodes, the only place where ATP consumption is required. The conduction through myelinated axons is also termed *saltatory conduction*.

BOX 4.4 Propagation of the Action Potential

The axon can be conceptually divided into several regions (a, b, c, etc.). If appropriate stimulation is provided to region *(a)* (see Fig. 4.27A), it will depolarize the axonal sector; thus the intracellular side of the membrane becomes positive with respect to the exterior and will cross the excitability threshold (–57 mV) and locally generate an action potential. This means that in *(a)*, the membrane will undergo a massive entrance of sodium that will diffuse in both directions toward the neighboring sectors *(b1)* and *(b2)*, which are at rest. This intracellular current of positive charges will be paralleled extracellularly by an opposite current from *(b1)* and *(b2)* toward *(a)*.

The arrival of sodium in *(b1)* and *(b2)* will create local suprathreshold depolarizations, leading to the generation of action potentials at the new sites. Thus *(b1)* and *(b2)* become new sources of action potentials with further entrance of sodium at *(b1)*, respectively *(b2)*. So far, the action potential generated by the stimulus in *(a)* has propagated until *(b1)* and *(b2)*. In the meantime, region *(a)* has entered the repolarization period (see Fig. 4.27B) and thus is still in an absolute refractoriness. Consequently, the sodium that diffuses back from *(b1)* (or *b2*) toward *(a)* cannot trigger a new action potential. However, sodium that diffuses from *(b1)* and *(b2)* toward *(c1)*, respectively *(c2)*, will find a resting membrane that is favorable to excitation and will trigger in *(c1)* and *(c2)* new action potentials (see Fig. 4.27B).

Synaptic Transmission

The synapse is the region where the activity is conveyed from one (presynaptic) neuron to another (postsynaptic). The transmission is generally mediated by a chemical substance called a *neurotransmitter*. Neurotransmitters can exert excitatory or inhibitory influences, depending on the receptors to which they bind. Typical excitatory neurotransmitters are glutamate, acetylcholine, and norepinephrine, and the inhibitory ones are gamma-aminobutyric acid (GABA) and glycine. Depending on the points where the synaptic communication is established, synapses can be axodendritic (an axon contacts a dendrite; the most common type, generally excitatory), axosomatic (axons contact the soma or the perisomatic region; generally inhibitory), or axoaxonal (quite rare). A peculiar type of synapse is dendrodendritic; this has been observed in few brain regions, such as the reticular nucleus of the thalamus.

The first discovered synapses were between a motor neuron and the muscular fiber it was innervating (called the *neuromuscular junction*). Eventually, synapses between neurons became well investigated, and more recent evidence has been gathered as to the existence of synapse-like communication between neurons and glial cells.

A classic neuroneuronal synapse is illustrated in Fig. 4.28. When the presynaptic axon approaches the postsynaptic cell it innervates, it loses its myelin sheath and divides into several terminals. Each of the terminals contains several vesicles with the neurotransmitter. The postsynaptic membrane forms several folds that increase the active surface of the membrane. Axonal terminals and postsynaptic buttons are separated by a space (synaptic cleft) with interstitial fluid.

The arrival of an action potential (see *step 1* in Fig. 4.28) into the axonal terminal of the presynaptic neuron activates (opens) voltage-gated calcium channels *(step 2)*. Because of its extremely high concentration gradient and favorable electric attraction, calcium ions cross the presynaptic membrane and trigger the exocytosis of the neurotransmitter in the synaptic cleft *(steps 3 and 4)*.

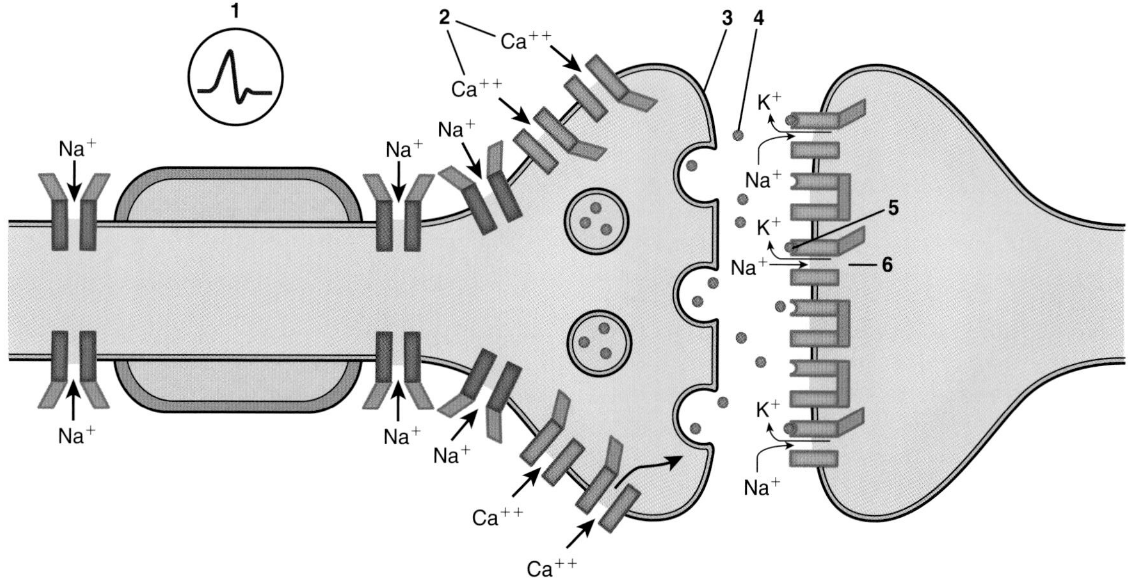

Fig. 4.28 Synaptic transmission with its consecutive phases: *(1)* arrival of the action potential, *(2)* opening of calcium channels by the action potential, *(3)* fusion of the vesicles, *(4)* exocytosis of the neurotransmitter, *(5)* binding of the neurotransmitter on the specific receptor sites, and *(6)* opening of the receptor channels and production of the excitatory postsynaptic potential.

Vesicles loaded with neurotransmitter freely move in the cytoplasmic fluid of the axonal terminal. Their membrane is identical with the external membrane of the axon. It is not uncommon that vesicles occasionally hit the presynaptic membrane and fuse with it, thus releasing their contents into the synaptic cleft. This spontaneous exocytosis constitutes a basal synaptic activity with no significant impact (below noise level) on the postsynaptic membrane. In contrast, the transient increase in cytoplasmic calcium levels triggered by the arrival of an action potential imposes a convergent docking of neurotransmitter-loaded vesicles to the presynaptic membrane, leading to massive exocytosis of the neurotransmitter *(step 4)*.

The postsynaptic membrane contains several specialized proteins (some channels, some not) that display on their extracellular domain-specific receptor sites for the neurotransmitter released by the presynaptic terminal. If one takes the example of a channel receptor (e.g., glutamate receptors in Fig. 4.28), the binding of the neurotransmitter to the receptor triggers the opening of the channel through which sodium and potassium ions are allowed to cross the membrane. Because sodium is attracted intracellularly by both electric and concentration gradients, whereas potassium exits the neuron only by its chemical gradient, the electric one retaining the ion in the cell, the net input of positive sodium charges overwhelms the countermovement of potassium *(step 5)*. This net depolarization of the postsynaptic membrane is called an *excitatory postsynaptic potential (EPSP)* *(step 6)*.

Once generated, an EPSP travels passively from the dendritic button toward the soma, losing much of its amplitude and sharpness. It is possible that the depolarizing EPSP that arrives at the axon hillock of the postsynaptic neuron has little excitatory effect on bringing the membrane potential over the firing threshold. Thus it is generally accepted that a single EPSP generated somewhere remotely in a dendrite has little chance to trigger a postsynaptic action potential. This situation occurs only at the healthy neuromuscular junction, where one action potential in the motor neuron is always followed by an action potential in the muscular fiber and a consecutive muscle contraction. However, it is rather the exception at the neuroneuronal synapse, where several concerted (synchronous) EPSPs need to be produced to relay the information through the postsynaptic neuron.

The inhibitory neuroneuronal synapse shares the same mechanism with the excitatory one, apart from the neurotransmitter used and the postsynaptic receptor it affects. The classic inhibitory neurotransmitter in the CNS is GABA. There are two main classes of receptors, $GABA_A$ and $GABA_B$. The former uses a channel permeable to chloride, the latter a second messenger that eventually increases the permeability to potassium. In both cases the net effect is a hyperpolarization of the postsynaptic membrane, generating an inhibitory postsynaptic potential. This effect is granted either by the influx of chloride in the postsynaptic terminal through $GABA_A$ channels (against its electric gradient but along its concentration gradient, which is dominant until reaching the −89 mV equilibrium potential for chloride) or the efflux of potassium after the activation of $GABA_B$ receptors. An interesting application corresponds to general anesthetics that often target GABA receptors to achieve enhanced hyperpolarization of neurons and a resultant reduced responsiveness (Box 4.5).

BOX 4.5 General Anesthesia

The principle of general anesthesia relies on the systemic diffusion of an anesthetic through the bloodstream to the brain. Here, general anesthetics act at synapses through several mechanisms. The most common act upon inhibitory synapses by increasing their permeability to chloride ions, which enter the neurons and produce a hyperpolarization of the cellular membrane. The overall inhibitory effect is achieved through two mechanisms: (1) The neuronal hyperpolarization impairs the ability of a neuron to respond to excitatory inputs, such as pain stimuli, by moving the membrane potential away from the excitability threshold (−57 mV); (2) through their perisomatic location, inhibitory synapses exert a shunting effect on incoming excitatory potentials originating at remote dendritic sites. Gamma-aminobutyric acid (GABA)-ergic agonists act at various sites within the GABA receptor and produce different effects. As an example, benzodiazepines increase the frequency of the channel opening, whereas barbiturates increase the duration of the channel opening. Another general anesthetic, propofol, also potentiates GABAergic synapses but acts by slowing the channel closing time. It has also been reported that it might block the sodium channel. The effect of halogenated anesthetics (isoflurane, sevoflurane) seems to rely on increasing the uptake of glutamate at excitatory synapses by glial cells that ensheathe them by stimulating the GLT1 transporter. Several anesthetics also modulate ion channels present on other cell types of the neurovascular unit, such as vascular smooth muscle cells, leading to changes in brain blood flow and neurovascular coupling pathways.

Glial cells participate in several ways in the synaptic function: (1) They ensheathe the synapse and isolate it against losing or spilling neurotransmitter outside the synaptic cleft. (2) They uptake neurotransmitters (e.g., glutamate) through specialized transporters (e.g., GLT1), thus regulating the amount of available transmitter in the synaptic cleft and contributing to the excitatory-inhibitory balance in neuronal networks. (3) Recently it has been demonstrated that glial cells can release neurotransmitters in the synaptic cleft that act on neuronal receptors; however, understanding the precise conditions upon which this occurs remains an intense area of investigation. This mechanism is calcium dependent and uses neurotransmitters that have been internalized by glia (see point 2). Thus glial cells become active partners in a tripartite synapse.

RECOMMENDED READING

Brew K, Nagase H: The tissue inhibitors of metalloproteinases (TIMPs): an ancient family with structural and functional diversity, *Biochim Biophys Acta* 1803:55–71, 2010.

Gordon MK, Hahn RA: Collagens, *Cell Tissue Res* 339:247–257, 2010.

Niessen CM, Gottardi CJ: Molecular component of the adherens junctions, *Biochim Biophys Acta* 1778:562–571, 2008.

Pollard TD, et al.: *Cell biology*, Philadelphia, PA, 2008, Saunders.

Singer SJ, Nicolson GL: The fluid mosaic model of the structure of cell membranes, *Science* 175:720–731, 1972.

Stuart GJ, Sakmann B: Active propagation of somatic action potentials into neocortical pyramidal cell dendrites, *Nature* 367:69–72, 1994.

Thomason HA, et al.: Desmosome: adhesive strength and signalling in health and disease, *Biochem J* 429:419–433, 2010.

5

Development of the Tooth and Its Supporting Tissues

Ophir Klein, Jimmy K. Hu, and Antonio Nanci

OUTLINE

The development of vertebrate teeth, known as *odontogenesis,* is a complex biologic process that is guided by well-defined, genetic signaling and cellular events. This chapter discusses the histologic aspect of tooth development and the coming together of the different tissues that form the tooth and its surrounding tissues. However, to better understand morphogenesis, the molecular signals that control cell growth, migration, and, ultimately, cell fate and differentiation also must be considered. The molecular aspect of tooth development is interesting in that its molecular aspects share many similarities with the development of a number of other organs (e.g., lung and kidney) and that of the limbs. Thus the tooth organ represents an advantageous system in which to study not only the formation of an organ that is key to dentistry but also developmental pathways in general. For every developmental event, whether of limb, kidney, or tooth, a complex and intricate cascade of gene expression takes place to direct the cells to self-organize, expand in number, and differentiate along the proper developmental trajectory. Five of the major conserved signaling pathways that coordinate these events are (1) bone morphogenetic protein *(BMP)*, (2) fibroblast growth factor *(Fgf)*, (3) sonic hedgehog *(Shh)*, (4) wingless-related integration site *(Wnt)*, and (5) ectodysplasin A *(Eda)*. Their importance in tooth development and for clinical translation is highlighted in Box 5.1.

In the case of mammalian development, most molecular analyses have been done in the mouse because it is readily amenable to genetic analysis and manipulations (knockout and transgenic animals) (Table 5.1). The temporal expression of some major molecules implicated in tooth crown development is presented in Fig. 5.1, and their action is detailed in the following paragraphs.

PRIMARY EPITHELIAL BAND

Chapter 3 explains how, after about 37 days of development in the human embryo, a continuous band of odontogenic epithelium forms around the mouth in the presumptive upper and lower jaws. These bands are roughly horseshoe shaped and correspond in position to the future dental arches of the upper and lower jaws (Figs 5.2 and 5.3). A long-standing theory suggested that the formation of these thickened epithelial bands from a simple monolayer to a stratified tissue is the result not so much of increased proliferative activity within the epithelium as it is a change in orientation of the mitotic spindle and cleavage plane of dividing cells. In this context, cells fated to form the dental band divide vertically relative to the plane of the oral surface, giving rise to suprabasal cells that now sit atop the initial single layer of epithelium, histologically identified as the basal layer. This gives the dental band a multilayered appearance. In contrast, epithelial cells outside the dental band predominantly divide horizontally relative to the oral surface, therefore remaining a simple epithelial structure at this early stage, although it eventually becomes stratified. More recently it has been proposed that tissue mechanical forces are also critical regulators of organ morphogenesis (see Bud Stage, later).

Each band of epithelium, called the *primary epithelial band,* quickly gives rise to two extensions that ingrow into the underlying mesenchyme that is colonized by neural crest (ectomesenchyme)–derived cells (Fig. 5.4). These are the dental lamina and the vestibular lamina, the latter of which is positioned just anterior to the dental lamina. The development of the two laminae is closely associated with each other. Depending on the location, both laminae can develop from the same epithelial thickening, which then bifurcate to become distinct structures. They can also develop independently with the vestibular lamina forming either before or after the dental lamina.

A key feature of the initiation of tooth development is the formation of localized thickenings or placodes within the primary epithelial bands (Fig. 5.5A and B; see also Fig. 5.1). Dental placodes are believed to initiate formation of the various tooth families. It is noteworthy that many ectodermal appendages, including teeth, hair, and salivary glands, develop morphologically similar placodes as they initiate their development. The

BOX 5.1 Molecular Regulation of Tooth Formation: From the Laboratory to the Clinic

The Molecular Program of Tooth Development

During the past 30 years, research using gene expression analyses, ex vivo explant cultures, and in vivo mouse models has gradually identified numerous genes that regulate tooth development and unraveled their expression patterns and functions during tooth morphogenesis. Most gene expression data on teeth come from mice, but studies in different mammals, including humans, as well as in several fish and reptile species indicate that the same groups of genes regulate tooth development across species.

The genes regulating tooth morphogenesis belong to the common toolbox of developmental regulatory genes that has been conserved to an astonishing extent during evolution. The signaling molecules mediating communication between cells constitute one of the key groups of molecules in this conserved toolbox. There are several major families of signal molecules that are essential for cell communication in all animals from flies to man as well as in all different organs, including teeth. These include bone morphogenetic protein *(BMP)*, fibroblast growth factor *(Fgf)*, hedgehog, and wingless homologue *(Wnt)*. In addition, ectodysplasin A *(Eda)*, a nuclear factor kappa B family signal, plays key roles in the development of teeth and other ectodermal appendages. These signals can be thought of as part of the language of interacting cells, and they regulate tooth development from initiation to root formation.

The toolbox also includes receptors for signals at the cell surface, mediators transmitting the signal in the cell, and transcription factors regulating gene expression in the nucleus. The transcription factors are of special importance because they regulate the fate of cells. In particular, specific combinations of transcription factors can determine the identities of different cell types. Knowledge of such transcription factor codes is essential for cellular reprogramming in regeneration studies. However, thus far the transcription factor codes of tooth-specific cells are not fully known.

The reciprocal and sequential interactions between dental mesenchyme and epithelium constitute the core of the molecular program. The interactions are mediated by the conserved signal molecules activating the expression of specific transcription factors, which, in turn, regulate the expression of numerous other genes important for advancing morphogenesis and cell differentiation in the developing tooth.

Initiation of Tooth Formation: Lessons From Missing Teeth in Transgenic Mice and Humans

The analysis of transgenic and mutant mice has revealed necessary functions of numerous genes for normal tooth development, and human genetics has pinpointed mutations causing dental aberrations. Interestingly, many of the targeted genes in mouse mutants and the identified human mutations are in genes associated with the signaling networks and include signaling molecules, signal mediators, and transcription factors. The fact that all genes in the networks regulate the development of many different organs and are not specific to teeth is of clinical importance in the diagnosis of patients with dental aberrations (most of which are genetic). The gene mutation behind a dental defect may have disturbed the development of other tissues and organs as well, and thus the tooth phenotype may be an indicator of a malformation syndrome.

Among the first genes in which mutations were shown to cause tooth agenesis in mice and humans were *Msx1* and *Pax9*. These genes encode transcription factors, which have essential functions in the mediation of *BMP*, *Wnt*, and *Fgf* signaling in early dental mesenchyme. Tooth development is arrested at the bud stage in *Msx1* and *Pax9* knockout mice, and in humans, heterozygous loss of function mutations in *Msx1* and *Pax9* genes cause tooth agenesis.

The list of genes associated with missing teeth in mice is long and growing, and in most cases these mice have serious defects in other organs, and they often die before birth. The list of mutations causing human hypodontia is shorter—likely because of embryonic lethality—and most of them are also implicated in mouse hypodontia. In addition to *Msx1* and *Pax9*, the genes that have been associated with nonsyndromic human hypodontia (i.e., no defects in other organs) include *Wnt10A*, *Axin2*, *Lrp6*, *Grem2*, *Spry2*, *Spry4*, and *Eda*. Notably all of these genes encode signals or inhibitors of signaling.

Human tooth agenesis is commonly associated with congenital defects in other organs, most often with ectodermal organs developing from the outer surface of the embryo. Conditions that affect two or more ectodermal organs are called ectodermal dysplasias. The most common of these is X-linked hypohidrotic ectodermal dysplasia (HED), caused by mutations in the *Eda* gene and characterized by oligodontia, hair loss, dry mouth, and inability to sweat. Identical phenotypes result from mutations in other components of the *Eda* signal pathway, including the receptor EDAR and signal mediator EDARADD.

Studies on the functions of human hypodontia genes in mouse models have increased the understanding of the pathogenesis of tooth agenesis as well as the genetic mechanisms of tooth initiation. Experimental work on the functions of the *Eda* and *Wnt* pathways provides examples of such approaches. The stimulation of *Eda* expression in transgenic mice induced the formation of extra teeth as well as mammary glands and stimulated the growth of hair, nails, and salivary glands. The *Eda* pathway is unique because it seems to be necessary, almost exclusively, for the formation of teeth and other ectodermal organs, unlike the other conserved signal pathways, which have more widespread functions.

Interestingly, *Wnt10A* has come up as the most common gene associated with human tooth agenesis, and mutations in *Wnt10A* have been shown to account for more than half of the nonsyndromic hypodontia cases. Based on mouse experiments, the *Wnt* pathway appears to be the most upstream signal pathway and the inducer of tooth initiation. The inhibition of *Wnt* signaling by overexpressing the *Wnt* inhibitor Dickkopf-1 *(Dkk1)* in transgenic mice prevents the formation of tooth placodes, and the initiation of teeth fails. Conversely, when the *Wnt* pathway was overactivated in the oral epithelium of transgenic mouse embryos (β-catex3K14/+), dozens of teeth were generated in succession. However, these supernumerary teeth are formed through epithelial evagination instead of invagination, suggesting that the timing and the level of *Wnt* signal is critical for tooth morphogenesis at early stages. These results also indicate that the capacity for continuous tooth formation, which was lost in the mouse (and humans) during evolution, could be unlocked by modulating *Wnt* signal activity in the oral epithelium.

Clinical Translation of Molecular Findings

Preventing Hypodontia

Understanding the developmental mechanisms underlying tooth morphogenesis and the exact roles that individual genes play in tooth development may form the basis for new ways to prevent and treat hypodontia and other dental defects. In addition, mouse models will help to elucidate pathogenesis and enable design of new treatments. There is already one potential treatment for the prevention and cure of X-linked HED, the ectodermal dysplasia syndrome caused by mutations in the *Eda* gene. The mouse model for this syndrome (*Eda*–/–) has similar phenotypic features as in human patients.

The fact that *Eda* is a soluble signal mediator makes this molecule an interesting candidate for the treatment of this syndrome. In fact, prenatal and neonatal injections of *Eda* protein rescued most of the tooth, hair, and sweat gland phenotypes of the *Eda* mutant mice. Interestingly, neonatal *Eda* protein injections had even more dramatic effects in dogs. *Eda*–/– dogs have a very severe tooth phenotype, characterized by absence of most permanent premolars and incisors, and *Eda* protein rescued the development of all these teeth completely. Remarkably, clinical trials have demonstrated that prenatal administration of *Eda* protein can ameliorate hypodontia and other congenital defects of human X-linked HED.

Building New Teeth

There are dreams that new teeth could be grown in the clinic to replace missing teeth in the future. This may become possible by novel cell-based technologies combining current genetic and stem cell technologies with accumulating knowledge on the mechanisms of tooth morphogenesis. As

BOX 5.1 Molecular Regulation of Tooth Formation: From the Laboratory to the Clinic—cont'd

described previously, we already understand much of the language that cells use for communication when they are building a tooth, and we also know in great detail the other components of the program underlying tooth development. In addition, it was demonstrated many decades ago that, once initiated, tooth development continues independently from the surrounding tissue.

As proof of principle, it has been shown that teeth can develop from dissociated cells derived from mouse tooth germ epithelium and mesenchyme. The cells were aggregated, and the epithelial and mesenchymal cells were recombined, grown in organ culture for a few days, and subsequently transplanted to the adult mouse jaw where they formed functional teeth. They were vascularized and innervated, and the erupted teeth could even be moved orthodontically. However, it is obvious that more research is needed, at least concerning programming of dental cells and controlling the timing, growth, and size of the tooth before the bioengineering of a whole new set of teeth can become feasible.

Irma Thesleff (Retired)
Professor
Institute of Biotechnology
University of Helsinki
Helsinki, Finland

Recommended Reading

Andl T, et al.: WNT signals are required for the initiation of hair follicle development, *Dev Cell* 2:643–653, 2002.

Arte S, et al.: Candidate gene analysis of tooth agenesis identifies novel mutations in six genes and suggests significant role for WNT and EDA signaling and allele combinations, *PLoS ONE* 8(8):e73705, 2013.

Bei M: Molecular genetics of tooth development, *Curr Opin Genet Dev* 19:504–510, 2009.

Casal ML, et al.: Significant correction of disease after postnatal administration of recombinant ectodysplasin A in canine X-linked ectodermal dysplasia, *Am J Hum Genet* 81:1050–1056, 2007.

Jarvinen E, et al.: Continuous tooth generation in mouse is induced by activated epithelial Wnt/beta-catenin signaling, *Proc Natl Acad Sci USA* 103:18627–18632, 2006.

Jussila M, Thesleff I: Signaling networks regulating tooth organogenesis and regeneration, and the specification of dental mesenchymal and epithelial cell lineages, *Cold Spring Harb Perspect Biol* 4(4):a008425, 2012. (Review).

Lefebvre S, Mikkola ML: Ectodysplasin research—where to next? *Semin Immunol* 26:220–228, 2014.

Mustonen T, et al.: Stimulation of ectodermal organ development by ectodysplasin-A1, *Dev Biol* 259:123–136, 2003.

Oshima M, Tsuji T: Whole tooth regeneration as a future dental treatment, *Adv Exp Med Biol* 881:255–269, 2015.

Thesleff I: Molecular genetics of tooth development. In Moody SA, editor: *Principles of developmental genetics*, ed 2, London, 2014, Elsevier Academic Press.

van den Boogaard MJ, et al.: Mutations in Wnt10A are present in more than half of isolated hypodontia cases, *J Med Genet* 49:327–331, 2012.

Yin W, Bian Z: Gene network underlying hypodontia, *J Dent Res* 94:878–885, 2015. (Review).

TABLE 5.1 Major Tooth Development Mouse Mutants and Associated Tooth Phenotypes

Gene Name	Type of Molecule	Type of Deletion	Mutant Tooth Phenotype
Apc	Intracellular: scaffold protein	Epithelial cKO	Deformed supernumerary teeth
Barx1	Transcription factor	KO	Reduced molar size
BMP4	Secreted ligand	Mesenchymal cKO	Bud- or cap-stage arrest
BMPr1a	Receptor	Epithelial cKO	Bud-stage arrest
Ctnna1	Cell adhesion protein	Epithelial cKO	Cap-stage arrest
Ctnnb1	Cell adhesion protein	Epithelial cKO	Early bud-stage arrest
Dlx1	Transcription factor	Double KO	Placode-stage arrest
Dlx2	Transcription factor	Double KO	Placode-stage arrest
Eda	Secreted ligand	KO	Reduced number and size of cusps of the first and second molars
Edar	Receptor	KO	Reduced cusp numbers and tooth size
Edaradd	Intracellular: scaffold protein	KO	Severe agenesis, cone/peg-shaped teeth
Fgfr2	Receptor	KO	Bud-stage arrest
Gli2	Transcription factor	Double KO	Initiation-stage arrest
Gli3	Transcription factor	Double KO	Initiation-stage arrest
Klk4	Protease	KO	Amelogenesis imperfecta
Lef1	Transcription factor	KO	Late bud-stage arrest
Lhx6	Transcription factor	Double KO	Initiation-stage arrest
Lhx8	Transcription factor	Double KO	Initiation-stage arrest
Msx1	Transcription factor	KO	Bud-stage arrest
Msx2	Transcription factor	KO	Misshaped teeth, enamel hypoplasia
Pax9	Transcription factor	KO	Bud-stage arrest
Perp	Cell adhesion protein	KO	Amelogenesis imperfecta
Pitx2	Transcription factor	KO	Bud-stage arrest
Runx2	Transcription factor	KO	Late bud-stage arrest, extra budding
Shh	Secreted ligand	Epithelial cKO	Cap-stage arrest
Sostdc1	Secreted ligand	KO	Change in cusp pattern, supernumerary teeth
Sp6	Transcription factor	KO	Reduction of cusp number, supernumerary teeth
Spry2	Intracellular: scaffold protein	KO	Slight change in cusp pattern, supernumerary teeth
Spry4	Intracellular: scaffold protein	KO	Slight change in cusp pattern, supernumerary teeth
Tp63	Transcription factor	KO	Placode-stage arrest
Wnt10a	Secreted ligand	KO	Abnormal cusp patterning, smaller and supernumerary teeth

cKO, Conditional knockout; *KO*, knockout.
From Hallikas O, et al.: System-level analyses of keystone genes required for mammalian tooth development, *J Exp Zoolog B Mol Dev Evol* 336:7–17, 2021.

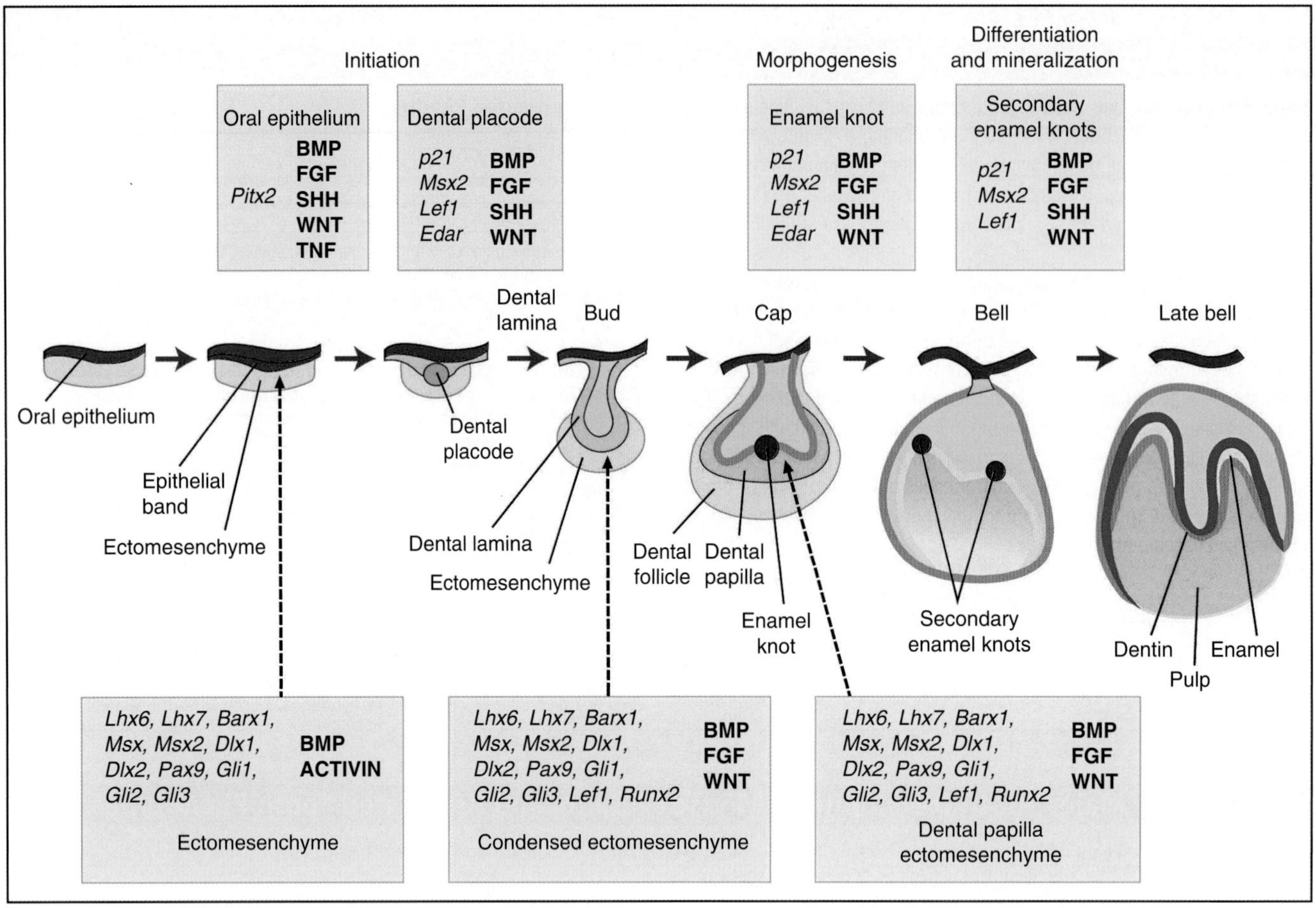

Initiation

Oral epithelium: *Pitx2* — **BMP FGF SHH WNT TNF**

Dental placode: *p21 Msx2 Lef1 Edar* — **BMP FGF SHH WNT**

Morphogenesis

Enamel knot: *p21 Msx2 Lef1 Edar* — **BMP FGF SHH WNT**

Differentiation and mineralization

Secondary enamel knots: *p21 Msx2 Lef1* — **BMP FGF SHH WNT**

Dental lamina
Bud
Cap
Bell
Late bell
Oral epithelium
Epithelial band
Ectomesenchyme
Dental placode
Dental lamina
Ectomesenchyme
Dental follicle
Dental papilla
Enamel knot
Secondary enamel knots
Dentin
Pulp
Enamel

Ectomesenchyme: *Lhx6, Lhx7, Barx1, Msx, Msx2, Dlx1, Dlx2, Pax9, Gli1, Gli2, Gli3* — **BMP ACTIVIN**

Condensed ectomesenchyme: *Lhx6, Lhx7, Barx1, Msx, Msx2, Dlx1, Dlx2, Pax9, Gli1, Gli2, Gli3, Lef1, Runx2* — **BMP FGF WNT**

Dental papilla ectomesenchyme: *Lhx6, Lhx7, Barx1, Msx, Msx2, Dlx1, Dlx2, Pax9, Gli1, Gli2, Gli3, Lef1, Runx2* — **BMP FGF WNT**

Fig. 5.1 Molecular signaling during tooth crown development. Expression sites of transcription factors *(italic)* and signaling molecules **(bold)** are listed.

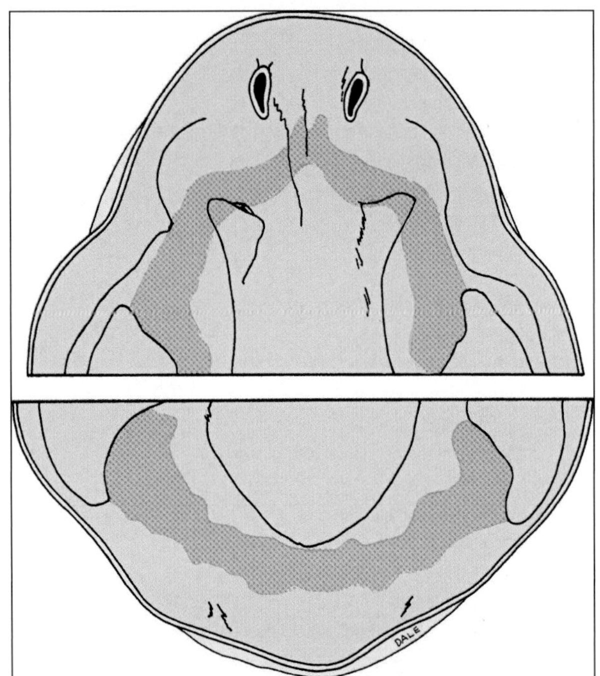

Fig. 5.2 Schematic representation of the early oral cavity showing the internal surface of the upper and lower jaws and illustrating the position of the primary epithelial band. (From Nery EB, et al.: Timing and topography of early human tooth development, *Arch Oral Biol* 15:1315–1326, 1970.)

basic mechanisms and genes involved in the formation and function of all placodes are similar. The balance between stimulatory *(Fgf, Wnt)* and inhibitory *(BMP)* signals is important in determining the site of placodes (see Fig. 5.1). Formation and growth of placodes are believed to involve the transcription factor p63 (a member of the *Tp53* tumor suppressor gene family), tumor necrosis factor, and *Eda*, among others. Defects in these pathways lead to ectodermal dysplasias characterized by missing teeth (oligodontia), misshapen teeth (see Fig. 5.5C), and abnormal development of other ectodermal organs. On the other hand, overactivation of the *Eda* receptor leads to extra teeth with aberrant morphology. Inhibition of *Wnt* signaling (such as by overexpressing the *Wnt* inhibitor Dickkopf 1 *(Dkk1)* in mice) prevents the formation of tooth placodes and the initiation of teeth fails, pointing to *Wnt* as one of the most upstream signals and the inducers of tooth initiation. In conclusion, placode formation is a determinant event in tooth development. Smaller-than-normal placodes lead to missing and smaller teeth, whereas larger placodes induce supernumerary and larger teeth.

Dental Lamina

On the anterior aspect of the downgrowing dental lamina, continued and localized proliferative activity leads to the formation of a series of epithelial outgrowths into the neighboring mesenchyme at sites corresponding to positions of the future deciduous teeth. Ectomesenchymal cells concurrently undergo the process of mesenchymal condensation to accumulate and become densely populated around these epithelial outgrowths. From this point, tooth development proceeds in three stages: bud, cap, and bell. These terms are descriptive of the morphology of the developing tooth germ as it undergoes morphogenesis and histodifferentiation. Note

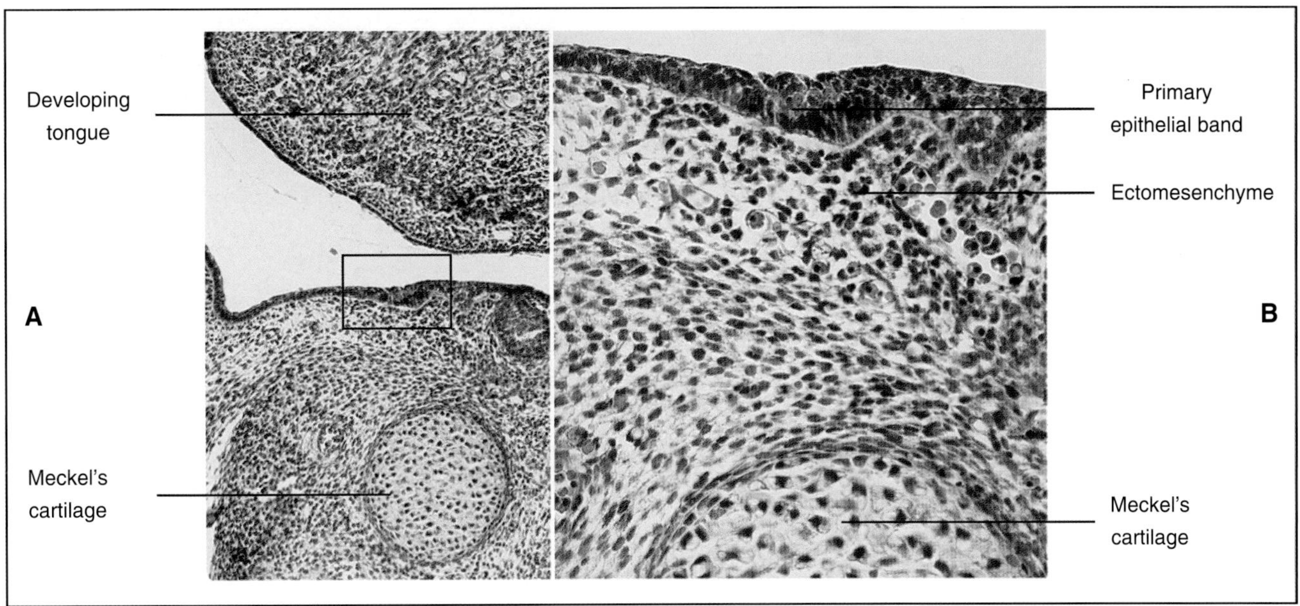

Fig. 5.3 Sagittal section through the head of an embryo. (A) The thickened epithelium of the primary epithelial band. (B) The same structure at higher magnification.

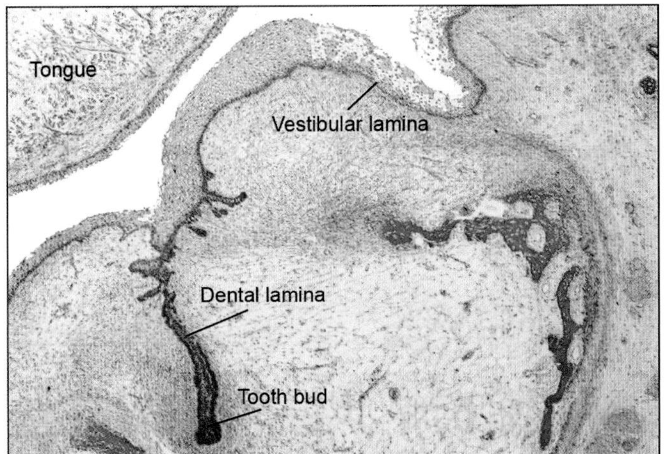

Fig. 5.4 Section through the anterior portion of the developing head illustrating the positions of the dental and vestibular laminae. The vestibular lamina is situated anteriorly, and its cells degenerate to create the vestibular furrow.

also that because development is a continuous process, clear distinction between the transition stages is not possible. Adding to this, histologic sections may possibly pass a particular angle or orientation such that they mimic tooth germs of a different developmental stage.

Vestibular Lamina

If a coronal section through the developing head region of a human embryo at 6 weeks of development is examined, no vestibule or sulcus can be seen between the cheek and tooth-bearing areas (see Fig. 5.4). The vestibule forms as a result of the proliferation of the vestibular lamina into the ectomesenchyme closely matching the formation of the dental lamina. The cells of the vestibular lamina rapidly enlarge and then undergo programmed cell death to form a cleft that becomes the vestibule between the cheek and the tooth-bearing area.

INITIATION OF THE TOOTH

An intriguing question is how dental development is initiated. When murine (mouse) first branchial arch epithelium from embryos at day 9 or 10 of gestation (E9 or E10) is isolated and combined with caudal or cranial neural crest and then grafted in the anterior chamber of the adult mouse eye, teeth form (Fig. 5.6). Epithelium from other sources, such as a limb bud or the second arch, does not elicit this response (Table 5.2). However, after E12, first arch epithelium loses this odontogenic potential, which then is assumed by the ectomesenchyme near the tooth germ; thereafter ectomesenchyme can induce tooth formation when combined with a variety of epithelia. For example, recombination of late first arch ectomesenchyme with embryonic plantar (foot) epithelium changes the developmental direction of the epithelium so that an enamel organ is formed. Conversely, if the epithelial enamel organ is recombined with skin mesenchyme, the organ loses its dental characteristics and assumes those of epidermis. What these experiments indicate is that odontogenesis is initiated first by factors resident in the first arch epithelium, influencing ectomesenchyme but that with time, this potential is transferred to and is assumed by the ectomesenchyme. These experimental findings are mirrored by the expression pattern of transcription and growth factors in these tissues, where factors important for inducing tooth development are first expressed by the epithelium and then in the ectomesenchyme.

The earliest histologic indication of tooth development in mice is at E11, which is marked by a thickening of the epithelium where tooth formation will occur on the oral surface of the first branchial arch. The genes that are implicated in the ensuing molecular cascade of events are illustrated in Fig. 5.1, and the nature of some of them is denoted in Table 5.3. To date, the earliest mesenchymal markers for tooth formation are the Lim-homeobox *(Lhx)* domain genes (transcription factors) *Lhx6* and *Lhx8* (previously *Lhx7*). Both of these genes are expressed broadly in the neural crest–derived ectomesenchyme of the oral (rostral) portion of the first branchial arch as early as on day 9 of gestation but absent in the aboral (caudal) arch mesenchyme. Experimental data demonstrate that the expression of *Lhx6* and *Lhx8* results from a signaling molecule originating from the oral epithelium of the first branchial arch. If first branchial arch oral epithelium is recombined with second arch mesenchyme, *Lhx6* and *Lhx8* expression will be induced in the mesenchyme. However, if first branchial arch mesenchyme (which expresses *Lhx6* and *Lhx8*) is recombined with second branchial arch epithelium, expression of both genes will be downregulated quickly. A prime candidate

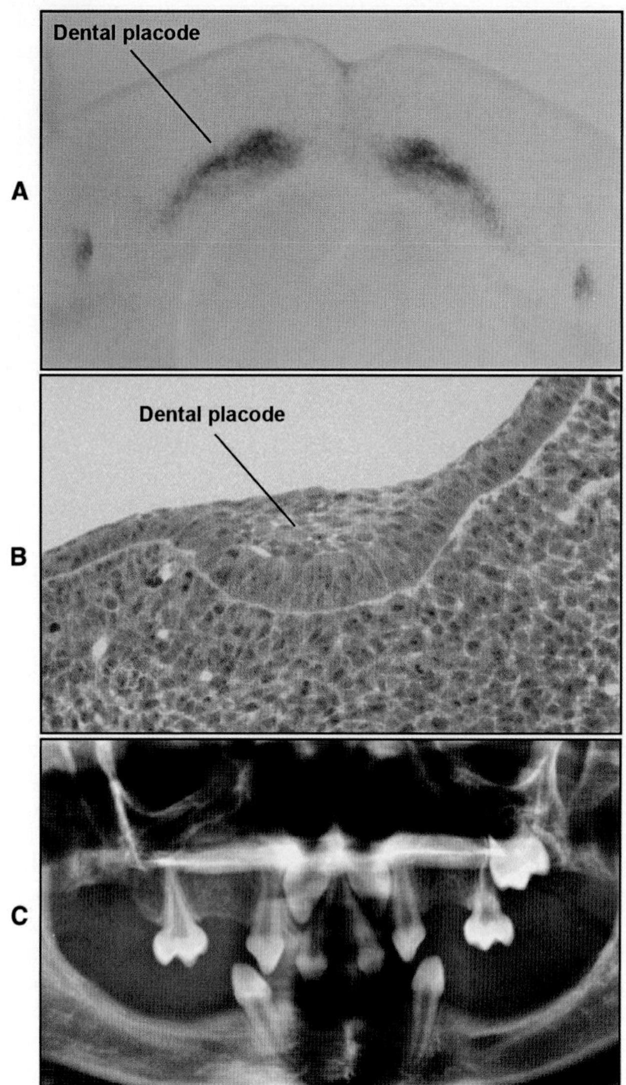

Fig. 5.5 (A) Whole-mount in situ hybridization of an E12 mouse embryo showing the expression of the signal molecule sonic hedgehog in the dental placodes of incisors and molars. (B) Histologic appearance of the dental placode. (C) Oligodontia (severe hypodontia) in a patient with loss of function of the signal molecule ectodysplasin-regulating placode formation. (Courtesy I. Thesleff.)

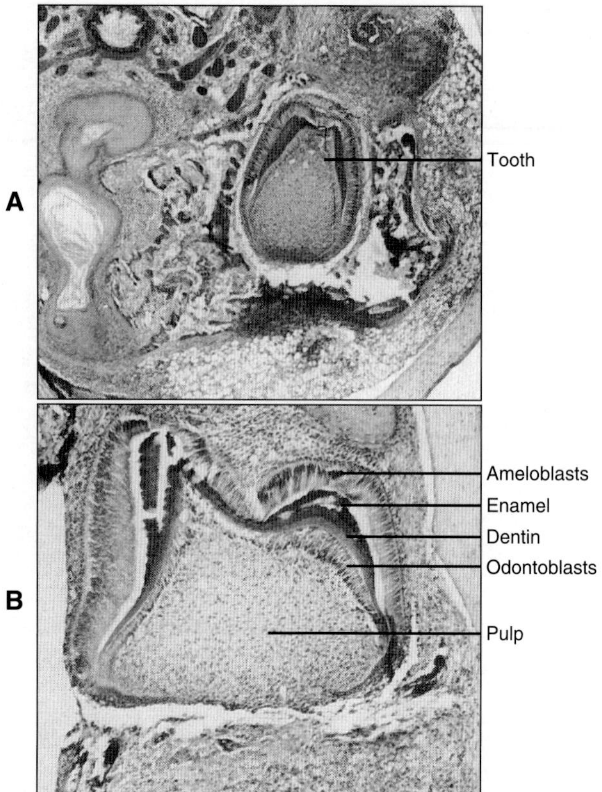

Fig. 5.6 Intraocular recombination of neural crest cells and dental epithelium. (A) Tooth formed from the combination of neural crest cells expanded from the neural folds and mandibular epithelium but not from combination with limb bud epithelium. (B) Tooth formed from the combination of neural crest expanded from the trunk level and mandibular epithelium. This indicates that tooth formation is initiated by factors residing in the oral epithelium. (Courtesy AGS Lumsden.)

for the induction of *Lhx* genes is secreted *Fgf8*; this growth factor is expressed at the proper place and time in the first branchial arch and is able to induce *Lhx6* and *Lhx8* expression in in vitro experiments. In mouse embryos with *Fgf8* deletion, expression of *Lhx6* (but not *Lhx8*) is also lost.

Specific expression of inducing signals from the oral epithelium thus explains in rather simple terms the establishment of the oral-aboral axis. The next question in terms of developmental signals is what controls the position and the number of tooth germs along the oral surface? Again, from the experimental data available, the signals for these aspects appear to originate from the oral epithelium. *Fgf8* has already been shown to play a role in the oral-aboral axis and seems to have one in determining the positions in which the tooth germs will form. The paired-box 9 *(Pax9)* homeotic gene is one of the earliest mesenchymal genes that define the localization of the tooth germs. *Pax9* gene expression colocalizes with the exact sites where tooth germs appear. *Pax9* is induced by *Fgf8* and is repressed by *BMP2* and *BMP4*. *Fgf8, BMP2,* and *BMP4* are expressed in nonoverlapping areas of the oral epithelium, with *Pax9* being expressed at sites where *Fgf8* is but *BMP* is not. Of course, a number of other genes are also expressed in oral epithelium at the same time. Whether they directly regulate the expression of *Fgf8* or *BMP* is not clear at this time.

Signaling molecules often regulate the expression of transcription factors that turn out to regulate the expression of those same signaling molecules. There is still much to be learned about the regulatory mechanisms of signaling molecules, and untangling the network of regulatory events can be difficult. To date, at least 14 transcription factors are found expressed in odontogenic mesenchyme, and some have redundant roles. More than 100 genes have also been identified in the oral epithelium, dental epithelium, and dental mesenchyme during the initiation of tooth development. The reader is directed to FaceBase (https://www.facebase.org/) for a more complete list. The level of complexity becomes evident quickly in that generating a single knockout mutant often is not sufficient to produce a phenotype that can help determine the role played by specific genes, especially when they are members of a large family. For example, distal-less homologues in vertebrae *(Dlx1, Dlx2)* show a tooth phenotype only in double-knockout mutant mice, and not all the teeth are affected. This may be explained by the compensatory action of other *Dlx* genes (e.g., *Dlx5* and *Dlx6*). Thus the evidence from experimental embryology, recombinant DNA technology, and immunocytochemistry indicates that first arch epithelium is essential for the initiation of tooth development.

In mice, expression of *Shh* is localized to the presumptive dental epithelium at E11 and is thus another good signaling candidate for tooth

TABLE 5.2 Outcome of Various Recombinations of Epithelium and Neural Crest

Combination	Teeth	Bone	Cartilage	Neural Crest
Neural crest and mandibular epithelium	+	+	+	+
Neural crest and limb epithelium	–	+	+	+
Neural crest alone	–	–	+	+
Mandibular epithelium alone	–	–	–	–

From Lumsden AGS. In Mederson PFA, editor: *Development and evolutionary aspects of the neural crest,* New York, NY, 1987, John Wiley & Sons.

TABLE 5.3 Genes Expressed During Tooth Development

Abbreviation	Gene Name
Barx	BarH-like homeobox genes (TF)
BMP	Bone morphogenetic proteins (SP)
Cbfa1	Core binding factor A1 (TF)
Dlx	Distal-less homologue in vertebrates (TF)
Eda	Ectodysplasin A (TP)
Fgf	Fibroblast growth factor (SP)
Gli	Glioma-associated oncogene homologue (zinc finger protein) (TF)
Hgf	Hepatic growth factor (SP)
Isl1	Islet1 (TF)
Lef	Lymphoid enhancer-binding factor 1 (TF)
Lhx	Lim-homeobox domain gene (TF)
Msx	Msh-like homeobox genes (TF)
Osf2	Osteoblast specific factor 2 (TF)
Otlx	Otx-related homeobox gene (TF)
Pax	Paired-box homeotic gene (TF)
Pitx	Transcription factor named for its expression in the pituitary gland
Ptc	Patched cell-surface receptor for sonic hedgehog (SP)
Shh	Sonic hedgehog (SP)
Slit	Homologous to Drosophila slit protein (SP)
Smo	Smoothed PTC coreceptor for sonic hedgehog (SP)
Wnt	Wingless homologue in vertebrates (SP)

SP, Secreted protein; *TF,* transcription factor; *TP,* transmembrane protein.

initiation (Fig. 5.7). *Shh* knockout mice have little development of facial processes, thus any role in tooth initiation cannot be identified from these. Deletions of glioma-associated oncogene homologue *(Gli)* genes that encode downstream transcriptional mediators of *Shh* action suggest a role in early tooth development, because *Gli2–/–* and *Gli3–/–* double mutant mouse embryos do not produce any recognizable tooth buds. Addition of *Shh*-soaked beads to oral epithelium can induce local epithelial cell proliferation to produce invaginations that are reminiscent of tooth buds. *Shh* thus appears to have a role in stimulating epithelial cell proliferation, and its local expression at the sites of tooth development implicates *Shh* signaling in tooth initiation. Runt-related transcription factor 2 *(Runx2),* also referred to as *core-binding factor A1* or *osteoblast specific factor 2,* is a transcription factor that plays a critical role during bone formation (see Chapter 6). Its expression in dental mesenchyme is associated with the early signaling cascades regulating tooth initiation. It regulates key epithelial-mesenchymal interactions that control advancing morphogenesis and histodifferentiation of the enamel organ. Lack of *Runx2* expression causes the syndrome cleidocranial dysplasia, which is characterized by bone defects and multiple supernumerary teeth.

Paired-like homeodomain transcription factor 2 (*Pitx2*) is a key player in pattern formation and cell fate determination during

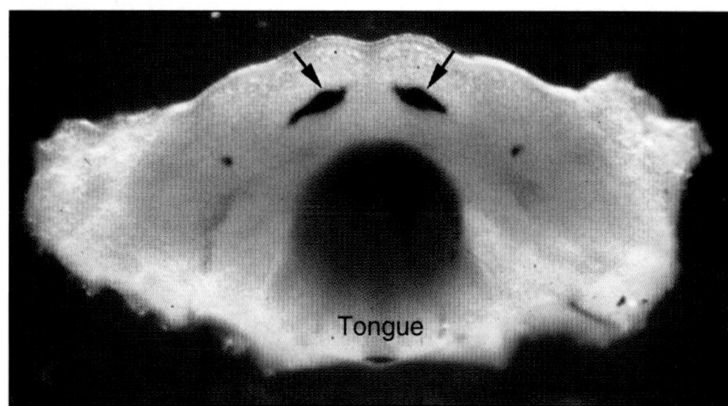

Fig. 5.7 Expression of sonic hedgehog in an isolated mouse embryonic jaw primordium at E11.5, showing expression in the dental epithelium at the future sites of tooth formation *(arrows).*

embryonic development. *Pitx2* is one of the earliest tooth markers in the dental epithelium and continues to be expressed through crown formation. It regulates early signaling molecules and transcription factors necessary for tooth development. Another factor is lymphoid enhancer–binding factor 1 *(Lef1),* a member of the high-mobility group family of nuclear proteins that includes the T-cell factor proteins, known to be nuclear mediators of *Wnt* signaling. *Lef1* is first expressed in dental epithelial thickenings, and during bud formation it shifts to being expressed in the condensing mesenchyme. In *Lef1* knockout mice, all dental development is arrested at the bud stage; recombination assays, however, have identified the requirement for *Lef1* in the dental epithelium as occurring earlier, before bud initiation. Ectopic expression of *Lef1* in the oral epithelium also results in ectopic tooth formation. These experiments highlight the importance of *Wnt* signaling in inducing tooth development.

Expression of several genes in ectomesenchyme marks the sites of tooth germ initiation. These include *Pax9* and activin A, both of which are expressed beginning around E11 in mice within small, localized groups of cells corresponding to where tooth epithelium will form buds. In the case of *Pax9,* antagonistic interactions between *Fgf8* and *BMP4* from oral epithelium, similar to those found to regulate BarH-like homeobox 1 *(Barx1)* expression (see next section), have been shown to possibly regulate localization of *Pax9* expression. Activin A expression is not regulated by the same mechanism, suggesting additional signaling pathways are involved to directly initiate tooth development.

Mutation in genes, such as *Pitx2, Shh,* and *Pax9,* are implicated in syndromes that result in tooth agenesis (missing teeth), a heterogeneous condition that affects various combinations of teeth. Tooth agenesis is a common developmental anomaly in humans, affecting 2% to 10% of the population, excluding third molars.

After the ability to initiate tooth development has been acquired by ectomesenchyme, dental papillary cells maintain it. Thus, if early tooth germs are cultured for an extended period, the cells dedifferentiate, and the morphology of the germs is lost completely; yet if these dedifferentiated epithelial and ectomesenchymal cells are harvested and recombined in vivo, they form a tooth. This tells us that the program for tooth formation is not lost. Of particular interest is that, while

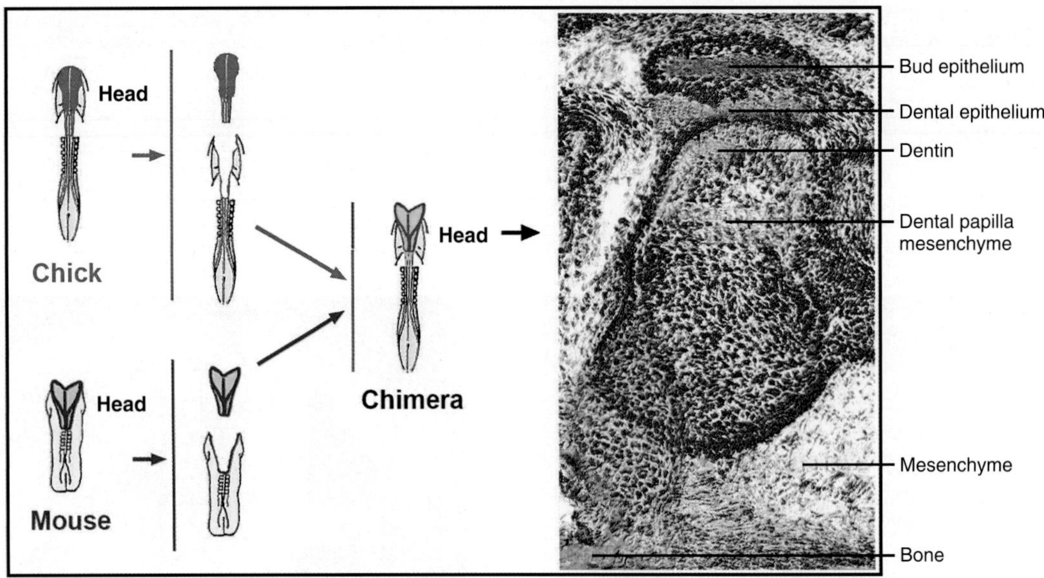

Fig. 5.8 Mouse neural tube transplantation (E8.4–6 somites) into chick host embryos equivalent to the mouse stage (6–7 somites). The resulting chick/mouse chimera leads to the formation of dental structures at 14 days posttransplantation. (Adapted from Mitsiadis TA, et al.: Development of teeth in chick embryos after mouse neural crest transplantations, *Proc Natl Acad Sci* 100:6541–6545, 2003.)

chickens do not have teeth, in chick/mouse chimera avian oral epithelium is able to induce a tooth developmental program in mouse neural crest–derived ectomesenchyme (Fig. 5.8). Avian oral epithelium has maintained the competence to form a dental organ, a competence last expressed some 100,000 years ago.

TOOTH TYPE DETERMINATION

The determination of specific tooth types at their correct positions in the jaws is referred to as *patterning* of the dentition. The determination of crown pattern is a remarkably consistent process. Although in some animals, teeth are all the same shape (homodont), in most mammals they are different (heterodont), falling into three families: incisiform, caniniform, and molariform. Two hypothetic models—the field (Fig. 5.9) and clone models (Fig. 5.10)—have been proposed to explain how these different shapes are determined, and evidence exists to support both.

Field Model

The field model proposes that the factors responsible for tooth shape reside within the ectomesenchyme in distinct graded and overlapping fields for each tooth family (see Fig. 5.9). The homeobox code (field) model for dental patterning is based on observations of the spatially restricted expression of several homeobox genes in the jaw primordial ectomesenchymal cells before E11 that results in differing combinations of patterning genes. The early expression of Msh-like *(Msx1, Msx2)* homeobox genes before the initiation of tooth germs is restricted to distal, midline ectomesenchyme in regions where incisors (and canines in human beings), but not multicuspid teeth, will develop, whereas *Dlx1* and *Dlx2* are expressed in ectomesenchymal cells where multicuspid teeth, but not incisors (or canines), will develop. These expression domains are broad and do not exactly correspond to specific tooth types. Rather, they are considered to define broad territories. Expression of *Barx1* overlaps with *Dlx1* and *Dlx2* and corresponds closely to ectomesenchymal cells that will develop into molars in mice.

The homeobox code model thus proposes that the overlapping domains provide the positional information for tooth-type morphogenesis, which is achieved by the expression of differing combinations of patterning homeobox genes in each of the fields. Functional support for this model is provided by the dental phenotype of *Dlx1−/−* and *Dlx2−/−* double-knockout mice in which development of maxillary molar teeth is arrested at the epithelial thickening stage. The normal development of mandibular molars (not predicted by the code) results from functional redundancy with other *Dlx* genes, such as *Dlx5* and *Dlx6*, which are expressed in ectomesenchyme in the mandibular primordium. Finally, as predicted by the code model, incisor development is normal in these double-knockout mice.

Additional functional support for the code model comes from misexpression of *Barx1* in distal ectomesenchymal cells, which results in incisor tooth germs developing as molars. *Barx1* expression is normally localized to proximal ectomesenchyme (molar) by a combination of positive and negative signals from the oral ectoderm. *Fgf8* localized in proximal ectoderm induces *Barx1* expression, whereas *BMP4* in the distal ectoderm represses *Barx1* expression. Ectopic expression of *Barx1* in distal (presumptive incisor) ectomesenchyme as a result of experimental inhibition of *BMP* signaling has the effect of repressing *Msx1* gene expression, which is otherwise induced in distal ectomesenchyme by *BMP4*. The transformation of incisors into molars thus may require a combination of loss of incisor genes *(Msx1)* and gain of molar genes *(Barx1)*.

It has also been reported that the transcriptional regulator islet 1 *(Isl1)*, a LIM homeodomain–containing protein, plays a role in incisor formation and patterning. This protein is found in epithelium of the mouse incisors but not of the molars, suggesting that it may be involved in tooth-type specification. Functionally, *Isl1* and *BMP4* act in a positive feedback loop and induce the expression of each other within the presumptive incisor field.

Clone Model

The clone model proposes that each tooth class is derived from a clone of ectomesenchymal cells programmed by epithelium to produce teeth of a given pattern (see Fig. 5.10). In support of this contention, isolated presumptive first molar tissues have been shown to continue development to form three molar teeth in their normal positional sequence.

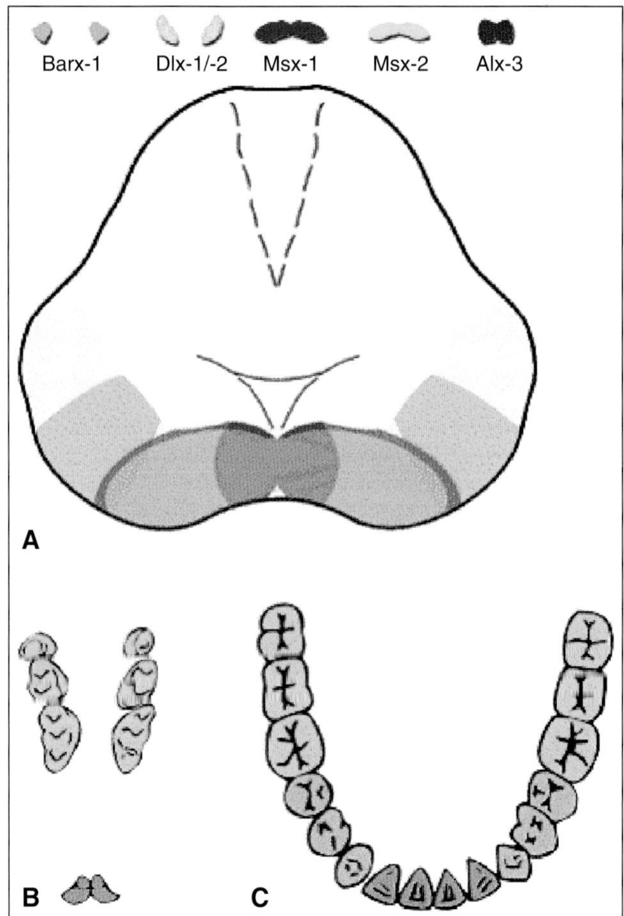

Fig. 5.9 Odontogenic homeobox code model of dental patterning. Epithelial Fgf8 and BMP4 expressed during early initiation induce the mesenchymal expression of a number of homeobox-containing genes in the underlying mesenchyme as overlapping domains that provide the spatial information necessary to determine tooth type. (A) Domains of *Barx1* and *Dlx1/2* expression overlap in the mesenchyme of the presumptive molar region, whereas domains of *Msx1, Msx2,* and *Alx3* overlap in presumptive incisor mesenchyme. (B) Mouse dental pattern. Incisors derive from *Msx1* and *Alx3*-expressing cells; molars derive from *Barx1* and *Dlx1/2*-expressing cells. (C) Human dental pattern. Premolars and canines can be derived from the same odontogenic code as that observed in mice by virtue of the overlapping domains of gene expression. Thus canines and premolars may be derived from cells expressing *Dlx1/2* and *Msx1*, for example. (From McCollum MA, Sharpe PT: Developmental genetics and early hominid craniodental evolution, *Bioessays* 23:481–493, 2001.)

Both Field and Clone Models

Possibly both models can be invoked because temporal factors may play a role. For instance, the coded pattern of homeobox gene expression in the ectomesenchyme might be expressed after an epithelial signal, as was the case for tooth initiation. Furthermore, as with tooth initiation, ectomesenchyme eventually assumes the dominant role in crown pattern formation. Recombination of molar papilla with the incisor enamel organ results in molar development; conversely, recombination of incisor papilla with the molar enamel organ results in incisor development.

INSTRUCTIVE SIGNALS FOR PATTERNING

Recombinations of incisor and molar epithelium with mesenchyme from young mouse embryos (~E10) showed that when molar epithelium was recombined with incisor mesenchyme, a molar tooth formed; when incisor epithelium was recombined with molar mesenchyme, an incisor formed. This led to the conclusion that the early-stage dental epithelium was responsible for determining the type and shape of a tooth. Other recombinations with older embryos (~E14), however, produced different results in which molar epithelium recombined with incisor mesenchyme resulted in incisor teeth, and incisor epithelium recombined with molar mesenchyme resulted in molar teeth. Further experiments used tissue from the hairless (plantar) surface of the foot in combination with dental tissues. At around E14, dental epithelium, when recombined with foot mesenchyme, showed no tooth development; however, when plantar epithelium was combined with dental mesenchyme, tooth development occurred.

The apparent conflict produced by these experiments of whether the ectoderm or ectomesenchyme provides the instructive information for patterning now has been resolved by studying the temporal regulation of homeobox gene expression in ectomesenchyme by ectodermal signals. Removal of the ectoderm from E10 mandibular arch explants results in loss of expression of ectomesenchymal homeobox gene expression within 6 hours, indicating that expression requires signals produced by the ectoderm. Expression can be restored by implantation of beads soaked in *Fgf8*, a factor expressed in oral ectoderm at this time. Expression of *Dlx1, Dlx2, Msx1,* and *Barx1* is seen around the implanted beads regardless of their position in the explant, indicating that all ectomesenchymal cells at this time are competent to respond to *Fgf8*. When this experiment was repeated at E10.5, ectomesenchymal gene expression again was lost after removal of ectoderm, but this time implantation of *Fgf8* beads only restored expression in the original domains. Thus at E10.5, ectomesenchymal cell competence to express homeobox genes in response to *Fgf8* has become restricted to those cells that expressed the gene at E10. By E11, removal of ectoderm had no effect on ectomesenchymal gene expression, showing that by this stage, expression is independent of ectodermal signals. These results provide a molecular understanding of the control of dental patterning and an explanation for the conflicting recombination results. The distoproximal (incisor-molar) spatial domains of homeobox gene expression (homeobox code) are produced in response to spatially restricted ectodermal signals acting on pluricompetent ectomesenchymal cells. Recombinations carried out before E10.5, therefore, will show the instructive influence of ectoderm on tooth shape, whereas those carried out after E10.5 will show an instructive influence of ectomesenchyme because by this stage expression is independent of ectodermal signals.

REGIONALIZATION OF ORAL AND DENTAL ECTODERM

Because regionally restricted expression of signaling protein genes in oral ectoderm controls dental initiation and patterning, it follows that the mechanisms that control the regional restriction of ectodermal signals need to be understood. During insect segmentation, interactions between hedgehog *(HH)* and wingless signaling *(Wg/Wnt)* are involved in ectodermal cell boundary specification. Several *Wnt* genes are expressed during tooth development, and one, *Wnt7b*, has a reciprocal expression pattern to *Shh* in oral ectoderm. *Wnt7b* is expressed throughout the oral ectoderm except for presumptive dental ectoderm where *Shh* is expressed. Misexpression of *Wnt7b* in presumptive dental ectoderm results in loss of *Shh* expression and failure of tooth bud formation. This shows that *Wnt7b* represses *Shh* expression in oral ectoderm, and thus the boundaries between oral and dental ectoderm are maintained by an interaction between *Wnt* and *Shh* signaling, similar to ectodermal boundary maintenance in segmentation in insects.

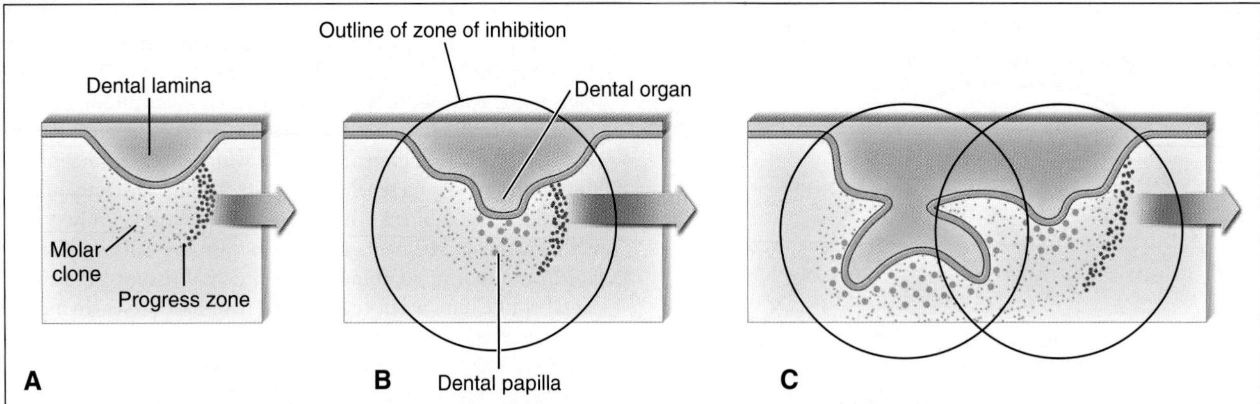

Fig. 5.10 Clone theory. (A) The molar clone ectomesenchyme has induced the dental lamina to begin tooth development. The clone and dental lamina progress posteriorly. (B) When a clone reaches the critical size, a tooth bud is initiated at its center. (C) The next tooth bud is not initiated until the progress zone of the clone escapes the influence of a zone of inhibition surrounding the tooth bud. (From Osborn JW, Ten Cate AR: *Advanced dental histology*, ed 3, Oxford, UK, 1983, Elsevier.)

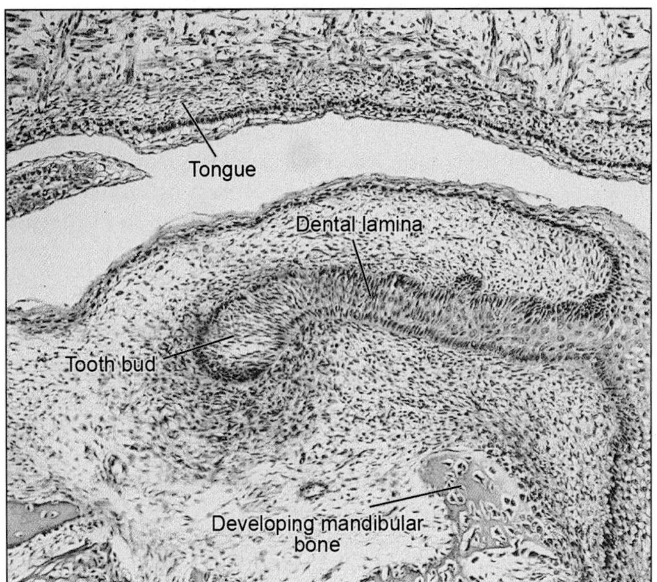

Fig. 5.11 Bud stage of tooth development seen in sagittal section.

BUD STAGE

The bud stage is represented by the first epithelial incursion into the ectomesenchyme of the jaw (Fig. 5.11). By directly visualizing live the development of mouse teeth under a microscope, we now know that active cell movement and cell-cell adhesion produce the contraction force necessary to narrow the epithelial region of the forming tooth bud near the oral surface (Box 5.2). In this context, suprabasal cells migrate toward the center of the placode and intercalate with one another. The suprabasal cells at the edge of the placode are, in turn, tightly attached to the basal cells via E-cadherin. As a result, the contracting force generated by cell intercalation is transmitted to the basal cells that are anchored to the basement membrane and pulls the basal cells at the border of the placode toward the center. This effectively buckles the epithelium toward the mesenchyme and progressively morphs the placode into a bud shape. These findings thus highlight that, in addition to biochemical signals, tissue mechanical forces are critical regulators of organ morphogenesis.

BOX 5.2 Force Generation by Cytoskeletons

Actin microfilaments are dynamic cytoskeletal structures in cells and are composed of two intertwined strands of polymerized actin subunits called *globular actin*. While actin microfilaments are involved in many different cellular processes, one of its key functions is to generate cellular forces via its interaction with the motor protein, nonmuscle myosin II (MyoII). MyoII has a head domain and a tail domain. While the head domain binds to filamentous actin, the tail domains of individual MyoII interact with each other to facilitate MyoII dimerization. As multiple MyoII dimers connect with multiple actin filaments, actin filaments are cross-linked into larger bundles, and this provides structural integrity to cells. When activated under the right signaling environment, the head domain of MyoII also converts energy from adenosine triphosphate hydrolysis into a power stroke that allows MyoII to walk on the actin filament. As the two head domains of dimerized MyoII walk in opposite directions, actin filaments also slide against each other in opposite directions, thus generating contractile forces. These forces propel various cellular processes, including cell migration, cell shape changes, and mechanical stability. They are also responsible for the active cellular movements observed in the developing tooth bud.

In epithelial tissues, including the tooth germ, cells are joined to each other via cell-cell adhesion complexes, such as the adherence junctions (AJs). AJs are composed of the membrane-spanning cadherins and associated cytoplasmic proteins, which connect actomyosin (actin filaments and MyoII) cables to AJs. Such setup allows cells to be mechanically linked at the supracellular level where actomyosin bundles within each cell are joined between neighboring cells to form a singular cable across multiple cells. In the tooth germ, these cables are visible in the suprabasal layer closer to the oral surface and are aligned in the same direction as the tissue tension. Suprabasal cells are similarly attached to basal cells that are anchored to the basement membrane. Consequently, as suprabasal cells migrate and intercalate toward the center of the tooth germ (as facilitated by actomyosin contraction), this generates an overall tissue tension that is transmitted via cadherins and actins between cells and ultimately to the basal layer. Analogous to a purse string, basal cells at the upper edge of the tooth placode are drawn toward the center of the placode in response to this tissue contraction, narrowing the epithelium at the neck region of the tooth germ. The bud shape of the tooth is thus formed.

At this same stage, the supporting ectomesenchymal cells are packed closely beneath and around the epithelial bud. As the epithelial bud continues to proliferate and invaginate into the ectomesenchyme, cellular density increases immediately adjacent to the epithelial outgrowth. This process is classically referred to as *condensation of the ectomesenchyme*. In mice, *Fgf8* secreted from the epithelial bud acts as a chemoattractant to draw ectomesenchymal cells toward the bud. As ectomesenchymal cells accumulate, individual cells experience increased crowding and cell constraint, which functions as a mechanical signal (as opposed to the biochemical signal provided by secreted ligands) to promote the ectomesenchyme toward the dental fate. Cell crowding during condensation also induces the expression of collagen VI, which adds mechanical stiffness to the extracellular matrix that surrounds cells. This change in the material property of the matrix reciprocally supports mesenchymal condensation and mechanically further stimulates the ectomesenchyme to differentiate along the odontogenic pathway.

BUD-TO-CAP TRANSITION

The transition from bud to cap marks the onset of morphologic differences between tooth germs that give rise to different types of teeth. Because signaling cues stimulate cell proliferation only in certain parts of the epithelium, differential cellular division in the epithelial bud initiates a change in shape from bud to cap. Now the epithelial outgrowth assumes a more complex outline with a flattened internal portion corresponding to regions with reduced proliferation, along which the mesenchymal condensation densifies (Fig. 5.12). Molecularly, *Msx1* is expressed with *BMP4* in the mesenchymal cells that condense around tooth buds. It should be noted that *BMP4* is initially expressed in the epithelium during tooth initiation but is induced in the mesenchyme shortly thereafter. In *Msx1−/−* embryos, tooth development is arrested at the bud stage, and *BMP4* expression is lost from the mesenchyme, suggesting that *Msx1* is required for *BMP4* expression. *BMP4* is able to maintain *Msx1* expression in wild-type tooth bud mesenchyme, indicating that *BMP4* induces its own expression via *Msx1*. Tooth development can be rescued in *Msx1−/−* embryos by addition of exogenous *BMP4*.

BMP4 expressed in the bud mesenchyme is required to maintain *BMP2* and *Shh* expression in the epithelium. Loss of *BMP4* expression in *Msx1* mutants is accompanied by loss of *Shh* expression at E12.5, which can be restored by exogenous *BMP4*. Blocking *Shh* function with neutralizing antibodies also results in loss of *BMP2* expression, suggesting *Shh* and *BMP2* may be in the same pathway and that downregulation of *BMP2* in *Msx1* mutants may be downstream of the loss of *Shh*.

Removal of *Shh* signaling at different stages of tooth development has enabled identification of distinct time-dependent requirements for *Shh*. Blocking *Shh* signaling using neutralizing antibodies or forskolin shows that, at E11 to E12, *Shh* is required for dental epithelium proliferation to form tooth buds, whereas blocking at E13 affects tooth bud morphology, but these buds still can form teeth. Genetic disruption of *Shh* signaling from E12.5 by Cre-mediated excision of targeted *Shh* conditional alleles results in a disruption of molar tooth morphology, but cytodifferentiation appears normal, suggesting that *Shh* has a major role at the cap stage of development.

Another homeobox gene with a role in the bud-to-cap transition is *Pax9*. *Pax9* is expressed in bud stage mesenchyme and earlier in domains similar to activin βA and *Msx1* in patches of mesenchyme that mark the sites of tooth formation. *Pax9−/−* mutant embryos have all teeth arrested at the bud stage. Despite being coexpressed, early activin βA expression is not affected in *Pax9−/−* embryos, and *Pax9* expression is not affected in activin βA−/− embryos. These two genes are essential for tooth development to progress beyond the bud stage and thus appear to function independently; however, changes occur in expression of other genes, such as *BMP4*, *Msx1*, and *Lef1* in *Pax9−/−* tooth bud mesenchyme.

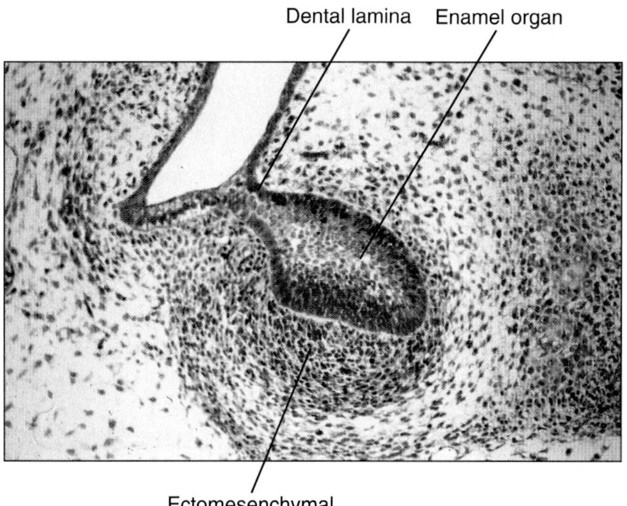

Fig. 5.12 Early cap stage of tooth development. A condensation of the ectomesenchyme associated with the epithelial cap is identified easily.

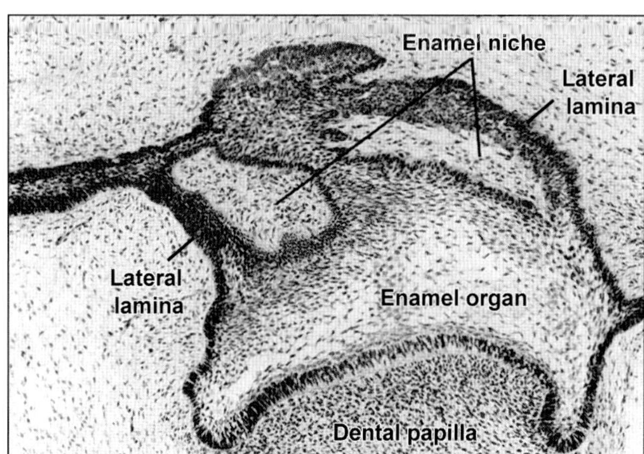

Fig. 5.13 Enamel niche. This structure is created by the plane of a section cutting through a curved lateral lamina so that mesenchyme appears to be surrounded by dental epithelium.

CAP STAGE

As the tooth bud grows larger, it drags along part of the dental lamina; thus from that point on, the developing tooth is tethered to the dental lamina by an extension called the *lateral lamina* (Fig. 5.13). At this early stage of tooth development, identifying the formative elements of the tooth and its supporting tissues is already possible. The epithelial outgrowth, which superficially resembles a cap sitting on a ball of condensed ectomesenchyme (Fig. 5.14; see also Fig. 5.13), is still referred to widely as the dental organ, although a better name is the enamel organ because it eventually will form the enamel of the tooth. Henceforth the term *enamel organ* is used.

The enamel niche is an apparent structure in histologic sections, created because the dental lamina is a sheet rather than a single strand and often contains a concavity filled with connective tissue. A section through this arrangement creates the impression that the tooth germ has a double attachment to the oral epithelium by two separate strands (see Fig. 5.13).

The ball of condensed ectomesenchymal cells, called the *dental papilla*, will form the dentin and pulp (see Figs. 5.13 and 5.14). The condensed

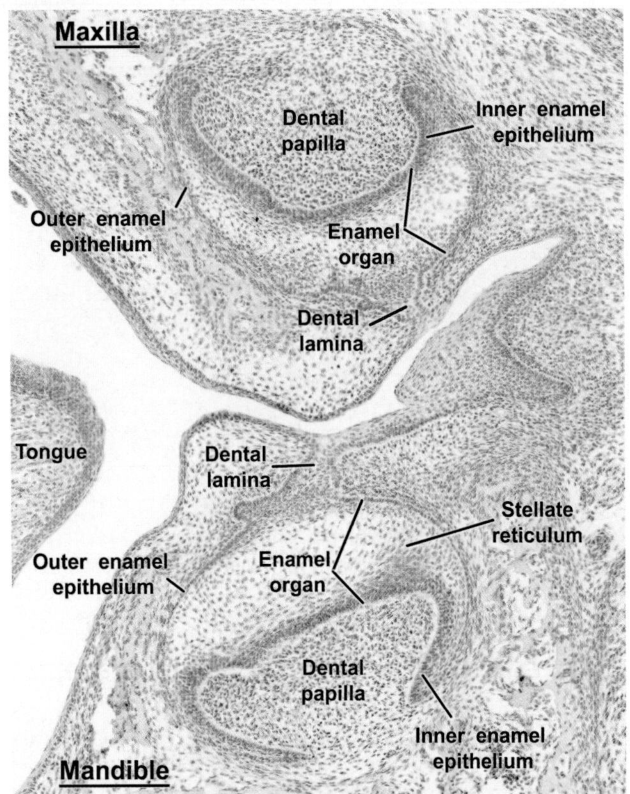

Fig. 5.14 Cap stage of tooth development. The epithelial enamel organ sits over a mass of ectomesenchymal cells, the dental papilla. (Courtesy Y. Zhang.)

ectomesenchyme limiting the dental papilla and encapsulating the enamel organ—the dental follicle or sac—gives rise to the supporting tissues of the tooth. Because the enamel organ sits over the dental papilla like a cap, this stage of tooth development is known as the *cap stage* (see Fig. 5.13). In mouse embryos, ectomesenchyme is initially a homogeneous population at the bud stage, but its fate subsequently bifurcates during the cap stage such that cells in the future pulp region become the dental papilla, and cells encapsulating the tooth germ become the dental follicle.

The enamel organ, dental papilla, and dental follicle together constitute the dental organ, or tooth germ. Early in the ontogeny (life history) of the tooth, those structures giving rise to the dental tissues (enamel, dentin-pulp, and supporting apparatus of the tooth) can be identified as discrete entities. Important developmental changes begin late in the cap stage and continue during the transition of the tooth germ from cap to bell. Through these changes (histodifferentiation), a mass of similar epithelial cells transforms itself into morphologically and functionally distinct components. The cells in the center of the enamel organ synthesize and secrete glycosaminoglycans into the extracellular compartment between the epithelial cells. Glycosaminoglycans are hydrophilic and so pull water into the enamel organ. The increasing amount of fluid increases the volume of the extracellular compartment of the enamel organ, and the central cells are forced apart. Because they retain connections with each other through their desmosomal contacts, they become star shaped (Fig. 5.15). The center of the enamel organ thus is termed the *stellate reticulum.*

SIGNALING CENTERS

There are three sets of transient signaling centers in the dental epithelium that produce more than a dozen different signaling molecules belonging to the *BMP, Fgf, Shh,* and *Wnt* families. First come the initiation knots, which appear in the dental placode and initiate budding of the tooth epithelium. Then appear the primary and secondary enamel knots that initiate the bud-to-cap stage transition and tooth crown formation. Precursor cells of these two knots are first detected at the tip of the tooth buds by expression of the *p21* gene, followed shortly after by *Shh*. The primary enamel knots become visible histologically as clusters of nondividing epithelial cells in sections of molar cap-stage tooth germs (Fig. 5.16). These clusters express genes for several signaling molecules, including *BMP2, BMP4, BMP7, Fgf4, Fgf9, Wnt10b, Slit1,* and *Shh* (Fig. 5.17). Three-dimensional reconstructions of the expression of these genes have revealed highly dynamic spatial and temporal nested patterns in the enamel knot. On the whole, receptors for the enamel knot signals are localized in the epithelial cells surrounding the enamel knot, and signals from the primary enamel knot promote their continued proliferation and tissue growth. Each cap-stage molar tooth germ has a single primary enamel knot that has been proposed to induce formation of secondary enamel knots at the tips of the future cusps and thereby regulate crown patterning. In monocuspid teeth, such as incisors, only the primary enamel knot is formed. *Fgf4* and *Slit1* may be the best molecular markers for enamel knot formation because they have been observed in both primary and secondary knots.

In summary, the enamel knot represents an organizational center that orchestrates cuspal morphogenesis. The enamel knot shares many similarities with the apical ectodermal ridge of developing limbs: both consist of nondividing cells; both express *Fgf, BMP,* and *Msx2*; and both act as signaling centers.

In some planes of section, one can see cells extending from the enamel knot across the stellate reticulum to the outer enamel epithelium (Fig. 5.18). This structure is referred to as the enamel cord; although it could be part of the enamel knot organizational center, it could also be related anatomically to the site where the lateral lamina attaches to the enamel organ cap and would only be visible in certain planes of section.

BELL STAGE

Continued growth of the tooth germ leads to the next stage of tooth development, the bell stage (Figs. 5.19 and 5.20; see also Fig. 5.15), so called because the enamel organ comes to resemble a bell as the undersurface of the epithelial cap deepens. By the start of this stage the shape of the tooth has already been decided (morphodifferentiation). During this stage, the cells that will be making the hard tissues of the crown (ameloblasts and odontoblasts) acquire their distinctive phenotype (histodifferentiation), and the crown completes its morphodifferentiation and attains its full size.

At the periphery of the enamel organ, the cells assume a low cuboidal shape and form the outer enamel epithelium (see Fig. 5.15A). The cells bordering on the dental papilla assume a short columnar shape and are characterized by high glycogen content (see Fig. 5.14B and C); they form the inner enamel epithelium. The outer and inner enamel epithelia are continuous; the inner epithelium begins at the point where the outer epithelium bends to form the concavity into which the cells of the dental papilla accumulate. The region where the inner and outer enamel epithelia meet at the rim of the enamel organ is known as the *zone of reflexion* or *cervical loop* (see Fig. 5.14A and D). Cells within the cervical loop express the transcription factor, sex determining region Y-box 2 *(Sox2)*, a common stem cell marker, and they continue to divide until the tooth crown attains its full size. After crown formation, these cells finally differentiate and give rise to the epithelial component of the tooth root. In the bell stage, some epithelial cells between the inner enamel epithelium and the stellate reticulum differentiate into a layer called the *stratum intermedium.* The cells of this layer soon are characterized by an exceptionally high activity of the

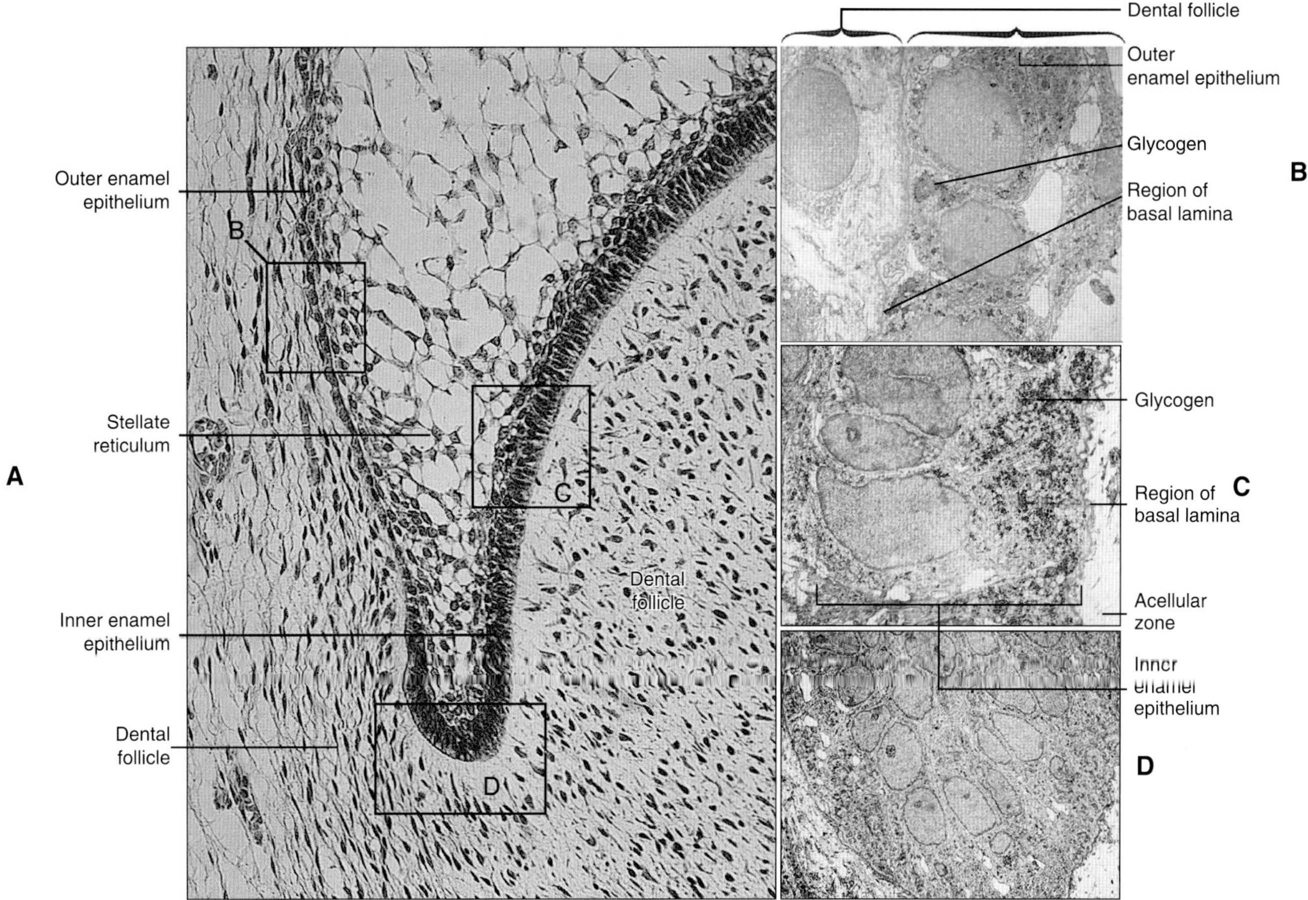

Fig. 5.15 Structure of a tooth germ at the early bell stage. (A) The enamel organ in the region of the cervical loop as seen with light microscopy. (B) The outer enamel epithelium; its cells are separated from the follicle by a basal lamina. Their cytoplasm contains few organelles, accumulations of glycogen, and a large nucleus. (C) The short columnar cells of the inner enamel epithelium are separated from the acellular zone of the dental papilla by a basal lamina. (D) The cervical loop region of the enamel organ; the difference between the follicle and the acellular zone in (C) is apparent. The latter area has few collagen fibrils in the extracellular compartment where dentin formation eventually will occur. (B–D, From Egawa I: Electron microscopy of human enamel organ, *Shikwa Gakuho* 70:803–836, 1970.)

enzyme alkaline phosphatase (see Fig. 5.19B). Although these cells are histologically distinct from the cells of the inner enamel epithelium, both layers work synergistically and have been considered as a single functional unit responsible for the formation of enamel.

Fine Structure of the Enamel Organ at the Very Early Bell Stage

The fine structure of the tooth germ at the bell stage (see Fig. 5.15B–D) is uncomplicated but must be understood to appreciate the changes occurring to prepare for the formation of the dental hard tissue enamel and dentin. The enamel organ is supported by a basal lamina around its periphery. The outer enamel epithelial cells are low cuboidal and have a high nuclear/cytoplasmic ratio (little cytoplasm). Their cytoplasm contains free ribosomes, a few profiles of rough endoplasmic reticulum, some mitochondria, and a few scattered tonofilaments. Junctional complexes join adjacent cells. The star-shaped cells of the stellate reticulum are connected to each other, to the cells of the outer enamel epithelium, and to the stratum intermedium by desmosomes. Their cytoplasm contains all of the usual organelles, but these are distributed sparsely. The cells of the stratum intermedium are connected to each other and to the cells of the stellate reticulum and inner enamel epithelium also by desmosomes. Their cytoplasm also contains the usual complement of organelles and tonofilaments. The cells of the inner enamel epithelium have a centrally placed nucleus and a cytoplasm that contains free ribosomes, a few scattered profiles of rough endoplasmic reticulum, evenly dispersed mitochondria, some tonofilaments, a poorly developed Golgi complex situated toward the stratum intermedium, and high glycogen content.

Dental Papilla and Follicle

The dental papilla is separated from the enamel organ by a basal lamina from which a mass of fine aperiodic fibrils extends into an acellular zone (see Fig. 5.15C). These fibrils correspond to the lamina fibroreticularis of the basal lamina, and the first secreted enamel matrix proteins accumulate there (see Chapters 7 and 8). The cells of the dental papilla appear as undifferentiated mesenchymal cells, having an uncomplicated structure with all the usual organelles in sparse amount. A few fine scattered collagen fibrils occupy the extracellular spaces. The dental papilla is referred to as the *tooth pulp* when the first calcified matrix appears at the cuspal tip of the bell-stage tooth germ.

The dental papilla extends around the rim of the enamel organ to form the dental follicle (see Figs. 5.15A and 5.16). The dental follicle is distinguished clearly from the dental papilla in that many more collagen fibrils occupy the extracellular spaces between the follicular

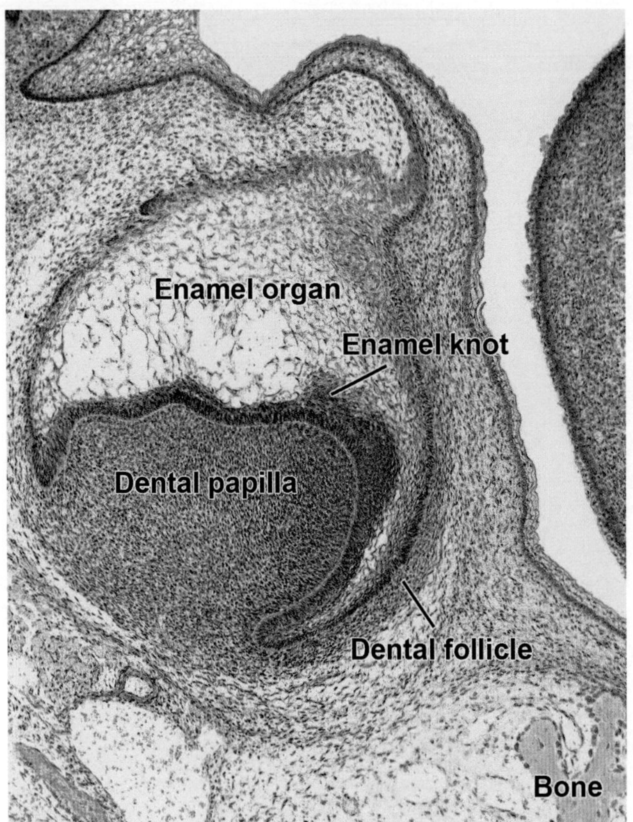

Fig. 5.16 Advanced cap-stage tooth germ showing the position of the enamel knot. The dental papilla extends around the rim of the enamel organ to form the dental follicle. (Courtesy Y. Zhang.)

fibroblasts; these generally are oriented circularly around the dental organ and dental papilla.

Breakup of the Dental Lamina and Crown Pattern Determination

Two other important events occur during the bell stage (see Fig. 5.20). First, the dental lamina (and the lateral lamina) join the tooth germ to the oral epithelium fragments, eventually separating the developing tooth from the oral epithelium. Second, the inner enamel epithelium completes its folding, making it possible to recognize the shape of the future crown pattern of the tooth.

Fragmentation of the dental lamina results in the formation of discrete clusters of epithelial cells, some of which persist and are given the name *epithelial pearls.* These clusters of cells may form small cysts (eruption cysts) over the developing tooth and delay eruption, may give rise to odontomas, or may be activated to form supernumerary teeth. The ability to form teeth suggests that these structures have been exposed to all necessary signals and retain memory. By analogy, sharks have a perpetual dental lamina and continuously regenerate teeth and, as demonstrated by their ability to form supernumerary teeth, the epithelial pearls may hold the key to tooth regeneration.

An important consequence of the fragmentation of the dental lamina is that the tooth continues its development within the tissues of the jaw divorced from the oral epithelium. Thus before the tooth can function, it must reestablish a connection with the oral epithelium and penetrate it to reach the occlusal plane. This penetration of the lining epithelium by the tooth is a unique example of a natural break in the epithelial barrier of the body. Integrity is reestablished by formation of a special seal around the tooth, the junctional epithelium. The causative factors responsible for gingivitis, and most likely periodontal disease, pass through this junction when integrity is compromised.

The folding that occurs as the crown develops results from intrinsic growth caused by differential rates of mitotic division within the inner enamel epithelium. The cessation of mitotic division within cells of the inner enamel epithelium helps determine the shape of a tooth. When the tooth germ is growing rapidly during the cap-to-bell stage, cell division occurs throughout the inner enamel epithelium. As development continues, division ceases at a particular point because the cells are beginning to differentiate and assume their eventual function of producing enamel. The point at which inner enamel epithelial cell differentiation first occurs represents the site of future cusp development. Because the inner enamel epithelium is constrained between the cervical loop and cusp tip, continued cell proliferation causes the inner enamel epithelium to buckle and form a cuspal outline (Fig. 5.21). Thus the future cusp is pushed up toward the outer enamel epithelium.

Eventually differentiation of inner enamel epithelium and papilla cells sweeps down along the cusp slopes and is followed by the deposition of dentin and enamel first at the cusp tip. These two matrices are deposited face to face, thereby defining the dentinoenamel junction. The occurrence of a second zone of cell differentiation within the inner enamel epithelium leads to the formation of a second cusp, a third zone leads to a third cusp, and so on until the final cuspal pattern of the tooth is determined. As discussed previously, these zones are determined by molecular signals in the primary and secondary enamel knots.

VASCULAR AND NERVE SUPPLY DURING EARLY DEVELOPMENT

Much attention has been directed to the vascular and nerve supplies of the developing tooth because either or both somehow may be involved in the induction of teeth. The few existing studies on the development of vascular and nerve supplies to teeth in primates tend to agree with similar studies on smaller mammals. Thus the ensuing account is generalized across species.

Vascular Supply

Clusters of blood vessels are found ramifying around the tooth germ in the dental follicle and entering the dental papilla during the cap stage. Their number in the papilla increases, reaching a maximum during the bell stage when matrix deposition begins. Interestingly, the vessels entering the papilla are clustered into groups that coincide with the position where the roots will form. With age, the volume of pulpal tissue diminishes, and the blood supply becomes progressively reduced, affecting the viability of the tissue. Angiogenesis, which is essential for organ development and survival, has not been studied extensively during the process of tooth development. Many studies describe the vasculature of the tooth, but expression of angiogenic factors responsible for the development of blood vessels has received little attention. This area of research undoubtedly will further improve our understanding of the role of angiogenesis in tooth development.

The enamel organ is avascular, although a heavy concentration of vessels in the follicle exists adjacent to the outer enamel epithelium.

Nerve Supply

Pioneer nerve fibers approach the developing tooth during the bud-to-cap stage of development. The target of these nerve fibers clearly is the dental follicle; nerve fibers ramify and form a rich plexus around the tooth germ in that structure. Not until dentinogenesis begins, however, do the nerve fibers penetrate the dental papilla (pulp). Although a possible relationship has been assumed between the developing nerve

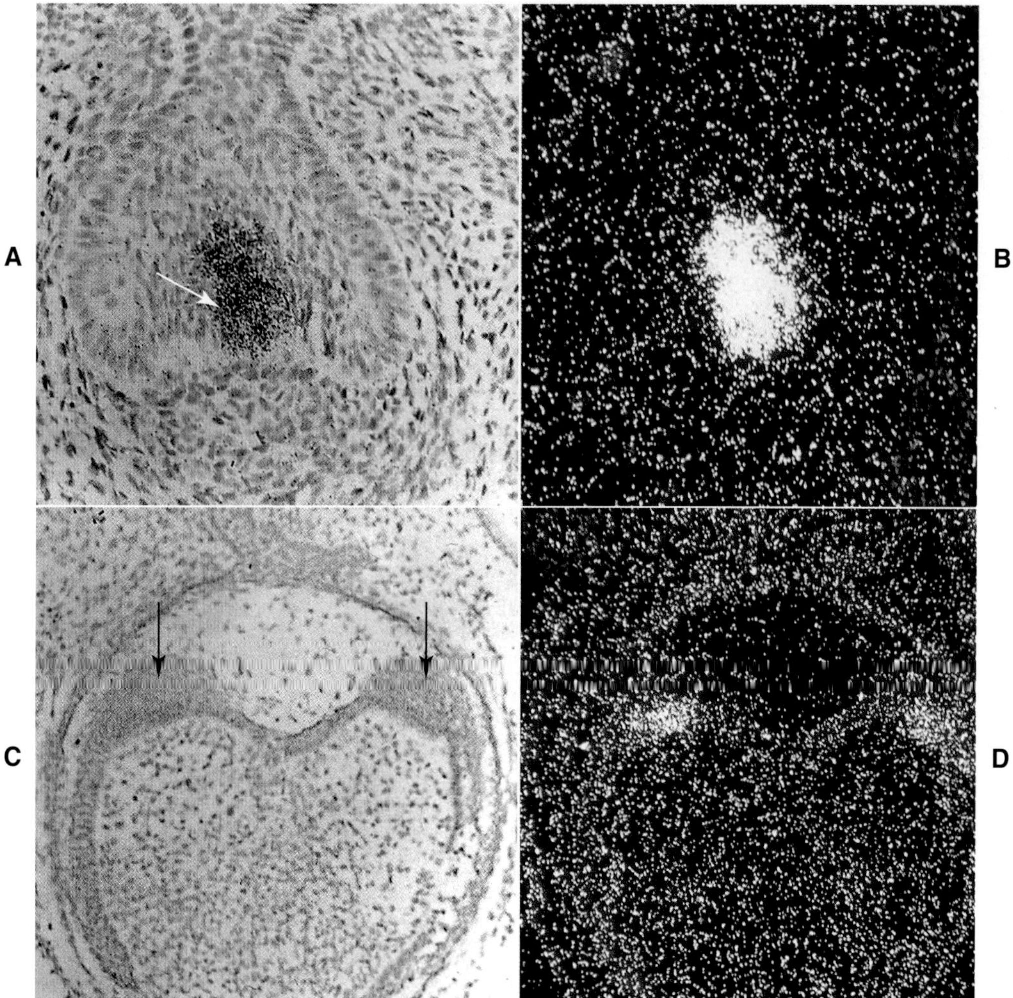

Fig. 5.17 Expression of *Fgf4* visualized by radioactive in situ hybridization technology in bright (A, C) and darkfield (B, D) light microscopy. Expression occurs in the enamel knot *(arrows)* at the cap (A, B) and early bell (C, D) stages of tooth development, indicating a relationship to crown pattern formation. (From Thesleff I, et al.: Regulation of organogenesis. Common molecular mechanisms regulating the development of teeth and other organs, *Int J Dev Biol* 39:35–50, 1995.)

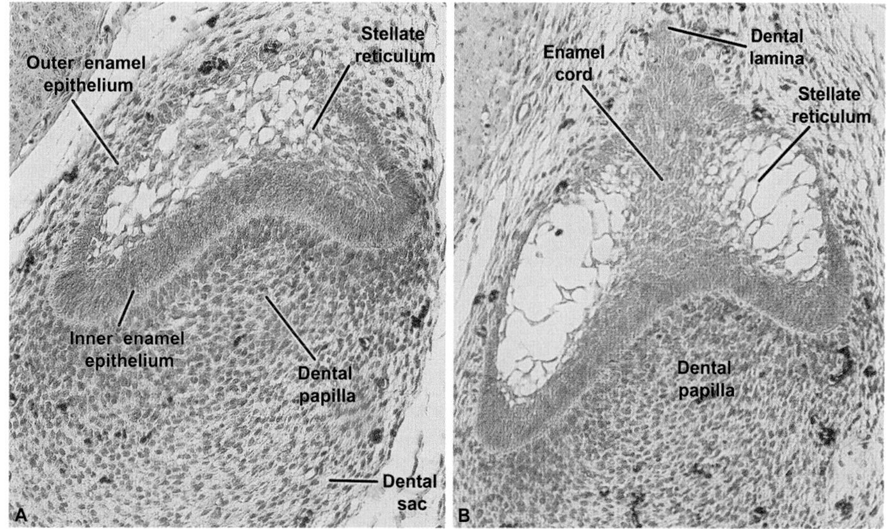

Fig. 5.18 (A, B) Histologic sections from a same cap-stage tooth organ. In some planes of section, the enamel organ seems to be divided by the enamel cord.

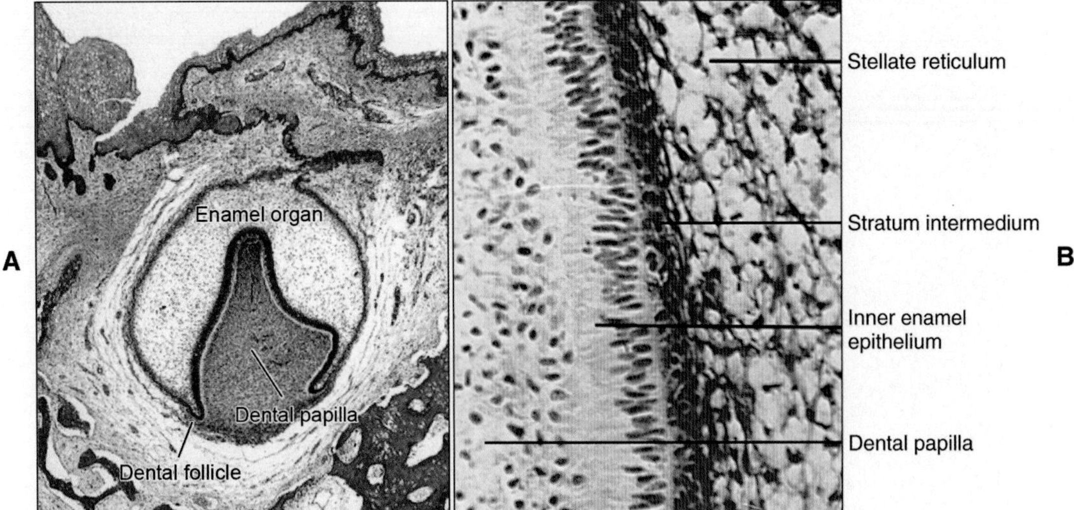

Fig. 5.19 Early bell stage of tooth development. (A) The undersurface of the enamel organ has deepened, giving the organ its bell shape. The dental papilla and dental follicle are evident. (B) The distribution of alkaline phosphatase in the early tooth germ is shown. Enzyme activity is demonstrated by the black precipitate localized largely in the stratum intermedium.

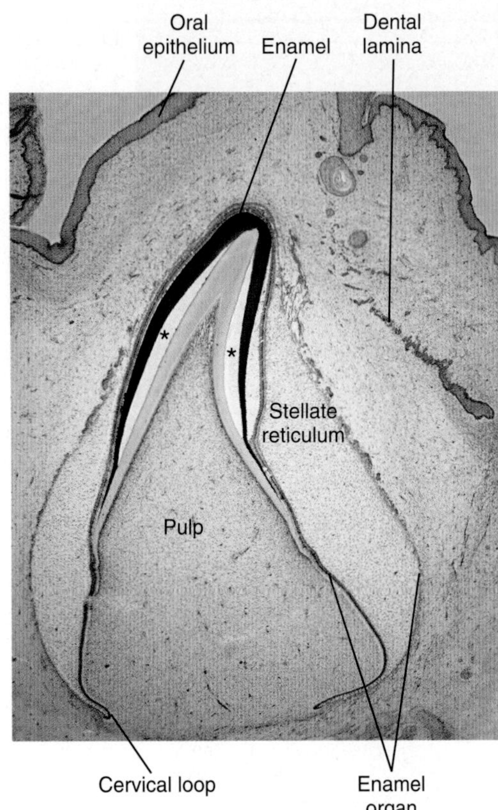

Fig. 5.20 Bell stage of tooth development. The dental lamina is disintegrating, so the tooth now continues its development divorced from the oral epithelium. The crown pattern of the tooth has been established by folding of the inner enamel epithelium. This folding has reduced the amount of stellate reticulum over the future cusp tip. Dentin and enamel have begun to form at the crest of the folded inner enamel epithelium. The space indicated by *asterisks* results from the artifactual detachment of the enamel from the dentin by tissue processing. (Courtesy B. Kablar.)

and blood supplies (i.e., that the nerves might supply the vessels), the timing differs in establishment of the papillary vascular and neural supplies. Furthermore, histochemical studies show that autonomic nerve fibers are absent from the makeup of the pioneer nerve fibers approaching the tooth germ. Thus the initial innervation of the developing teeth is concerned with the sensory innervation of the future periodontal ligament and pulp. At no time do nerve fibers enter the enamel organ.

The nerve growth factors neurotrophin, glial cell line–derived growth factor, and semaphorin are among the few nerve-related signaling molecules that have been studied during the process of tooth development. Interestingly, they seem to be expressed in a pattern that supports an early implication of innervation in tooth development. Just as multiple molecules are capable of stimulating axonal growth or migration, multiple molecules are likely involved in the early innervation of the tooth germ.

FORMATION OF THE PERMANENT DENTITION

So far, only the initial development of the deciduous (or primary) dentition has been described. The permanent (secondary) dentition also arises from the dental lamina. The tooth germs that give rise to the permanent incisors, canines, and premolars form as a result of further proliferative activity within the dental lamina at its deepest extremity. This increased proliferative activity leads to the formation of another tooth bud on the lingual aspect of the deciduous tooth germ (Figs. 5.22 and 5.23), which remains dormant for some time. Because mice are monophyodont and form only one set of teeth, they are not ideal models to study the formation of replacement teeth. However, other mammals, such as miniature pigs and house shrews, are diphyodonts that develop successional teeth just like humans. Recent experiments using these new models have thus shed light on the regulation of tooth replacement. In particular, it was noticed that because deciduous teeth grow faster than the expansion of the surrounding alveolar sockets, mesenchymal cells of the tooth experience compressive forces. This compression acts as a mechanical signal and modulates downstream *Wnt* signaling to suspend the development of the permanent tooth

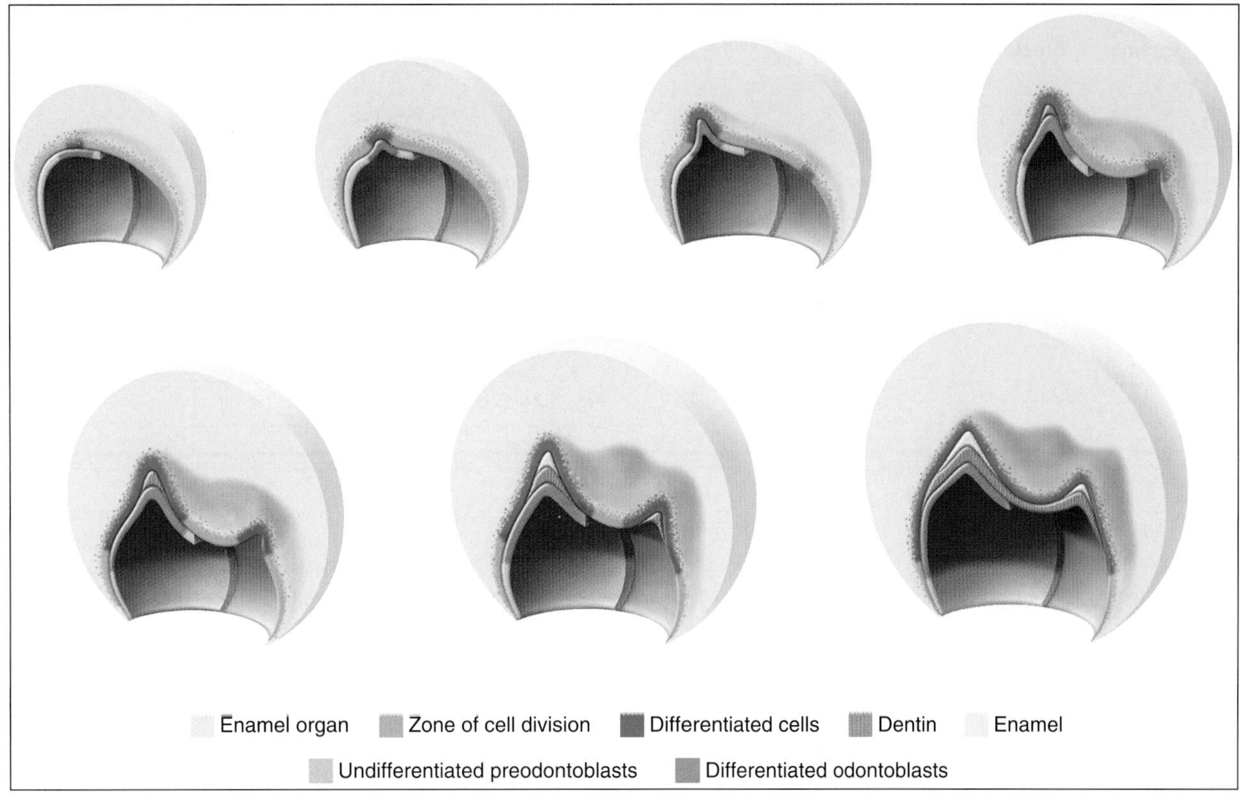

Fig. 5.21 Summary of crown pattern formation in the inner enamel epithelium.

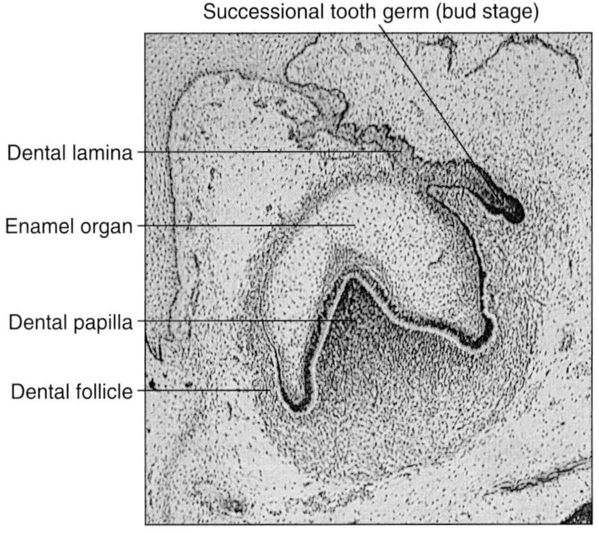

Fig. 5.22 Photomicrograph of the cap stage of tooth development. Further epithelial proliferation from the dental lamina at its deepest extremity forms the tooth bud of the successional tooth germ. This situation occurs only in relation to primary or deciduous tooth germs. (Courtesy E.B. Brain.)

germ in an arrested state. However, after the eruption of the deciduous tooth, the compression is released, and the permanent tooth germ resumes to develop. As a result, mechanical forces that arise due to differential growth between the primary tooth and the alveolar bone play an important role in determining the timing of permanent tooth development. In diphyodonts, the molars of the permanent dentition have no deciduous predecessors, so their tooth germs do not originate in the same way. Instead, when the jaws have grown long enough, the dental lamina burrows posteriorly beneath the lining epithelium of the oral mucosa into the ectomesenchyme. This backward extension successively gives off epithelial outgrowths that, together with the associated ectomesenchymal response, form the tooth germs of the first, second, and third molars (Figs 5.24 and 5.25). Because of this backward extension of the dental lamina of the forming mandible, on occasion teeth occur in the flattened, bony ramus of the adult mandible. The same biochemical and mechanical signaling cues regulating primary tooth development are, however, likely present during the initial formation of the permanent tooth as well.

Thus the teeth of the primary and secondary dentitions form in essentially the same manner, although at different times (see Fig. 5.25). The entire primary dentition is initiated between 6 and 8 weeks of embryonic development, the successional permanent teeth between week 20 in utero and 10 months after birth, and the permanent molars between week 20 in utero (first molar) and 5 years of age (third molar). Aberrations in this pattern of development result in missing teeth or the formation of extra teeth.

HARD TISSUE FORMATION

The next step in the development of the tooth is terminal differentiation of ameloblasts and odontoblasts and formation of the two principal hard tissues of the tooth, the dentin (the specialized hard connective tissue forming the bulk of the tooth) and the enamel, a process called *histodifferentiation.*

Fig. 5.26 provides a summary of key histologic features leading to the formation of enamel and dentin, and Table 5.4 provides an approximate timeline of tooth development up to the crown stage. Until the crown assumes its final shape during the cap to early bell stage, all cells

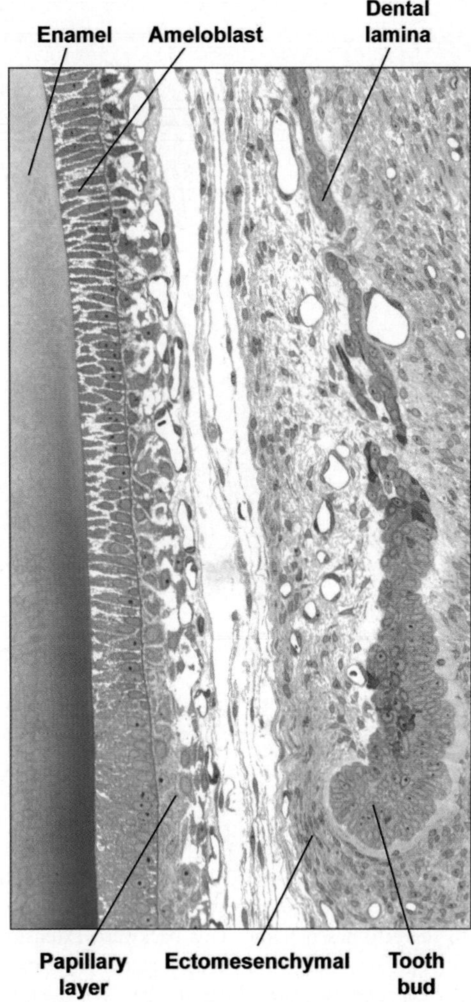

Fig. 5.23 Histologic section showing a higher magnification of the permanent tooth bud at the extremity of the fragmenting dental lamina adjacent to a primary tooth at an advanced stage of crown formation. Note the clear space separating the bud from the surrounding mesenchymal cells.

of the inner enamel epithelium continually divide. Thereafter, until the tooth crown attains its full size, only cells at the cervical margin of the enamel organ divide. At the sites of the future cusp tips, where a layer of dentin will first appear, mitotic activity ceases, and the short columnar cells of the inner enamel epithelium elongate and reverse polarity, becoming taller with their nuclei aligned adjacent to the stratum intermedium and the Golgi complex facing the dental papilla. A second junctional complex develops apically above the Golgi, thereby separating the differentiating ameloblast into a cell body and an apical cell extension above the complex. By definition, the base of a cell lies against the basal lamina. Hence before inner epithelial cells change polarity, the base of the cell faces the dental papilla (a basal lamina separates the inner enamel epithelium and dental papilla), and the apex faces the stratum intermedium. When they reverse polarity, the embryonic base becomes the functional apex, and the embryonic apex becomes the functional base; hence the apical portions of ameloblasts now face the papilla.

As these morphologic changes occur in the cells of the inner enamel epithelium, changes also occur within the adjacent dental papilla.

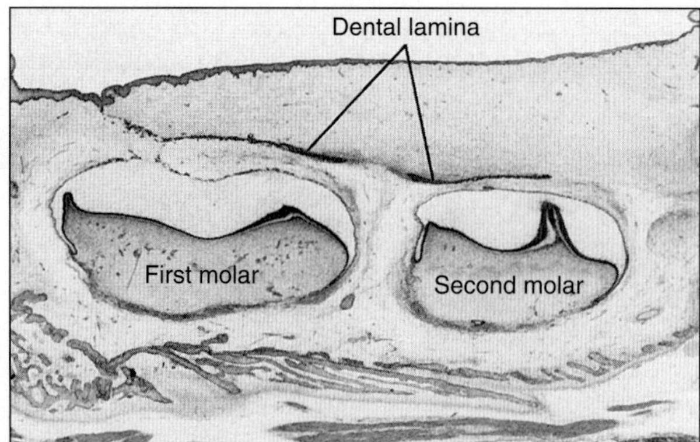

Fig. 5.24 Sagittal section through the distal part of a developing jaw showing the incipient permanent molar tooth germs.

The undifferentiated ectomesenchymal cells increase rapidly in size and ultimately differentiate into odontoblasts, the dentin-forming cells. This increase in size of the papillary cells eliminates the acellular zone between the dental papilla and the inner enamel epithelium. Tissue culture experiments have established that the differentiation of odontoblasts from the undifferentiated ectomesenchyme of the dental papilla is initiated by an organizing influence from the cells of the inner enamel epithelium. In the absence of epithelial cells, no dentin develops. The epithelial cells of the inner enamel epithelium are inductive and have been shown to express and secrete several growth factors. The ectomesenchymal cells of the dental papilla assume competence only after a set number of cell divisions, after which they presumably express the appropriate cell-surface receptors able to capture the growth factors.

As development continues, progressive differentiation of the cells of the inner enamel epithelium down the cusp slopes and differentiation of odontoblasts in the papilla take place. The odontoblasts, as they differentiate, begin to elaborate the organic matrix of dentin, which ultimately mineralizes. As the organic matrix is deposited, the odontoblasts move toward the center of the dental papilla, leaving behind a cytoplasmic extension around which dentin is formed. In this way the tubular character of dentin is established. Chapter 8 gives a full account of dentin formation (dentinogenesis).

Just before the first layer of dentin forms (mantle dentin), differentiating inner enamel epithelium cells (ameloblasts) secrete some enamel proteins, which do not accumulate as a layer (discussed in Chapter 7). These first proteins, together with other molecules (including growth factors), may play a role in the epithelial-mesenchymal signaling that leads to the terminal differentiation of odontoblasts, possibly by interacting with components of the basal lamina that separates them. Differentiating inner enamel epithelium and dental papilla cells transiently expresses proteins from the other cell types before assuming fully their own secretory activity. The reason for this transient secretory output still is not understood but may be part of the process for phenotype acquisition. Inner enamel epithelium cells continue their differentiation into ameloblasts that produce organic matrix against the newly formed dentinal surface. Almost immediately, this organic matrix mineralizes and becomes the initial enamel layer of the crown. Thus, although enamel protein secretion occurs before mantle dentin is visible on the crown, these proteins do not assemble as a layer until dentin forms. The enamel-forming cells, the ameloblasts, move away from the dentin, leaving behind an ever-increasing thickness of enamel. Chapter 7 deals fully with the process of enamel formation (amelogenesis).

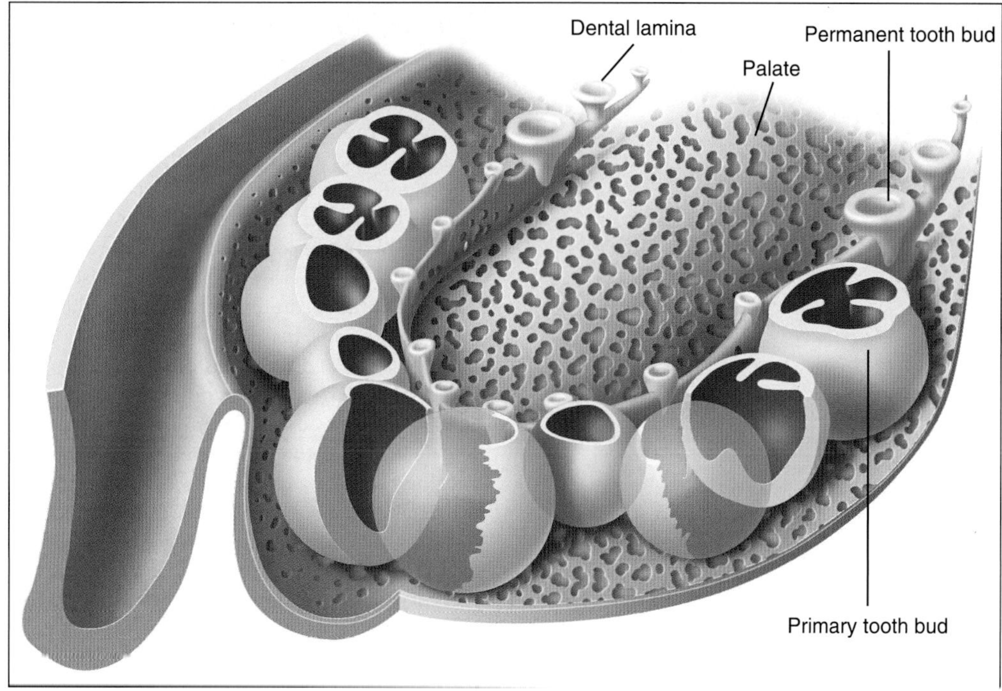

Fig. 5.25 Schematic representation of tooth development in situ. Tooth germs of the primary and permanent dentition are shown in the maxilla.

For these events to take place normally, differentiating odontoblasts must receive signals from differentiating ameloblasts (inner enamel epithelium), and vice versa—an example of reciprocal signaling.

Before formation of the first dentin, cells of the enamel organ and, in particular, those of the inner enamel epithelium receive nourishment from two sources: blood vessels located in the dental papilla and vessels situated along the periphery of the outer enamel epithelium. When the dentin is formed, it cuts off the papillary source of nutrients, causing a drastic reduction in the amount of nutrients reaching the enamel organ. This reduction occurs when the cells of the inner enamel epithelium are about to actively secrete enamel, and thus the demand for nutrients increases. The demand is satisfied by an apparent collapse of the stellate reticulum and invagination of the outer enamel epithelium by blood vessels lying outside.

ROOT FORMATION

The root of the tooth consists of dentin covered by cementum. Two aspects of dentinogenesis have already been explained: (1) how the differentiation of odontoblasts from cells of the dental papilla is initiated by cells of the inner enamel epithelium and (2) how these cells initiate formation of crown dentin. It follows that epithelial cells also may be required to initiate the odontoblast, which eventually will form the dentin of the root. Once crown formation is completed, epithelial cells of the inner and outer enamel epithelium proliferate from the cervical loop of the enamel organ to form a transient bilayered epithelial structure known as *Hertwig epithelial root sheath*. Mesenchymal *BMP* signals are important for this process, as deletion of *Smad4*, a transcription factor downstream of *BMP* signals, maintains the cervical loop structure and *Sox2*-expressing dental epithelial stem cells. This sheath of epithelial cells extends around the dental pulp between the latter and the dental follicle until it encloses all but the basal portion of the pulp. The rim of this root sheath, the epithelial diaphragm, encloses the primary apical foramen. As the inner epithelial cells of the root sheath progressively enclose more and more of the expanding dental pulp, they initiate the differentiation of odontoblasts from ectomesenchymal cells at the periphery of the pulp, facing the root sheath. These cells eventually form the dentin of the root. In this way a single-rooted tooth is formed (Fig. 5.27).

Multirooted teeth are formed in essentially the same way. To picture multiple root formation, one must imagine the root sheath as a skirt hanging from the enamel organ. Visualizing two opposing tongues of epithelium folding into the pulp and growing toward each other from this collar allows an appreciation of how a primary apical foramen is bisected into two secondary apical foramina and how, if three tongues are formed, three secondary apical foramina arise (Fig. 5.28). Hertwig epithelial root sheath extends around each apical foramen, forming as many epithelial tubes that evolve similarly as in single-rooted teeth. Aberrations in this splitting of the primary apical foramen can lead to the formation of pulpoperiodontal canals at the sites of fusion of the epithelial tongues.

An intact root sheath extending from the cervical loop to the apical foramen can be demonstrated in histologic sections only at the initial stages of root formation. In fact, the root sheath disintegrates as root formation progresses, and it remains intact only at the advancing root edge where cell division takes place, and the process of root induction continues until the root is complete. As the root sheath fragments, it leaves behind a number of discrete clusters of epithelial cells, separated from the surrounding connective tissue by a basal lamina, known as the *epithelial cell rests of Malassez* (Fig. 5.29). In adults these epithelial cell rests persist next to the root surface within the periodontal ligament. Although apparently functionless, there is now growing evidence that these cell rests play an active role and can be activated to participate in periodontal repair and regeneration. They also represent a potential source to extract dental epithelial cells for tooth bioengineering.

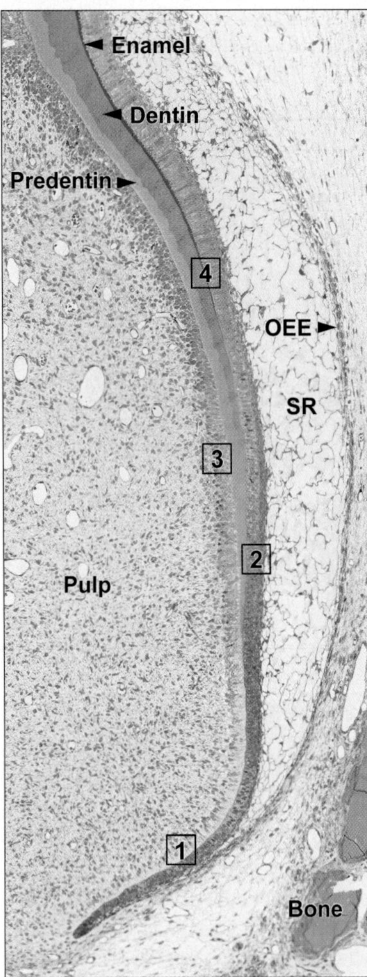

Fig. 5.26 Photomicrograph illustrating some key features of tooth crown formation. At *1,* the epithelium is separated from the dental papilla by an acellular zone. At *2,* the cells of the inner enamel epithelium have elongated, and the acellular zone begins to be eliminated as odontoblasts differentiate from ectomesenchymal cells in the tooth pulp. At *3,* the odontoblasts retreat toward the center of the pulp, leaving behind formed dentin. At *4,* the cells of the inner enamel epithelium, now ameloblasts, begin to migrate outward and leave behind formed enamel. *OEE,* Outer enamel epithelium; *SR,* stratum reticulum.

TABLE 5.4 Timeline of Human Tooth Development

Age	Developmental Characteristics
42–48 Days	Dental lamina formation
55–56 Days	Bud stage: deciduous incisors, canines, and molars
14 Weeks	Bell stage for deciduous teeth; bud stage for permanent teeth
18 Weeks	Dentin and functional ameloblasts in deciduous teeth
32 Weeks	Dentin and functional ameloblasts in permanent first molars

The histologic features of root development and of formation of the associated hard tissues are well established and are considered in detail in Chapter 9. However, the molecular signaling and regulatory mechanisms leading to root morphogenesis and development are still not fully elucidated. Current information indicates that, like in the crown, the *Tgfβ/BMP, Wnt, Fgf,* and *Shh* signaling pathways are also implicated.

TOOTH ERUPTION

Tooth development occurs within the bone of the developing jaw in bony crypts separate from the oral epithelium. Soon after formation of the root is initiated, the tooth begins to erupt (i.e., move in an axial direction) until it assumes its final position in the mouth with its occlusal surface in the occlusal plane. The possible mechanisms of tooth eruption are discussed in Chapter 10; for this discussion, it is necessary only to recognize the axial movement of the tooth.

In erupting, the crown of the tooth must escape from its bony crypt and pass through the lining mucosa of the oral cavity. As eruptive movement begins, the enamel of the crown is still covered by a layer of ameloblasts and remnants of the other three layers of the enamel organ. These are sometimes difficult to distinguish, and, together, the ameloblasts and adjacent cells form the reduced enamel epithelium (Fig. 5.30). The bone overlying the erupting tooth soon is resorbed, and the crown passes through the connective tissue of the mucosa, which is broken down in advance of the erupting tooth. The reduced dental epithelium and the oral epithelium fuse and form a solid mass of epithelial cells over the crown of the tooth. The central cells in this mass degenerate, forming an epithelial canal through which the crown of the tooth erupts (Fig. 5.31) and leaving cellular debris on the crown. In this way, tooth eruption is achieved without exposing the surrounding connective tissue and without hemorrhage.

As the tooth pierces the oral epithelium, another significant development occurs: The dentogingival junction forms from epithelial cells of the oral epithelium and the reduced enamel epithelium (Fig. 5.32). The importance of this junction already has been stressed (its histologic appearance is discussed in detail in Chapter 12).

FORMATION OF SUPPORTING TISSUES

While roots are forming, the supporting tissues of the tooth also develop. At the bell stage, the tooth germ consists of the enamel organ, dental papilla, and dental follicle; this last component is a fibrocellular layer investing the dental papilla and enamel organ. The supporting tissues of the tooth are traditionally believed to arise from the dental follicle. As the root sheath fragments, ectomesenchymal cells of the dental follicle penetrate between the epithelial fenestrations and become apposed to the newly formed dentin of the root (Fig. 5.33). In this situation, these cells differentiate into cementum-forming cells (or cementoblasts). Chapter 9 also discusses the alternate possibility that some cells from Hertwig epithelial root sheath may transform directly into cementoblasts and may give rise to other periodontal components. These cells elaborate an organic matrix that becomes mineralized and in which collagen fiber bundles of the periodontal ligament become anchored. The cells of the periodontal ligament and the fiber bundles also differentiate from the dental follicle. Some recent evidence indicates that the bone in which the ligament fiber bundles are embedded also is formed by cells that differentiate from the dental follicle.

In conclusion, this chapter has described the formation of the teeth and their supporting tissues in straightforward terms (Fig. 5.34). Although there has been significant progress in understanding tooth crown formation, the molecular biology of root development has only recently been described in molecular terms. The root likewise undergoes morphogenesis, and the molecular events regulating this aspect are the subject of great interest. The role of nerves and of angiogenesis in tooth development also needs more attention. Progress in these areas is fundamental for achieving tooth regeneration.

The histology and cell biology of the various tooth components and of its supporting structural tissues are further discussed in subsequent chapters.

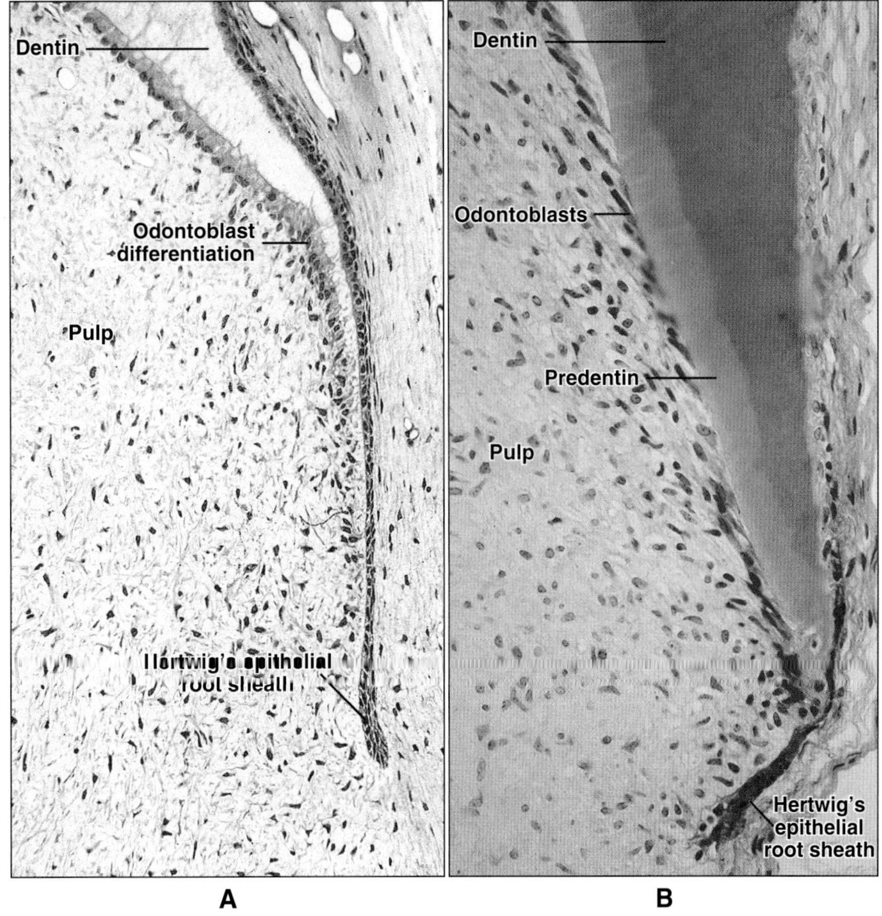

Fig. 5.27 Photomicrographs summarizing root formation. (A) The root is beginning to form as an extension of the inner and outer enamel epithelia in the cervical loop region, which form a bilayered structure (Hertwig epithelial root sheath). The root sheath will induce differentiation of odontoblasts from the radicular pulp. (B) The differentiation of odontoblasts and the formation of root dentin are shown.

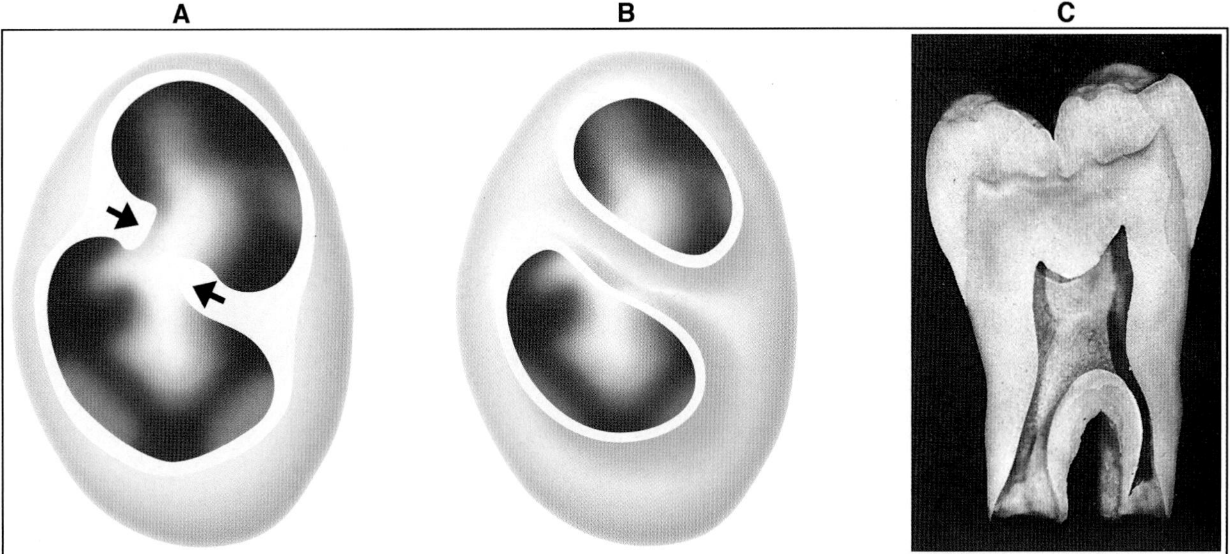

Fig. 5.28 (A, B) Root formation of a two-rooted tooth as seen on the undersurfaces of developing tooth germs. (C) Section of a tooth with developing root. The roots have not finished forming, and the division into two roots is clearly visible.

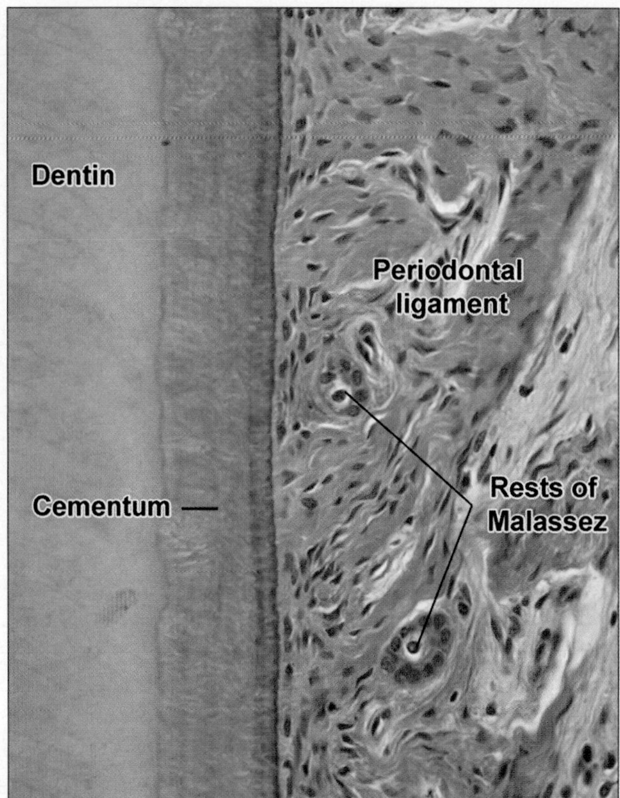

Fig. 5.29 Photomicrograph of the periodontal ligament showing the epithelial cell rests of Malassez (remnants of Hertwig epithelial root sheath) situated along cementum.

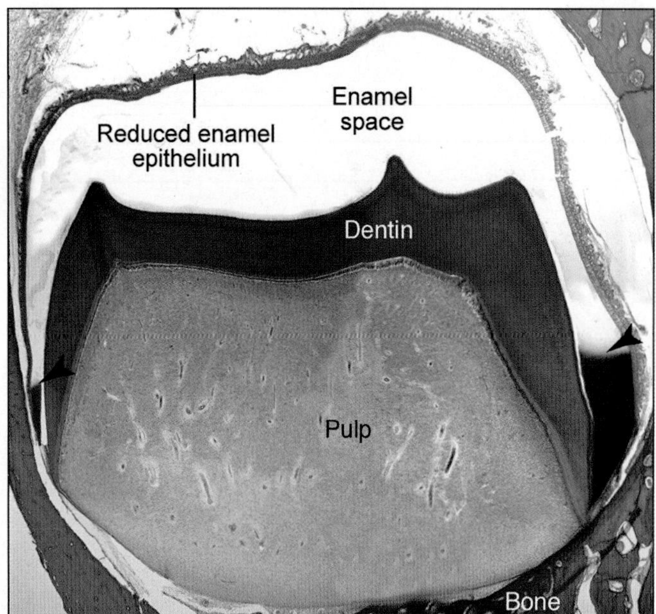

Fig. 5.30 Tooth bud in which crown formation is almost completed. The formation of hard tissues is well advanced. Because of demineralization during section preparation, the enamel has been lost from this specimen, except at the cervical margin *(arrowheads)*.

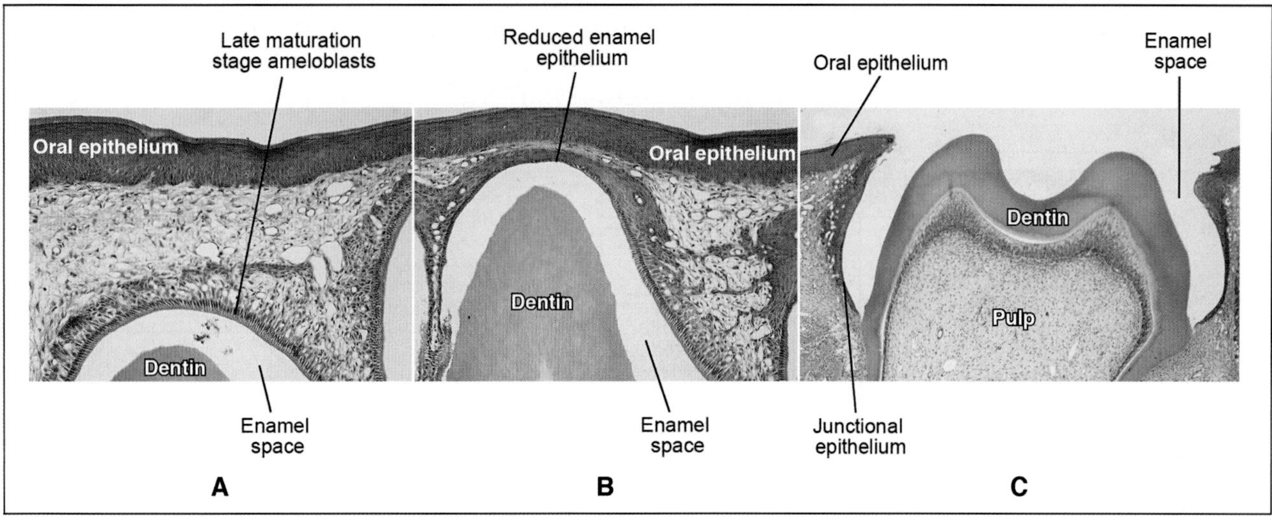

Fig. 5.31 Erupting tooth. (A) As the tooth approaches the oral epithelium, a thin layer of connective tissue separates the enamel organ from the oral epithelium. (B, C) As the connective tissue is lost, the two epithelia come in contact and will fuse along the lateral aspect of the tooth crown. This lateral fusion allows epithelial continuity to be maintained at all times as the central part of the crown pierces the oral epithelium.

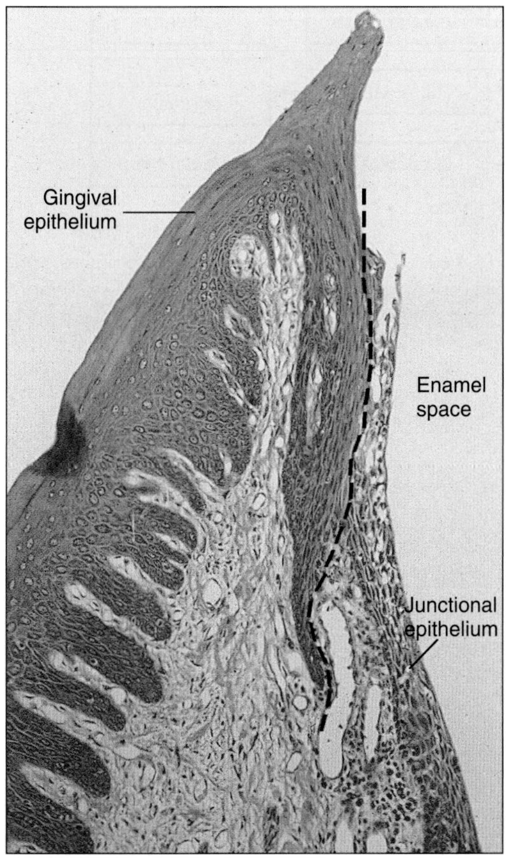

Fig. 5.32 Formation of the dentogingival junction from the oral and dental epithelia. The dashed line separates junctional epithelium from oral epithelium.

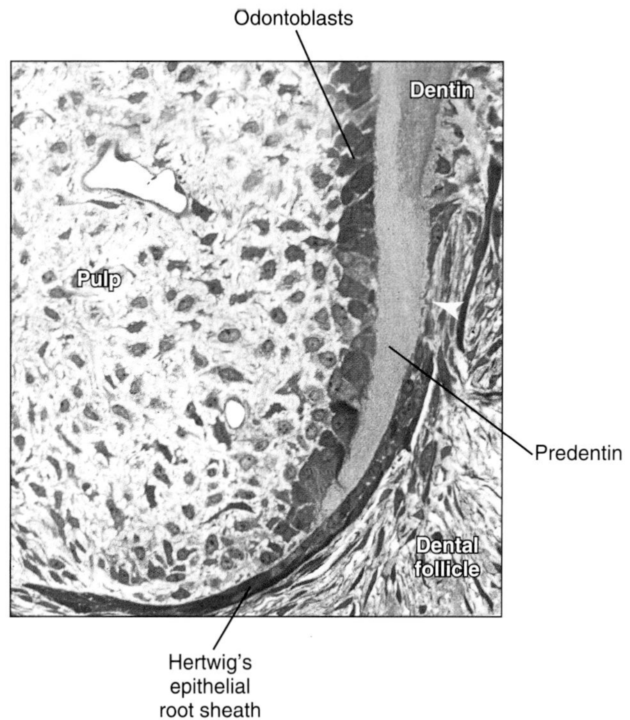

Fig. 5.33 Fragmentation of the root sheath and the formation of cementum. Follicular cells have been proposed to migrate through the break area *(arrowhead)*.

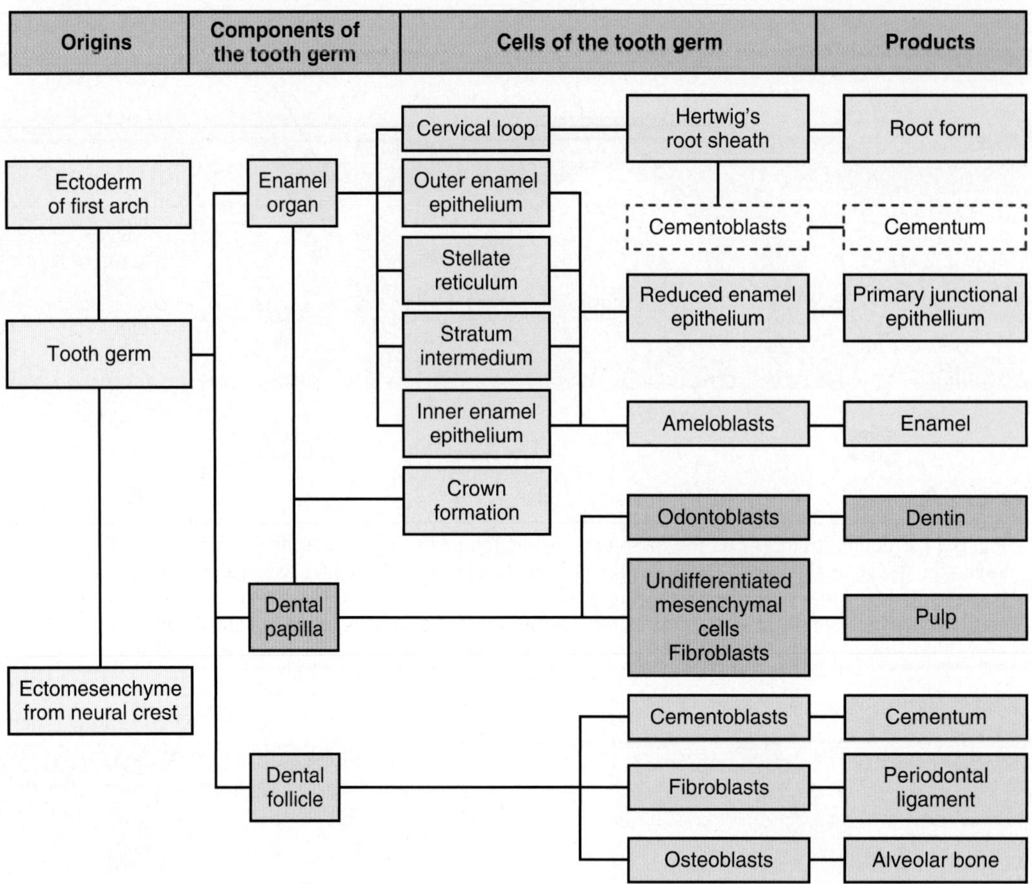

Fig. 5.34 Summary of tooth formation.

RECOMMENDED READING

Cobourne MT, Sharpe PT: Making up the numbers: the molecular control of mammalian dental formula, *Semin Cell Dev Biol* 21:314–324, 2010.

Li J, et al.: Cellular and molecular mechanisms of tooth root development, *Development* 144:374–384, 2017.

Mitsiadis TA, Luder H: Genetic basis for tooth malformations: from mice to men and back again, *Clin Genet* 80:319–329, 2011.

Thesleff I: Molecular genetics of tooth development. In Moody SA, editor: *Principles of developmental genetics*, ed 2, London, 2015, Elsevier Academic Press.

Bone

Antonio Nanci and Pierre Moffatt

OUTLINE

Bone is a mineralized connective tissue consisting by dry weight of about 67% mineral and 33% organic matrix (Fig. 6.1). The organic matrix contains about 28% type I collagen and 5% noncollagenous matrix proteins. The major noncollagenous matrix proteins and their general function are listed in Table 6.1. This organic matrix is permeated by substituted hydroxyapatite ($Ca_{10}[PO_4]_6[OH]_2$) in the form of small platelets, which lodge in the holes and pores of collagen fibrils as well as within the interfibrillar spaces (see Chapter 1).

The structural organization and composition of bone reflect the activity of the cells involved in the formation of the organic matrix. Bone from different anatomic sites, developmental stages, and species exhibits different bulk biochemical properties, organizations, and relative proportions of collagenous and noncollagenous components. Variations also exist at the microenvironmental level in the proportion of noncollagenous matrix proteins; indeed, regions containing a paucity or an abundance of these proteins can be found next to each other, reflecting local tissue dynamics.

In addition to its obvious functions of support, protection, and locomotion, bone constitutes an important reservoir of minerals. Systemically, hormonal factors control the bone physiology; locally, mechanical forces (including tooth movement), growth factors, and cytokines also have regulatory functions. Also, there is now evidence that there is central nervous system control of bone mass mediated by a neuroendocrine mechanism. Bone resists compressive forces best and tensile forces least. Fractures of bone thus occur most readily because of tensile and slicing stresses.

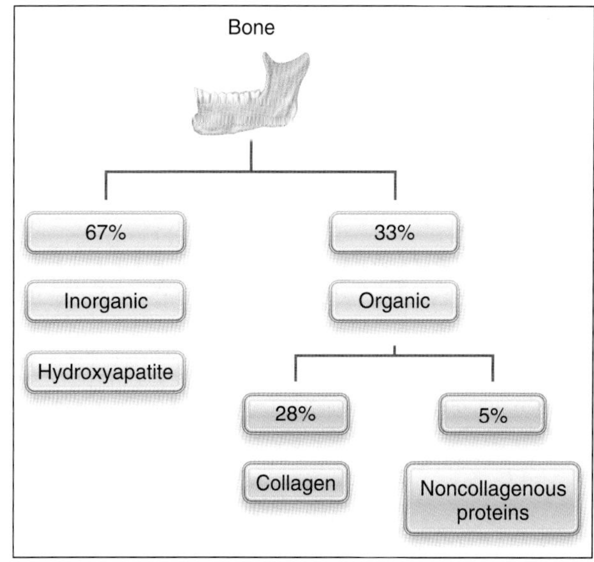

Fig. 6.1 Chemical composition of dry bone.

GROSS BONE HISTOLOGY

Bones have been classified as long or flat based on their gross appearance and on their physical characteristics (Table 6.2). Long bones include the bones of the limbs (tibia, femur, radius, ulna, and humerus) and of the axial skeleton (vertebrae). Flat bones include all bones of the skull plus the sternum, ribs, scapula, and pelvis. Other types of bones, called *sesamoids,* are embedded in tendons (e.g., patella [kneecap]).

Characteristic of all bones are a dense outer sheet of compact bone and a central, medullary cavity. This cavity is filled with red or yellow bone marrow that is interrupted, particularly at the extremities of long bones, by a network of bone trabeculae. Terms used to describe this network include *trabecular, cancellous,* and *spongy bone* (Fig. 6.2). Compact and trabecular bone behave differently and have different metabolic responses.

Mature or adult bones, whether compact or trabecular, are histologically identical in that they consist of microscopic layers (lamellae). Three distinct types of layering are recognized: circumferential, concentric, and interstitial (Figs. 6.3, 6.4, and 6.5). Circumferential lamellae enclose the entire adult bone, forming its outer and inner perimeters. Concentric lamellae make up the bulk of compact bone and form the basic metabolic unit of bone, the osteon (also called the *Haversian system*) (see Fig. 6.4). The osteon is a cylinder of bone, generally oriented parallel to the long axis of the bone. In the center of each is a canal, the Haversian canal, which is lined by a single layer of

TABLE 6.1 Major Noncollagenous Proteins Found in Bone

Type	General Function
Glycosaminoglycan-Containing Molecules	
Aggrecan	Matrix organization
Biglycan	Binds to collagen
Decorin	Binds to collagen
Glycoproteins	
Alkaline phosphatase	Increases local phosphate concentration
Osteonectin	Collagen organization
Periostin	Collagen organization and mechanical signals
Tenascin	Cell-matrix interactions
Small Integrin-Binding Ligand, N-Glycosylated Protein	
Bone sialoprotein	Involved in initial mineralization and bone resorption
Dentin sialophosphoprotein	Regulates mineralization
Dentin matrix protein 1	Regulates osteocyte function
Matrix extracellular phosphoprotein	Regulates phosphaturic hormone activity
Osteopontin	Regulates mineralization
Arginine-Glycine-Aspartic Acid–Containing Glycoproteins	
Fibronectin	Cell attachment
Thrombospondins	Cell attachment
Vitronectin	Cell attachment
Gamma-Carboxy glutamic Acid-Containing Proteins	
Matrix-Gla protein	Negative regulator of mineralization
Osteocalcin	Hormone, bone remodeling
Serum Proteins	
Albumin	Inhibitor of crystal growth
α2HS-glycoprotein	Inhibits calcification

From Robey PG, Boskey AL: The composition of bone. In Rosen CJ, et al., editors: *Primer on the metabolic bone diseases and disorders of mineral metabolism,* ed 8, Washington, DC, 2013, American Association for Bone and Mineral Research.

bone cells that cover the bone surface; each canal houses a capillary. Adjacent Haversian canals are interconnected by Volkmann's canals; these channels, like Haversian canals, contain blood vessels, thus creating a rich vascular network throughout compact bone. Interstitial lamellae are interspersed between adjacent concentric lamellae and fill the spaces between them. Interstitial lamellae are fragments of preexisting concentric lamellae from osteons created during remodeling that can take a multitude of shapes. It should be noted that the structure of the osteon, with its elaborate network of concentric rings and canals typically observed in human bone, is much less developed and even absent in other species such as rodents.

Surrounding the outer aspect of every compact bone is a connective tissue membrane, the periosteum, which has two layers. The outer layer of the periosteum consists of a dense, irregular connective tissue

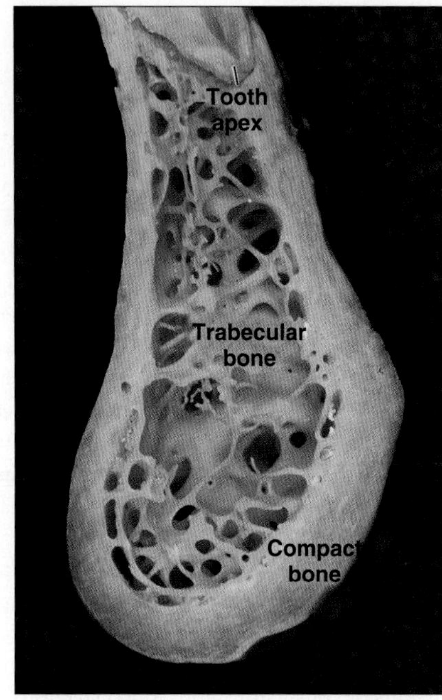

Fig. 6.2 Body of the mandible. The outer layer of compact bone and an inner supporting network of trabecular bone can be distinguished clearly.

TABLE 6.2 Bone Terminology

Appearance	Bone Type	Example
Gross appearance	Flat	Skull, pelvis, scapula
	Long	Appendicular skeleton
Macroscopic appearance	Compact	Mature bone; flat bones and shaft of long bones
	Spongy/cancellous/trabecular	Early embryonic bone; interior of extremities of long bones
Development/formation	Intramembranous	Direct transformation of mesenchyme
	Endochondral	From a cartilage model
Regions	Diaphysis	Shaft
	Metaphysis	Transitional portion of the shaft leading to the growth plate zone
	Epiphysis	Extremities of long bones
Microstructure	Embryonic/woven	Irregular collagen network
	Lamellar	Collagen arranged in concentric layers
Disposition of lamellae	Circumferential	Found on periosteal and endosteal surfaces
	Osteonic	Concentric lamellae forming osteons
	Interstitial	Residual fragments between osteons
Types of osteons	Primary	The first formed Haversian systems (osteons) consisting of poorly organized lamellae
	Definitive	Higher orders of osteons formed after remodeling of primary osteons

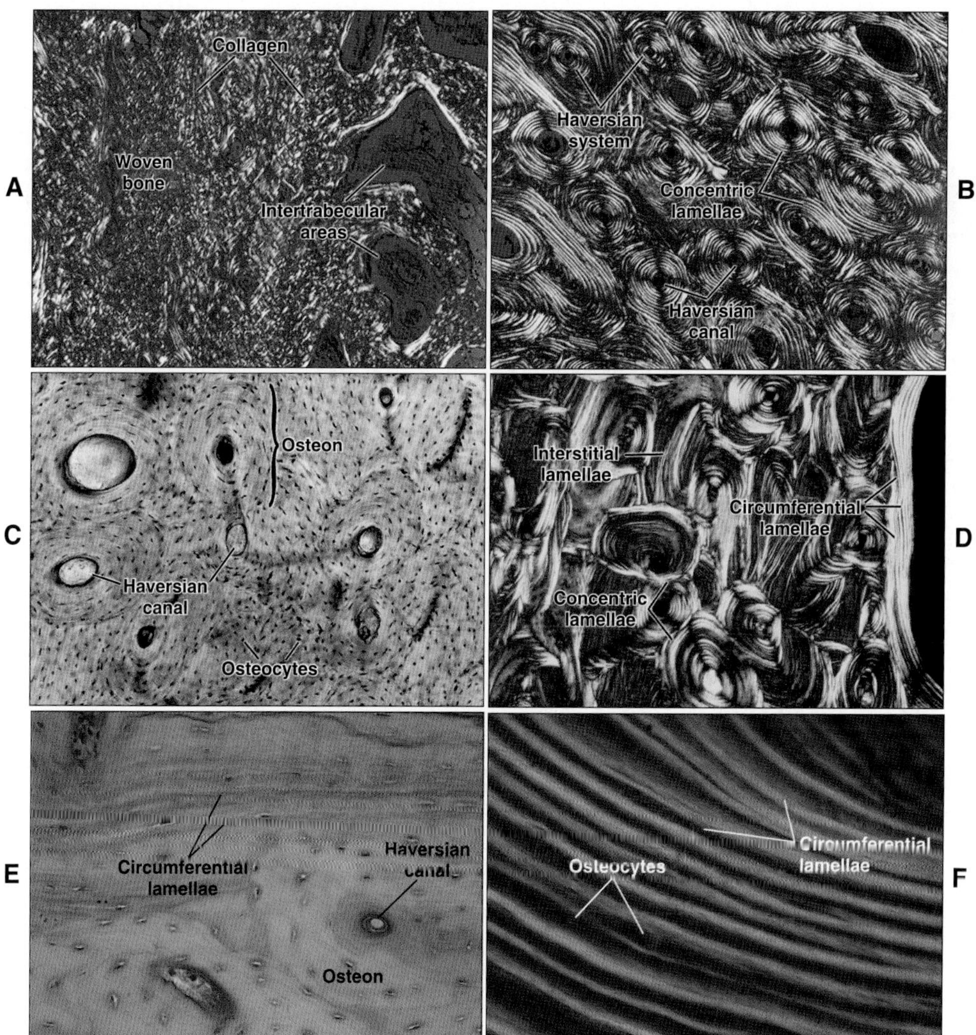

Fig. 6.3 The organization of collagen and the various lamellae are seen readily using phase-contrast microscopy (A, B, D). (A) Embryonic (woven) bone is characterized by randomly oriented collagen fibrils. (B–F) Collagen fibrils in lamellar bone assume a layered organization, including circumferential, concentric, and interstitial lamellae. Interstitial lamellae are interspersed between osteons, these represent fragments of preexisting concentric lamellae. Circumferential lamellae enclose the inner (D) and outer (E, F) aspects of bone. (Courtesy P. Tambasco de Oliveira.)

termed the *fibrous layer*. The inner layer of the periosteum, next to the bone surface, consists of bone cells, their precursors, and a rich microvascular supply. The internal surfaces of compact and cancellous bone are covered by endosteum. However, this layer is not well demarcated and consists of loose connective tissue containing osteogenic cells, which physically separates the bone surface from the marrow within. In general, the periosteal surface of bone is more active in bone formation than the endosteal one.

BONE CELLS

Different cells are responsible for the formation, resorption, and maintenance of osteoarchitecture. Two cell lineages are present in bone, each with specific functions: (1) osteogenic cells, which form and maintain bone, and (2) osteoclasts, which resorb bone (Figs. 6.6, 6.7, and 6.8). Osteogenic cells have variable morphology (including osteoprogenitors, preosteoblasts, osteoblasts, osteocytes, and bone-lining cells) representing different maturational stages. The differentiation sequence from osteoprogenitor to preosteoblast shows no distinctive morphologic features, and much research interest is focused on finding molecular markers for the various stages of the osteogenic life cycle. Yet, there are known markers that are expressed at different stages of differentiation/maturation, and these play sequential roles in the process. Mutations in gene expressed in such a cell-type–specific context have been found to disrupt the normal function of many key proteins, causing either loss of function or gain of function, and consequently cause a variable spectrum of skeletal syndromes in humans (Table 6.3).

Osteoblasts

Osteoblasts are mononucleated cells that synthesize the organic matrix of bone. Osteoblasts arise from pluripotent stem cells, which are of mesenchymal origin in the axial and appendicular skeleton and of ectomesenchymal origin (neural crest cells that migrate in mesenchyme) in the head. Although osteoblasts are differentiated cells, both preosteoblasts and osteoblasts can undergo mitosis during prenatal development and occasionally during postnatal growth. Both cell types exhibit high levels of alkaline phosphatase activity on the outer surface of their plasma membrane (Fig. 6.9). Functionally, the enzyme cleaves inorganically bound phosphate. The liberated phosphate likely contributes to the initiation and progressive growth of bone mineral crystals (hydroxyapatite). However, the function of alkaline phosphatase in bone-forming cells is likely complex and is not yet defined completely. It has been shown that active osteoblasts express the bone-restricted interferon-inducible transmembrane (IFITM)–like (BRIL) membrane protein, a member of the IFITM protein family (Fig. 6.10). Like alkaline phosphatase, the precise function of BRIL is not yet fully defined, but this protein is a marker of sites where bone is actively forming, and a mutation in this protein has been associated with a type of osteogenesis imperfecta.

Osteoblasts are plump, cuboidal cells (when very active) or slightly flattened cells that are primarily responsible for the production of the organic matrix of bone (Fig. 6.11; see also Figs. 6.7 and 6.8). They exhibit abundant and well-developed protein synthetic organelles. At the light microscopic level, the Golgi complex characteristically appears as a clear, paranuclear area that can be defined easily after cytochemical reactions for Golgi-resident enzymes (see Figs. 6.8A and 6.11A and B). The secretory matrix products of osteoblasts include type I collagen, the dominant component of the organic matrix; small amounts of other collagens, including types V and XII; proteoglycans; and several noncollagenous proteins. The type I collagen molecule is formed and assembled, as in fibroblasts and odontoblasts (see Chapters 4 and 8), within the rough endoplasmic reticulum (rER) and Golgi compartments. Complex II–coated vesicles are implicated in the translocation of secretory cargo from the rER to the Golgi. Research suggests that, because of the large size of the procollagen fibrils (300–400 nm), these fibrils may use larger

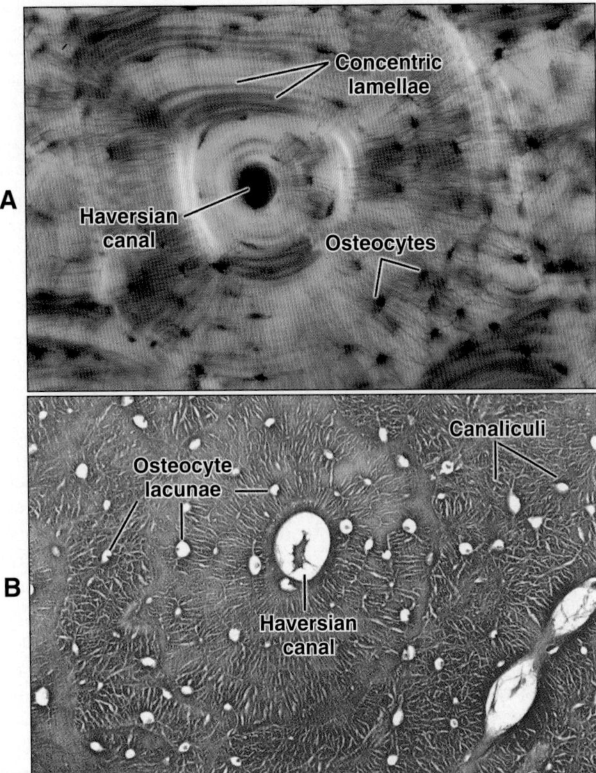

Fig. 6.4 As seen here with two different imaging modalities (A, polarized light and B, bright light), the osteon is the basic organizational unit in lamellar bone and is particularly evident in compact bone. It consists of concentric lamellae that form a cylinder of bone with a vascular canal—the Haversian canal—at its center. Numerous osteocytes are entrapped in these lamellae. These cells reside in lacunae and their processes in interconnecting canaliculi that form an extensive network for the diffusion of nutrients and the transduction of local bone status. (Courtesy P. Tambasco de Oliveira.)

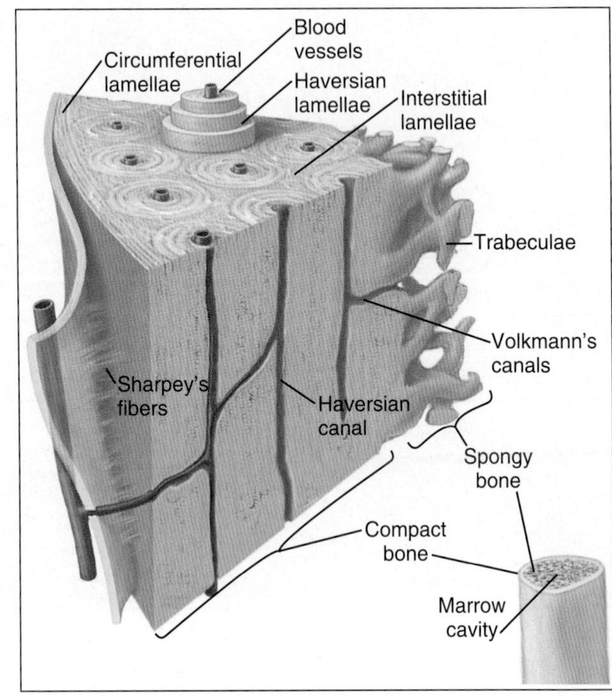

Fig. 6.5 Organizational components of bone. (From Pollard TD, Earnshaw WC: *Cell biology*, Philadelphia, PA, 2002, Saunders.)

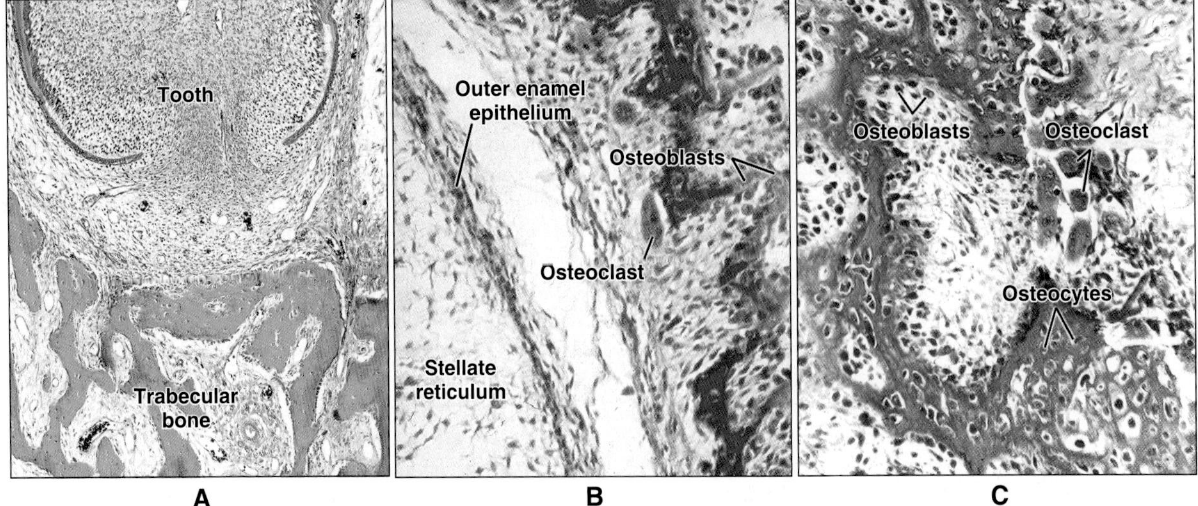

Fig. 6.6 Light microscopic views of embryonic mandibular bone. (A) The bone forms by intramembranous ossification and initially assumes a trabecular organization. (B) Plump-looking osteoblasts line forming bone surfaces. (C) The abundance of large osteocytes entrapped in the bone and the presence of numerous osteoclasts indicate that the bone trabeculae are being formed and turned over rapidly.

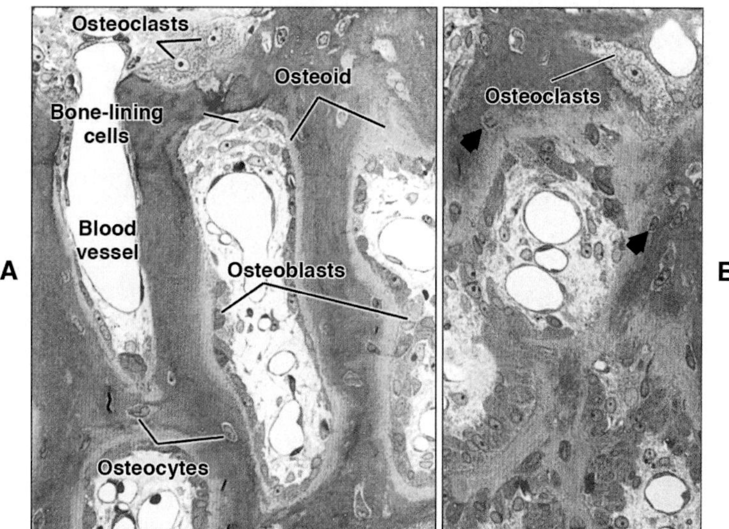

Fig. 6.7 (A) Mandibular bone soon after birth. By this time the bone has undergone substantial turnover and appears more compact (compare with Fig. 6.6). Bone-forming surfaces are covered by plump osteoblasts or flattened, less active cells. Quiescent areas are covered by bone-lining cells. Osteoclasts usually are found opposite actively forming bone surfaces. (B) Osteocytes *(arrows)* are present within the calcified matrix *(dark blue)* and in some cases within osteoid *(pale blue)*.

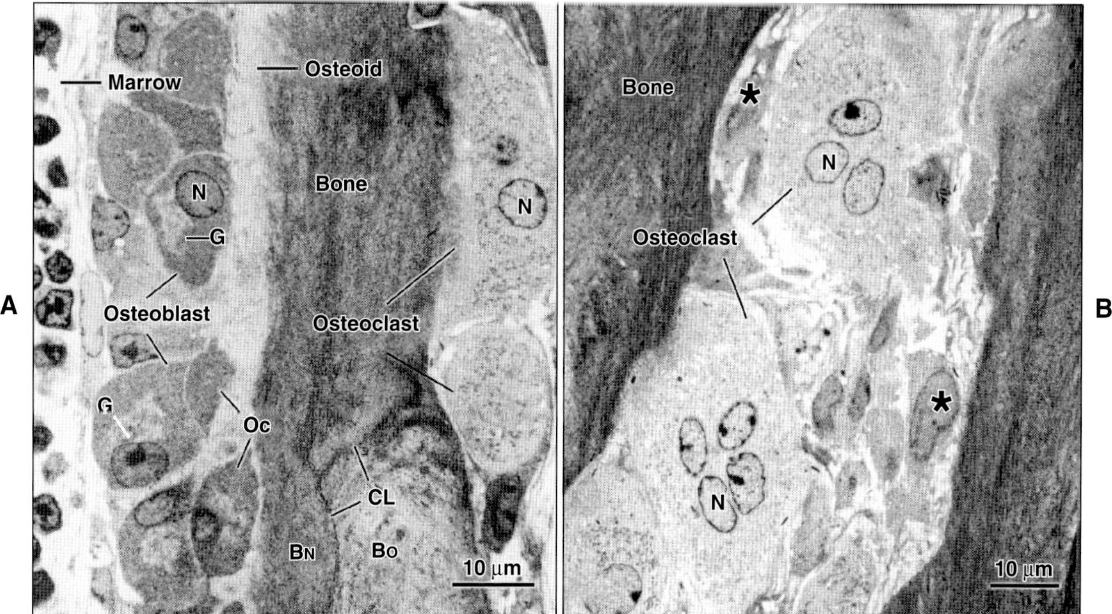

Fig. 6.8 Immunohistochemical preparation for osteopontin process for imaging by backscatter electron imaging in the scanning electron microscope. Such preparation results in the formation of fine, dark peppery precipitates over bone that denote the site and concentration of this noncollagenous matrix protein. (A) Bone trabecula being formed along one surface by osteoblasts and resorbed by osteoclasts on the other. Osteoblasts form a layer of cuboidal cells, with an eccentric nucleus *(N)* and a large paranuclear Golgi complex (*G*; which appears as a clear cytoplasmic region) apposed to osteoid. Some of the osteoblasts are entrapped in osteoid as osteocytes *(Oc)*. Osteopontin is not distributed uniformly throughout the calcified bone matrix; one site where osteopontin is concentrated is in cement lines *(CL)* at the interface between old *(BO)* and new *(BN)* bone. (B) Osteoclasts are large, multinucleated cells that often work as groups to resorb bone. Mononucleated cells accompany them; some of these mononucleated cells *(asterisks)* eventually differentiate into osteoblasts to produce new bone on the resorbed surface.

complex II–coated tubules (tunnels) for translocation from the ER to the *cis*-Golgi. The spheric and cylindric distentions of the Golgi complex are believed to represent different stages of procollagen processing and packaging (see Fig. 6.11C). The typical elongated, electron-dense, collagen-containing secretory granules release their contents primarily along the surface of the cell apposed to forming bone. Without going into much detail, there are several steps of high complexity required for collagen assembly and secretion. Each requires a vast number of chaperones and accessory molecules along the secretory pathway, which are all essential for proper collagen

TABLE 6.3 Examples of Human Diseases Caused by Genetic Mutations in Different Bone Cells

Cell Type	Gene	Mutation	Inheritance	Syndrome	Main Characteristics	OMIM
Chondrocytes	*COL2A1*	LOF	AD	Achondrogenesis type II	Micromelic dwarfism, small chest, prominent abdomen, incomplete ossification of vertebral bodies, disorganization of the costochondral junction	200610
	SOX9	LOF	AD	Campomelic dysplasia	Short and bowed long bones, hypoplastic scapulae, narrow iliac wings, cleft palate	114290
Osteoblast precursors	*RUNX2*	LOF GOF	AD AD	Cleidocranial dysplasia Metaphyseal dysplasia and maxillary hypoplasia with brachydactyly	Open cranial sutures, dental anomalies, hypoplasia of clavicles, metaphyseal flaring of long bones, dysmorphism of the mandible, enlarged clavicles, brachydactyly	119600 156510
	SP7	LOF	AR	Osteogenesis imperfecta (type 12)	Low bone mass, fractures	613849
Mature osteoblast	*ALPL*	LOF	AD/AR	Hypophosphatasia	Hypomineralized skeleton dental anomalies	241510
	COL1A1/ COL1A2	LOF	AD	Osteogenesis imperfecta (type 1–4)	Low bone mass, bone fractures and bowing, dentinogenesis imperfecta, growth retardation	166200
	SERPINH1 (HSP47)	LOF	AR	Osteogenesis imperfecta (type 10)	Bone deformities and fractures, generalized osteopenia, dentinogenesis imperfecta	613848
	LRP5	LOF GOF	AR	Osteoporosis-pseudoglioma syndrome Osteopetrosis (OPTA1)	Low bone mass, fractures, blindness, osteosclerosis, cortical thickening of long bones/cranial vault hearing loss	259770 607634
Osteocytes	*PHEX*	LOF	XD	Hypophosphatemic rickets X-linked	Bone deformities, short stature, dental anomalies, phosphate wasting	307800
	SOST	LOF	AR	Sclerosteosis/Van Buchem disease	Sclerosing bone dysplasia, skeletal overgrowth, syndactyly	269500/ 239100
Osteoclasts	*TNFSF11 (RANKL)*	LOF	AR	Osteopetrosis (OPTB2)	Mandibular prognathism, genu valgum, anemia, tendency to fracture dental anomalies	259710
	ACP5 (TRAP)	LOF	AR	Spondyloenchondrodysplasia with immune dysregulation	Short stature, rhizomelic micromelia, increased lumbar lordosis, facial anomalies	607944

AD, Autosomal dominant; *AR*, autosomal recessive; *GOF*, gain of function; *LOF*, loss of function; *OMIM*, Online Mendelian Inheritance in Man; *XD*, X-linked dominant.

synthesis, proper modification, and final assembly. To a different extent, mutations found in genes encoding such accessory molecules (see Table 6.3, *SERPINH1*) significantly disrupt extracellular collagen matrix assembly and lead to low bone mass syndromes.

These molecules assemble extracellularly as fibrils and accumulate as a layer of uncalcified matrix called *osteoid (prebone)* (see Fig. 6.11D and E). Some debate still continues as to whether the noncollagenous proteins are contained within the collagen secretory granules or in a distinct population of granules. Irrespective of this aspect, noncollagenous proteins also are released mainly along the surface of osteoblasts apposed to osteoid and diffuse from the osteoblast surface toward the mineralization front where they participate in regulating mineral deposition. Near the mineralization front, mineralization foci can be seen within osteoid, and certain noncollagenous proteins, such as bone sialoprotein (BSP) and osteopontin (OPN), accumulate within them (Fig. 6.12).

In addition to structural matrix proteins, osteoblasts, their precursors, or both secrete a number of cytokines and growth factors that help regulate cellular function and bone formation. These include several members of the bone morphogenetic protein (BMP) superfamily, such as BMP2, BMP7, and transforming growth factor beta (TGF-β), in addition to insulin-like growth factors (IGF1 and IGF2), platelet-derived growth factor (PDGF), fibroblast growth factor (FGF), and wingless-related integration site (WNT). WNT molecules are small, secreted glycoproteins that act extracellularly to regulate different processes (development, growth, patterning, stemness, cancer). Although the timing of secretion and the complex interactions of these growth factors remain to be clarified, the combinations of IGF1, TGF-β, and PDGF increase the speed of bone formation and bone repair and are being considered for dental therapy. For instance, these combinations may be used to speed healing and bone growth after periodontal surgery or to prevent periodontal disease by the early treatment of periodontal pockets. Similarly, these factors may be used to enhance osseous integration after placement of dental implants. WNT is also showing promises in these regards.

The great importance of WNT signaling in bone biology is evolutionarily conserved and extraordinarily complex, deserving a more in-depth description. The complexity is illustrated by the presence of, depending on the context, tissue origin and cell-type specificity, 19 WNTs, 7 receptors (Frizzled [FZD]), 2 coreceptors (low-density lipoprotein receptor-related protein 5 [LRP5] or LRP6), 5 soluble FZD-related receptors (sFRP), and several secreted inhibitors (Dickkopfs [DKKs], sclerostin [SOST], SOST domain containing protein 1 [SOSTDC1], WNT inhibitory factor 1 [WIF1]). Secretion of WNT proteins in bone by osteoblasts and osteocytes is also highly coordinated

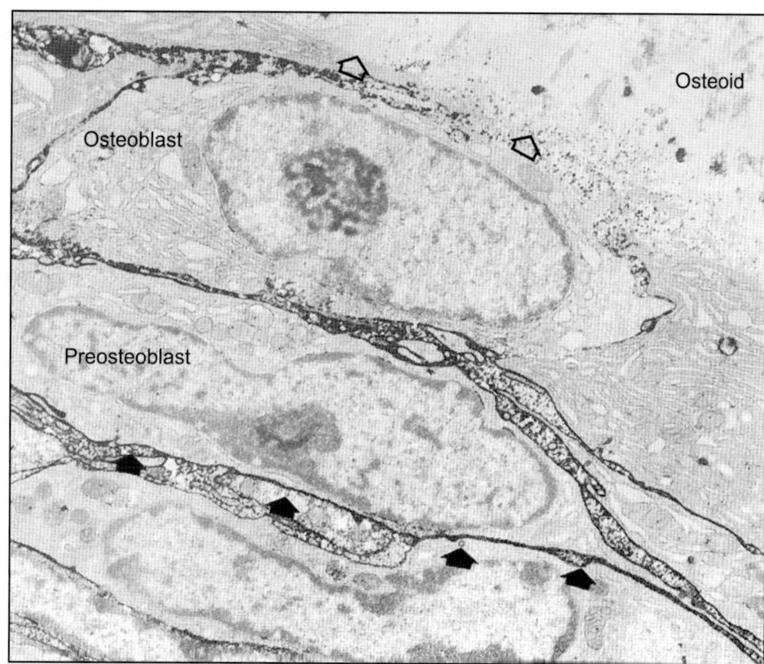

Fig. 6.9 Calvarial preosteoblasts and osteoblasts demonstrating histochemical localization of alkaline phosphatase along the plasma membrane *(solid arrows)*. The amount of enzyme on the secretory surface *(empty arrows)* of the osteoblasts is significantly less or is absent (direction of secretory surface, *empty arrows*). (Courtesy L. Watson.)

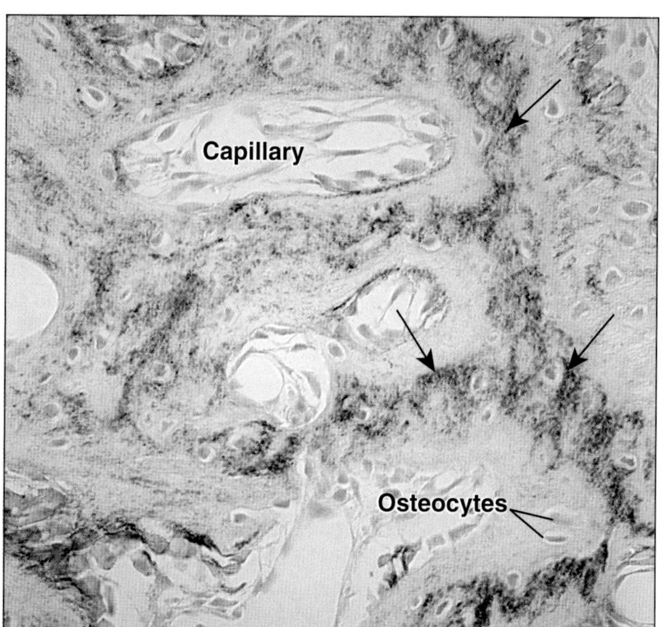

Fig. 6.10 Immunohistochemical localization of bone-restricted IFITM–like (BRIL) in rat alveolar bone. Labeling for BRIL is found on surfaces with active bone formation *(arrows)*.

and requires additional special intracellular machinery. Hence two transmembrane proteins (porcupine [PORCP] and WNTless [WLS]; or G protein–coupled receptor 177 [GPR177] in mammals) are necessary for this process to occur adequately. PORCP is an acyltransferase enzyme responsible for the covalent linkage of a monounsaturated form of palmitate (*cis*-Δ9-palmitoleate) onto a serine residue of WNT. Palmitoleoylated WNT is required for its interaction with GPR177, a chaperone that will escort WNTs during trafficking from the Golgi en route to the cell surface for secretion, and eventually for receptor binding and signaling. Lipidation imparts on WNT molecules a very hydrophobic nature that restricts their extracellular diffusion once secreted. Therefore WNTs have been known to not travel at great distance and to act mostly locally in an autocrine or paracrine fashion. Cells have devised shielding molecules (e.g., Secreted Wingless-interacting molecule [SWIM]) to increase WNT solubility and traveling distance capability. Once outside in the extracellular space, WNTs can also be inactivated through removal of the fatty acid moiety by a secreted hydrolase called NOTUM.

Active WNTs go on to bind receptors on neighboring cell surfaces where they initiate different signaling cascades depending on the receptor that is engaged. At least two such pathways can be elicited, either canonic or noncanonic. The canonic pathway requires recruitment of single-span transmembrane coreceptors (LRP5 or 6) that engage into a signalosome complex. Phosphorylation of the intracellular domain of LRP5/6 recruits a scaffolding complex comprising several different cytoplasmic molecules, including AXIN, disheveled, and glycogen synthase kinase-3 beta (GSK3β). Sequestration of GSK3β to the cytoplasmic tail of LRP5/6 will prevent it from phosphorylating β-catenin, culminating in its stabilization, accumulation, and translocation in the nucleus. In cells not exposed to WNT ligands, cytoplasmic levels of β-catenin are kept low through polyubiquitination and proteasomal degradation. Once in the nucleus, β-catenin interacts with transcription factors of the T-cell factor/lymphoid enhancer-binding factor family and activates transcription for a diverse set of target genes, such as *Myc, Axin,* and *Dkk1*. As discussed in Chapter 4, β-catenin is also implicated in molecular interactions defining adherens junctions.

The noncanonic branch of WNT signaling, known as *planar cell polarity,* also involves FZD receptors but interacting with another set of coreceptors, such as the tyrosine kinase ROR or RYK2. Depending on the accessory cytoplasmic proteins recruited, these can go on to trigger activation of several different intracellular cascades (RHO/ROCK, Ca^{2+}, JNK, PLC, PKC, PI3K/AKT, and mammalian target of rapamycin [mTOR]). In turn, many different phosphorylation events will

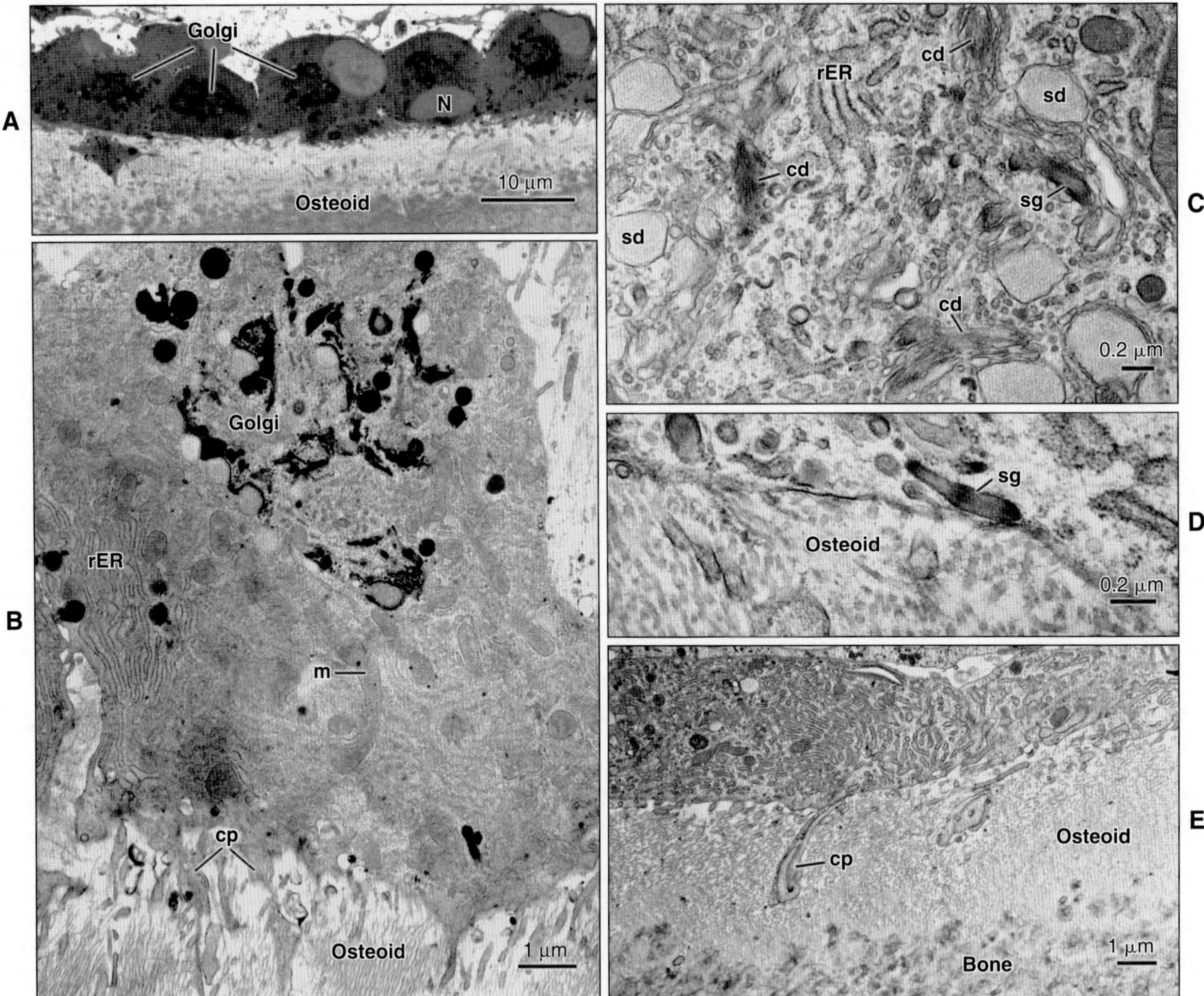

Fig. 6.11 Light level (A) and electron microscope (B–D) micrographs of active osteoblasts. (A) and (B) are cytochemical preparations for pH-dependent phosphatase activity in the Golgi complex. (B–D) These cells contain an extensive Golgi complex surrounded by abundant rough endoplasmic reticulum *(rER)* profiles. (C) The Golgi saccules exhibit spheric *(sd)* and cylindric *(cd)* distentions characteristic of collagen-producing cells. (D) The cylindric distentions bud off from the Golgi complex to form secretory granules *(sg)*. These collagen-containing granules are typically elongated structures with regions of increased electron density. (E) As osteoblasts reduce their synthetic activity, they flatten, and protein synthetic organelles, particularly the Golgi complex, become reduced. *cp,* Cell process; *m,* mitochondria; *N,* nucleus.

be initiated that affect nuclear transcription factor activity and gene expression. Among others, the noncanonic pathway will influence cell movement and polarity, and thereby tissue patterning.

WNT signaling will also evoke many feedback and feedforward mechanisms to either terminate or enhance its own signaling; this can be accomplished in many different ways. For instance, many sFRP have been identified that act as decoys in the extracellular space to capture and neutralize WNTs before they can reach and trigger cell-surface receptors/coreceptors. Other secreted proteins are also involved through different mechanisms in quenching WNT signaling activity, such as WIF1, SOST, SOSTDC1, and DKKs.

However, many components have clearly been identified as key to the maintenance of a healthy skeleton in humans. Among others (see Table 6.3), inactivating mutations in the WNT coreceptor LRP5 causes the low bone mass osteoporosis pseudoglioma syndrome, whereas gain-of-function mutations cause the opposite, osteosclerosis. Furthermore, mutations in the *SOST* gene were found to be causative for the high bone mass in sclerosteosis and Van Buchem disease. More recently, multiple inactivating mutations found in WNT1 were associated with early-onset osteoporosis and osteogenesis imperfecta, giving rise to poorly mineralized and brittle bones.

All these studies have paved the way to many therapeutic approaches, whether for early-onset (childhood) brittle bone diseases or later (adult) postmenopausal osteoporosis. Although several potential targets within the WNT pathway are being scrutinized for drug development, SOST has by far been exploited most successfully in preclinical studies and now under clinical settings. Given the negative inhibitory role of SOST, one strategy was to generate a monoclonal neutralizing antibody against it. Inhibiting the inhibitor proved to be a successful approach to increase WNT signaling in bone and to favor a positive balance toward formation. Although investigated first in the context of adult osteoporosis, this therapeutic intervention is now turning to pediatric cases for the treatment of osteogenesis imperfecta. The advantage of SOST as a target is that its expression is confined to bones, being expressed almost exclusively by osteocytes, and its effects are believed to be local, not systemic. Therefore the likelihood of the therapy affecting other organs is

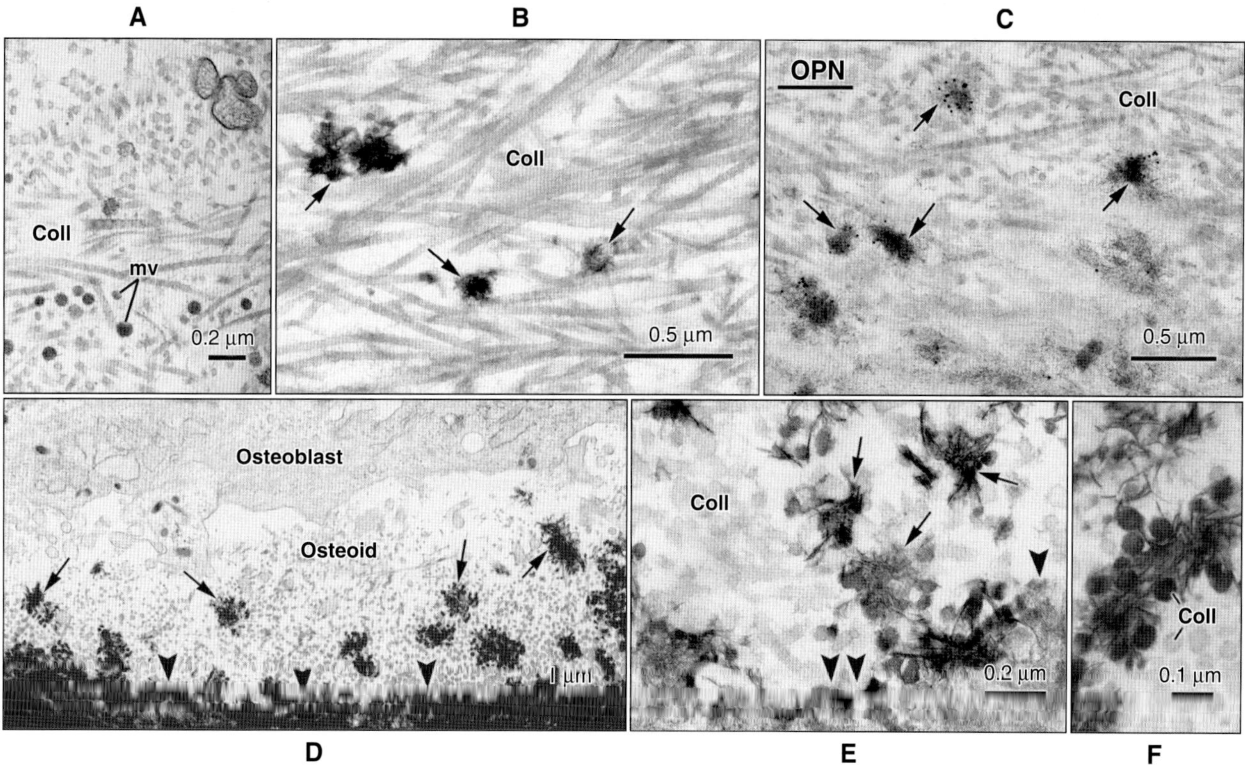

Fig. 6.12 (A–E) Osteoid is a layer of nonmineralized matrix that gradually transforms into mineralized bone, a transformation that takes place at the mineralization front *(arrowheads)*. With an electron microscope, (A) matrix vesicles *(mv)* sometimes can be seen among the nonmineralized collagen fibrils *(Coll)*, and (C–E) mineralization foci *(arrows)* are found within osteoid near the mineralization front. (C) Immunolabeling *(black dots)* reveals the presence of osteopontin *(OPN)*, among other noncollagenous proteins, in these foci. (F) The linear profiles among the calcified collagen fibrils are mineral crystals.

minimized. Caution must be exercised nevertheless, as rare occurrence of extraskeletal effects of the antibody treatment have been observed, increasing the risk of cardiovascular events.

Not surprisingly, newer exciting molecular studies worthy of mention include the global effect WNT has on cellular metabolism independent of the usual known routes. As alluded previously, the extremely high synthetic capacity of osteoblasts to produce the extracellular collagen building blocks must be met with correspondingly high energetic requirements. It has been shown that WNT influences osteoblast activity through a parallel, β-catenin–independent, mTOR complex 1 (mTORC1) pathway. mTORC1 is known to sense nutrient status, and its activation stimulates protein synthesis. It has been uncovered that WNT/mTORC1 is a central and integral decision-making system for an energy consumption source in osteoblasts. It overall reprograms osteoblasts to enhance its translational capacity, much needed for the energetically costly process of very high collagen and for extracellular matrix component synthesis demand.

The hormones most important in bone metabolism are parathyroid hormone (PTH), 1,25-dihydroxyvitamin D, calcitonin, estrogen, and glucocorticoids. The actions of PTH and vitamin D are dual, enhancing bone resorption at high (pharmacologic) concentrations but supporting bone formation at lower (physiologic) concentrations. Calcitonin and estrogen inhibit resorption, whereas the glucocorticoids inhibit resorption and formation (but primarily formation). Importantly, it is the action of FGF23 that regulates phosphate wasting. The hormones affecting bone most likely work primarily through altering the secretion of cytokines and growth factors. Evidence is increasing that centrally mediated mechanisms also are involved in bone metabolism. Leptin, a circulating hormone produced by adipocytes, inhibits the release of brainstem-derived serotonin, which favors bone mass accrual and appetite through its action on hypothalamic neurons. This hormone acts on the hypothalamus and, through involvement of the sympathetic nervous system, can promote and inhibit the differentiation of osteoclasts. Some evidence also indicates that leptin may work locally to promote the differentiation of osteoprogenitor cells and stimulate osteoblasts to make new bone. Noteworthy, hormones produced in bone (e.g., osteocalcin, lipocalin) can affect distant organs such as the pancreas, testis, and brain. Furthermore, bone is considered to regulate whole-body energy expenditure.

Osteoblasts form a cell layer over the forming bone surface and have been proposed to act as a barrier to control ion flux into and out of bone. Although there are no junctional complexes between cells, gap junctions do form and functionally couple adjacent cells. When bone is no longer forming, osteoblasts flatten substantially, extending along the bone surface (Fig. 6.13; see also Fig. 6.7A). These bone-lining cells contain few synthetic organelles, suggesting that they are less implicated in the production of matrix proteins. Bone-lining cells cover most surfaces in the adult skeleton. It has been postulated that bone-lining cells retain their gap junctions with osteocytes, creating a network that functions to control mineral homeostasis and ensure bone vitality. Such quiescent bone surfaces are believed to be the primary site for mineral exchange between blood and bone.

Another critical aspect of the bone formation that has been appreciated and scrutinized in recent years is the extremely high energetic demand it requires. Indeed, many studies have revealed that osteoblast differentiation and function require a complex metabolic demand that can change and adapt depending on fuel availability in health and disease. The major nutrients essential for and the many different pathways controlling adequate bone formation have been identified. Those studies illustrate the great importance and need for the osteoblasts to tightly control the fuel sources and their metabolism to generate adenosine triphosphate (ATP). This is achieved through a closely interconnected network integrating metabolism of glucose, fatty acids, and amino acids through glycolysis, beta-oxidation, and amino acid metabolism.

Osteocytes

As osteoblasts form bone, some become trapped in the matrix they secrete, whether mineralized or unmineralized; these cells then are called *osteocytes* (Figs. 6.14 and 6.15; see also Figs. 6.4, 6.6, and 6.7). The number of osteoblasts that become osteocytes varies depending on the rapidity of bone formation; the more rapid the formation, the more osteocytes are present per unit volume. As a general rule, embryonic (woven) bone and repair bone have more osteocytes than lamellar bone (Fig. 6.16; see also Fig. 6.6C). Approximately 5% to 20% of all osteoblasts will eventually be entombed in the bone matrix and change phenotype to become osteocytes, the most abundant cell type in an adult bone, comprising up to 95% of all bone cells. The process by which an osteoblast will turn into an osteocyte is still poorly understood. But once osteocytes are formed, they are long lived, being present for several decades. Most osteocytes will eventually die by apoptosis.

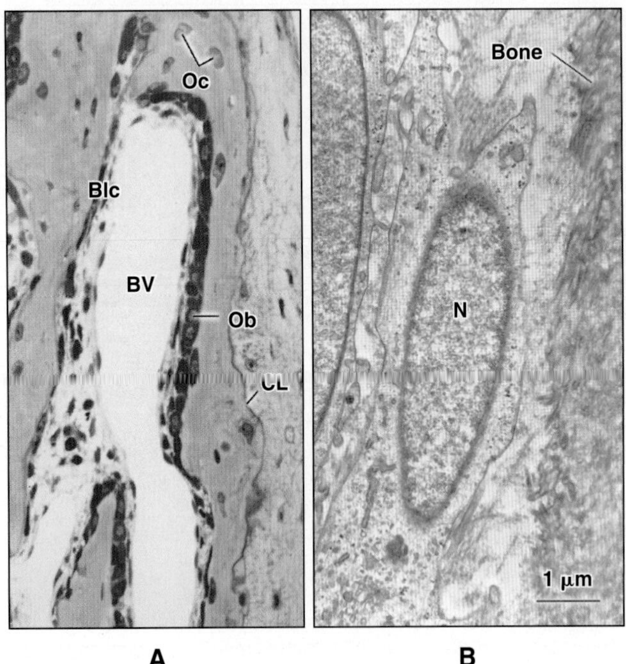

Fig. 6.13 (A) Light micrograph showing active and quiescent bone surfaces. Plump osteoblasts *(Ob)* line the surface where bone is actively being formed while bone-lining cells *(Blc)* cover the quiescent surface. (B) Electron micrograph of area labeled *Blc* in (A). Bone-lining cells are flattened osteoblasts with poorly developed protein synthetic organelles. *BV,* Blood vessel; *CL,* cement line; *N,* nucleus; *Oc,* osteocyte.

After their formation, osteocytes become reduced in size. The space in the matrix occupied by an osteocyte is called the *osteocytic lacuna* (see Figs. 6.4B and 6.15). Narrow extensions of these lacunae form enclosed channels (canaliculi) that house radiating osteocytic processes (see Figs. 6.4B and 6.15E). Through these channels, osteocytes maintain contact with adjacent osteocytes and with the osteoblasts (see Fig. 6.15C) or lining cells on bone surfaces. This places osteocytes in an ideal position to sense the biochemical and mechanical environments and to respond themselves or to transduce signals that affect the response of the other cells involved in bone remodeling to maintain bone integrity and vitality, particularly for the repair of microcracks. Osteocytes secrete SOST; this phosphoprotein acts on the WNT signaling pathway to inhibit osteoblast activity and decrease bone formation. SOST production is inhibited by PTH and mechanical loading, among other factors. Its expression is increased by the hormone calcitonin produced in the thyroid gland. Exercise-induced loading of bones also results in a global change in gene expression, to shut down the inhibitor SOST, and favors activators of osteoblast activity and bone deposition. A number of WNT-secreted molecules (WNT7b, WNT10a) are upregulated and activate osteoblasts through cell-surface receptors and downstream gene expression (Fig. 6.17). Osteocytes have also been identified as a major source of receptor activator of nuclear factor kappa B ligand (RANKL), influencing osteoclast differentiation and eventually bone matrix resorption (Fig. 6.18). The osteocyte is thus an important player for the maintenance of bone homeostasis. Failure of any part of this interconnecting system may result in hypermineralization (sclerosis) and death of the bone. This nonvital bone then may be resorbed and replaced during the process of bone turnover. Although osteocytes gradually reduce most of their matrix-synthesizing machinery, they

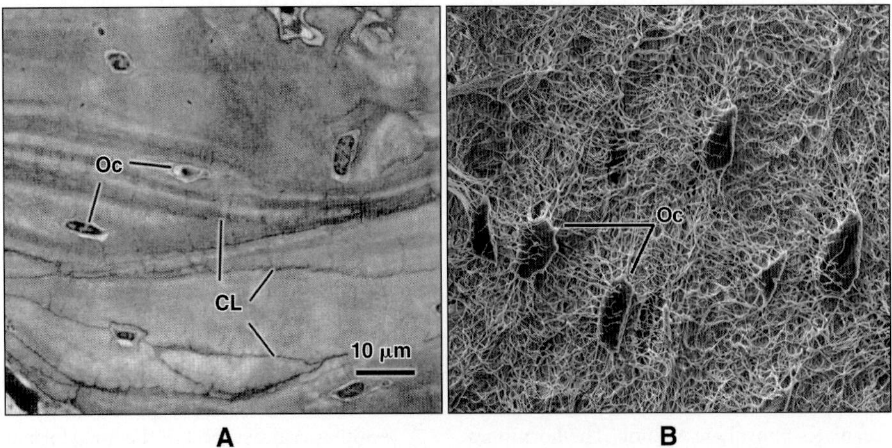

Fig. 6.14 (A) Light-level micrograph of rat mandibular bone. Osteocytes *(Oc)*, residing in lacunae, populate the bone. Note the abundant cement lines *(CL)*. (B) Scanning electron microscope view of the extensive meshwork of osteocyte cell processes. *BV,* Blood vessel. (B, Courtesy J. Feng.)

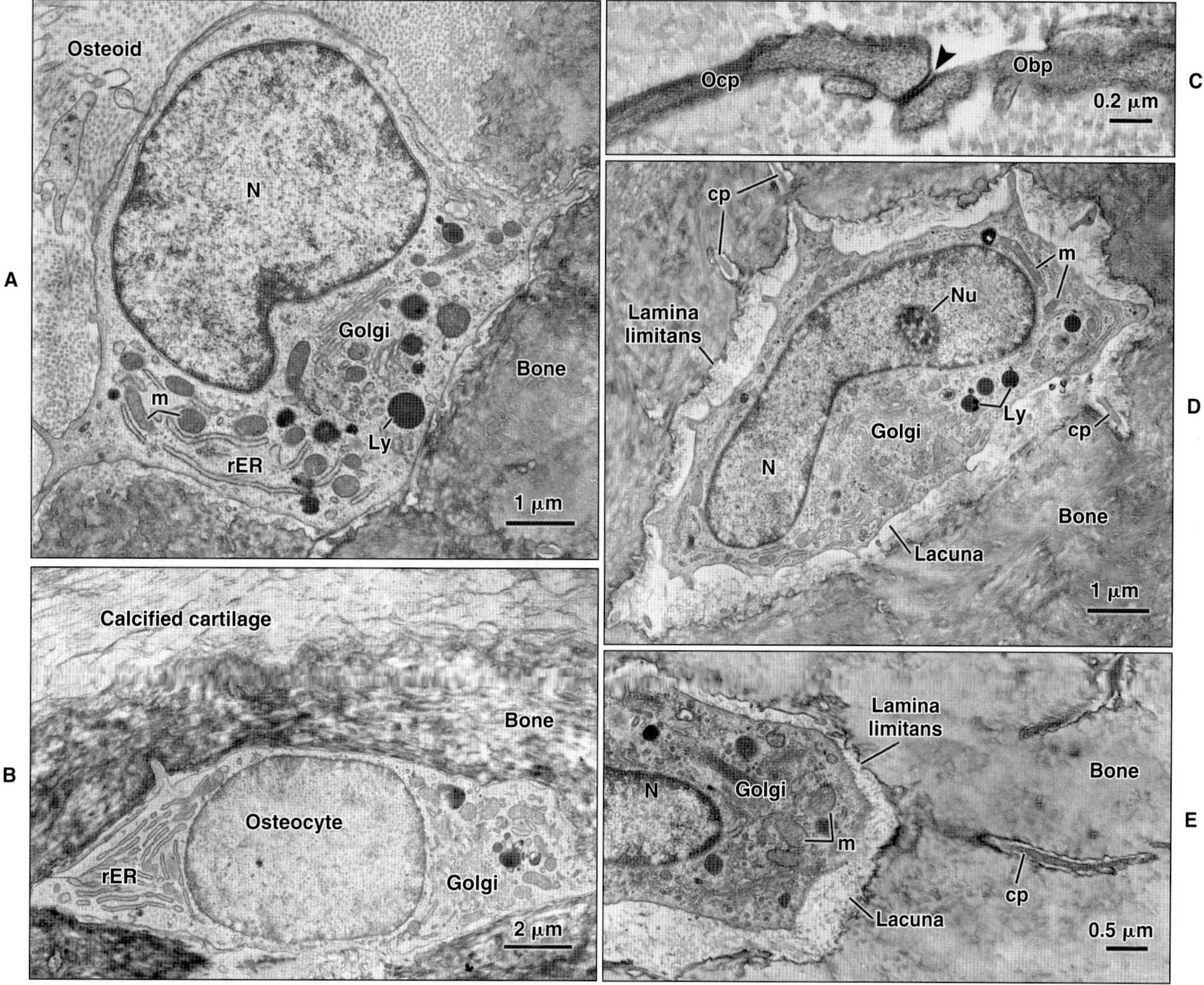

Fig. 6.15 Electron micrographs illustrating various osteocyte morphologies. (A) Young osteocyte is entrapped partly in osteoid and bone. (B) An osteocyte recently surrounded by bone and still near the surface. (C) Gap junction *(arrowhead)* between an osteoblast process *(Obp)* and an osteocyte process *(Ocp)*. (D, E) Older osteocytes deep in bone sit in lacunae delimited by a lamina limitans; these cells have numerous processes *(cp)* that ramify from the cell through bone in canaliculi. Although osteocytes have a reduced matrix-synthesizing machinery, they still are able to synthesize and secrete matrix proteins. They also occasionally exhibit numerous lysosomes *(Ly)*, supporting their participation in the local degradation of bone. *m*, Mitochondria; *N*, nucleus; *Nu*, nucleolus; *rER*, rough endoplasmic reticulum.

still are able to produce matrix proteins. Osteocytes also have been proposed to participate in the local degradation of bone (osteocytic osteolysis), thus influencing the structure of the perilacunar matrix.

Osteoclasts

Compared with all other bone cells and their precursors, the multinucleated osteoclast is a much larger cell. Because of their size, osteoclasts can be identified easily under the light microscope and often are seen in clusters (see Figs 6.6–6.8, 6.16B; also see Figs. 6.36, and 6.37, later). The osteoclast is characterized cytochemically by possessing tartrate-resistant acid phosphatase within its cytoplasmic vesicles and vacuoles (Fig. 6.19), which distinguishes it from multinucleated giant cells. Different osteoclast morphologies occur; however, unequivocally determining whether the cell is about to initiate or terminate resorption based solely on appearance is difficult.

Typically, osteoclasts are found against the bone surface, occupying hollowed-out depressions (Howship lacunae) that they have created. Scanning electron microscopy of bone-resorbing surfaces shows that Howship lacunae are often shallow troughs with an irregular shape (Fig. 6.20), reflecting the activity and mobility of osteoclasts during active resorption.

Under the transmission electron microscope, multinucleated osteoclasts exhibit a unique set of morphologic characteristics (Figs. 6.21, 6.22, and 6.23). Adjacent to the tissue surface, the cell membrane of the osteoclast is thrown into myriad deep folds that form a ruffled border (see Figs. 6.21 and 6.22). At the periphery of this border, the plasma membrane is apposed closely to the bone surface, and the adjacent cytoplasm, devoid of cell organelles, is enriched in actin, vinculin, and talin (proteins associated with integrin-mediated cell adhesion). This clear or sealing zone not only attaches the cells to the mineralized surface but also (by sealing the periphery of the ruffled border) isolates a microenvironment between them and the bone surface. An electron-dense, interfacial matrix layer (lamina limitans) often is observed between the sealing zone and calcified tissue surface (Fig. 6.24A; see also Fig. 6.21). Several mechanisms bind the osteoclasts to surfaces; among these, the concentration of arginine-glycine-aspartic acid–containing molecules, such as BSP, and OPN on bone surfaces (lamina limitans) may facilitate osteoclast

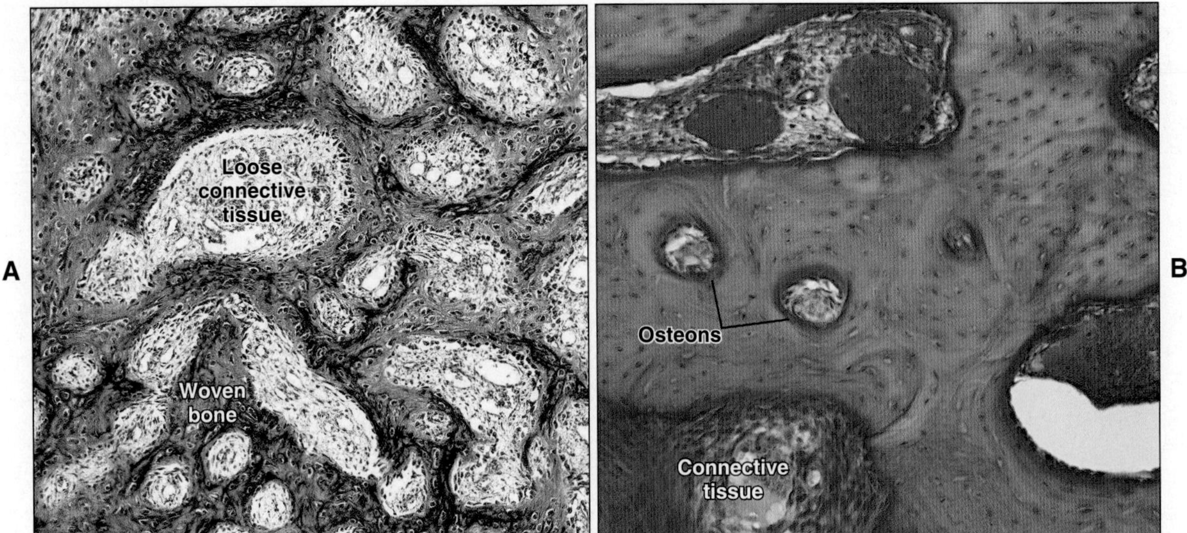

Fig. 6.16 (A) Light micrograph of woven bone. This bone exhibits high vascularity, soft tissue content, and bone cellularity. (B) Light micrograph of older alveolar bone. This section exhibits primary osteons, less bone cellularity, and loose connective tissue.

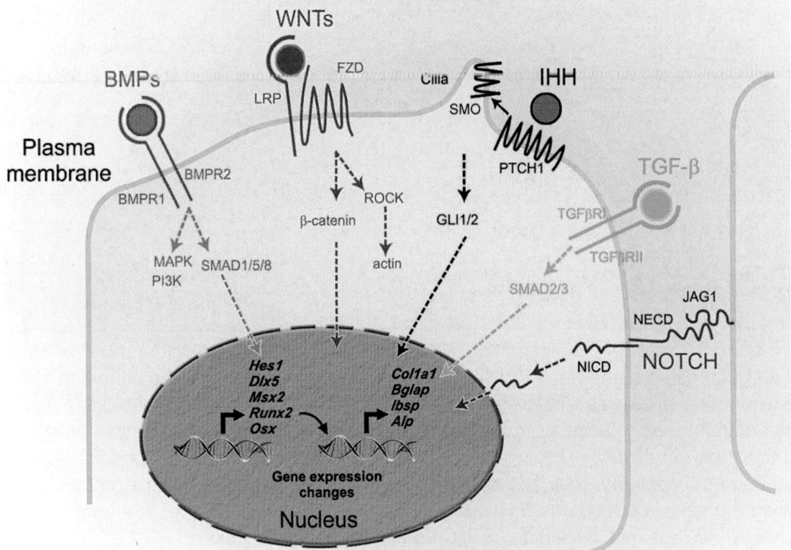

Fig. 6.17 Schematic representation of some signaling pathways affecting gene expression in osteoblasts. Five different signaling mechanisms crucial to instruct proper osteoblast function are represented by the different colors. Extracellular ligands bind their respective transmembrane receptors at the cell surface. Activation of receptors transmit a cascade of intracellular events (phosphorylation, protein stabilization, cleavage) that are distinct for each ligand-receptor pair. Ultimately, the intracellular effectors culminate in the nucleus to alter expression of master transcriptional regulators (*Hes1*, distal-less homeobox 5 [*Dlx5*], Msh homeobox 2 [*Msx2*], runt-related transcription factor 2 [*Runx2*], osterix [*Osx*]). These further modulate expression of secondary genes *(Col1a1, Bglap, Ibsp, Alp)* that encode proteins of the extracellular matrix essential for bone formation and mineralization. Ligands: *BPMs,* Bone morphogenetic proteins; *IHH,* Indian hedgehog; *JAG1,* jagged 1; *TGF-β,* transforming growth factor beta; *WNTs,* wingless-type MMTV integration site family. Receptors: *BMPR1/2,* Bone morphogenetic protein receptors; *FZD,* frizzled; *LRP,* low-density lipoprotein; *NOTCH,* NOTCH Drosophila homologue; *PTCH1,* patched 1; *SMO,* smoothened. Intracellular effectors: *GLI1/2,* Glioma-associated oncogene homolog; *MAPK,* mitogen-activated protein kinase; *NICD,* NOTCH intracellular domains; *ROCK,* RHO-associated coiled-coil-containing protein kinase; *SMAD,* mothers against decapentaplegic homologue of Drosophila.

adhesion and formation of the sealing zone by means of an integrin $\alpha_v\beta_3$-mediated mechanism (see Fig. 6.24A). The cell organelles consist of many nuclei, each of which is surrounded by multiple Golgi complexes, mitochondria, rER, and numerous vesicular structures situated between the Golgi complex and resorption surface (see Figs. 6.21–6.23). For years, osteoclasts have been known to be rich in acid phosphatase and other lysosomal enzymes. These enzymes, however, are not concentrated in the lysosomal structures as in most other cells. Instead, the enzymes are synthesized in the rER, transported to the Golgi complexes, and moved to the ruffled border in transport

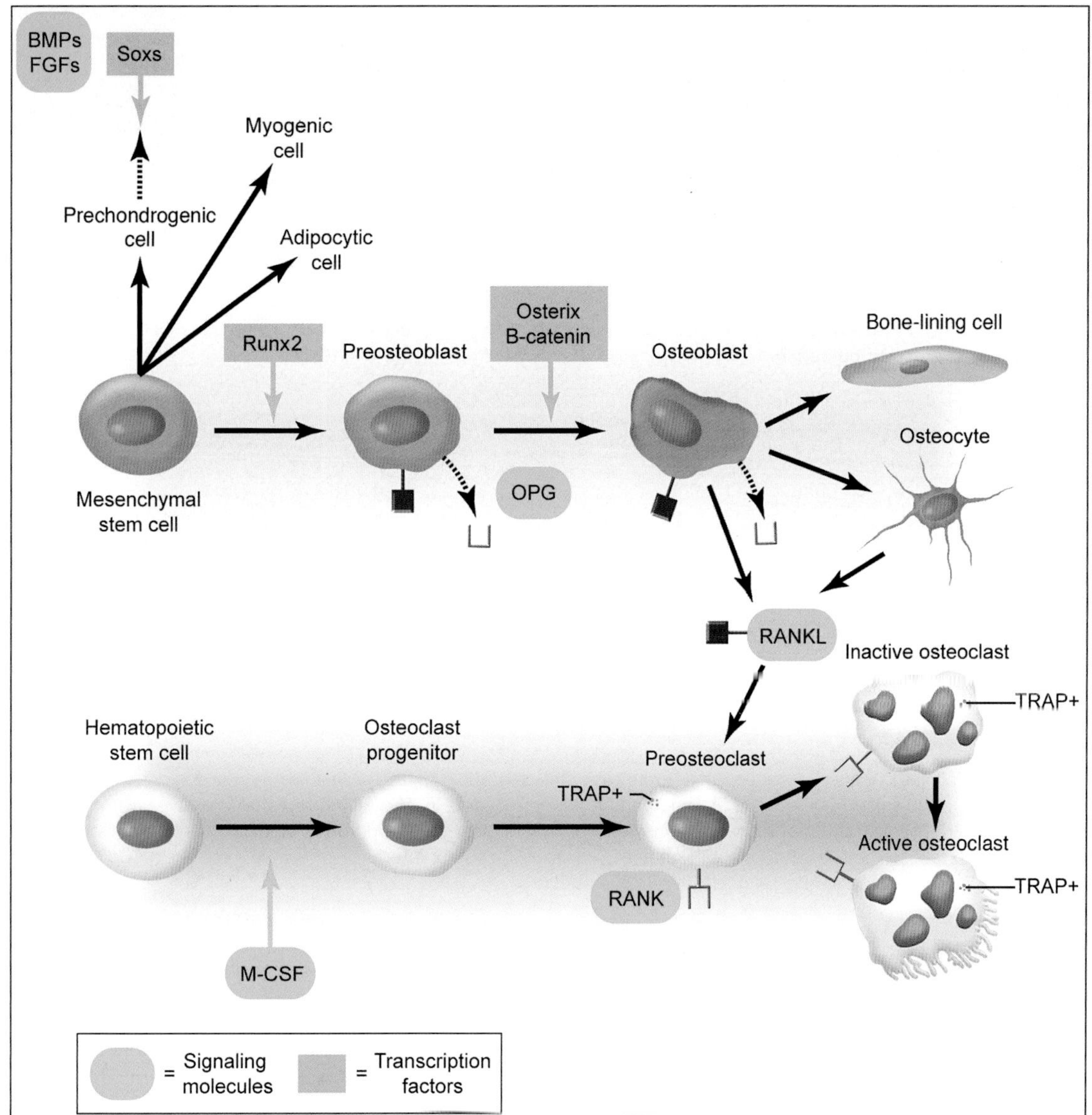

Fig. 6.18 Origin of bone cells. *BMPs,* Bone morphogenetic proteins; *FGFs,* fibroblast growth factors; *M-CSF,* macrophage colony–stimulating factor; *OPG,* osteoprotegerin; *RANK,* receptor activator of nuclear factor kappa B; *RANKL,* receptor activator of nuclear factor kappa B ligand; *RUNX2,* runt-related transcription factor 2; *SOX,* Sry-related high-mobility group box; *TRAP,* tartrate-resistant acid phosphatase.

vesicles where they release their content into the sealed compartment adjacent to the bone surface, essentially creating an extracellular lysosome (see Fig. 6.24B). Another feature of osteoclasts is a proton pump associated with the ruffled border that pumps hydrogen ions into the sealed compartment. Thus the sequence of resorptive events is considered to be as follows:

1. Attachment of osteoclasts to the mineralized surface of bone
2. Creation of a sealed acidic microenvironment through action of the proton pump, which demineralizes bone and exposes the organic matrix
3. Degradation of the exposed matrix by the action of released enzymes, such as acid phosphatase and cathepsin B
4. Endocytosis at the ruffled border of organic degradation products
5. Translocation of degradation products in transport vesicles and extracellular release along the membrane opposite the ruffled border (transcytosis)

Regulation of Bone Cell Formation

Large numbers of cells must be recruited continuously to maintain the structural integrity of bone. Interference with recruitment mechanisms can cause pathologic conditions. Bone-forming cells have a mesenchymal origin, whereas that of osteoclasts is hematopoietic. Differentiation of both cell types is a multistep process that is stimulated by a unique set of cytokines, growth factors, and hormones that are part of complex signal transduction pathways. Fig. 6.18 summarizes the current concepts concerning the origin of bone cells.

Two transcription factors have been identified as essential for osteoblast differentiation from mesenchymal stem cells and their function; these are runt-related transcription factor 2 (RUNX2, also known as *CBFA1*) and osterix (OSX, also known as *SP7*). The RUNX (runt-related) family of transcription factors is an important regulator of cell fate during embryogenesis and tissue differentiation. Only RUNX2

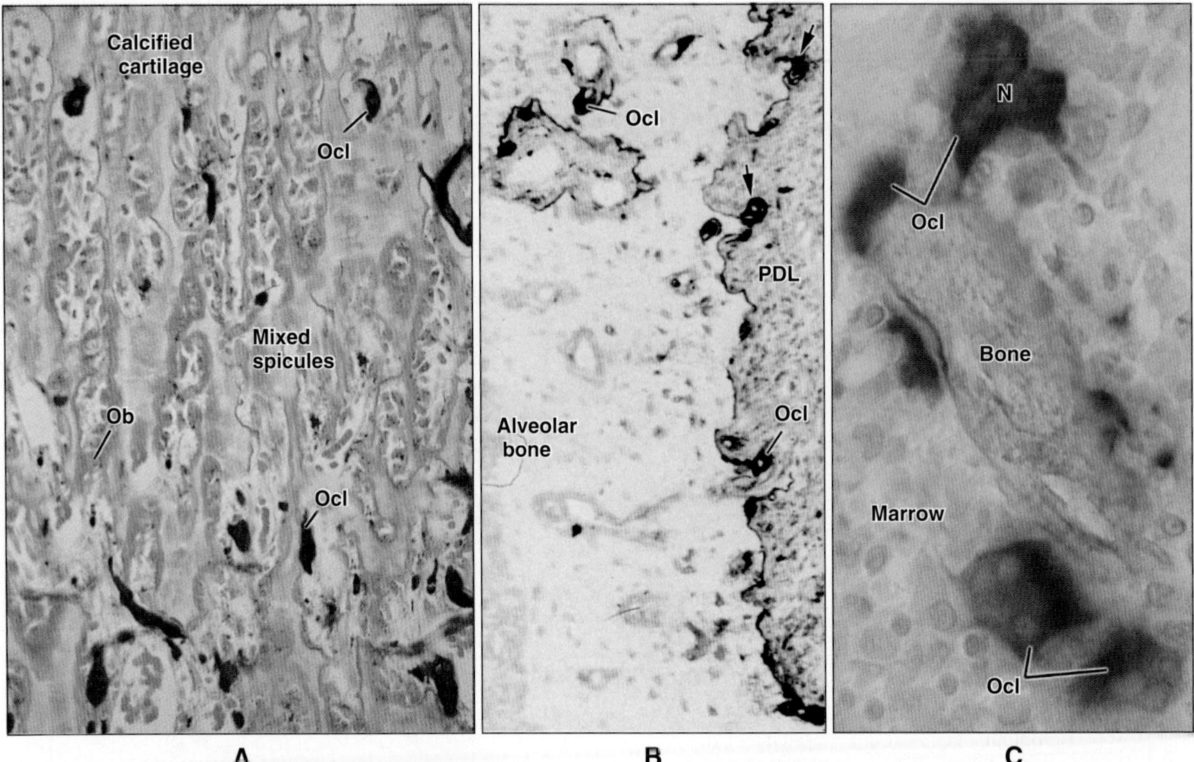

Fig. 6.19 Histochemical detection of tartrate-resistant acid phosphatase activity, a marker for osteoclasts *(Ocl)*, in rat tibia (A), alveolar bone (B), and human trabecular bone (C). (A) Osteoclasts progressively remove the mixed spicules of the primary spongiosa of the growth plate. (B) Numerous osteoclasts are seen along some surfaces where the periodontal ligament *(PDL)* attaches and, internally, in vascular channels. (C) Several nuclei *(N)* are present in osteoclasts. *Ob*, Osteoblasts.

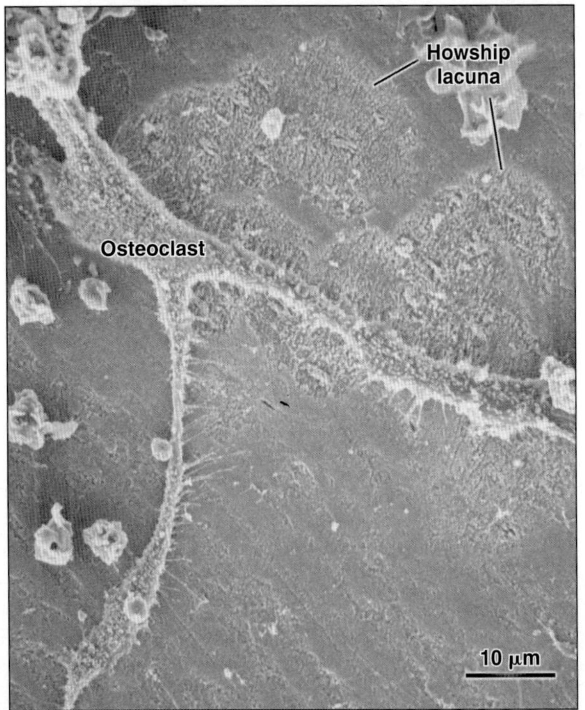

Fig. 6.20 Scanning electron micrograph of a Howship lacuna created by an osteoclast grown on a dentin slice.

is involved in osteoblast differentiation, whereas all family members (RUNX1 to RUNX3) seem to participate in chondrogenesis. RUNX2 acts as a master regulatory switch that mediates the temporal activation and/or repression of cell growth and phenotypic genes as osteoblasts progress through stages of differentiation. RUNX2 triggers the expression of major bone matrix proteins such as BSP, OPN, osteocalcin, and type I collagen, and it seems to control the maturation of osteoblasts and their transition into osteocytes. OSX, which contains zinc-finger motifs, belongs to the specific protein family of transcription factors, hence named *SP7*. OSX may play an important role in directing precursor cells away from the chondrocyte lineage and toward osteoblast lineage.

Both genes are critical for bone formation; mice that do not express RUNX2 or OSX show a complete absence of intramembranous and endochondral ossification. Also, differentiation of osteoblasts during development and remodeling depends on the activity of the WNT signaling pathway. The mechanism whereby this occurs is not fully understood, but there is evidence that the β-catenin pathway and BMP2 signaling are involved. Finally, various nonbone-specific transcription factors also have been demonstrated to affect osteoblast differentiation and function; these include, among others, genes from the *Dlx* and *Msx* families that, as described previously, are involved in embryogenesis and tooth development (see Chapters 3 and 5).

Important advances also can be expected from the realization that pluripotent mesenchymal cells are found in the postnatal bone marrow stroma. Some cells from this stroma can generate a broad range of skeletal tissues, such as cartilage, bone, adipocytes, and hematopoietic

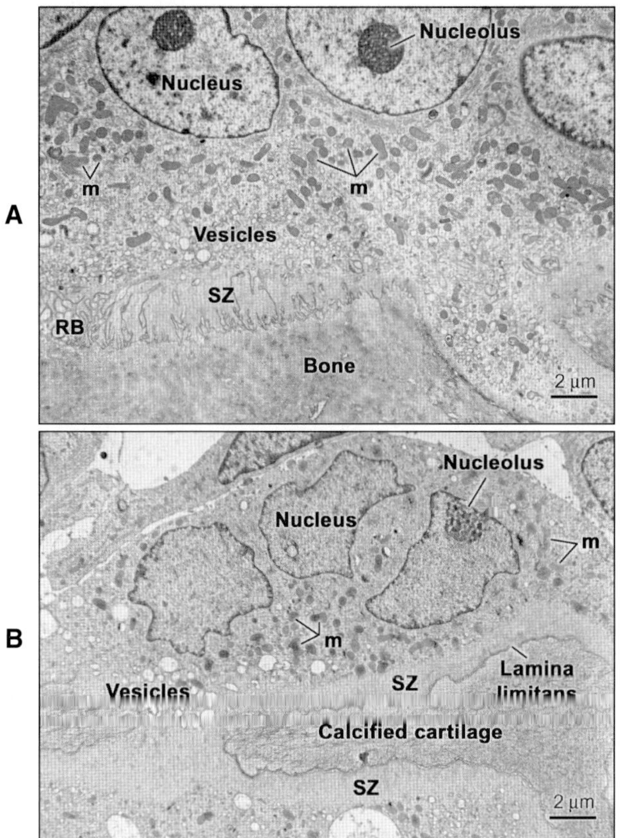

Fig. 6.21 Transmission electron micrographs of osteoclasts attached to (A) bone and (B) calcified cartilage. Osteoclasts are large, multinucleated cells with abundant mitochondria. Attachment occurs via the sealing zone *(SZ)* and resorptive activity along the ruffled border *(RB)*. An electron-dense, interfacial matrix layer (lamina limitans) often is observed between the sealing zone and calcified tissue surface. Abundant vesicles in the cytoplasm face the site of resorption (see also Fig. 6.22B). *m*, Mitochondria.

stroma. Other stem cells with the capacity to differentiate in osteogenic cells have been found in adipose, umbilical cord, pulp, and periodontal tissues. Cells from these sources could be induced to form bone, and their use may form the basis for developing novel therapeutic approaches such as for augmentation of alveolar bone and repair of the temporomandibular articulation.

The multinucleated osteoclasts arise from hematopoietic precursors of the monocyte/macrophage lineage. Stromal cells in the marrow cavity and osteoblasts modulate the differentiation of osteoclasts via secreted molecules and via direct cell-to-cell interaction. The signaling pathway implicating RANK and RANKL plays a major role in controlling osteoclastogenesis. RANKL is expressed by osteoblasts and osteocytes. It can either be localized on the plasma membrane of stromal and osteoblastic cells or be shed as a soluble mediator. This implies that RANKL can affect either through cell-to-cell interactions or over longer distance where it binds to RANK expressed on the plasma membrane of osteoclast progenitors to induce a signaling cascade leading to the differentiation and fusion of osteoclast precursor cells and the promotion of the survival and activity of mature osteoclasts. Osteoblasts also secreted a soluble decoy for RANKL, called *osteoprotegerin,* which blocks the interaction between RANKL and RANK and interferes with osteoclast formation. All three—osteoprotegerin, RANKL, and RANK—belong to the tumor necrosis factor/receptor superfamily. Several autocrine/paracrine factors influence osteoprotegerin and RANKL production; some of these are proinflammatory cytokines that, under normal physiologic conditions, help to maintain a proper balance between bone formation and resorption but in pathologic conditions, such as periodontal disease, favor bone loss.

In the process of physiologic bone remodeling it should also be noted that osteoclasts also secrete molecules that signal back to osteoblasts to attract them to sites of resorption.

Because the bone marrow stroma includes direct progenitors of osteoblasts and regulates the differentiation of osteoclast progenitors, the bone marrow stroma is a tissue of critical importance for skeletal physiology. The main cell type in the bone marrow stroma is a cell with a reticular morphology, which expresses alkaline phosphatase and resides at the abluminal side of sinusoids and arterioles.

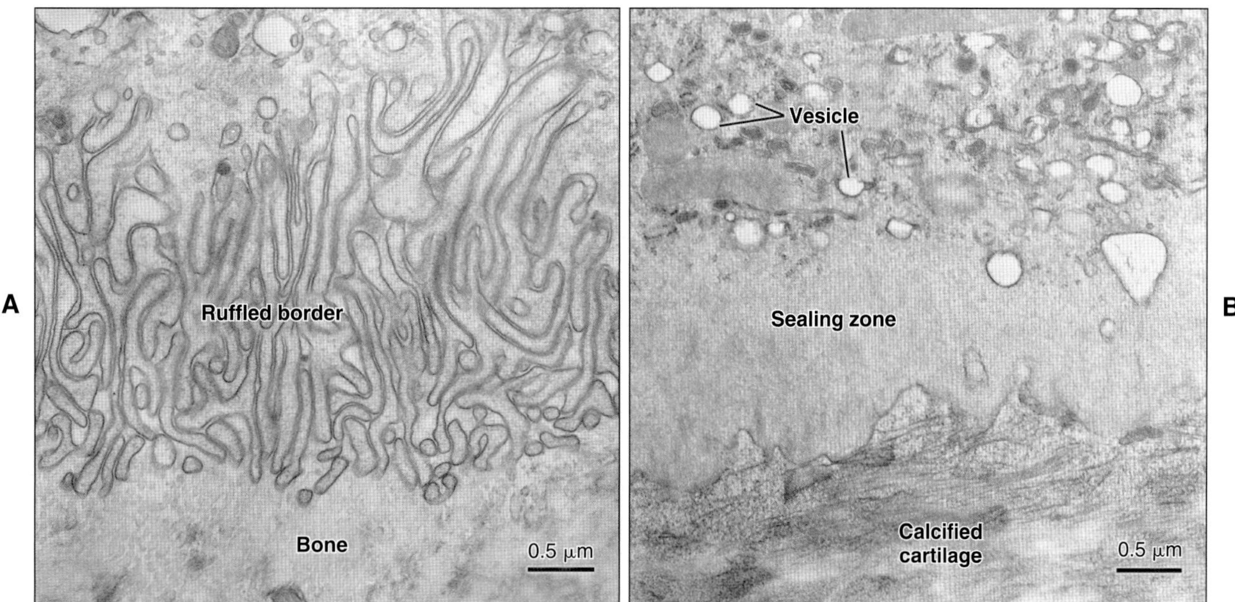

Fig. 6.22 High-magnification views of (A) the myriad membrane infoldings making up the ruffled border and (B) the sealing zone of an osteoclast in which contractile proteins concentrate.

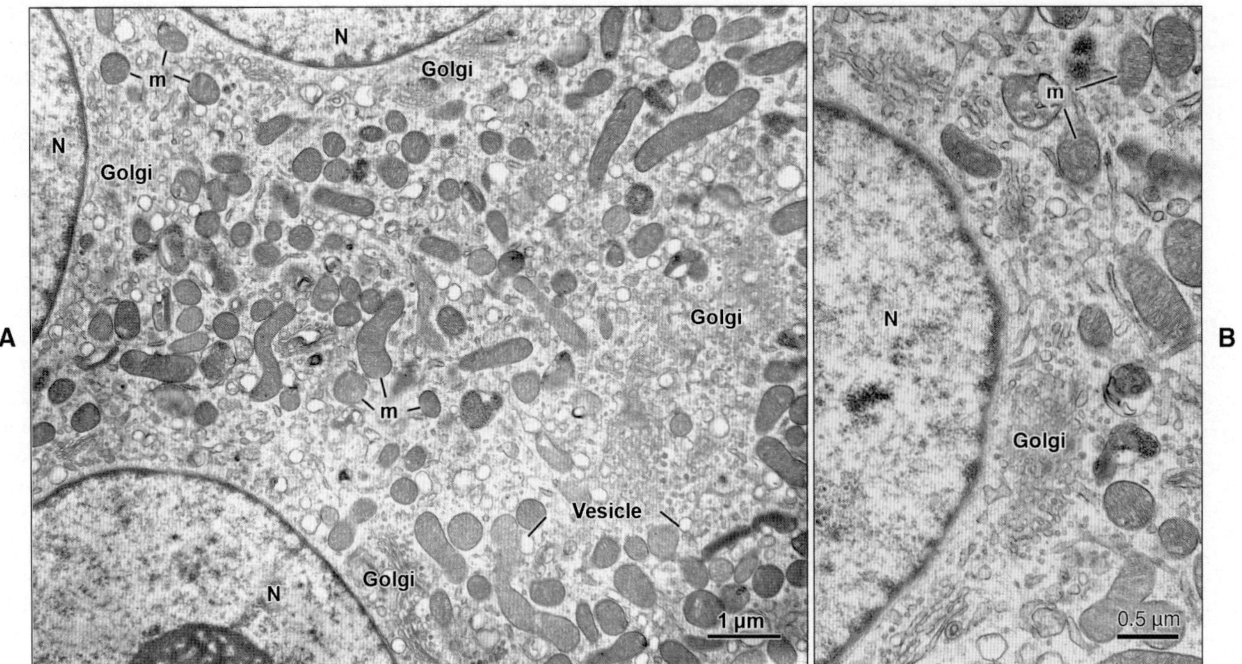

Fig. 6.23 (A) Osteoclasts possess numerous Golgi complexes. (B) Golgi bodies occupy a perinuclear position. *m*, Mitochondria; *N*, nucleus.

BONE DEVELOPMENT AND FORMATION

Although histologically one bone is no different from another, bone formation occurs by three main mechanisms: endochondral, intramembranous, and sutural. Endochondral bone formation takes place when cartilage is replaced by bone. Intramembranous bone formation occurs directly within mesenchyme. Bone formation along sutural margins is a special case.

Endochondral Bone Formation

Endochondral bone formation occurs at the extremities of all long bones, in vertebrae, in ribs, at the articular extremity of the mandible, and at the base of the skull. Early in embryonic development a condensation of mesenchymal cells occurs. Some of the sex-determining region Y (SRY)-related high-mobility group box (SOX) family of transcription factors (SOX9, SOX5, SOX6) govern the induction of cartilage formation and the differentiation of chondrogenic cells from this condensed mesenchyme (see Fig. 6.18). SOX9 not only specifies chondrocyte lineage specification during embryogenesis, but it also acts as an inhibitor of late-stage growth plate and articular chondrocyte maturation, maintaining differentiation status, and preventing redifferentiation into osteoblasts. Perichondrium forms around the periphery of the forming cartilage, giving rise to a cartilage model that eventually is replaced by bone (Fig. 6.25). Rapid growth of this cartilage anlage ensues by interstitial growth within its core (as more and more cartilage matrix is secreted by each chondroblast) and by appositional growth through cell proliferation and matrix secretion within the expanding perichondrium.

In the case of long bones, as differentiation of cartilage cells proceeds toward the metaphysis, the cells organize roughly into longitudinal columns. These columns can be subdivided into three functionally different zones: the zone of proliferation, the zone of hypertrophy and maturation, and the zone of provisional mineralization (Fig. 6.26; see also Fig. 6.25). The cells in the zone of proliferation are smaller and somewhat flattened and primarily constitute a source of new cells.

The zone of maturing cartilage is the broadest zone (see Fig. 6.26); in this zone, chondrocytes hypertrophy and their secretory machinery changes. In the early stages of hypertrophy, the chondrocytes secrete mainly type II collagen, which forms the primary structural component of the longitudinal matrix septum. As hypertrophy proceeds, mostly proteoglycans are secreted; when chondrocytes reach their maximum size, they secrete type X collagen and noncollagenous proteins that, together with partial proteoglycan breakdown, create a matrix environment receptive for mineral deposition. Matrix mineralization begins in the zones of mineralization by elaboration of matrix vesicles (Fig. 6.27). These vesicles are small, membrane-bound structures that bud off from the cell to form independent units within the longitudinal septa of cartilage (they are not present in the transverse septa). The first morphologic evidence of crystallite formation occurs in association with the membrane of these vesicles. The matrix vesicle provides a microenvironment for initiation of mineralization. Thus the matrix vesicle contains alkaline phosphatase, pyrophosphatase, calcium-ATP, metalloproteinases, proteoglycans, and anionic phospholipids, which can bind to calcium and inorganic phosphate and thereby form calcium-inorganic phosphate phospholipid complexes. The longitudinal cartilage septa thus become calcified.

Concurrently, vascularization of the middle of the cartilage occurs. Within the perichondrium in the diaphysis, vascularization is increased, the perichondrium converts to a periosteum, and intramembranous bone begins to form. Centrally, the calcified cartilage disintegrates, and multinucleated cells (chondroclasts [similar to osteoclasts]) resorb most of the mineralized matrix to make room for further vascular ingrowth. Recent advancement in lineage tracing coupled to single-cell RNA sequencing has identified a potentially different kind of osteoclast that preferentially degrades the cartilage septum near the metaphyseal region. These have been called *septoclasts* and appear different than conventional osteoclasts in that they are not multinucleated, are not capable of resorbing bone matrix, and would be of mesenchymal origin. The septoclasts, marked by expression of fatty acid binding protein 5, would be a more prominent contributor to longitudinal bone

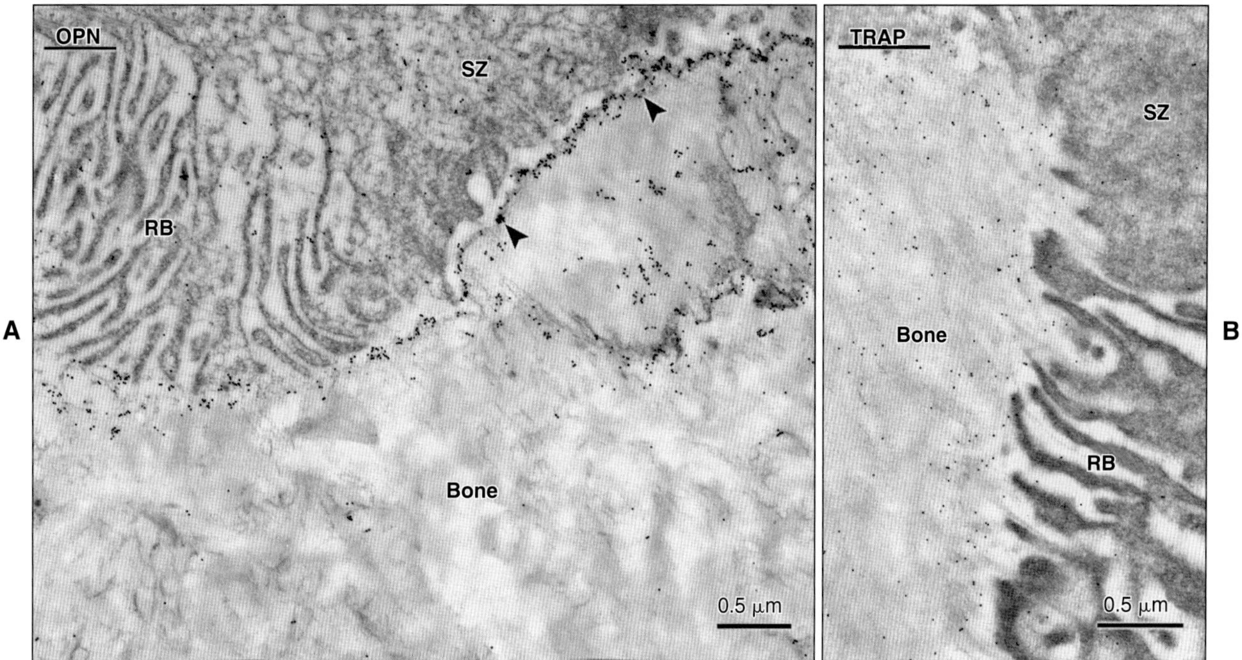

Fig. 6.24 Immunocytochemical preparations for (A) osteopontin *(OPN)* and (B) tartrate-resistant acid phosphatase *(TRAP)*. (A) The bone surface *(arrowheads)* onto which the sealing zone *(SZ)* attaches often shows a concentration of osteopontin *(black dots)*. (B) Enzymes can be detected in the extracellular matrix where resorption is taking place. *RB,* Ruffled border.

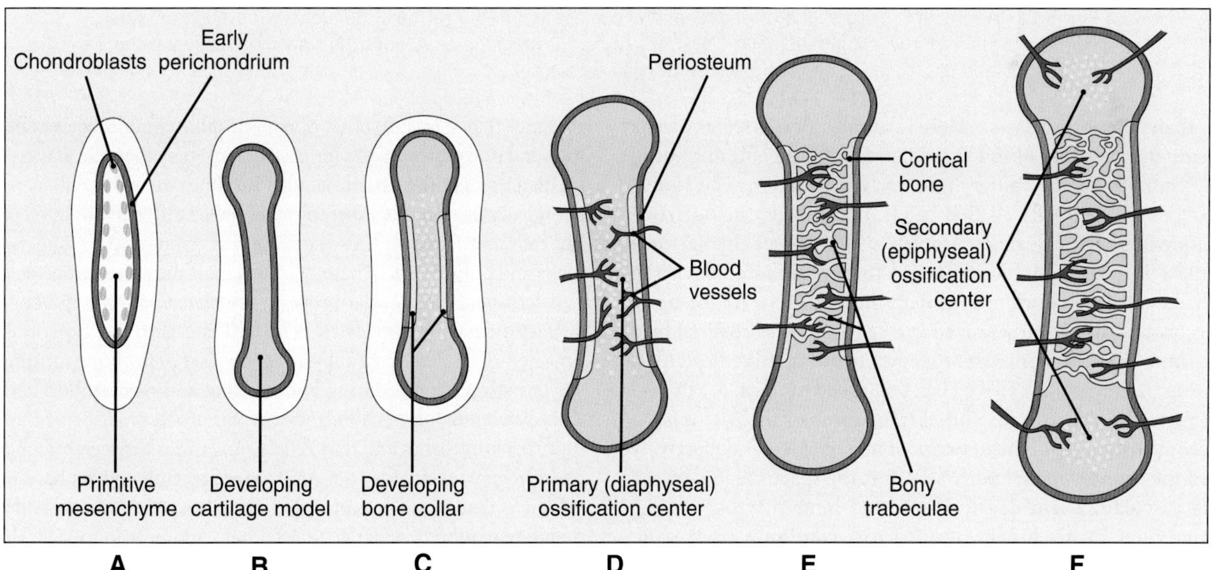

Fig. 6.25 Endochondral bone formation. (A) Chondroblasts develop in primitive mesenchyme and form an early perichondrium and cartilage model. (B) The developing cartilage model assumes the shape of the bone to be formed, and a surrounding perichondrium becomes identifiable. (C) At the midshaft of the diaphysis the perichondrium becomes a periosteum through the development of osteoprogenitor cells and osteoblasts, the osteoblasts producing a collar of bone by intramembranous ossification. Calcium salts are deposited in the enlarging cartilage model. (D) Blood vessels grow through the periosteum and bone collar, carrying osteoprogenitor cells within them. These cells establish a primary (or diaphyseal) ossification center in the center of the diaphysis. (E) Bony trabeculae spread out from the primary ossification center to occupy the entire diaphysis, linking up with the previously formed bone collar, which now forms the cortical bone of the diaphysis. At this stage the terminal club-shaped epiphyses are still composed of cartilage. (F) At about term (the precise time varies between long bones), secondary or epiphyseal ossification centers are established in the center of each epiphysis by the ingrowth along with blood vessels of mesenchymal cells, which become osteoprogenitor cells and osteoblasts. (From Stevens A, Lowe J: *Human histology*, ed 3, London, 2005, Mosby Elsevier.)

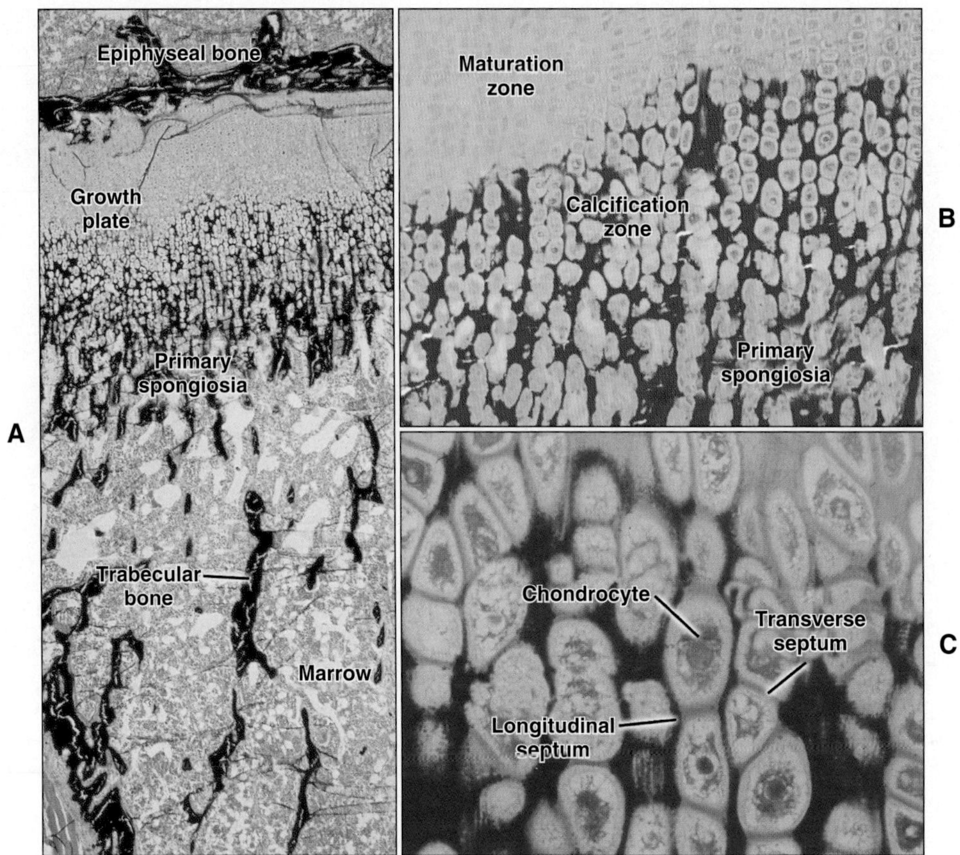

Fig. 6.26 (A–C) Light micrographs of endochondral ossification in the rat tibia. Sections were stained with von Kossa stain for revealing mineral (in *black*). (C) At higher magnification, note the transition between the maturation and calcification zones of the growth plate cartilage.

growth than the osteoclasts. Mesenchymal (perivascular) cells accompany the invading blood vessels, proliferating and migrating onto the remains of the mineralized cartilage matrix. The longitudinal septa are generally all that is left of cartilage, the horizontal septa having been resorbed completely. The mesenchymal cells differentiate into osteoblasts and begin to deposit osteoid on the mineralized cartilage columns and then mineralize it. As the bone matrix is produced, the mineralized cartilage becomes covered by a circular rim of new bone matrix, together forming mixed spicules, which hang in the marrow space (Fig. 6.28; see also Figs. 6.19A and 6.26). Bone matrix surrounds and entraps some of the osteoblasts; these become osteocytes. The network of mixed spicules collectively is termed the *primary spongiosa*. With time, the space created by the invading vascular system develops into red bone marrow. As the developing bone grows longer, the marrow continues to expand. Osteoclasts progressively remove the core of mineralized cartilage and the surrounding bone so that cartilage activity becomes restricted to extremities of the developing bone. This process occurs at approximately the same rate as cartilage formation so that the volume of the primary spongiosa remains relatively constant during growth. Osteoclasts also expand the marrow cavity radially by resorbing bone along the entire endosteal surface.

The classic account given previously of endochondral ossification holds that chondrogenesis and osteogenesis are closely linked but separate processes. Accordingly, chondrocytes undergo a differentiation cascade leading to hypertrophy and culminating by programmed cell death (apoptosis). Bone then forms on calcified cartilage by bone marrow–derived osteoprogenitor cells brought to the site by vascular invasion. Although, overall, the outcome of this classic view is correct, there is now growing evidence that at least a subset of hypertrophic chondrocytes evades apoptosis and transdifferentiates into osteoblasts; the others die. It was proposed by Bianco et al. (see Recommended Reading, later) that "all hypertrophic chondrocytes have the inherent potential to differentiate into osteoblast-like cells, but that only those at the border (transition zone) between cartilage and bone do so." These cells switch off their chondrogenic program and activate the molecular program associated with pluripotency; vascular factors may be implicated here. Cell lineage tracer experiments have now demonstrated that a substantial fraction of the bone forming cells in the growth plate and during bone healing and regeneration derive from transdifferentiation of chondrocytes. This process may be tied to the evolution of bony fishes and may reflect similarities between osteoblastic and chondrogenic regulatory networks. More recently, others have presented evidence that some hypertrophic chondrocytes undergo a process of dedifferentiation to generate skeletal stem and progenitor cells that adopt a reticular-[C-X-C motif chemokine ligand 12 (CXCL12)]-expressing signature. These were shown to serve as a source of multipotent progenitors for later differentiation into functional osteoblasts, either during embryogenesis, postnatal development, or adult stages.

In some bones (e.g., the tibia, but not the ramus of the mandible), a secondary invasion of blood vessels into the head (end) of the bone creates a secondary ossification center (see Fig. 6.25). This secondary bone growth proceeds in a fashion identical to that occurring in primary bone growth, resulting in a plate of growing cartilage remaining between the diaphysis and the end (epiphysis) of the bone. This plate is termed the *epiphyseal growth plate* (see Fig. 6.26). Longitudinal bone growth occurs as a result of cell division and interstitial growth in the plate. It ceases when the cartilage cells stop proliferating and the growth plate disappears. In addition, as longitudinal bone growth

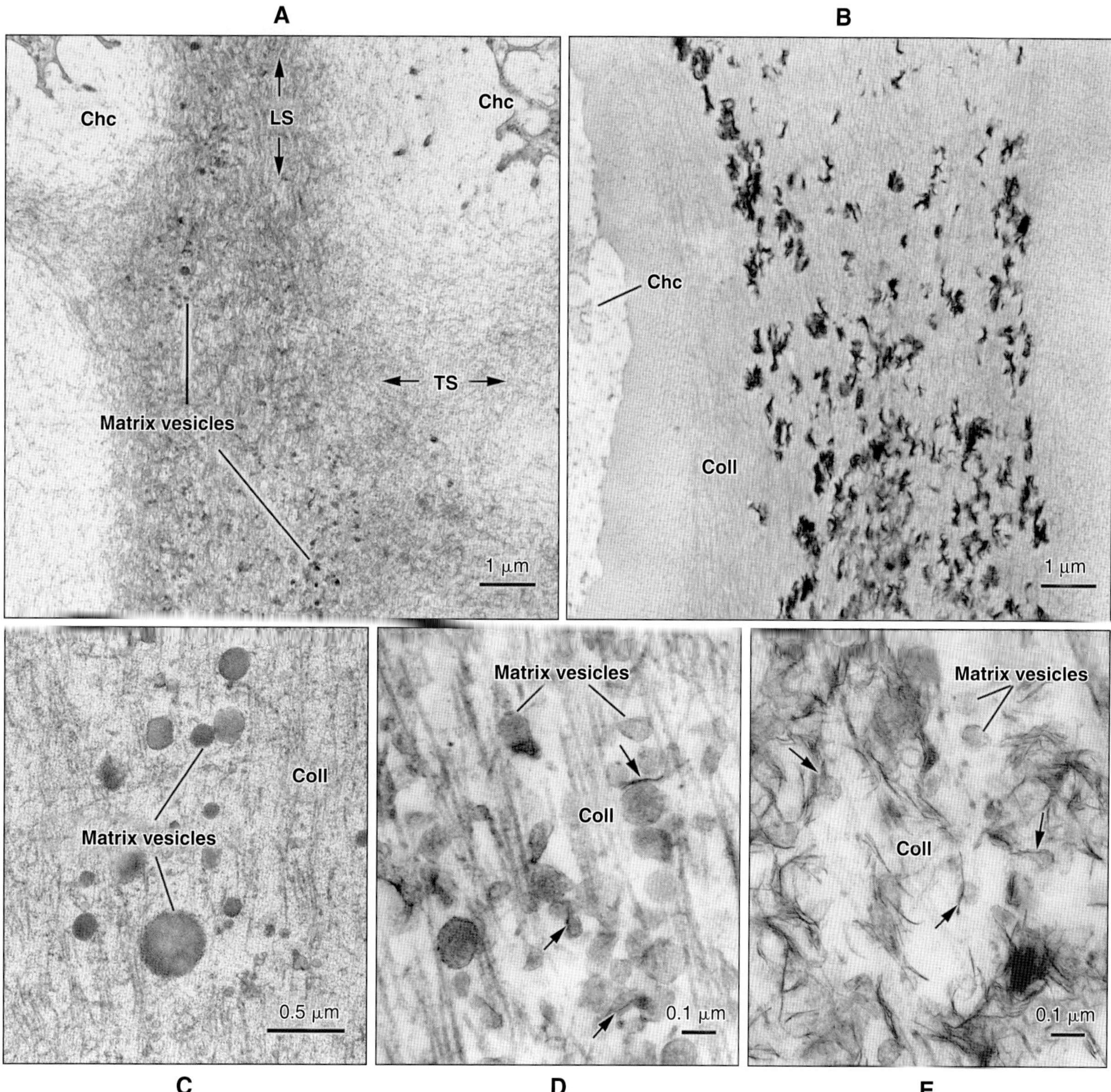

Fig. 6.27 Electron micrographs of rat tibia growth plate cartilage illustrating matrix events in (A) the zone of maturation and (B) the zone of mineralization and (C–E) the progression of matrix vesicles across these two zones. Matrix vesicles are small, membrane-bound structures that bud off from chondrocytes *(Chc)* and that provide a microenvironment favorable for mineral deposition. Crystal formation is believed to initiate in relation to the membrane of the vesicles. These first crystals *(arrows)* encourage the formation of more crystals around them, forming mineralization foci seen in (B) as irregular black deposits within the type II collagen matrix *(Coll)*. These foci gradually increase in size, transforming the organic matrix of the longitudinal septa *(LS)* into calcified cartilage. The transverse septa *(TS)* do not mineralize.

slows and ceases, so does the expansion of the marrow cavity. The bone-covered cartilage remaining in the primary spongiosa and in the secondary ossification centers is replaced by lamellar bone, thus creating the secondary spongiosa found throughout adult bone. The shaft grows in diameter as osteoblast differentiation and new bone deposition occur on the periosteal surface while old bone is removed on the endosteal surface by osteoclasts.

Intramembranous Bone Formation

Intramembranous bone formation was first recognized when early anatomists observed that the fontanels of fetal and newborn skulls were filled with a connective tissue membrane that was replaced gradually by bone during development and growth of the skull. In intramembranous bone formation, bone develops directly within the soft connective tissue. The mesenchymal cells proliferate and condense (Fig. 6.29A). Concurrent with an increase in vascularity at these sites of condensed mesenchyme, osteoblasts differentiate and begin to produce bone matrix (see Fig. 6.29B). As the mesenchymal cells differentiate into osteoblasts, they start exhibiting alkaline phosphatase activity (Fig. 6.30). This sequence of events occurs at multiple sites within each bone of the cranial vault, maxilla, body of the mandible, and midshaft of long bones.

After it is begun, intramembranous bone formation proceeds rapidly. This first embryonic bone is termed *woven bone* (Fig. 6.31;

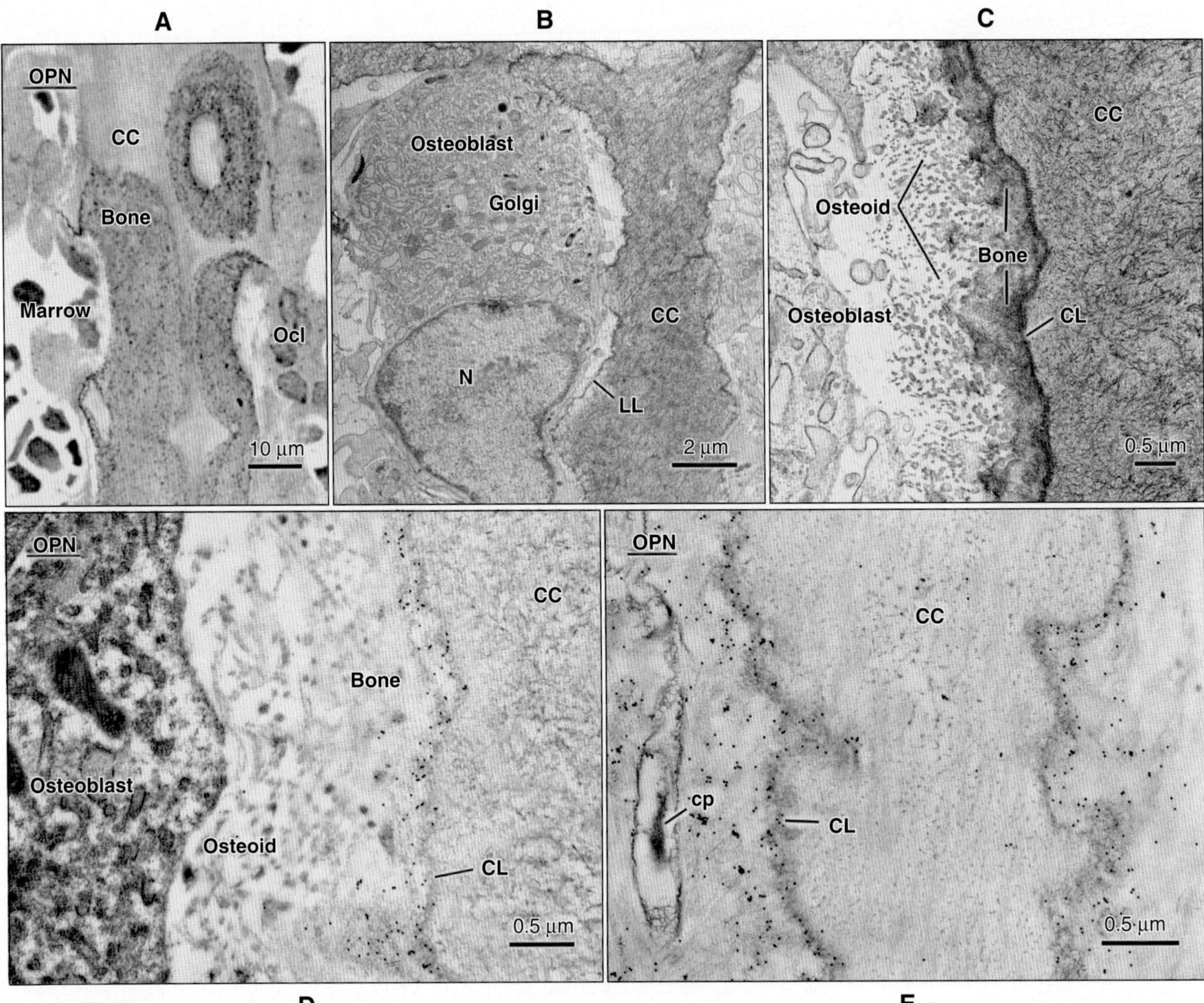

Fig. 6.28 Endochondral bone formation. (A) Light-level micrograph of a mixed spicule consisting of a calcified cartilage core *(CC)* onto which bone is deposited. The black deposits over bone represent immunocytochemical labeling for osteopontin *(OPN)*. (B, C) Electron micrographs that illustrate the sequence of bone deposition onto calcified cartilage. Osteoblasts surround the cartilage. First, an electron-dense surface coating appears on the cartilage; this coating is initially termed *lamina limitans (LL)* when osteoblasts are apposed to it and *cement line (CL)* when it is at the interface between bone and calcified cartilage. Subsequently, there is deposition of osteoid, which gradually transforms into calcified bone. (D, E) Electron microscope immunocytochemical preparations showing the distribution of osteopontin *(black dots)* in the newly formed bone. *cp,* Cell process; *N,* nucleus; *Ocl,* osteoclast.

see also Fig. 6.6). At first the woven bone takes the form of radiating spicules and trabecula, but progressively these fuse into thin bony plates. In the cranium, more than one plate may fuse to form a single bone. Early plates of intramembranous bone are structurally unsound not only because of poor fiber orientation and mineralization but also because many islands of soft connective tissue remain within the plates. Soon after plate formation in the skull or the establishment of intramembranous bone formation in the midshaft region, the bone becomes polarized. The establishment and expansion of the marrow cavity turn the endosteal surfaces of bone into primarily a resorbing surface, whereas the periosteum initiates the formation of most of the new bone. However, depending on adjacent soft tissues and their growth, segments of the periosteal surface of an individual bone may contain focal sites of bone resorption. For instance, growth of the tongue, brain, and nasal cavity and lengthening of the body of the mandible require focal resorption along the periosteal surface. Conversely, segments of the endosteum of the same bone simultaneously may become a forming surface, resulting in bone drift.

Woven bone of the early embryo and fetus turns over rapidly. As fetal bones begin to assume their adult shape, continued proliferation of soft connective tissue between adjoining bones brings about the formation of sutures and fontanels.

From early fetal development to full expression of the adult skeleton, a continual, slow transition occurs from woven bone to lamellar bone. This transition is rapid during late fetal development and the first years of life (see Figs. 6.16B and 6.31B) and involves the formation of primary osteons deposited around a blood vessel. The primary osteon tends to be small, with lamellae that are neither numerous nor well delineated. As more osteons are formed at the periosteal surface, they become more tightly packed so that eventually a higher percentage of compact bone consists of osteons.

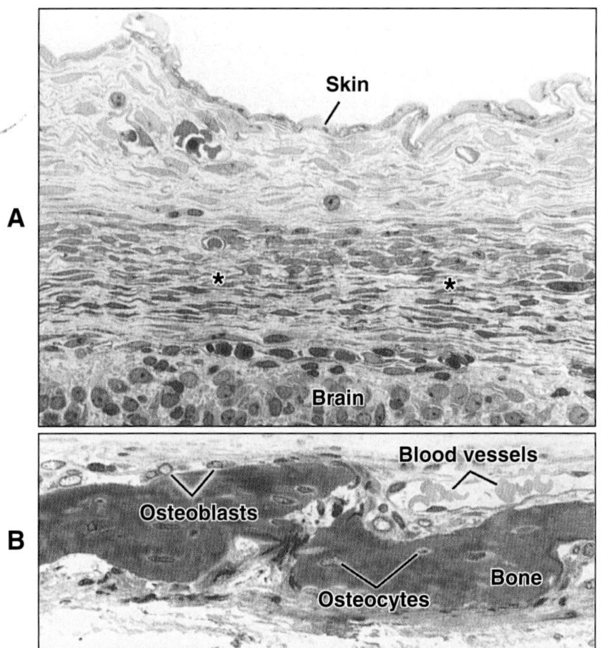

Fig. 6.29 Light micrographs of intramembranous bone formation in the rat calvaria. (A) Ectomesenchymal cells *(asterisks)* condense between the skin and developing brain. (B) These cells differentiate into osteoblasts that deposit bone directly as woven cancellous bone.

Woven bone is characterized by intertwined collagen fibrils oriented in many directions, showing wide interfibrillar spaces. Collagen fibrils in lamellar bone, however, are generally thicker and are arranged in ordered sheets consisting of aligned and closely packed fibrils. It follows from these structural features that the widely spaced collagen meshwork of woven bone will accommodate more noncollagenous matrix proteins.

Just like calcified cartilage, matrix vesicles are believed to be implicated in the initiation of mineral deposition during intramembranous bone formation. The relative importance of matrix vesicles versus secreted noncollagenous matrix proteins in the control of initial events in mineralization remains unclear, and both may be implicated independently or in succession. The sporadic observation of matrix vesicles in osteoid (Fig. 6.32A; see also Fig. 6.12A) and their increase in number under some altered physiologic conditions suggest that matrix vesicles may play a predominant role when mineralization needs to be intensely promoted.

Among noncollagenous bone matrix proteins, BSP and OPN have received particular attention because they are implicated in cellular and matrix events. They are part of a family of proteins (small integrin-binding ligand, N-linked glycoprotein [SIBLING]) believed to have evolved from the divergent evolution of a single ancestral gene. Because the site where a protein is present is suggestive of its function, the distribution of these two proteins has been studied extensively. In general, consensus exists that BSP and OPN codistribute. They are found in mineralization foci near the mineralization front, accumulate within the spaces between the calcified collagen fibrils, and are associated with cement lines (see Fig. 6.32). Depending on the antibody used for immunolocalization, OPN and occasionally BSP are immunodetected along the surface of osteocyte lacunae and canaliculi (lamina limitans). With respect to mineralization, the consensus of biochemical, functional, and immunolocalization studies is that BSP is a promoter and OPN an inhibitor. It has also been recently reported that BSP plays a role in both osteoclast formation and activity. Surprisingly, mice that do not express the genes for these proteins (knockouts) do not show overt bone alterations most likely because these proteins are part of a redundant system. In contrast, knockout mice for dentin matrix protein 1 and matrix extracellular phosphoprotein exhibit evident bone phenotypes. Studies underway aimed at determining how these proteins exert their effects and to characterize functional domains associated with mineral ion deposition, protein-to-protein interactions, and cell binding are important for the creation of therapeutic peptides derived from them.

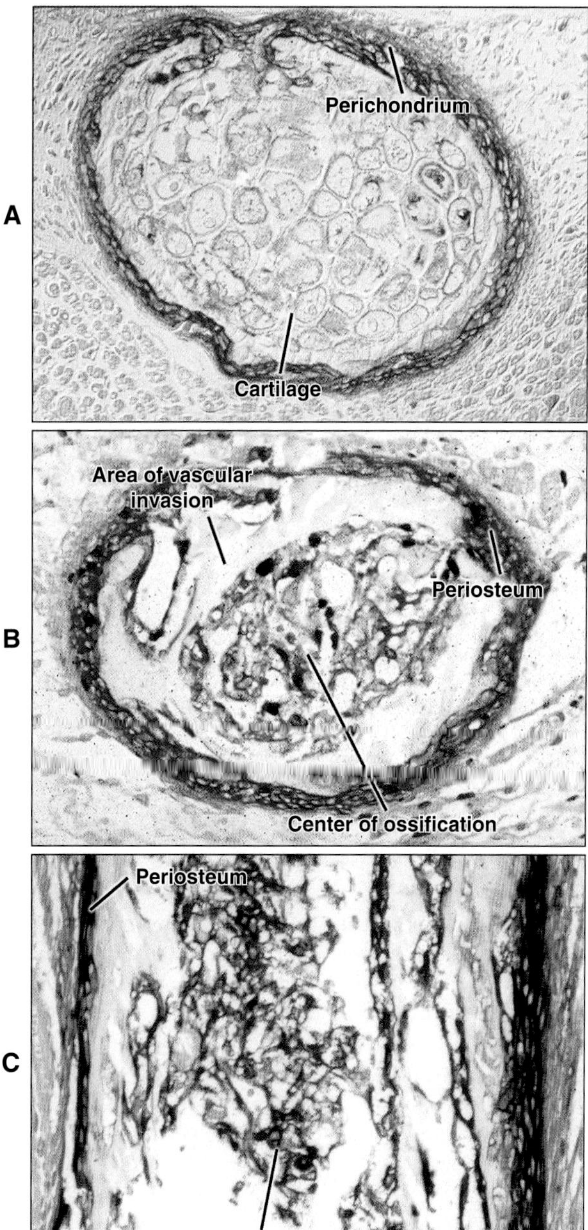

Fig. 6.30 Intramembranous bone formation around the cartilage model of digits. (A, B) Cross section. (C) Longitudinal section. The preparations are stained for alkaline phosphatase activity *(blue)*. Such activity is present in the perichondrium and periosteum and in areas of vascular invasion.

Sutural Bone Growth

Sutures play an important role in growing the face and skull. Found exclusively in the skull, sutures are the fibrous joints between bones; however, sutures allow only limited movement. Their function is to permit the skull and face to accommodate growing organs, such as the eyes and brain.

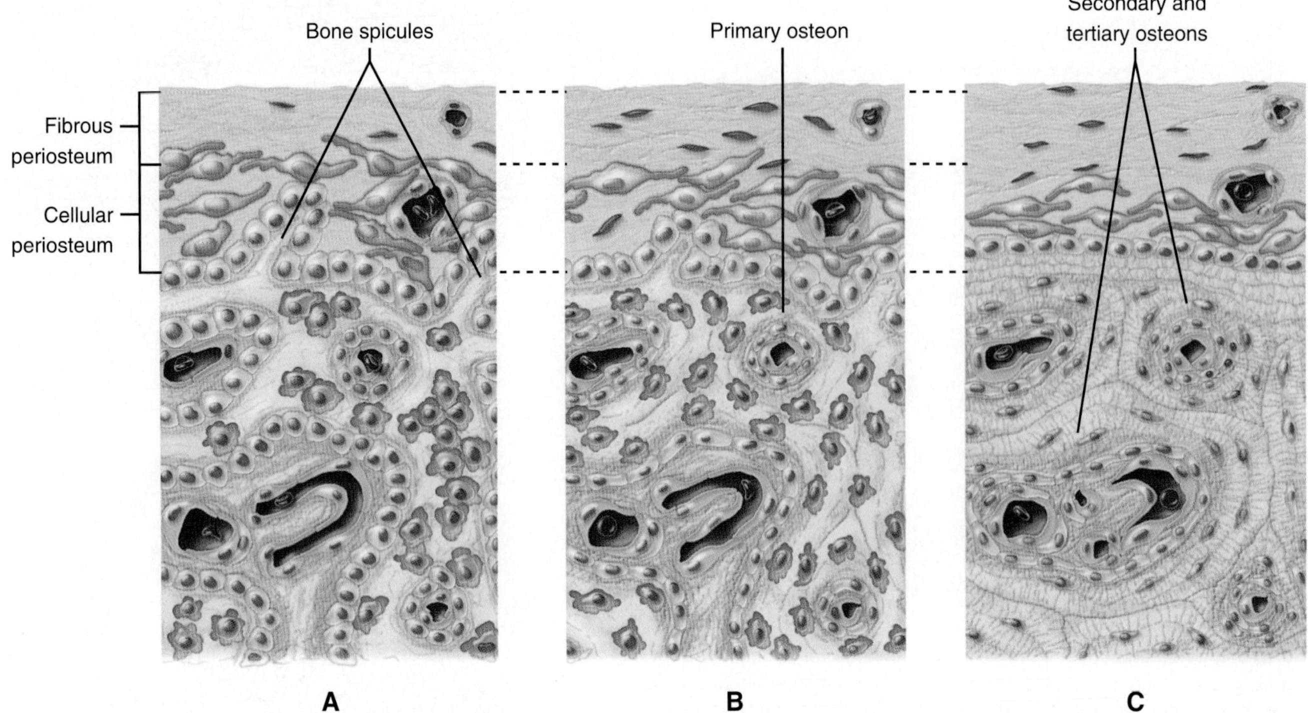

Fig. 6.31 Diagrammatic illustration of intramembranous bone formation. (A) Coarse woven bone. The bone is cellular and disorganized. (B) Immature bone. The bone is less cellular and slightly more organized; some primary osteons are forming. (C) Mature lamellar bone. The tightly packed osteons create an organized bone matrix; fewer cells and little loose connective tissue are apparent. As remodeling of the bone in its mature state takes place, the periosteal bone surface becomes more regular and eventually will be covered with circumferential lamellae.

Understanding the structure of a suture is based on the knowledge that the periosteum of a bone consists of two layers, an outer fibrous layer and an inner cellular or osteogenic layer. At the suture the fibrous layer separates into outer and inner portions. The outer portion runs across the gap of the suture to unite with the outer portion from the other side. On each side, the inner portion, together with the osteogenic layer of the periosteum, run down the suture along the surface of the bones involved in the joint. The osteogenic layer of the suture is called the *cambium,* and the inner portion is the *capsule.* Between these two layers is a loose cellular and vascular tissue (Fig. 6.33).

Sutures are best regarded as having the same osteogenic potential as periosteum. When two bones are separated (e.g., the skull bones are forced apart by the growing brain), bone forms at the sutural margins with successive waves of new bone cells differentiating from the cambium. Thus the histologic structure of the suture permits a strong tie between bones while providing a site for new bone formation. The two cambium layers are separated by a relatively inert middle layer so that growth can occur independently at each bony margin.

Bone Turnover (Remodeling)

The process by which the overall size and shape of bones is established is referred to as *bone modeling;* it extends from embryonic bone development to the preadult period of human growth. During this phase, bone is being formed rapidly, primarily (but not exclusively) on the periosteal surface. Simultaneously, bone is being destroyed along the endosteal surface, at focal points along the periosteal surface, and within the osteons of compact bone. Because bones increase greatly in length and thickness during growth, bone formation occurs at a much greater rate than bone resorption. This replacement of old bone by new is called *bone turnover (remodeling).* Bone turnover rates of 30% to 100% per year are common in rapidly growing children; most of the bone present today in a child will not be present a year from now. Bone turnover does not stop when adulthood is reached, although its rate slows. Indeed, the adult skeleton is broken down continuously and reformed by the coordinated action of osteoclasts and osteoblasts. In a healthy individual, this turnover is in a steady state; that is, the amount of bone lost is balanced by bone formed. In certain diseases (e.g., osteoporosis) and with age, the resorption exceeds formation, resulting in an overall loss of bone. Bone turnover occurs in discrete, focal areas involving groups of cells called *bone remodeling (basic multicellular) units.* The sequence of events at these temporary and evolving anatomic sites consists of five phases: activation, resorption, reversal, formation, and resting (Fig. 6.34). During the resorption phase, bone is removed, and a resorption lacuna is created. Factors produced by osteoclasts, mononuclear reversal cells, or liberated from the resorbed bone matrix trigger the formative phase during which the lacuna then is filled with new bone produced by osteoblasts recruited at the site. As these osteoblasts mature, they produce more osteoprotegerin and less RANKL, leading to a reduction in RANK/RANKL interactions. This results in an inhibition of osteoclast activity, thereby allowing osteoblasts to refill the resorption lacuna. The formation phase lasts substantially longer than the resorption and reversal phases together. Osteocytes are likely implicated in sensing the need for remodeling and transmitting signals via their extensive canalicular network to osteoclast and osteoblast compartments.

The rate of cortical bone turnover is approximately 5% per year, whereas turnover rates of trabecular bone and the endosteal surface of cortical bone can approach 15% per year. The release of mineral ions during bone turnover, together with the concerted action of the kidneys and intestine, is an integral part of the phosphocalcic homeostasis system.

Primary osteons of fetal bone eventually are resorbed by osteoclasts to make room for the expanding marrow cavity, or they undergo turnover; that is, a primary osteon is replaced by succeeding generations of

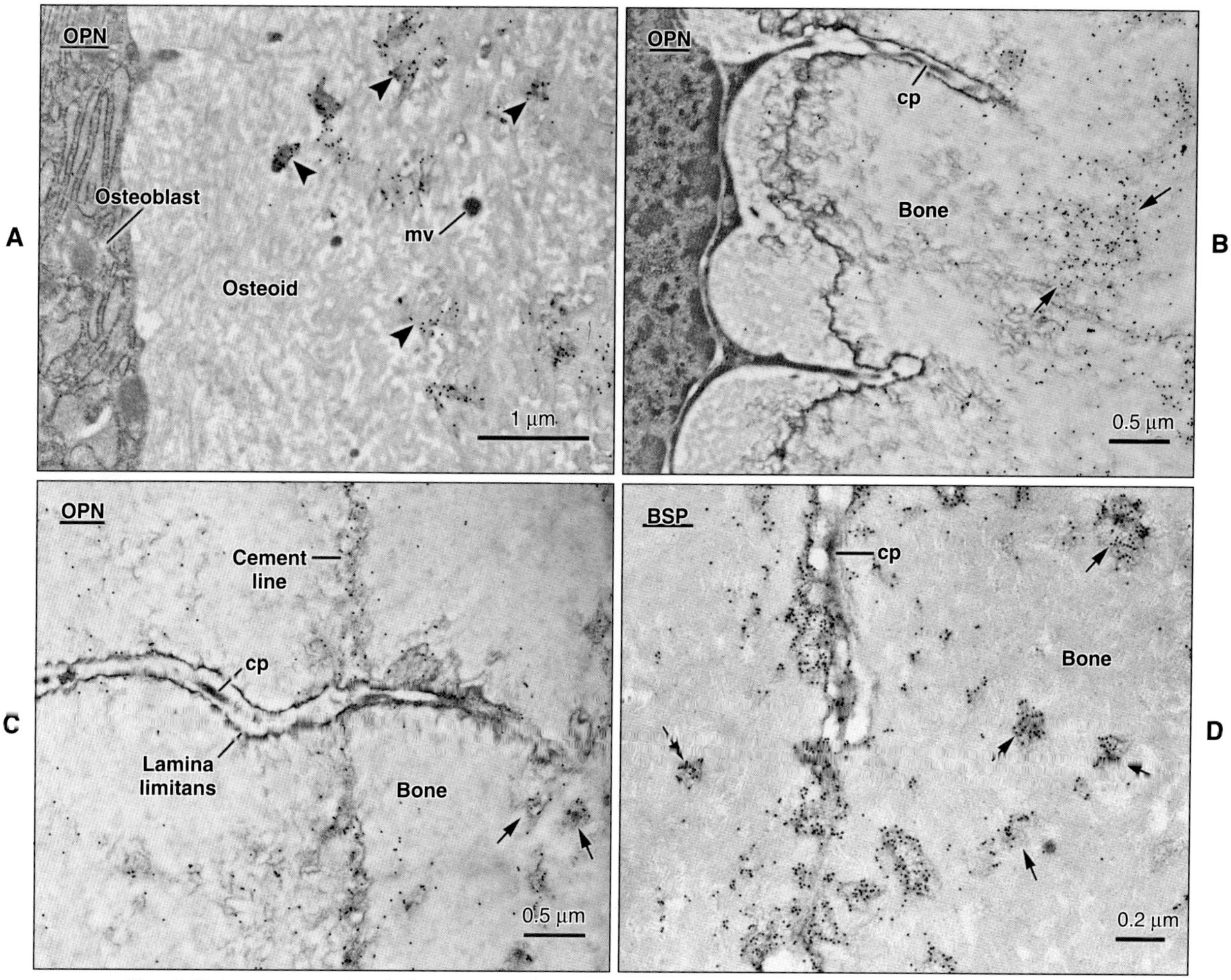

Fig. 6.32 Immunocytochemical preparations illustrating the distribution of (A–C) osteopontin (OPN) in rat bone and (D) bone sialoprotein (BSP) in human bone. Both proteins are essentially found at similar matrix sites, that is, mineralization foci *(arrowheads)*, diffusely or as patches between the calcified collagen fibrils *(arrows)*, and cement lines. *cp*, Cell process; *mv*, matrix vesicle.

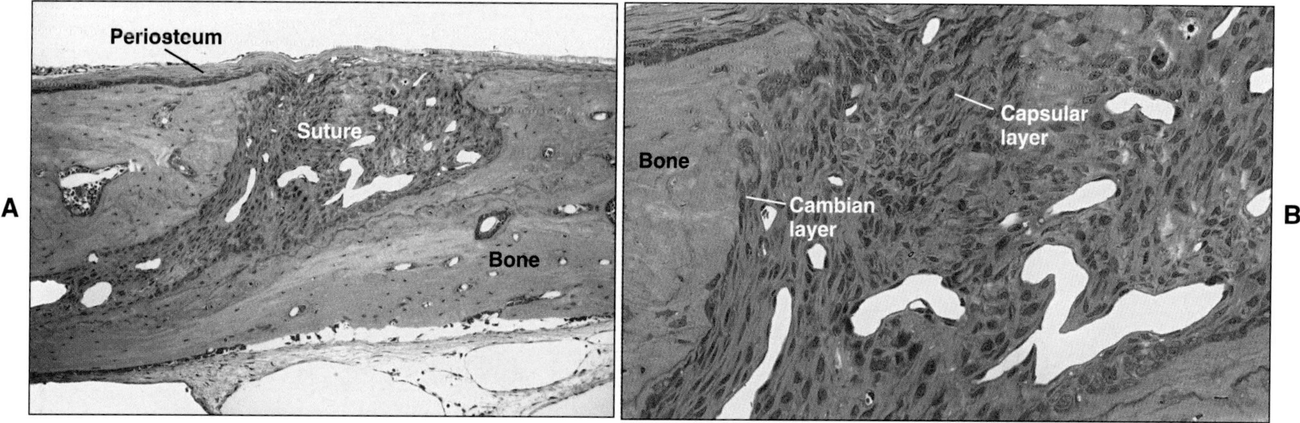

Fig. 6.33 Sutural growth. (A) Low-magnification light micrograph showing that the suture connects two periosteal surfaces. (B) A higher magnification shows the developing inner osteogenic or cambian layer and the central capsular layer.

higher-order osteons (e.g., secondary and tertiary). Each succeeding generation is slightly larger, functionally more mature, and therefore more lamellar (Fig. 6.35). Exactly what induces turnover is still poorly understood and likely involves local mechanisms in the bone microenvironment and systemic factors.

As osteoclasts move through compact bone, they create a resorption channel. The leading edge of resorption is termed the *cutting cone* and is characterized by a scalloped array of resorption (Howship) lacunae, each housing an osteoclast (Figs. 6.36 and 6.37). When a portion of an earlier osteon is not resorbed, it remains as interstitial lamellae (see Figs. 6.3

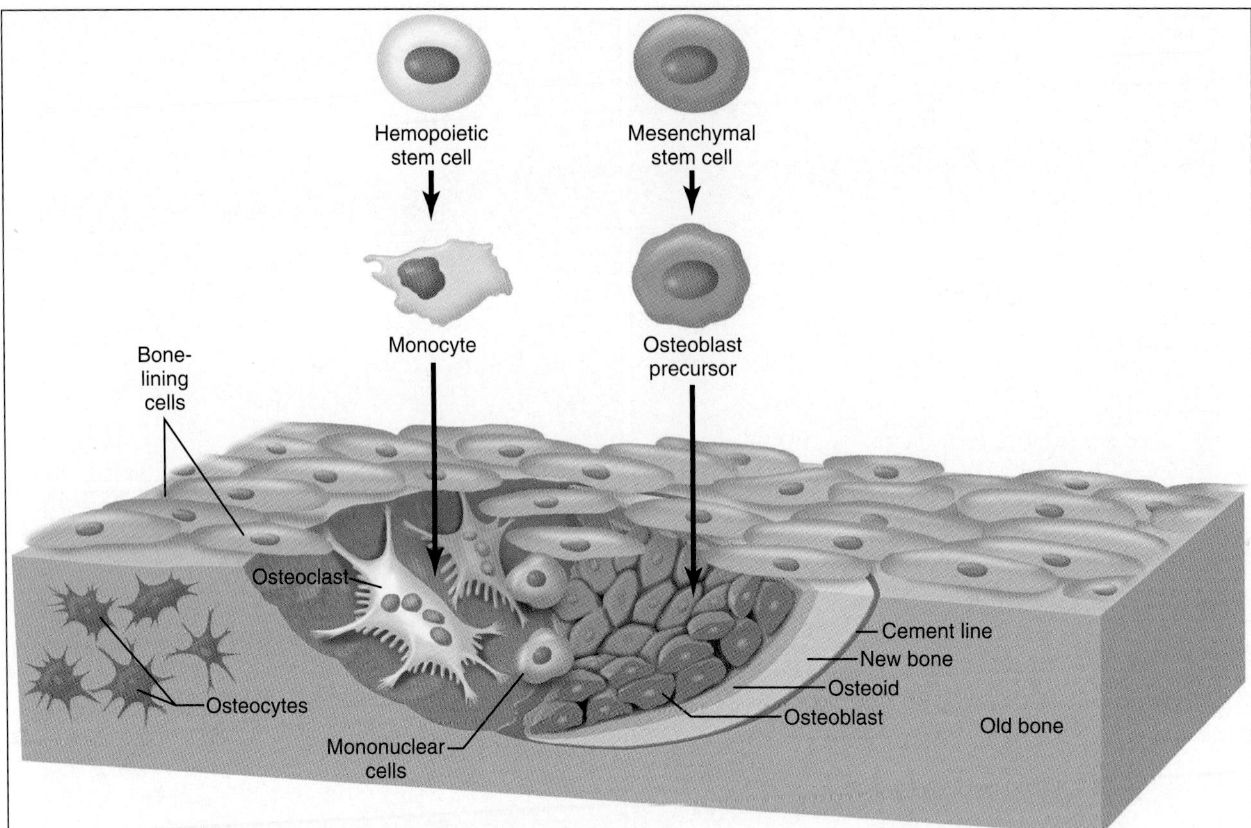

Fig. 6.34 Schematic representation of bone remodeling on the surface of trabecular (cancellous) bone as seen in longitudinal sequence. The process occurs through the cooperative activity of various cells that form a temporary functional compartment known as *basic multicellular (bone remodeling) unit*. The process begins with the activation of osteoclast formation, followed in order by (1) a resorption phase during which osteoclasts remove old bone and create the resorption lacuna, (2) reversal in which mononuclear cells (macrophage-like or osteoblast precursors) deposit a cement line, (3) a formation phase during which new bone is deposited, and (4) a resting phase during which osteoblasts become quiescent and become the flattened bone-lining cells. These cells are believed to persist as a canopy over the resorption lacuna during the bone remodeling cycle. (From Raiz LG: Pathogenesis of osteoporosis: concepts, conflicts, and prospects, *J Clin Invest* 115:3318–3325, 2005.)

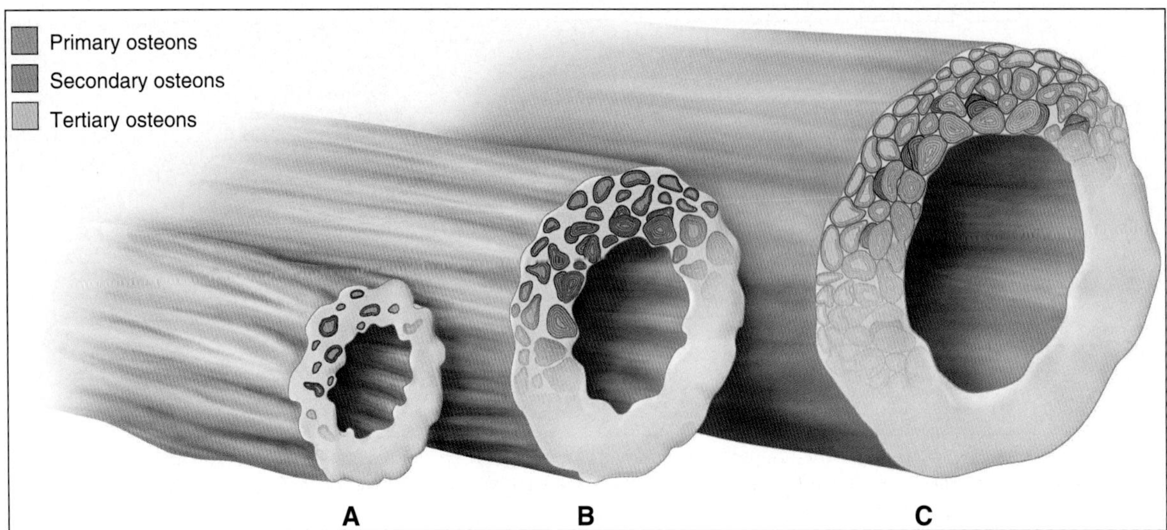

Fig. 6.35 Diagrammatic illustration of progressive bone growth and turnover. (A) Young immature bone is thin with few primary osteons. The periosteal surface is undulating and forms bone rapidly. The endosteal surface is primarily for resorption. (B) The immature bone thickens. The periosteal surface is not as undulating, and secondary osteons are now present. The primary osteons are resorbed, and the fragments are buried by new bone on the periosteal surface. (C) The bone becomes nearly mature. The bone is thicker still, its periosteal surface is less undulating, and tertiary osteons replace the secondary osteons. Fragments of primary and secondary osteons persist as interstitial lamellae. Eventually, circumferential lamellae smooth out the periosteal surface.

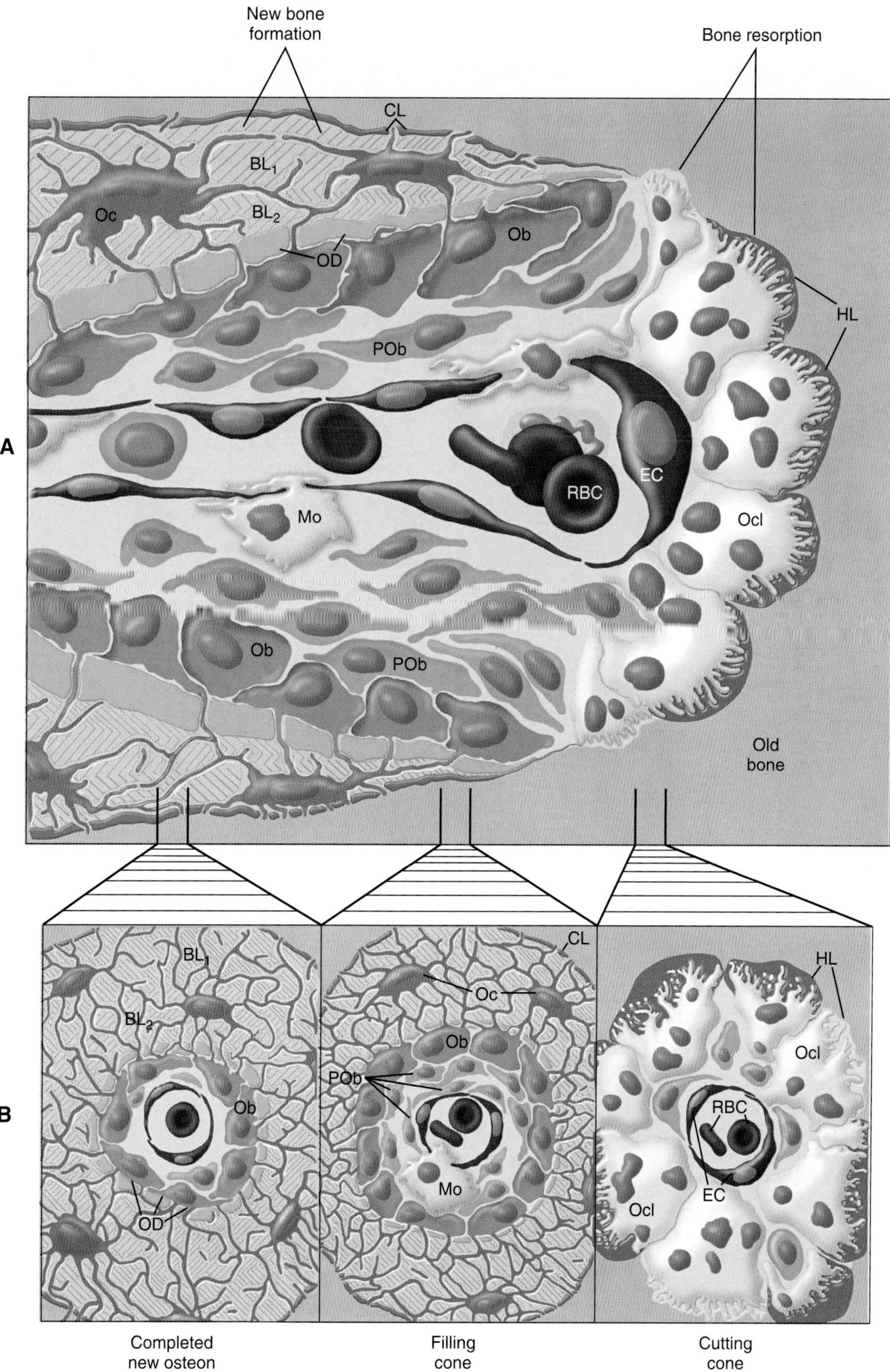

Fig. 6.36 Diagrammatic illustration of bone remodeling unit during compact (cortical) bone turnover in (A) longitudinal and (B) cross section. Turnover of old bone progresses from left to right as osteoclasts continue to resorb and osteoblasts continue to form new bone. Bloodborne monocytes migrate through the endothelial cells and fuse to form osteoclasts, which ream out the old bone, forming a frontal and a circular array of Howship lacunae *(HL)*. Collectively, they make up the cutting cone. Behind the osteoclasts, uninucleated cells (preosteoblasts) migrate onto the bone surface and differentiate into osteoblasts responsible for forming osteoid *(OD)* that mineralizes to become new bone (filling cone). Some osteoblasts become entrapped in the matrix they produce as osteocytes. A cement line forms at the interface between old and new bone. Collectively, osteoblasts form the filling cone; as they do, they change the orientation of collagen in succeeding lamellae (BL_1 and BL_2). *CL*, Cement line; *EC*, endothelial cell; *Mo*, monocyte; *Ob*, osteoblast; *Oc*, osteocyte; *Ocl*, osteoclast; *POb*, preosteoblast; *RBC*, red blood cells.

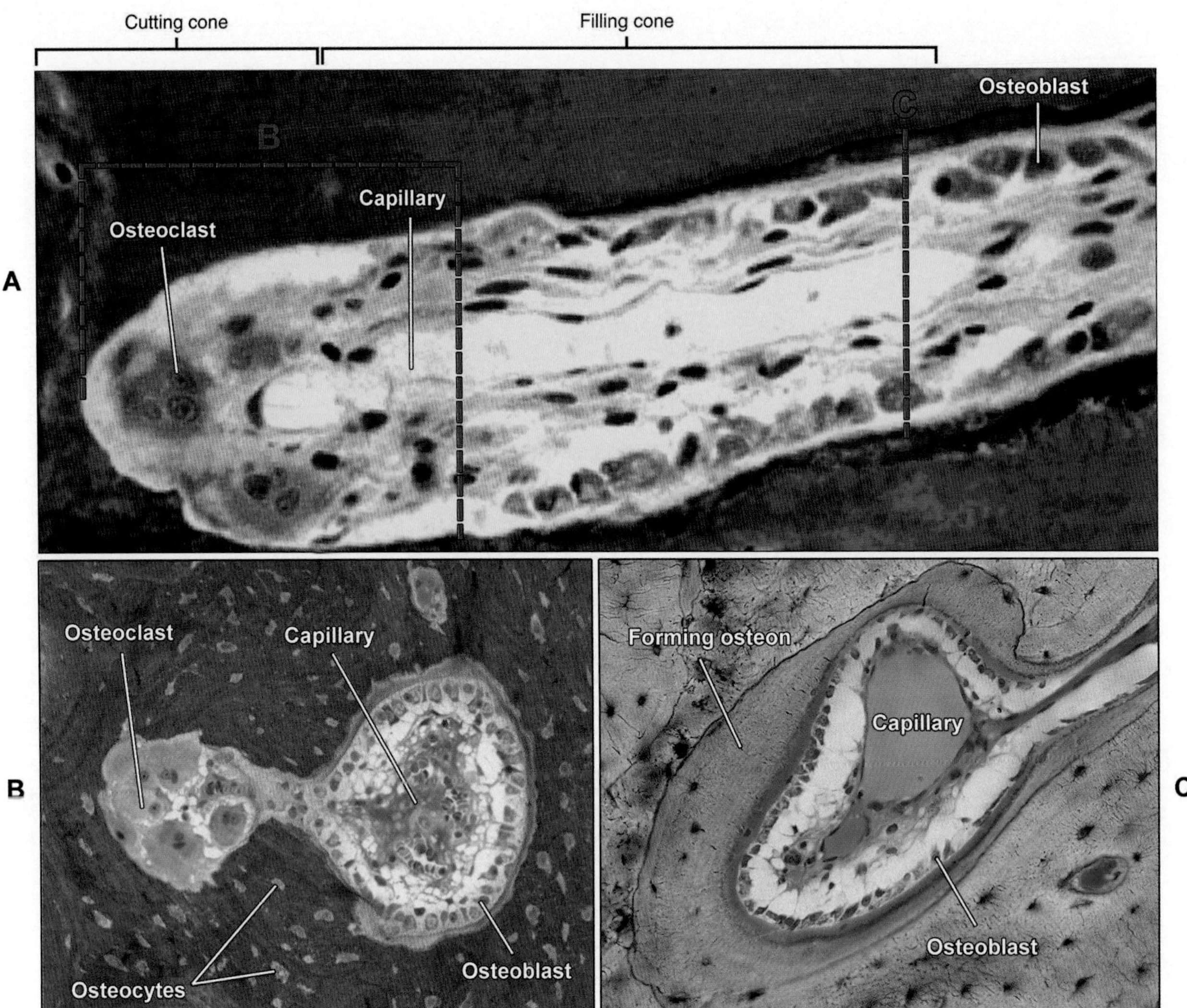

Fig. 6.37 Light micrographs showing resorption channels through compact bone in (A) longitudinal section and (B, C) cross section. (A) The leading edge of the channel (cutting cone) contains osteoclasts that resorb the old bone. The portion behind (filling cone) contains a central capillary and osteoblasts that will deposit bone in concentric lamellae, giving rise to a new osteon. (B) Several large multinucleated osteoclasts cluster in the cutting cone, each resorbing small packets of bone. The shallow resorption lacunae they create are Howship lacunae. (C) After resorption, uninucleated osteoblasts ring the eroded bone surface to form new bone onto it. (A, Coutersy R.K. Schenk; B, C, courtesy P. Tambasco de Oliveira.)

and 6.4). Behind the cutting cone is a migration of mononucleated cells (macrophages and/or preosteoblasts) onto the roughened surface of the bone channel. As the preosteoblasts differentiate into osteoblasts, they deposit onto the resorbed bone surface a thin coating of noncollagenous matrix proteins termed the *cement,* or *reversal line.* This layer is composed of at least BSP and OPN and acts as a cohesive, mineralized layer between the old bone and the new bone that will be formed on top of the cement line by these same osteoblasts (Fig. 6.38; see also Figs. 6.32, 6.34, and 6.36). The entire area of the osteon where active formation occurs is termed the *filling cone* (see Figs. 6.36 and 6.37). As formation proceeds, some osteoblasts become osteocytes. When formation is complete, the Haversian canal contains a central blood vessel and a layer of inactive osteoblasts, the lining cells that communicate by means of cell processes with the embedded osteocytes.

Lamellar cancellous or spongy bone (secondary spongiosa) also turns over (see Figs. 6.34 and 6.38). Osteoclasts create resorption cavities on quiescent trabecular surfaces covered by bone-lining cells that then are colonized by new osteoblasts that slowly fill in the cavities with new bone, as described earlier. The bone remodeling unit on trabecular bone surfaces can actually be viewed as a resorption channel in compact bone cut in half (compare Figs. 6.34 and 6.36).

This account indicates that a considerable amount of internal remodeling by means of resorption and deposition occurs within bone. How such remodeling is controlled is an intriguing problem. A key question is how the osteoclasts become targeted to reach specific sites. As previously stated, osteoblasts, appropriately stimulated by hormones (or perhaps by local environmental changes that occur in situations such as tooth movement), may provide the controlling mechanism for bone resorption. The controlling mechanism that arrests bone resorption also needs to be determined. Such a signal may be hormonal; alternatively, the process of resorption may be self-limiting.

The repeated deposition and removal of bone tissue accommodates the growth of a bone without losing function or its relationship to neighboring structures during the remodeling phase. Thus, for

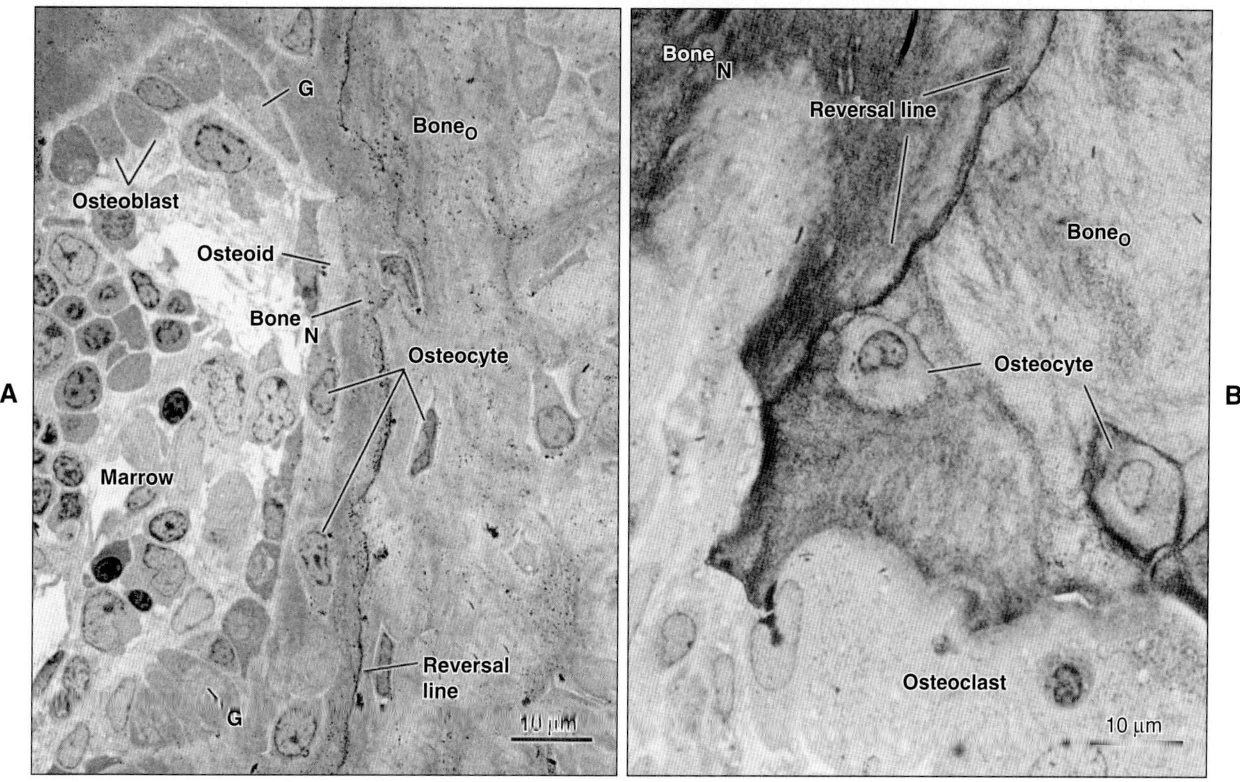

Fig. 6.38 Light-level preparations illustrating (A) deposition of new bone *(Bone$_N$)* onto the resorbed surface of older bone *(Bone$_O$)* and (B) newer and older bone with part of the older bone being resorbed by an osteoclast. The preparations are immunolabeled for osteopontin *(black deposits)*. At the interface between the two layers is a scalloped line, intensely immunoreactive for osteopontin. This scalloped appearance matches the concavities created by osteoclasts during bone resorption. The line is a cement line, or reversal line, created during the reversal from the resorptive to the formative phase. The pale regions in the cytoplasm of osteoblasts in (A) represent the Golgi complex *(G)*.

example, a significant increase in size of the mandible is achieved from birth to maturity largely by bone remodeling without any loss in function or change in its position relative to the maxilla. Any of the bone present in a 1-year-old mandible most likely is not present in the same bone 30 years later.

RECOMMENDED READING

Bianco P: The stem cell next door: skeletal and hematopoietic stem cell "niches" in bone, *Endocrinology* 152:2957–2962, 2011.

Bonewald LF: The role of the osteocyte in bone and nonbone disease, *Endocrinol Metab Clin North Am* 46:1–18, 2017.

Everts V, et al.: The bone lining cell: its role in cleaning Howship's lacunae and initiating bone formation, *J Bone Miner Res* 17:77–90, 2002.

Gorski JP: Is all bone the same? Distinctive distributions and properties of non-collagenous matrix proteins in lamellar vs woven bone imply the existence of different underlying osteogenic mechanisms, *Crit Rev Oral Biol Med* 9:201–223, 1998.

Karsenty G, et al.: Genetic control of bone formation, *Ann Rev Cell Dev Biol* 25:629–648, 2009.

Karsenty G, Oury F: The central regulation of bone mass: the first link between bone remodeling and energy metabolism, *J Clin Endocrinol Metab* 95:4795–4801, 2010.

Kobayashi T, Kronenberg H: Minireview: transcriptional regulation in development in bone, *Endocrinology* 146:1012–1017, 2005.

Martin TJ, Ng KW: Mechanisms by which cells of the osteoblast lineage control osteoclast formation and activity, *J Cell Biochem* 56:357, 1994.

Moffatt P, et al.: Bril: a novel bone-specific modulator of mineralization, *J Bone Miner Res* 23:1497, 2008.

Parfitt AM: The bone remodelling compartment: a circulatory function for bone lining cells, *J Bone Miner Res* 16:1583, 2001.

Quarles LD: Endocrine functions of bone in mineral metabolism regulation, *J Clin Invest* 118:3820–3828, 2008.

Raiz LG: Pathogenesis of osteoporosis: concepts, conflicts, and prospects, *J Clin Invest* 115:3318–3325, 2005.

Robey PG, Boskey AL: The composition of bone. In Rosen CJ, et al., editors: *Primer on the metabolic bone diseases and disorders of mineral metabolism*, ed 8, Washington, DC, 2013, American Association for Bone and Mineral Research.

Roger A, Eastell R: Circulating osteoprotegerin and receptor activator for nuclear factor κB ligand: clinical utility in metabolic bone disease assessment, *J Clin Endocrinol Metab* 90:6323–6331, 2005.

Roodman GD: Osteoclast differentiation and activity, *Biochem Soc Trans* 26:7–13, 1998.

Salo J, et al.: Removal of osteoclast bone resorption products by transcytosis, *Science* 276:270–273, 1997.

7

Enamel: Composition, Formation, and Structure

Antonio Nanci

OUTLINE

Enamel is the hardest calcified matrix of the body. The cells that are responsible for its formation, the ameloblasts, are lost as the tooth erupts into the oral cavity, and hence enamel cannot renew itself. To compensate for this inherent limitation, enamel has acquired a complex structural organization and a high degree of mineralization rendered possible by the almost total absence of organic matrix in its mature state. These characteristics reflect the unusual life cycle of the ameloblasts and the unique physicochemical characteristics of the matrix proteins that regulate formation of the extremely long crystals of enamel. Although enamel is structurally distinctive from collagen-based calcified tissues, there are fundamental similarities and common themes in the formation of all calcified tissues.

PHYSICAL CHARACTERISTICS OF ENAMEL

Enamel is translucent and varies in color from light yellow to gray-white. It also varies in thickness, from a maximum of approximately 2.5 mm over working surfaces to a feather edge at the cervical line in humans. This variation influences the color of enamel because the underlying yellow dentin is seen through the thinner regions.

Fully formed enamel consists of approximately 96% mineral and 4% organic material and water (Table 7.1). The inorganic content of enamel is a crystalline calcium phosphate (hydroxyapatite) substituted with carbonate ions, also found in bone, calcified cartilage, dentin, and cementum. Various ions (strontium, magnesium, lead, and fluoride), if present during enamel formation, may be incorporated into the crystals. The susceptibility of these crystals to dissolution by acid provides the chemical basis for dental caries.

The high mineral content renders enamel extremely hard; this is a property that, together with its complex structural organization, enables enamel to withstand the mechanical forces applied during mastication. This hardness also makes enamel brittle; therefore an underlying layer of more resilient dentin is necessary to maintain its integrity (Fig. 7.1A). If this supportive layer of dentin is destroyed by caries or improper cavity preparation, the unsupported enamel fractures easily.

STRUCTURE OF ENAMEL

Because of the highly mineralized nature of enamel, its structure is difficult to study. When conventional demineralized sections are examined, only an empty space can be seen in areas previously occupied by mature enamel because the mineral has been dissolved, and the trace organic material has been washed away.

The fundamental organizational units of mammalian enamel are the rods (prisms) and interrod enamel (interprismatic substance) (Fig. 7.2; also see Fig. 7.1B–D). The enamel rod was first described as hexagonal and prismlike in cross section, and the term *enamel prism* still is used frequently. This term is not used in this text because rods do not have a regular geometry and hence are not prismatic.

Enamel is built from closely packed and long, ribbonlike carbonate apatite crystals (Fig. 7.3; see also Fig. 7.2) measuring 60 to 70 nm in width and 25 to 30 nm in thickness. The crystals are extremely long; some investigators believe that the length of the crystals spans the entire thickness of the enamel layer. The calcium phosphate unit cell has a hexagonal symmetry and stacks up to impart a hexagonal

TABLE 7.1 Percentage Wet Weight Composition of Rat Incisor Enamel

Component	Secretory Stage (%)	Midmaturation (%)	Late Maturation (%)
Water	5	3	1
Mineral	29	93	95
Protein	66	4	4

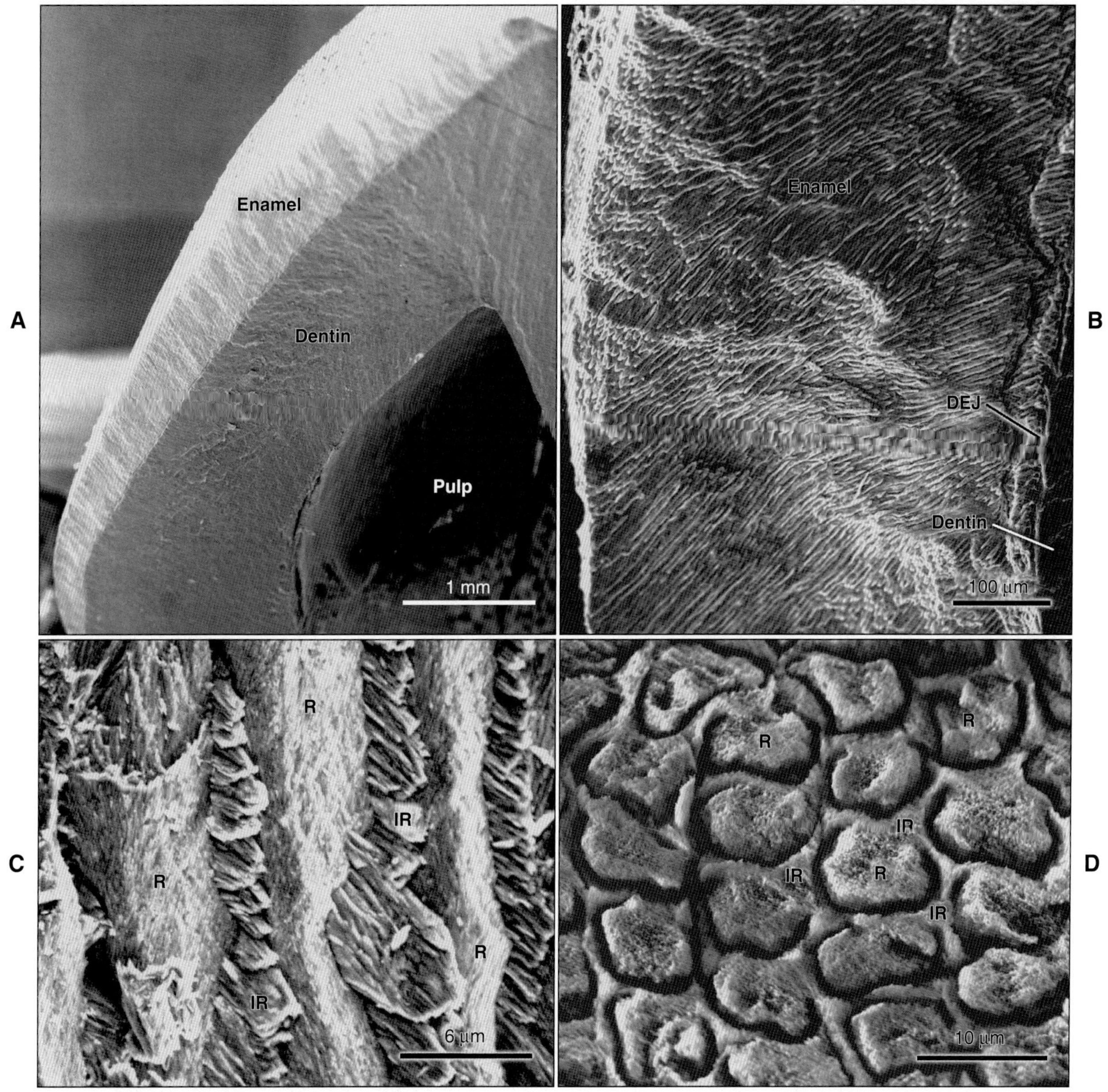

Fig. 7.1 Scanning electron microscope views of (A) the enamel layer covering coronal dentin, (B) the complex distribution of enamel rods across the layer, and (C, D) perspectives of the rod/interrod relationship when rods are exposed (C) longitudinally or (D) in cross section. Interrod enamel surrounds each rod. *DEJ,* Dentinoenamel junction; *IR,* interrod; *R,* rod.

outline to the crystal, which is clearly visible in cross-sectional profile in maturing enamel (Fig. 7.4). However, fully mature enamel crystals are no longer perfectly hexagonal but rather exhibit an irregular outline because they press against each other during the final part of their growth (Fig. 7.5). These crystals are grouped together as rod or interrod enamel (see Figs. 7.2 and 7.3).

In ground sections the orientation of rods may be misinterpreted because the crystalline nature of enamel leads to optical interference as the light passes through the section, and their outline is difficult to resolve. As a result, when the roughly cylindric enamel rods are sectioned, cut profiles that line up may be misinterpreted as rods viewed longitudinally, making assessment of rod direction under

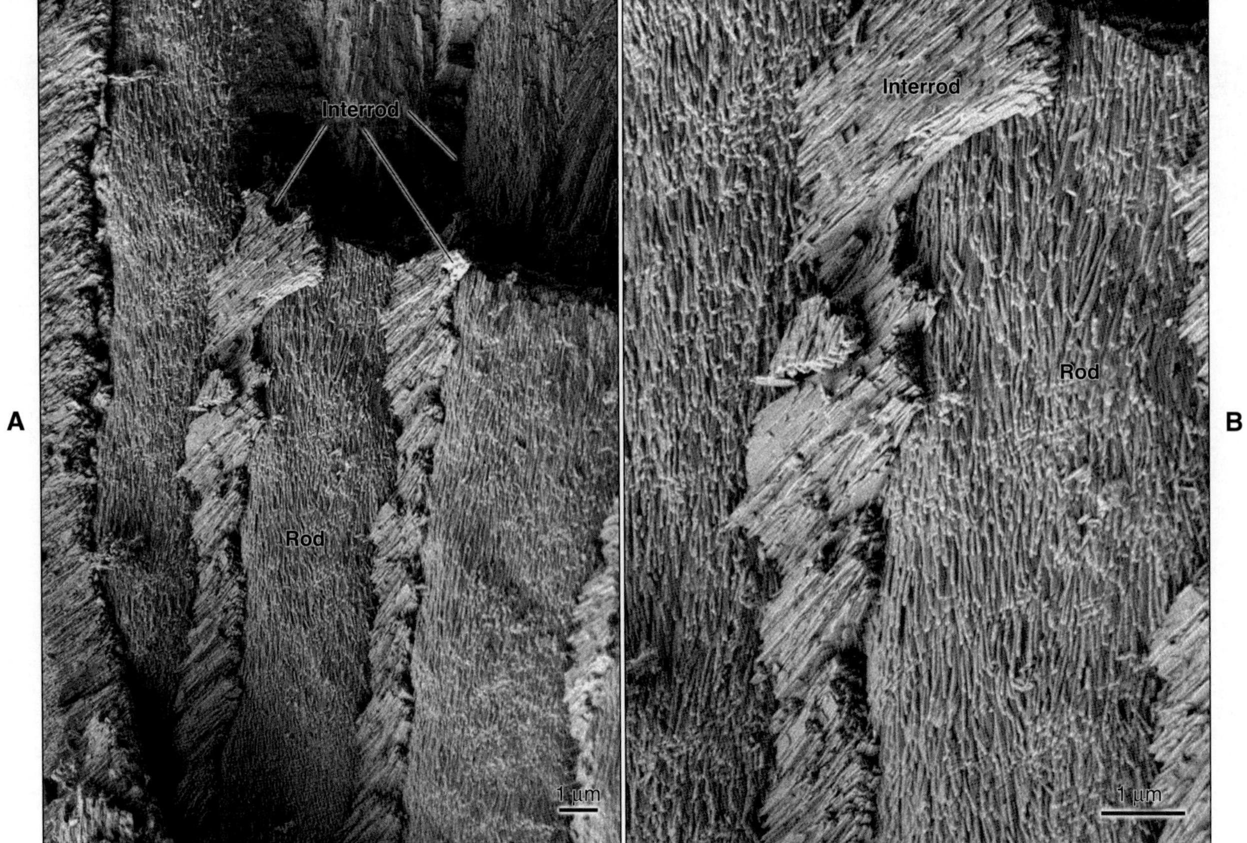

Fig. 7.2 (A, B) High-resolution scanning electron microscope images showing that crystals in rod and interrod enamel are similar in structure but diverge in orientation.

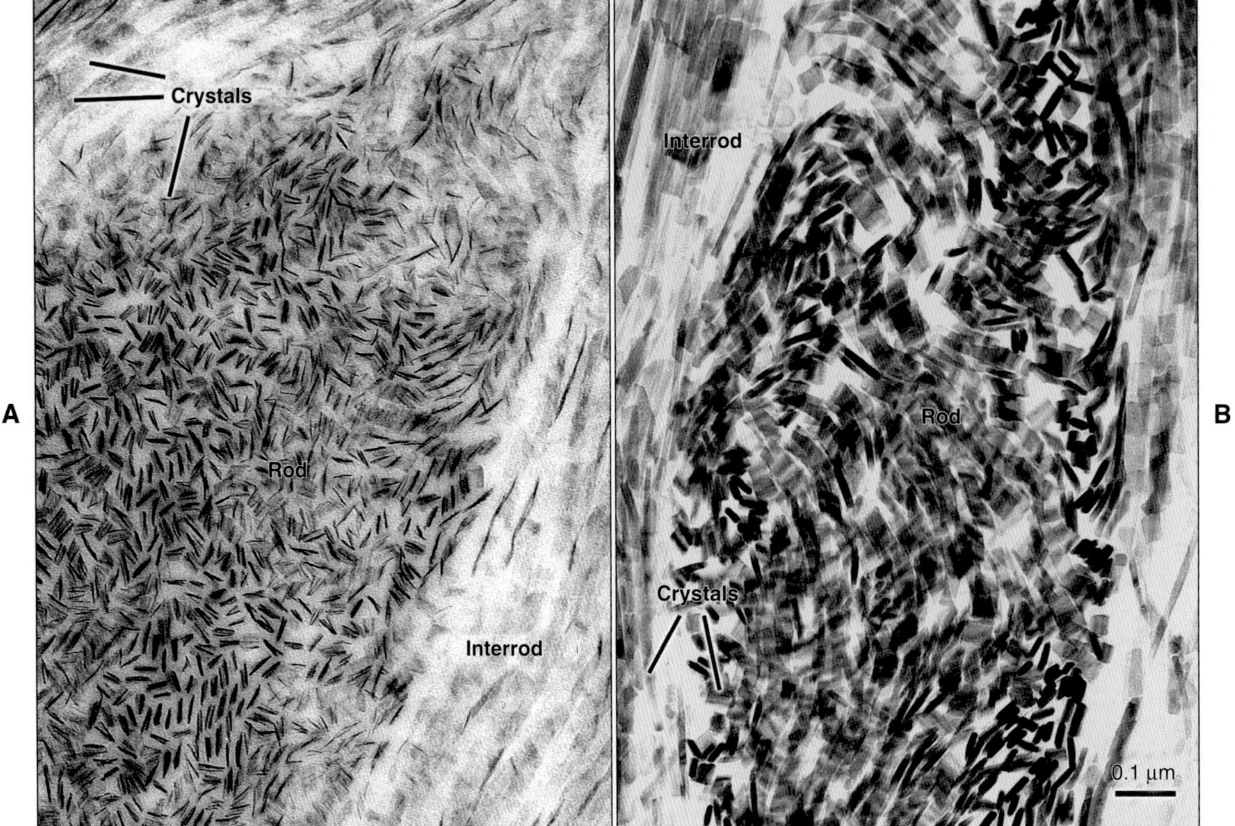

Fig. 7.3 Transmission electron microscope images of a rod surrounded by interrod enamel from (A) young and (B) older forming enamel of a rodent. The crystals that make up the rod and interrod enamel are long, ribbonlike structures that become thicker as enamel matures. They appear in different planes of sections because they have different orientations.

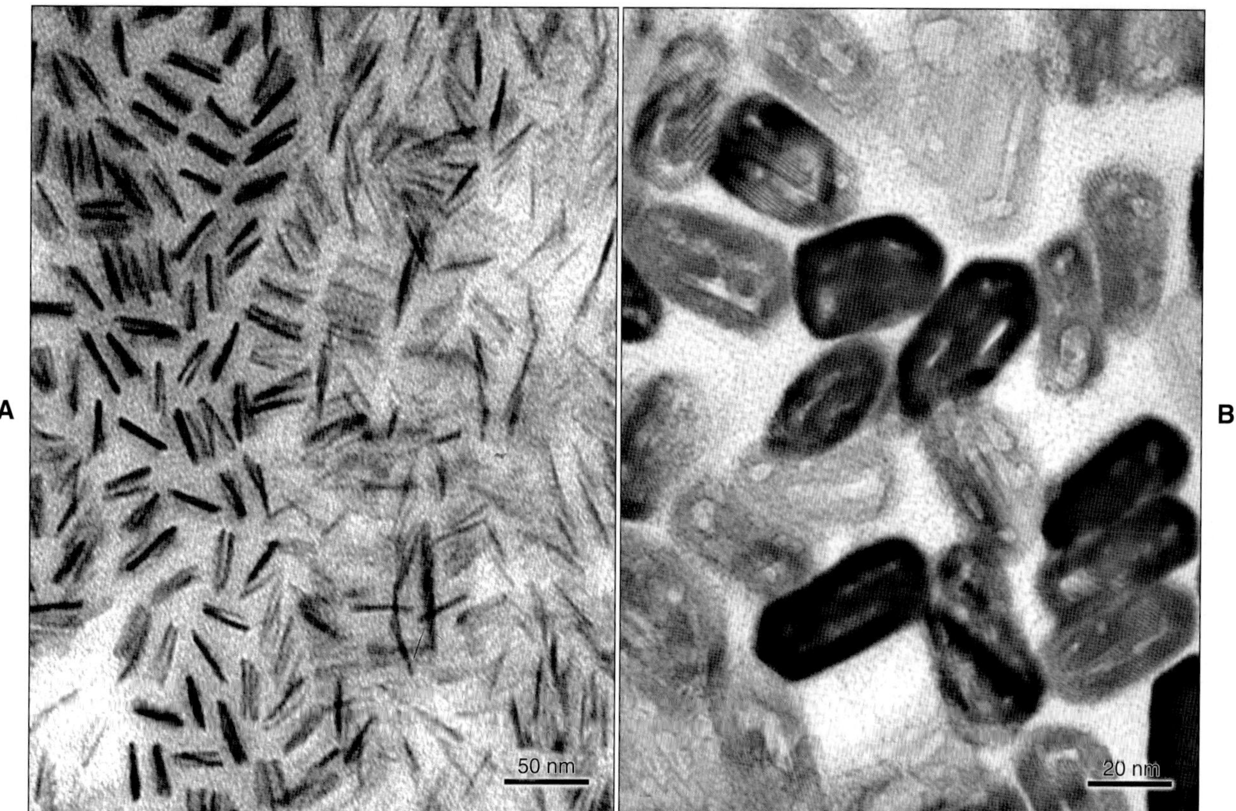

Fig. 7.4 Cross-sectional profiles of (A) recently formed, secretory-stage enamel crystals and (B) older ones from the maturation stage. Initially the crystals are thin; as they grow in thickness and width, their hexagonal contour becomes apparent. (B) The linear patterns seen in older crystals reflect their crystalline lattice.

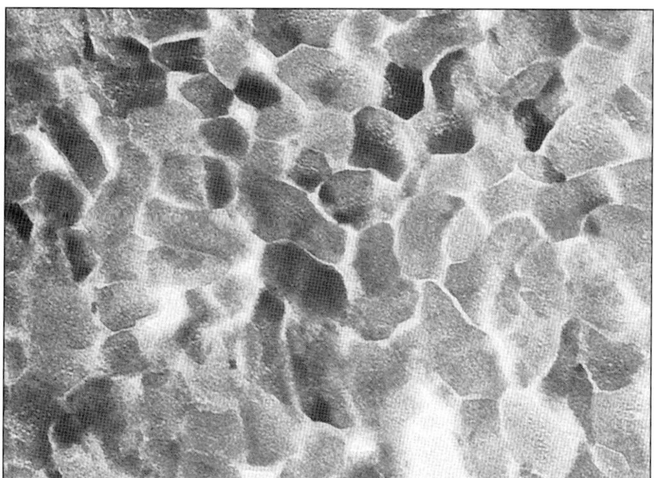

Fig. 7.5 Electron micrograph of mature enamel crystals. The outline is irregular as they press against each other. (Courtesy J.W. Simmelink et al.)

the light microscope difficult. Use of both the scanning and transmission electron microscopes has overcome these interpretative difficulties.

The rod is shaped somewhat like a cylinder and is made up of crystals with long axes that run, for the most part, in the general direction of the longitudinal axis of the rod (Fig. 7.6; see also Figs 7.1C and D, 7.2, and 7.3). The interrod enamel surrounds each rod, and its crystals are oriented in a direction different from those making up the rod (Fig. 7.7; see also Figs. 7.1C and D, 7.2, 7.3, and 7.6). The difference in orientation is significant at approximately three-fourths of the circumference of a rod. The boundary between rod and interrod enamel in this region is delimited by a narrow space containing organic material known as the *rod sheath* (Fig. 7.8; see also Figs. 7.1D and 7.7); the rod sheath is visualized more clearly in forming enamels of higher mammals (Fig. 7.9). Along a small portion of the circumference of the rod the crystals are confluent with those of interrod enamel (Fig. 7.10; see also Fig. 7.1D). In this region, rod and interrod enamel are not separated, and there is no space or rod sheath between them, and rod crystals can be seen to flare out into the interrod enamel (see Fig. 7.7). The cross-sectional outline of these two related components in humans has been compared with the shape of a keyhole; however, the keyhole analogy does not adequately account for some of the variations in the structural arrangement of the enamel components and is not consistent with the pattern of formation of enamel. The basic organizational pattern of mammalian enamel thus is described more appropriately as cylindric rods embedded in interrod enamel.

AMELOGENESIS

Amelogenesis (enamel formation) is a two-step process. When enamel first forms, it mineralizes only partially to approximately 30% (see Table 7.1). Subsequently, as the organic matrix breaks down and is removed, crystals grow wider and thicker. This process whereby organic matrix and water are lost and mineral is added accentuates after the full thickness of the enamel layer has been formed to attain greater than 96% mineral content.

Ameloblasts (the enamel forming cells) secrete matrix proteins and are responsible for creating and maintaining an extracellular

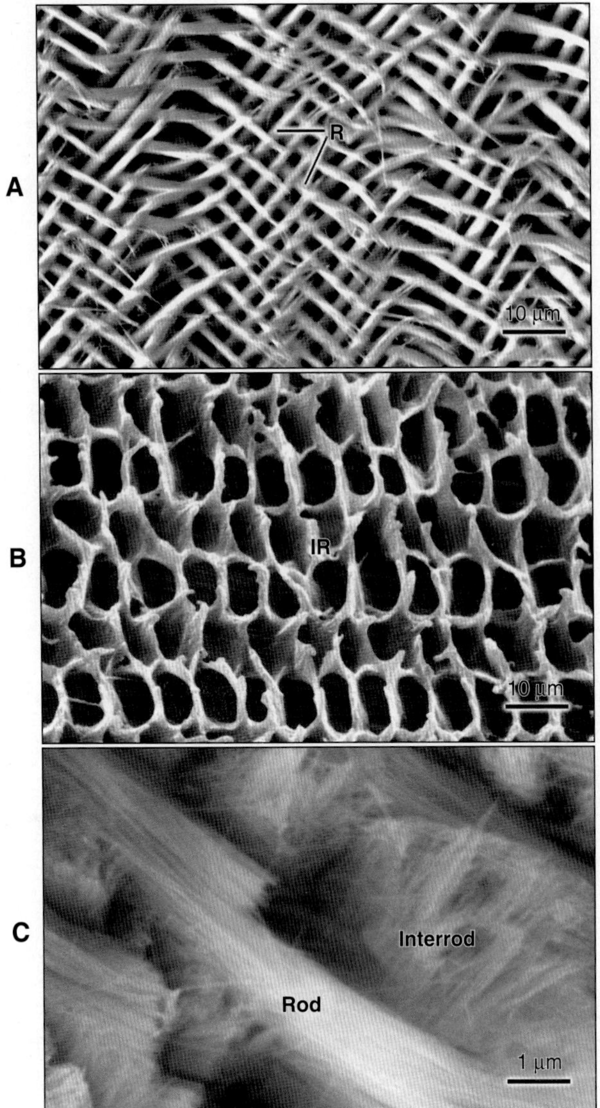

Fig. 7.6 Scanning electron microscope images showing various aspects of rat incisor enamel. (A) The enamel rods *(R)* are arranged in rows with alternating orientations. (B) The alternating row arrangement is also evident in the interrod *(IR)* cavities that accommodate the enamel rod. (C) Rod and interrod enamel are made up of thin and long apatite crystals.

environment favorable to mineral deposition. This epithelial cell exhibits a unique life cycle characterized by progressive phenotype changes that reflect its primary activity at various times of enamel formation (Figs. 7.11–7.18). Amelogenesis has been described in as many as six phases but generally is subdivided into three main functional stages referred to as the *presecretory, secretory,* and *maturation stages.* Classically, ameloblasts from each stage have been portrayed as fulfilling exclusive functions. First, during the presecretory stage, differentiating ameloblasts acquire their phenotype, change polarity, develop an extensive protein synthetic apparatus, and prepare to secrete the organic matrix of enamel. Second, during the secretory (or formative) stage, ameloblasts elaborate and organize the entire enamel thickness, resulting in the formation of a highly ordered tissue. Last, during the maturation stage, ameloblasts modulate and transport specific ions required for the concurrent accretion of mineral. Ameloblasts are now considered to be cells that carry out multiple activities throughout their life cycle and that upregulate or downregulate some or all of them, according to the developmental requirements.

Enamel formation begins at the early crown stage of tooth development and involves differentiation of cells of the inner enamel epithelium first at the tips of the cusp outlines formed in that epithelium (see Fig. 7.11). The process then sweeps down the slopes of the tooth crown until all cells of the epithelium have differentiated into enamel-forming ameloblasts (see Fig. 7.12). Another feature is notable: When differentiation of the ameloblasts occurs and dentin starts forming, these cells are distanced from the blood vessels that lie outside the inner enamel epithelium within the dental papilla. Compensation for this distant vascular supply is achieved by blood vessels invaginating the outer enamel epithelium and by reduction of the intervening stellate reticulum, which brings ameloblasts closer to the blood vessels (see Fig. 7.11C).

LIGHT MICROSCOPY OF AMELOGENESIS

At the late bell stage, most of the light microscopic features of amelogenesis can be seen in a single section (see Fig. 7.13). Thus in the region of the cervical loop, the low columnar cells of the inner enamel epithelium are clearly identifiable. Peripheral to the inner enamel epithelium lie the stratum intermedium, stellate reticulum, and outer enamel epithelium, the last closely associated with the many blood vessels in the dental follicle.

As the inner enamel epithelium is traced coronally in a crown-stage tooth germ, its cells become taller and columnar, and the nuclei become aligned at the proximal ends of the cells adjacent to the stratum intermedium. Shortly after dentin formation initiates, a number

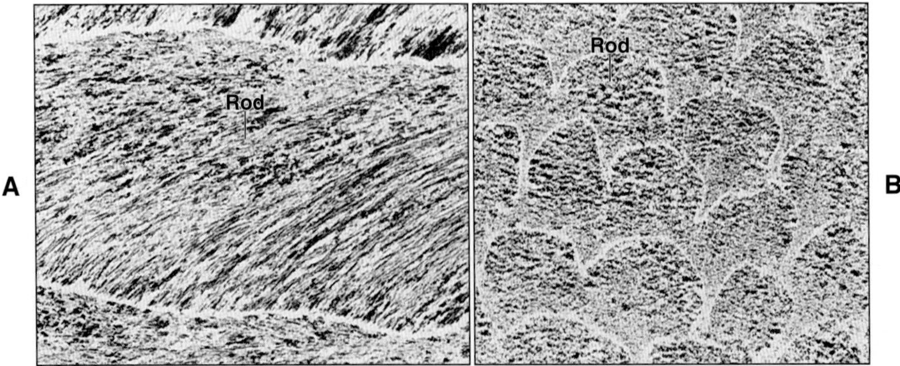

Fig. 7.7 Transmission electron micrograph of human enamel in the (A) longitudinal and (B) cross-section plane of the rods. (Courtesy A.H. Meckel.)

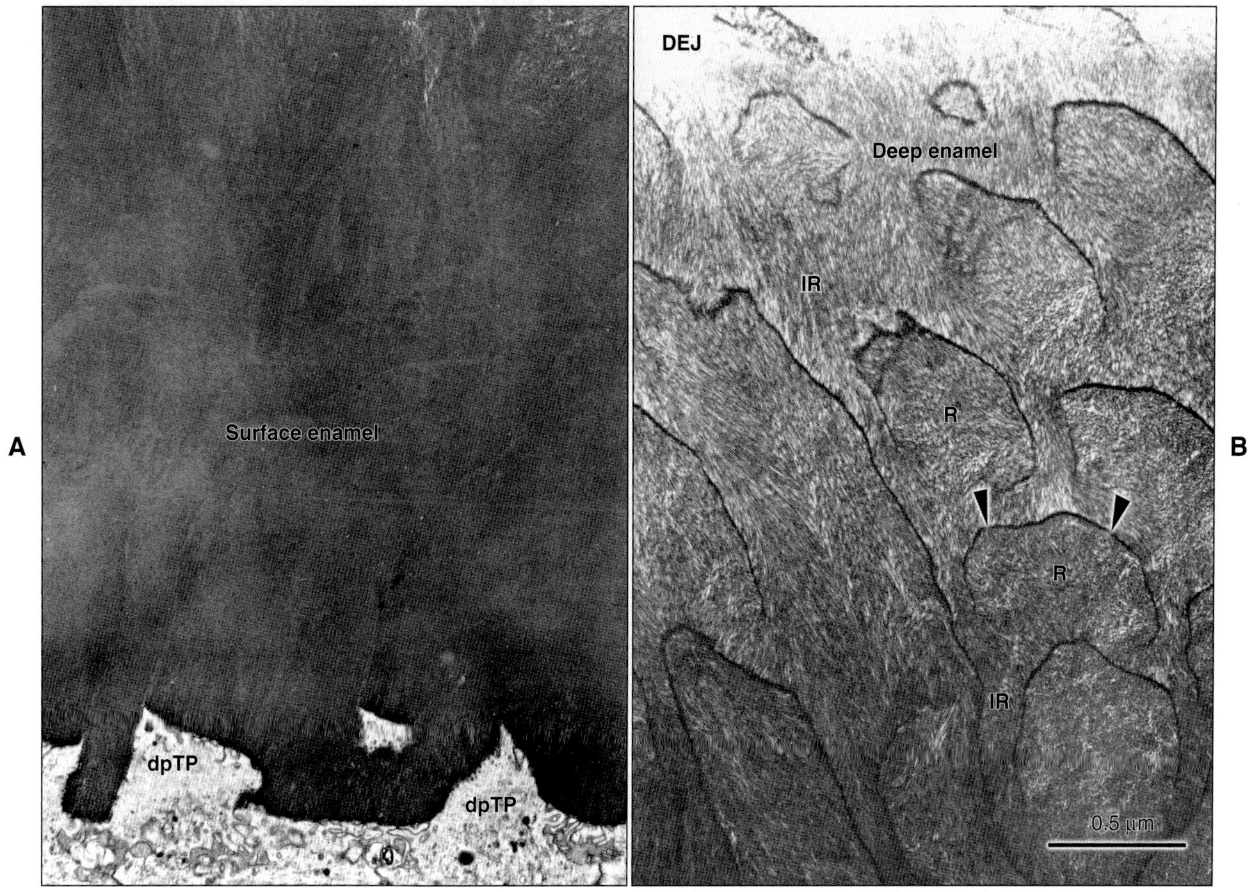

Fig. 7.8 Decalcified preparation of cat secretory-stage enamel. The organic matrix near the ameloblasts is younger and shows a uniform texture. No rod sheath is discernible in younger enamel near the surface where rods are structured. The distal portion of Tomes process *(dpTP)* penetrates into the enamel. In deeper areas, near dentin, matrix is older and partly removed. As enamel matures, matrix accumulates at the interface between rod *(R)* and interrod *(IR)* to form the rod sheath *(arrowheads)*. *DEJ,* Dentinoenamel junction.

of distinct and almost simultaneous morphologic changes associated with the onset of amelogenesis occur in the enamel organ (see Figs. 7.11C and 7.12). The cells of the inner enamel epithelium, now ameloblasts, begin to more actively secrete enamel proteins that accumulate and immediately participate in the formation of a partially mineralized initial layer of enamel, which does not contain any rods. As the first increment of enamel is formed, ameloblasts move away from the dentin surface. An important event for the production and organization of the enamel is the development of a cytoplasmic extension on ameloblasts, Tomes process (its formation and structure are described later in the chapter), that juts into and interdigitates with the newly forming enamel (see Figs. 7.14–7.16). In sections of forming teeth in higher mammals, Tomes processes give the junction between the enamel and the ameloblast a picket-fence or saw-toothed appearance (see Figs. 7.15C and 7.16).

When formation of the full thickness of enamel is complete, ameloblasts enter the maturation stage (see Figs 7.14 and 7.15). Typically this stage starts with a brief transitional phase during which significant morphologic changes occur. These postsecretory transition ameloblasts shorten and restructure themselves into squatter maturation cells (see Fig. 7.14). Cells from the underlying stratum intermedium, remaining stellate reticulum, and outer enamel epithelium reorganize so that recognizing individual cell layers is no longer possible. Blood vessels invaginate deeply into these cells, without disrupting the basal lamina associated with the outer aspect of the enamel organ, to form a convoluted structure referred to as the *papillary layer* (see Figs. 7.14 and 7.17).

Finally, when enamel is fully mature, the ameloblast layer and the adjacent papillary layer regress and together constitute the reduced enamel epithelium (see Fig. 7.18). The ameloblasts stop alternating appearance (modulation, see later), reduce their size, and assume a low cuboidal to flattened appearance. This epithelium, although no longer involved in the secretion and maturation of enamel, continues to cover it and has been proposed to have a protective function. In the case of premature breaks in the epithelium, connective tissue cells could come in contact with the enamel and deposit a cementum-like material on it. During this protective phase, however, the composition of enamel can still be modified. For instance, fluoride, if available, still can be incorporated into the enamel of an unerupted tooth, and evidence indicates that the fluoride content is greatest in those teeth that have the longest interregnum between the completion of enamel formation and tooth eruption (at which time, of course, the ameloblasts are lost). The reduced enamel epithelium remains until the tooth erupts. As the tooth passes through the oral epithelium, the part of the reduced enamel epithelium situated incisally is destroyed, whereas that found more cervically interacts with the oral epithelium to form the junctional epithelium (discussed in Chapter 12). Thus the contribution of enamel organ cells goes beyond enamel formation.

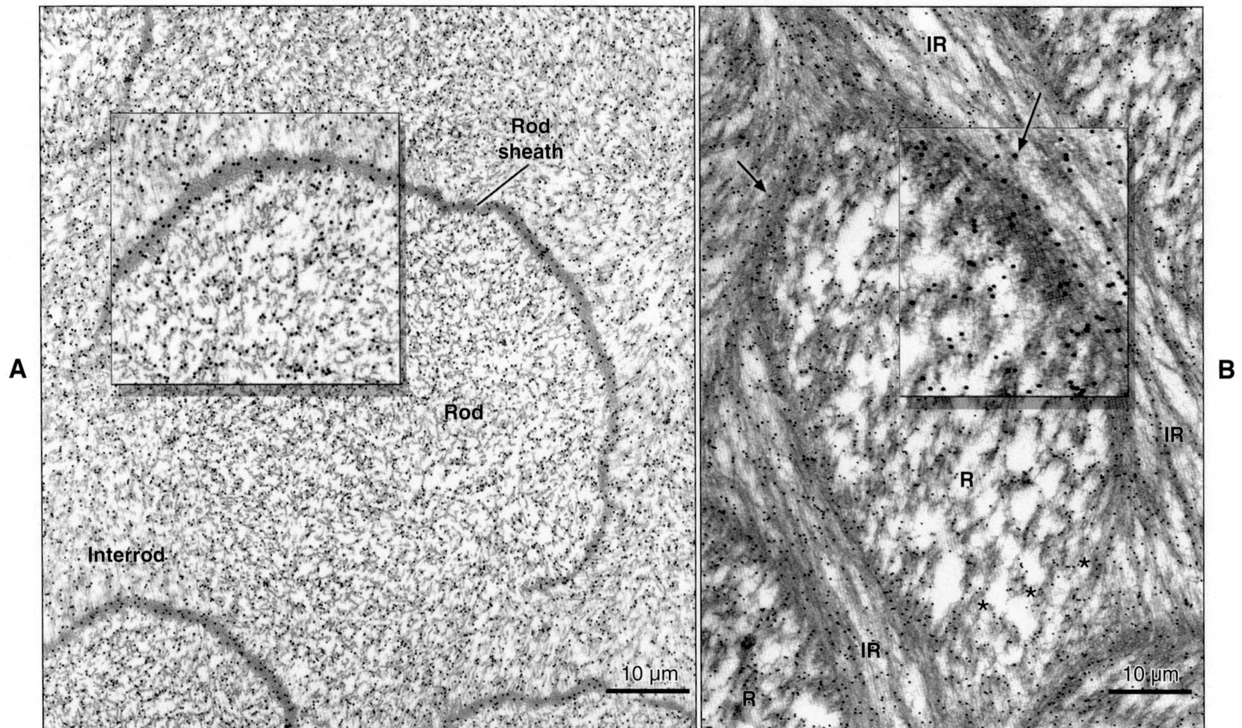

Fig. 7.9 The rod sheath has been proposed to be made up of sheath protein, now known as *ameloblastin.* (A) However, colloidal gold *(black dots)* immunocytochemical labeling of maturing cat enamel also reveals an abundant presence of amelogenin in the organic matrix that accumulates to form the rod sheath. (B) Rodents have no well-defined rod sheath; however, decalcified preparations of maturing enamel reveal a concentration of organic matrix *(arrows)* around most of the periphery of the rod *(R),* except at the zone of confluence *(*)* with interrod *(IR).* This matrix, like the one at other sites, is immunoreactive for amelogenin. It is thus likely that more than one protein accumulates in the thin space between rod and interrod as enamel matures.

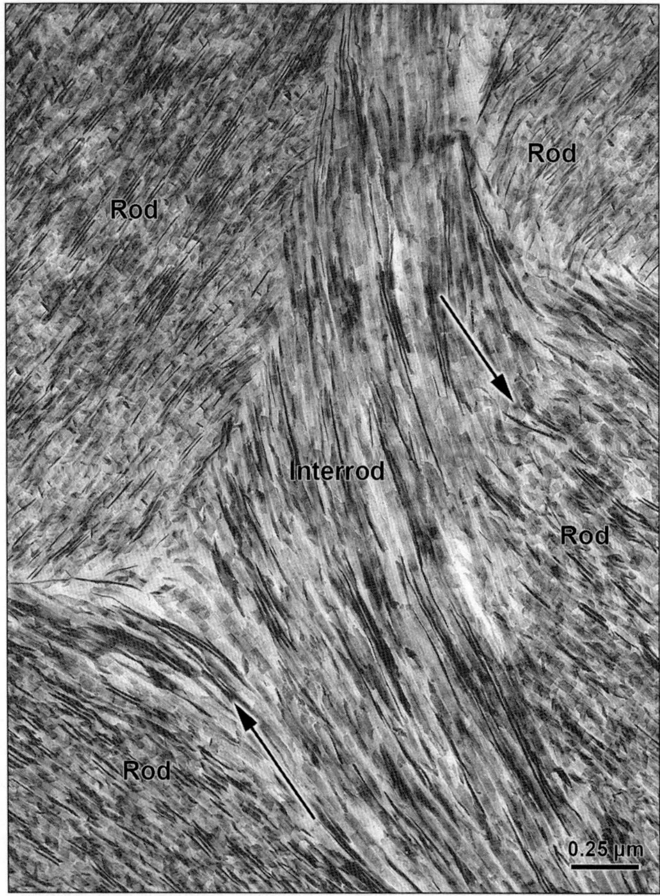

Fig. 7.10 Interrod partition associated with four rod profiles. At certain sites (*arrows,* zone of confluence), crystals from interrod enamel enter the rod.

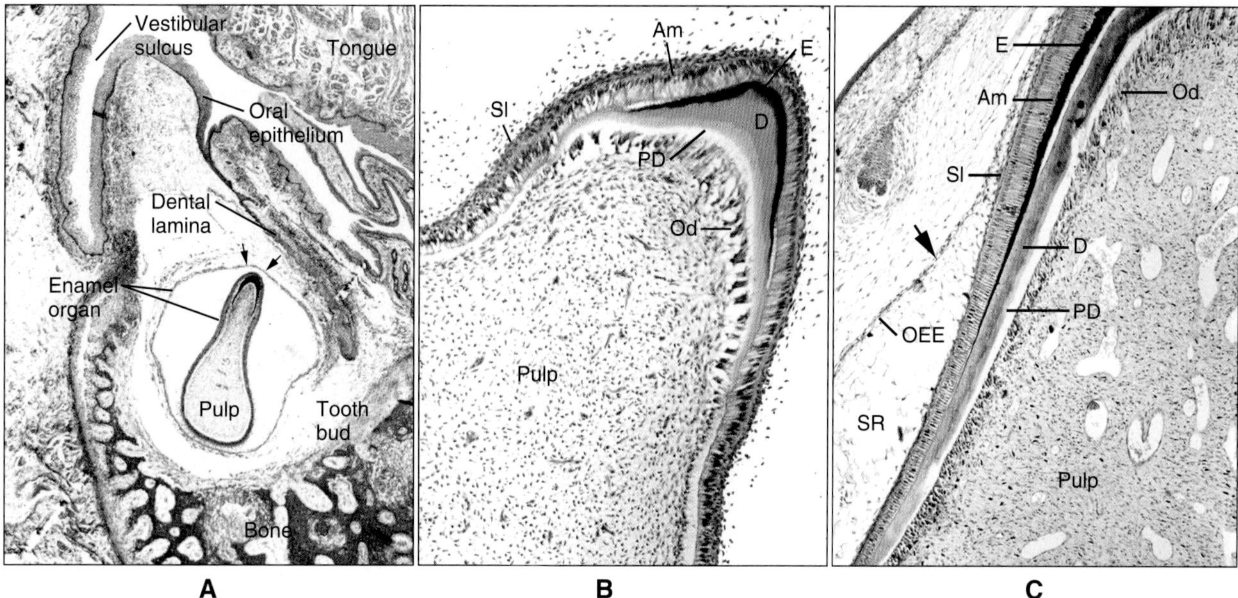

Fig. 7.11 Early bell stage of tooth development. (A, B) Dentin and enamel have begun to form at the crest of the forming crown, accompanied by a reduction in the amount of stellate reticulum *(SR)* over the future cusp tip (*arrows* in [A]). (C) Ameloblast *(Am)* and odontoblast *(Od)* differentiation and formation of enamel *(E)* and dentin *(D)* progress along the slopes of the tooth, in an occlusal-to-cervical direction. Note the reduction in the amount of *SR* above the arrow where the enamel is actively forming. *OEE,* Outer enamel epithelium; *PD,* predentin; *SI,* stratum intermedium. (B and C, Courtesy P. Tambasco de Oliveira.)

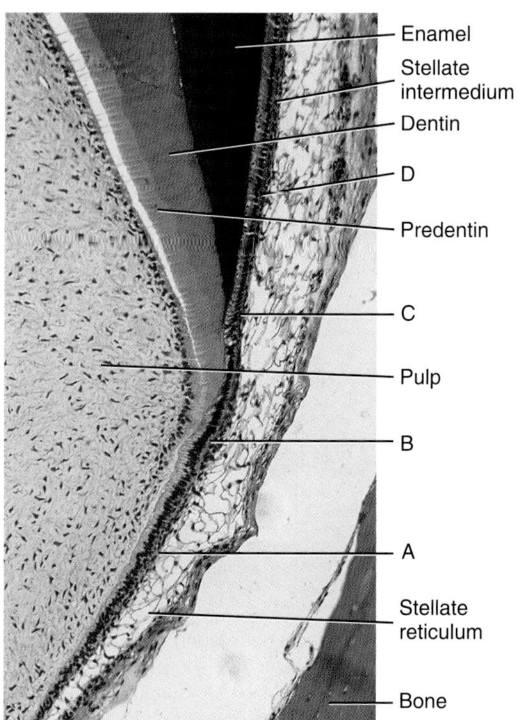

Fig. 7.12 Features of amelogenesis as seen through a light microscope. At *A,* the inner enamel epithelium consists of short, columnar undifferentiated cells. At *B,* these cells elongate and differentiate into ameloblasts that face differentiating odontoblasts and then begin to secrete enamel matrix *(C).* At *D,* ameloblasts are actively depositing enamel matrix.

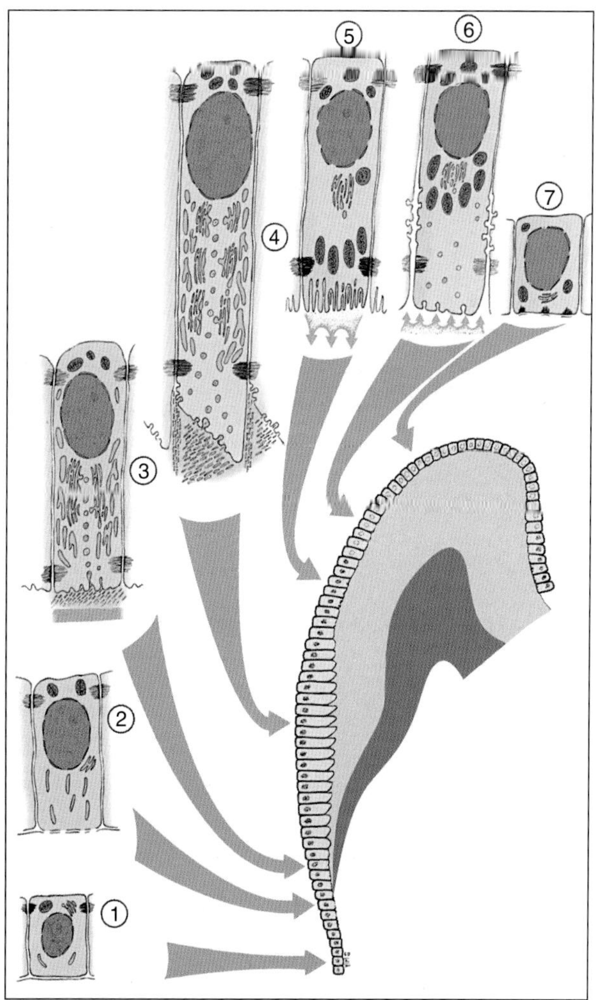

Fig. 7.13 Schematic representation of the various functional stages in the life cycle of ameloblasts as would occur in a human tooth: *1,* morphogenetic stage; *2,* histodifferentiation stage; *3,* initial secretory stage (no Tomes process); *4,* secretory stage (Tomes process); *5,* ruffle-ended ameloblast of the maturative stage; *6,* smooth-ended ameloblast of the maturative stage; *7,* protective stage.

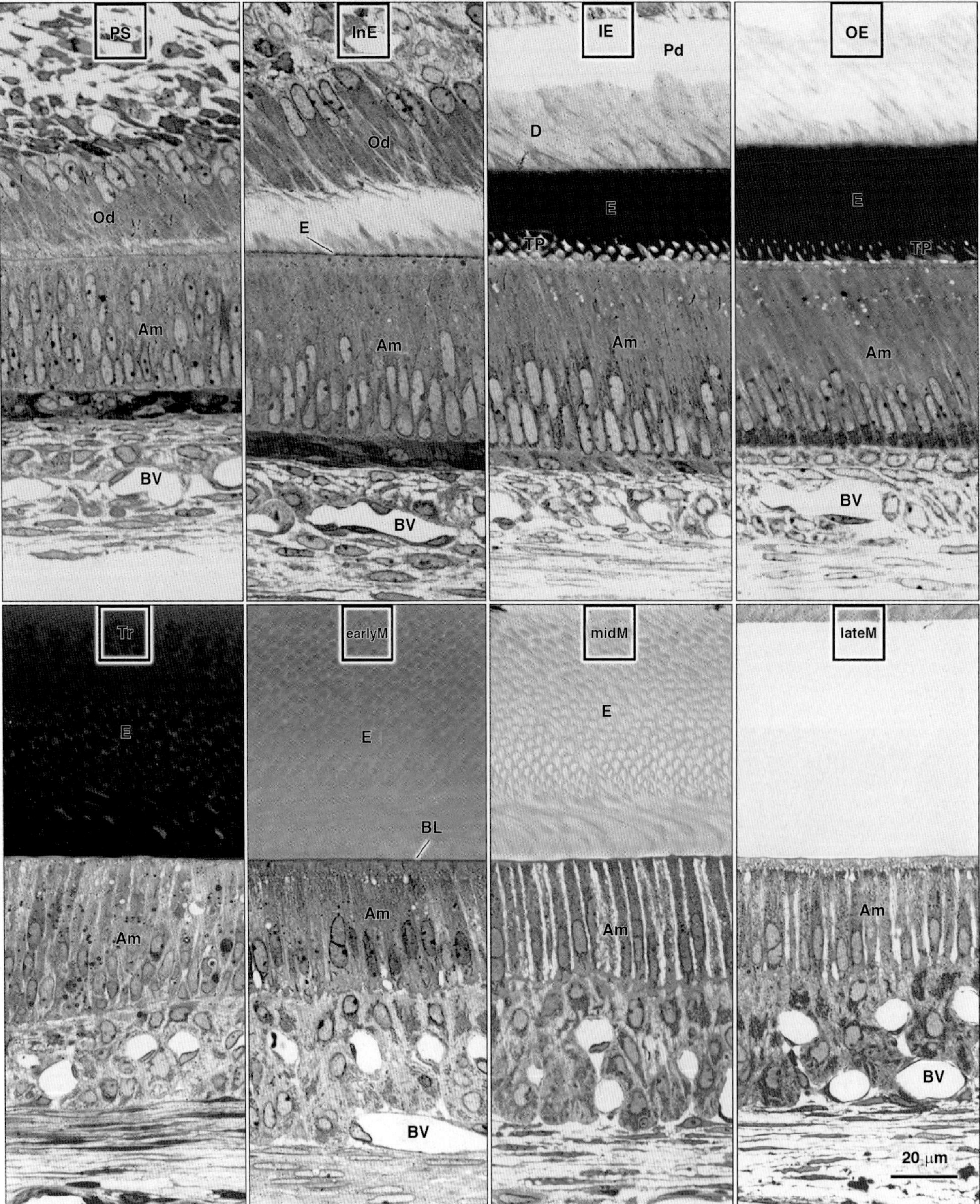

Fig. 7.14 Composite plate illustrating the morphologic changes that rat incisor ameloblasts undergo throughout amelogenesis. *Am,* Ameloblasts; *BL,* basal lamina; *BV,* blood vessel; *D,* dentin; *E,* enamel; *IE,* secretory-stage inner enamel; *InE,* secretory-stage initial enamel; *earlyM,* early maturation stage; *lateM,* late maturation stage; *midM,* midmaturation stage; *Od,* odontoblasts; *OE,* secretory-stage outer enamel; *Pd,* predentin; *PS,* presecretory stage; *TP,* Tomes process; *Tr,* maturation stage transition.

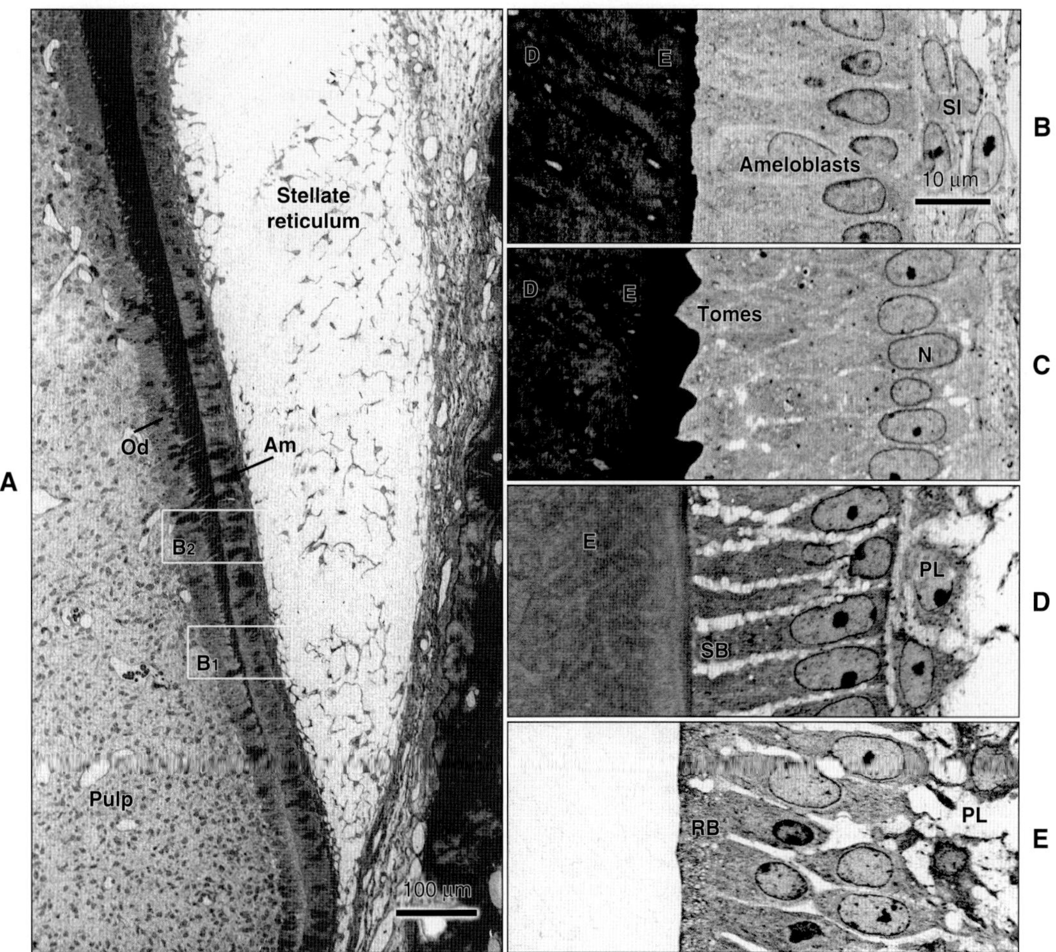

Fig. 7.15 Representative micrographs of amelogenesis in cats. (A) Tooth formation shows an occlusal-to-cervical developmental gradient so that on some crowns finding most of the stages of the ameloblast life cycle is possible. The panels on the right (B corresponds with B_1 and C with B_2) are enlargements of the boxed areas in (A). (B) Secretory stage, initial enamel formation. (C) Secretory stage, inner enamel formation. (D, E) From the incisal tip of the tooth (see Fig. 7.13). (D) Midmaturation stage, smooth-ended ameloblasts. (E) Late maturation stage, ruffle-ended ameloblasts. *Am,* Ameloblasts; *D,* dentin; *E,* enamel; *N,* nucleus; *Od,* odontoblasts; *PL,* papillary layer; *RB,* ruffled border; *SB,* smooth border; *SI,* stratum intermedium.

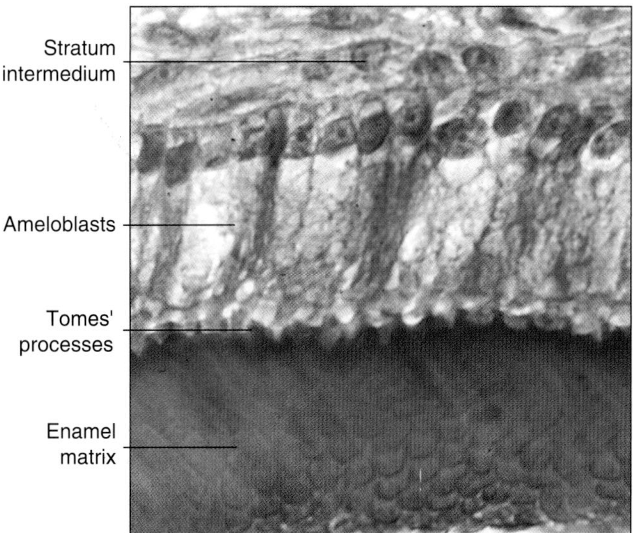

Fig. 7.16 Enamel matrix formation as seen with a light microscope. The Tomes processes of ameloblasts jut into the matrix visible after decalcification in certain planes of section, creating a picket-fence appearance in higher mammals.

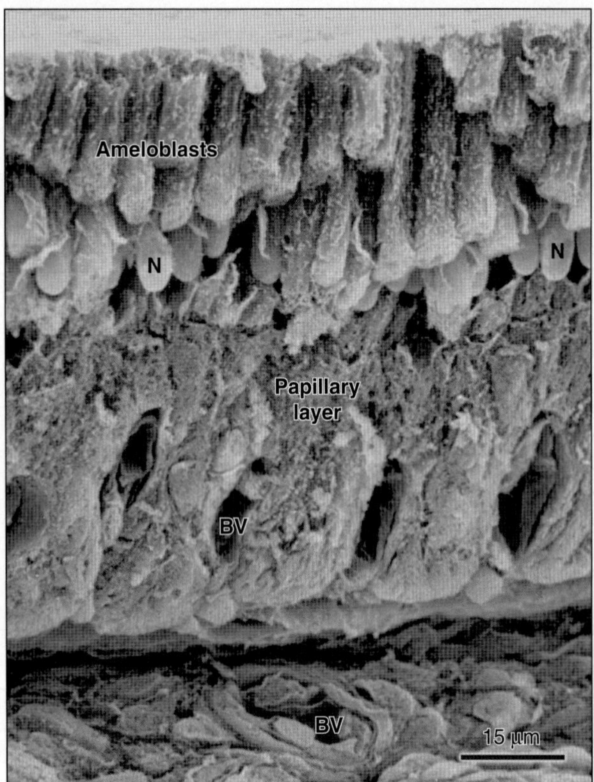

Fig. 7.17 Scanning electron microscope view of the enamel organ during the maturation stage. Cells from the stratum intermedium, stellate reticulum, and outer enamel epithelium amalgamate into a single layer. Blood vessels invaginate deeply into this layer to form a convoluted structure referred to as the *papillary layer*. *BV,* Blood vessel; *N,* nucleus.

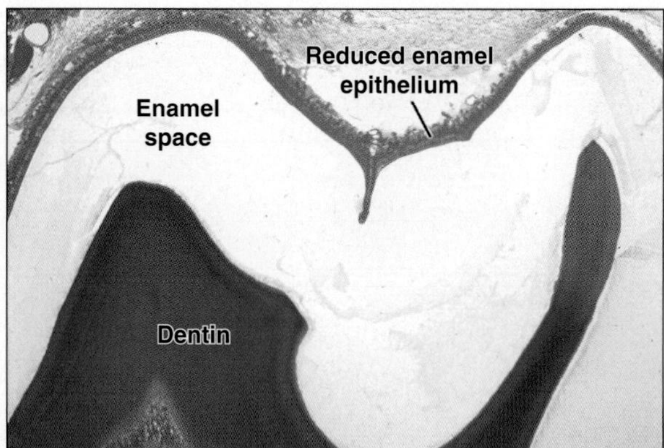

Fig. 7.18 When enamel maturation is completed, the ameloblast layer and the adjacent papillary layer together constitute the reduced enamel epithelium. Only an enamel space is visible in this histologic preparation because, at this late developmental stage, enamel is heavily calcified and therefore any residual matrix is lost during decalcification.

ELECTRON MICROSCOPY OF AMELOGENESIS

Ultrastructural studies of enamel formation by electron microscopy have added greatly to the understanding of this complex process. Such studies often have used the continuously erupting rat incisor as a model because all developmental stages can be found in a single tooth and because it has been demonstrated that the various stages of enamel formation bear an overall similarity to those in human teeth. In continuously erupting rodent incisors, the various stages of amelogenesis are disposed sequentially along the length of the tooth (Fig. 7.19). In such a system, position represents developmental time, and one can look predictably at the various stages of amelogenesis by sampling at different positions from the apical end, where cell renewal occurs, to the incisal tip, where occlusal attrition balances the continuous, apically initiated tooth-forming activity.

Presecretory Stage

Morphogenetic Phase

During the bell stage of tooth development, the shape of the crown is established. A basal lamina is present between cells of the inner enamel epithelium and dental papilla (Figs. 7.20 and 7.21A). At this stage the dentin is not yet mineralized, as evidenced by the presence of intact matrix vesicles in it (Fig. 7.22; see also Figs. 7.20 and 7.21A). The cells of the inner enamel epithelium still can undergo mitotic division throughout the bell initially and eventually limited to the cervical portion of the tooth. These cells are cuboidal or low columnar with large, centrally located nuclei and poorly developed Golgi elements in the proximal portion of the cells (facing the stratum intermedium), where a junctional complex exists. Mitochondria and other cytoplasmic components are scattered throughout the cell.

Differentiation Phase

As the cells of the inner enamel epithelium differentiate into ameloblasts, they elongate and their nuclei shift proximally toward the stratum intermedium. The basal lamina supporting them is fragmented by cytoplasmic projections and is then degraded during mantle predentin formation (see Fig. 7.20). In each cell the Golgi complex increases in volume and migrates distally from its proximal position to occupy a major portion of the supranuclear cytoplasm. The amount of rough endoplasmic reticulum (rER) increases significantly, and in some species mitochondria cluster in the infranuclear compartment, with only a few scattered through the rest of the cell. A second junctional complex develops at the distal extremity of the cell (facing differentiating odontoblasts), compartmentalizing the ameloblast into a body and a distal extension (Tomes process) against which enamel forms (see Fig. 7.21B and C). Thus the ameloblast becomes a polarized cell, with the majority of its organelles situated in the cell body distal to the nucleus. These cells can no longer divide.

Although in the past these differentiating ameloblasts have been regarded as nonsecreting cells, it has been now clearly demonstrated that production of some enamel proteins starts much earlier than anticipated, even before the basal lamina separating preameloblasts and preodontoblasts is lost (see Fig. 7.21A). Surprisingly, preameloblasts also express some odontoblast products such as dentin sialoprotein, albeit transiently. This reciprocal expression of opposing matrix proteins as cells differentiate, as well as the production of typical (ecto)mesenchymal proteins by enamel organ–derived cells at later stages (see Chapter 9), is consistent with the common ectodermal origin (oral epithelium/neural crest) of all hard tissue–forming cells in the craniofacial region.

From this point to the end of the secretory stage (see the next section), ameloblasts are aligned closely with each other, and attachment specializations (junctional complexes) between them maintain the alignment. These complexes encircle the cells at their distal (adjacent to enamel) and proximal (adjacent to the stratum intermedium) extremities. Fine actin-containing filaments radiate from the junctional complexes into the cytoplasm of the ameloblasts and can be distinguished as forming distal and proximal terminal webs (Fig. 7.23). These junctional complexes play an important role in amelogenesis by

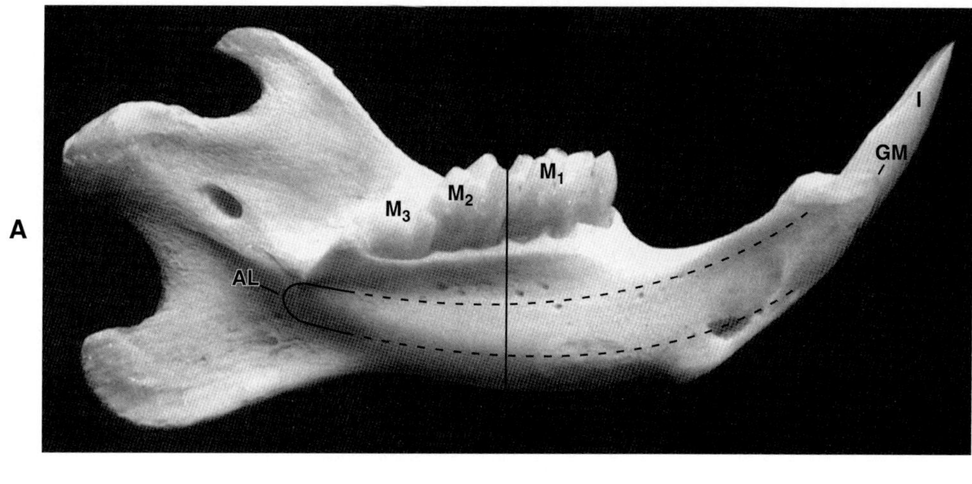

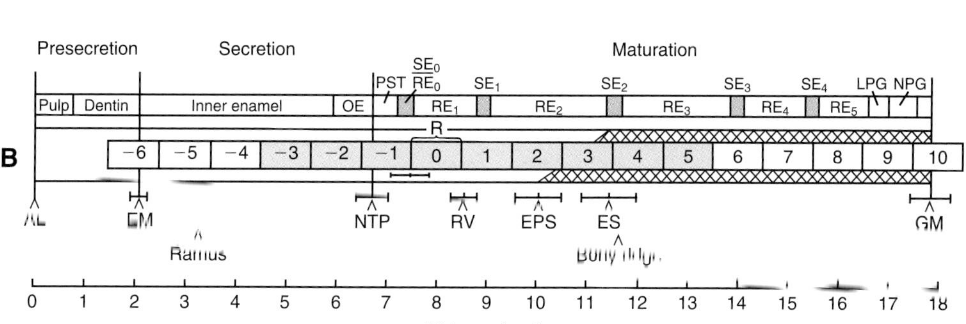

Fig. 7.19 (A) Mesial view of the left rat hemimandible. The dashed line outlines the approximate position of the incisor within the bone. The solid line perpendicular to the labial surface of the incisor and passing between the first *(M_1)* and second molar *(M_2)* demarcates the secretory and maturation stages. Enamel formation progresses sequentially from the apical to the incisal end *(I)* of the tooth. (B) Schematic representation of the curvilinear length of the labial surface of the incisor from the apical loop *(AL)* to the gingival margin *(GM)*, and mapping of the respective lengths occupied by the various stages and regions of amelogenesis. *EM,* Start of enamel matrix secretion; *EPS,* enamel partially soluble during decalcification; *ES,* enamel completely soluble; *LPG,* region where ameloblasts accumulate large pigment granules; *NPG,* region where ameloblasts show no pigment granules; *NTP,* point marking the location of loss of Tomes process; *OE,* region of outer enamel secretion; *PST,* region of postsecretory transition; *RE,* band of ruffle-ended ameloblasts; *RV,* rods visible; *SE,* band of smooth-ended ameloblasts. (From Smith CE, Nanci A: A method for sampling the stages of amelogenesis on mandibular rat incisors using the molars as a reference for dissection, *Anat Rec* 225:257–266, 1989.)

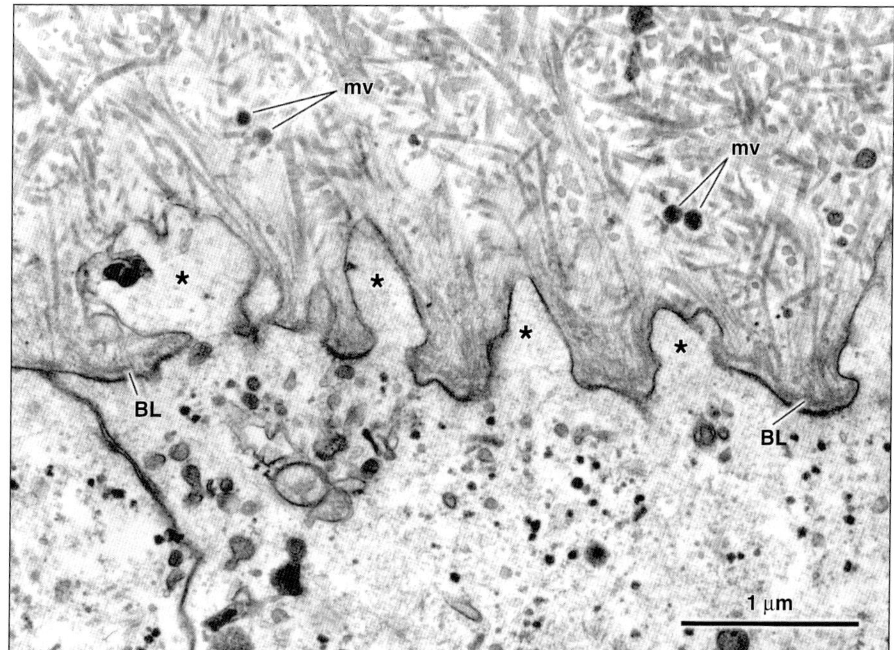

Fig. 7.20 Differentiating ameloblasts extend cytoplasmic projections *(*)* through the basal lamina *(BL)*, separating them from the forming mantle predentin. The basal lamina is fragmented and is removed before the active deposition of enamel matrix. *mv,* Matrix vesicle.

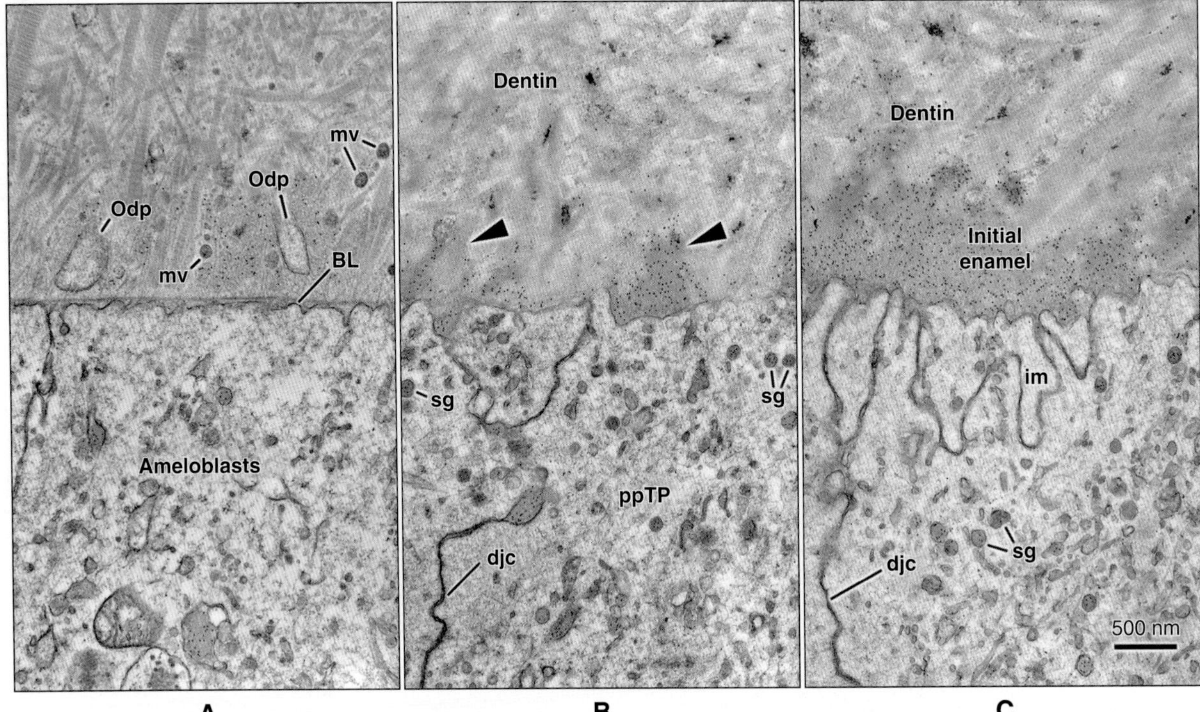

Fig. 7.21 Colloidal gold immunocytochemical preparations illustrating the expression of amelogenin by differentiating ameloblasts. (A) Amelogenin molecules are immunodetected *(black dots)* extracellularly early during the presecretory stage, before the removal of the basal lamina *(BL)* separating ameloblasts from the developing predentin matrix. Thereafter, enamel proteins (B) accumulate first as patches *(arrowheads)* at the interface with dentin and then (C) as a uniform layer of initial enamel that in mineralized preparations is seen to contain numerous crystallites. *djc,* Distal junctional complex; *im,* infolded membrane; *mv,* matrix vesicle; *Odp,* odontoblast process; *ppTP,* proximal portion of Tomes process; *sg,* secretory granule.

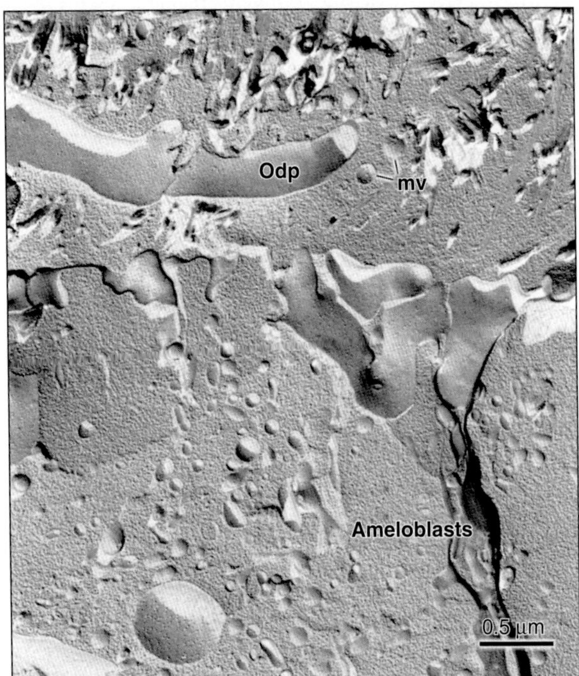

Fig. 7.22 Freeze-fracture preparation illustrating a three-dimensional view of presecretory stage ameloblasts, similar to those in Fig. 7.21A, and an odontoblast process *(Odp)* and matrix vesicles *(mvs)* in the region of forming mantle predentin where the first enamel proteins are deposited.

tightly holding together ameloblasts and determining at different times what may, and what may not, pass between them to enter or leave the enamel.

Secretory Stage

The fine structure of secretory stage ameloblasts reflects their intense synthetic and secretory activity. The Golgi complex is extensive and forms a cylindric organelle surrounded by numerous cisternae of rER, occupying a large part of the supranuclear compartment (Figs. 7.24–7.27A). The mRNA for enamel proteins is translated by ribosomes on the membrane of the rER, and the synthesized proteins then are translocated into its cisternae. The proteins then progress through the Golgi complex for continued posttranslational modification (mainly for nonamelogenins) and are packaged into membrane-bound secretory granules. These granules migrate to the distal extremity of the cell (i.e., into Tomes process) (Fig. 7.28B; see also Figs. 7.23A, 7.26, and 7.27B). Secretion by ameloblasts is constitutive (i.e., continuous), and secretory granules are not stored for prolonged periods, as is the case for salivary gland acinar cells, for example.

When enamel formation begins, Tomes process comprises only a proximal portion (Fig. 7.29; see also Fig. 7.21). The content of secretory granules is released against the newly formed mantle dentin along the surface of the process to form an initial layer of enamel that does not contain enamel rods. Little if any time elapses between the secretion of enamel matrix and their participation in mineralization. The first hydroxyapatite crystals formed interdigitate with those of dentin (Fig. 7.30).

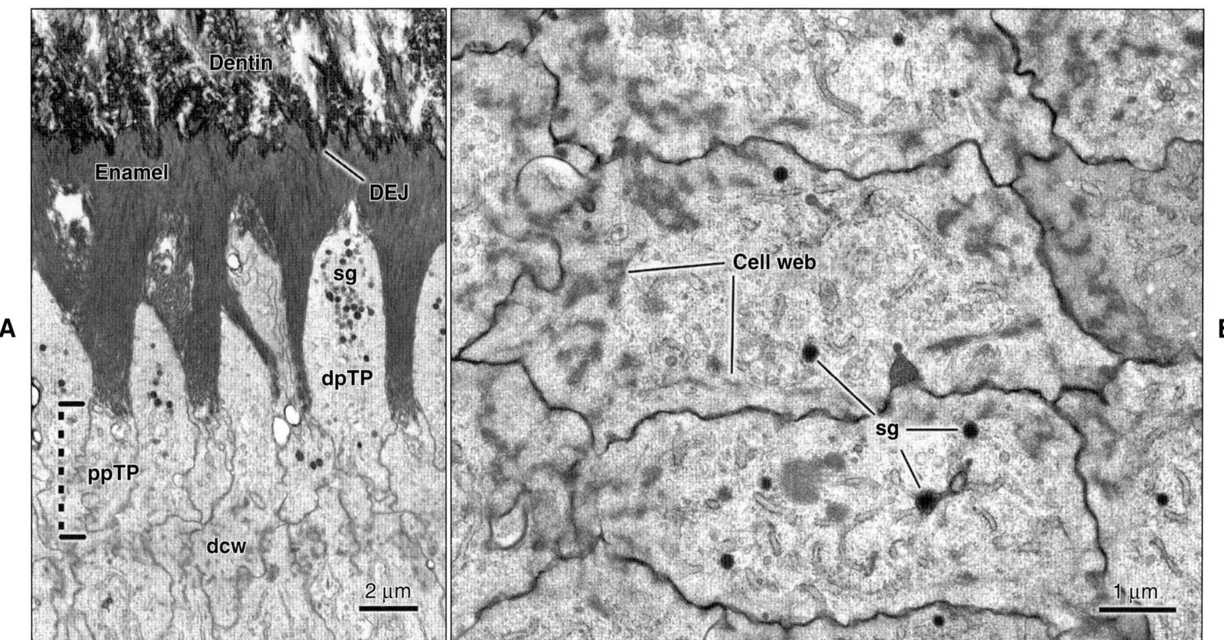

Fig. 7.23 (A) Differentiated ameloblasts, here from the early secretory stage, develop a junctional complex at their distal extremity. The cell extension above the complex is Tomes process and is divided into two parts. The proximal portion of Tomes process *(ppTP)* extends from the junctional complex to the surface of the enamel layer, whereas the more distal portion *(dpTP)* penetrates into enamel. (B) Cross-sectional view of ameloblasts at the level of the distal junctional complex. This beltlike complex extends around the entire circumference of the ameloblast and tightly holds the cells together. Bundles of microfilaments *(Cell web)* concentrate and run along the cytoplasmic surface of the complex. *dcw,* Distal cell web; *DEJ,* dentinoenamel junction; *sg,* secretory granule.

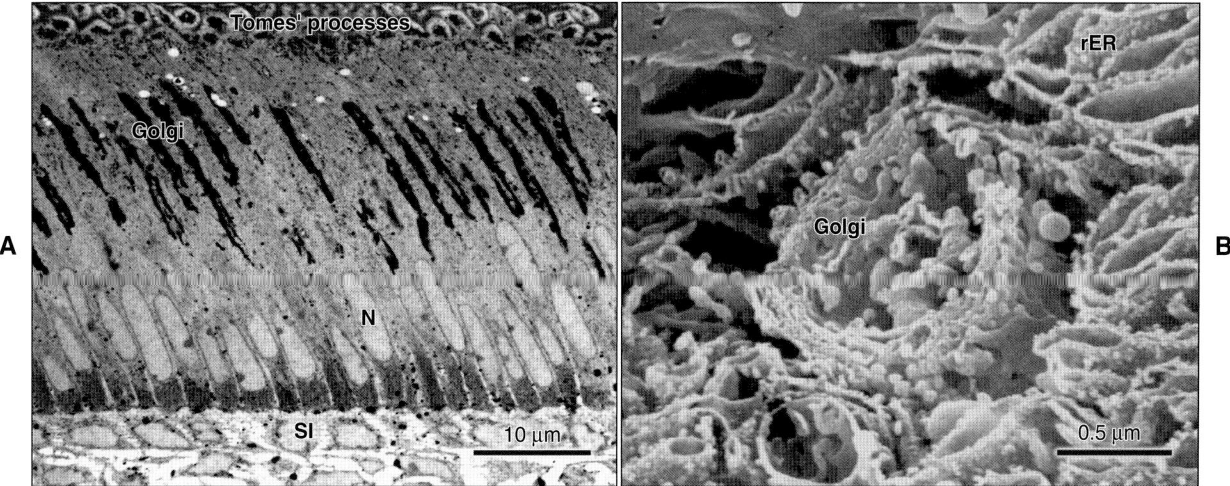

Fig. 7.24 (A) Cytochemical preparation for an enzyme resident in the Golgi complex showing the extent of this organelle throughout the supranuclear compartment of secretory stage ameloblasts. (B) Scanning electron microscope image of a cross-fractured ameloblast. The Golgi complex has a cylindric configuration and is surrounded by rough endoplasmic reticulum *(rER)*. *N,* Nucleus; *SI,* stratum intermedium.

As the initial enamel layer is formed, ameloblasts migrate away from the dentin surface and develop the distal portion of Tomes process as an outgrowth of the proximal portion. The proximal portion extends from the distal junctional complex to the surface of the enamel layer, whereas the distal portion penetrates into and interdigitates with the enamel beyond the initial layer (Fig. 7.31; see also Figs. 7.23A, 7.26, and 7.27B). The cytoplasm from both portions of Tomes process is continuous with that of the body of the ameloblast. The rod/interrod configuration of enamel crystals is a property of the ameloblasts and their Tomes processes. The organizational framework of rod/interrod is similar in all species, but their size and outline vary to reflect the geometry of the cell.

When the distal portion of Tomes process is established, secretion of enamel proteins becomes staggered and is confined to two sites (see Figs. 7.26 and 7.31). The sites where enamel proteins are released extracellularly can be identified by the presence of abundant

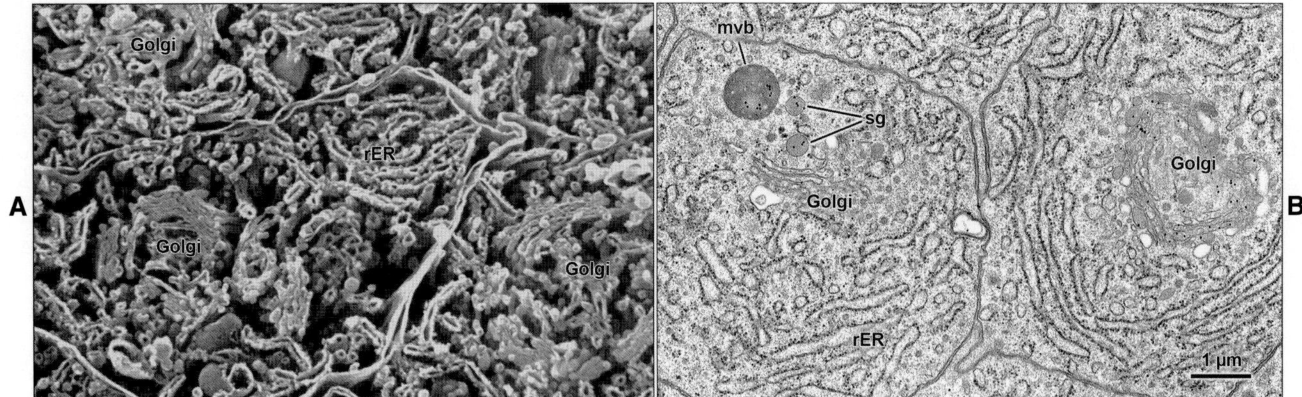

Fig. 7.25 Comparative (A) scanning and (B) transmission electron microscope views of cross-cut secretory stage ameloblasts. The Golgi complex is located centrally and surrounded by cisternae of rough endoplasmic reticulum *(rER)*. The preparation in (B) is immunolabeled *(black dots)* for amelogenin. Labeling is found not only in the Golgi complex and secretory granules *(sg)* but also in organelles involved in protein degradation, such as multivesicular bodies *(mvbs)*.

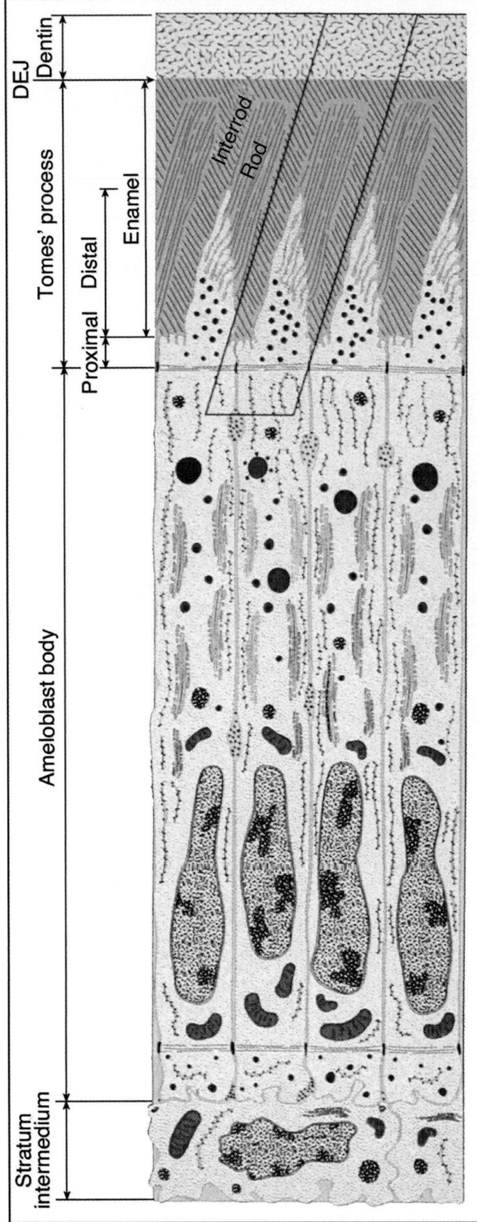

Fig. 7.26 Schematic representation of the organization of secretory stage ameloblasts as would be revealed in a section along their long axis. *DEJ*, Dentinoenamel junction.

membrane infoldings (Fig. 7.32; see also Fig. 7.31). These infoldings are believed to form to accommodate the excess membrane brought about by the rapid fusion of many secretory granules at these sites. Secretion from the first site (on the proximal part of the process, close to the junctional complex, around the periphery of the cell), along with that from adjoining ameloblasts, results in the formation of enamel partitions that delimit a pit (Fig. 7.33; see also Fig. 7.6B) in which resides the distal portion of Tomes process. These partitions are not distinct units and in effect form a continuum throughout the enamel layer called the *interrod enamel.* Secretion from the second site (along one face of the distal portion of Tomes process) provides the matrix that participates in formation of the enamel rod that later fills a pit. Formation of interrod enamel is always a step ahead because the cavity into which an enamel rod is formed must first be defined. In fact, the interrod matrix secretion site abuts against the growing front of the enamel layer, and that for rod matrix is deeper in the enamel layer. At both sites the enamel is of identical composition, and rod/interrod enamel differ only in the orientation of their crystallites (Fig. 7.34; see also Figs. 7.1C, 7.2, 7.3, and 7.10).

The distal portion of Tomes process is believed to lengthen as the enamel layer thickens and becomes gradually thinner as the rod growing in diameter presses it against the wall of the interrod cavity (see Fig. 7.34). The distal Tomes process eventually is squeezed out of existence, creating a narrow space along most of the circumference between rod and interrod enamel that fills with organic material, and (as indicated previously) forms the rod sheath that is prominent in higher mammals. The secretory surface on the distal portion of Tomes process faces the region where there is no rod sheath. Rod crystals formed in relation to the secretory surface are created directly against the interrod partition; consequently, over a narrow area, rod and interrod crystals are confluent (see Fig. 7.34). When the outer portion of the enamel layer is being formed, the shape of the distal portion of Tomes process is altered, and its orientation to the cell body changes (Fig. 7.35; see also Fig. 7.14). As a result, enamel rods in the outer third of the enamel layer have a slightly different profile and have a more rectilinear trajectory (Fig. 7.36; see also Fig. 7.1B). Eventually, the ameloblast becomes shorter and loses its distal portion of Tomes process; the cell now has the same overall appearance as when it was forming initial enamel (see Figs. 7.14 and 7.35). Because rods form in relation to the distal portion of Tomes process (which no longer exists), the final few enamel increments (final enamel), just as the first few, do not contain rods (Fig. 7.37). The enamel layer is thus composed of a rod/interrod-containing (prismatic) layer that is sandwiched between thin,

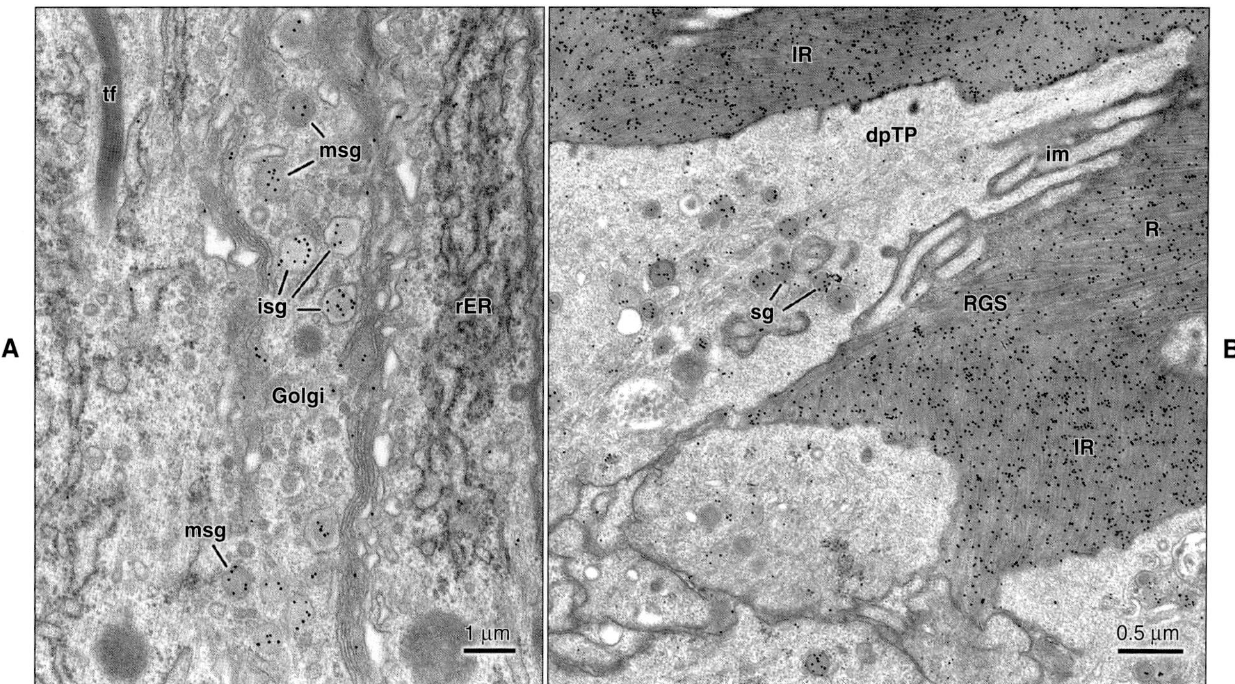

Fig. 7.27 Immunocytochemical preparations for amelogenin. (A) Immature *(isg)* and mature *(msg)* secretory granules are found on the mature face of the Golgi complex. (B) Secretory granules are translocated into Tomes process and accumulate near secretory surfaces, recognized by the presence of membrane infoldings *(im)*. *dpTP,* Distal portion of Tomes process; *IR,* interrod; *R,* rod; *rER,* rough endoplasmic reticulum; *RGS,* rod growth site; *sg,* secretory granule; *tf,* tonofilaments.

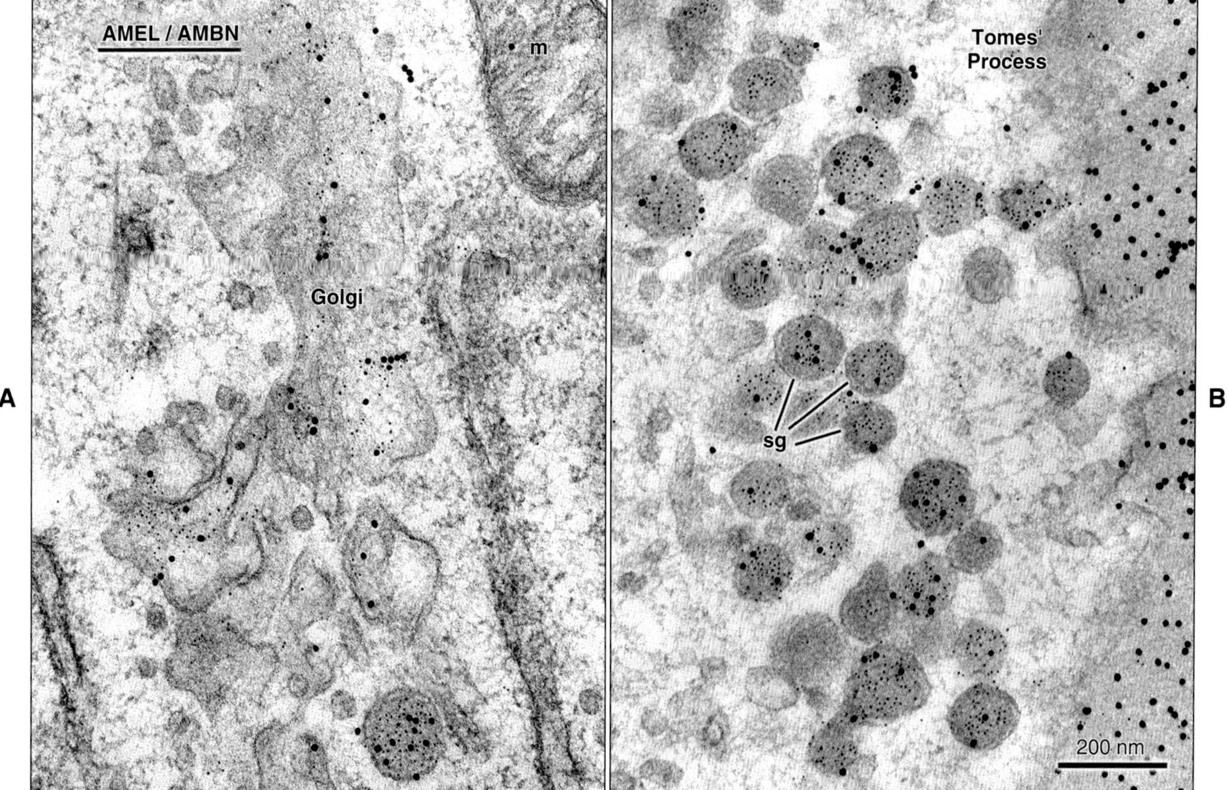

Fig. 7.28 Double-labeled immunocytochemical preparations; the fine black dots indicate the presence of ameloblastin *(AMBN),* whereas the larger ones indicate that of amelogenin *(AMEL).* (A) Both proteins are processed simultaneously in the Golgi complex. (B) The majority of secretory granules *(sg)* in Tomes process contains both proteins, indicating they are cosecreted. *m,* Mitochondria.

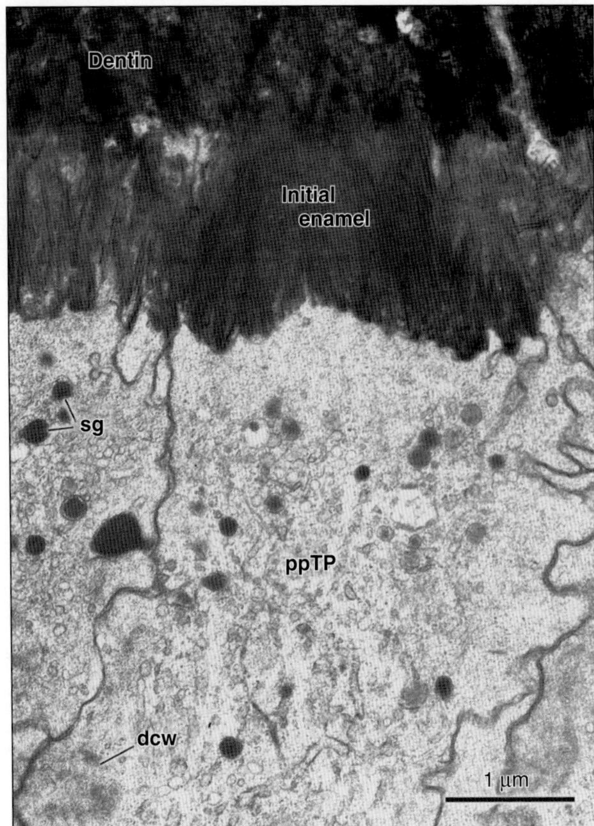

Fig. 7.29 When initial enamel forms, the ameloblast only has a proximal portion of Tomes process *(ppTP)*. The distal portion develops as an extension of the proximal one slightly later when enamel rods begin forming. *dcw,* Distal cell web; *sg,* secretory granules.

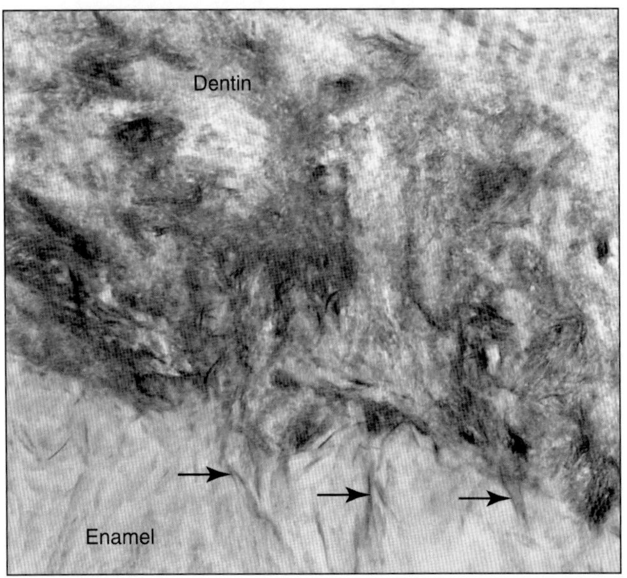

Fig. 7.30 Transmission electron micrographs of initial enamel formation showing the close intermingling of the mineralized dentin collagen with the thinner ribbonlike crystals of enamel.

rodless (aprismatic) initial and final enamel layers. Notably, the initial, interrod, and final enamel are formed from the same secretory surface on ameloblasts (i.e., on the proximal portion of Tomes process) and indeed are believed to constitute a continuum.

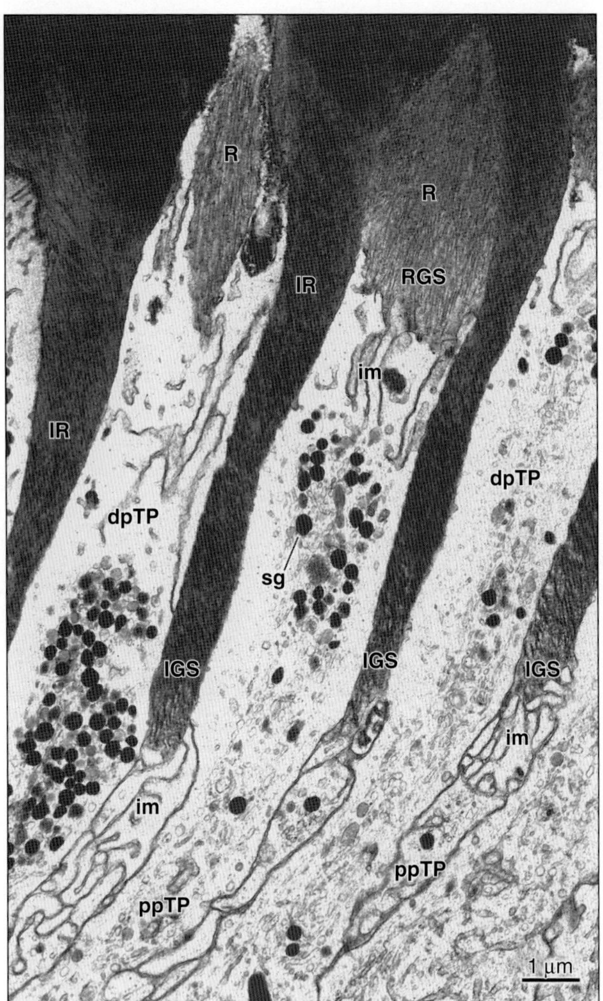

Fig. 7.31 Interrod *(IR)* enamel surrounds the forming rod *(R)* and the distal portion of Tomes process *(dpTP)*; this portion is the continuation of the proximal portion *(ppTP)* into the enamel layer. The interrod *(IGS)* and rod *(RGS)* growth sites are associated with membrane infoldings *(im)* on the proximal and distal portions of Tomes process, respectively. These infoldings represent the sites where secretory granules *(sg)* release enamel proteins extracellularly for growth in length of enamel crystals that results in an increase in thickness of the enamel layer.

Maturation Stage

Before the tooth erupts in the oral cavity, enamel hardens. This change in physicochemical properties results from growth in width and thickness of preexisting crystals seeded during the formative phase of amelogenesis and not because additional crystals are created de novo (see Figs. 7.3 and 7.4). Crystal growth during the maturation stage occurs at the expense of matrix proteins and enamel fluid that are largely absent from mature enamel. Amelogenesis is a rather slow developmental process that can take as long as 5 years to complete on the crowns of some teeth in the permanent dentition in humans; up to about two-thirds of the formation time can be occupied by the maturation stage. Maturation stage ameloblasts seem to carry out small, repeated developmental increments with a cumulative effect of great change.

Although maturation stage ameloblasts generally are referred to as *postsecretory cells,* they still synthesize and secrete proteins (see Fig. 7.35). These ameloblasts still exhibit a prominent Golgi complex, a structural feature consistent with such activity (Fig. 7.38). Surprisingly, in some species the ameloblasts still temporarily produce some enamel matrix proteins during this stage (amelogenin and ameloblastin, see

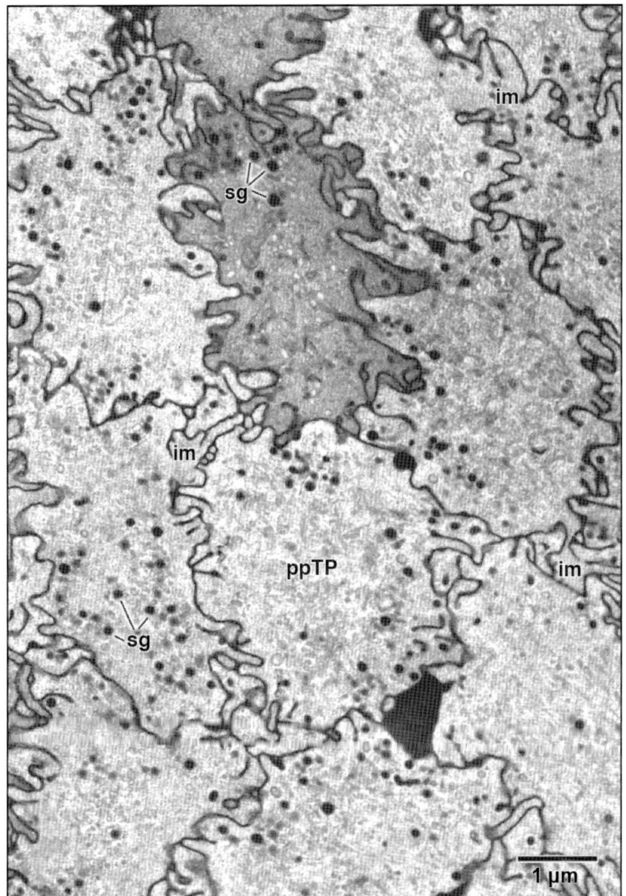

Fig. 7.32 Cross-sectional view of the proximal portion of Tomes process *(ppTP)* of ameloblasts at the level of the interrod secretory surface. Membrane infoldings *(im)* are present around the circumference of the cells and outline the edge of each of the interrod cavities shown in Fig. 7.6B. *sg,* Secretory granule.

later) (see Fig. 7.38). Although amelogenin signals are found only in the early maturation stage, curiously those for ameloblastin continue to be expressed until later. The significance of this continued production while major matrix removal occurs is unclear. Maturation stage ameloblasts also, however, normally produce other proteins (see later).

Transitional Phase

After the full thickness of immature enamel has formed, ameloblasts undergo significant morphologic changes in preparation for their next functional role, that of maturing the enamel. A brief transitional phase involving a reduction in height of the ameloblasts and a decrease in their volume and organelle content occurs (see Figs. 7.14 and 7.35C).

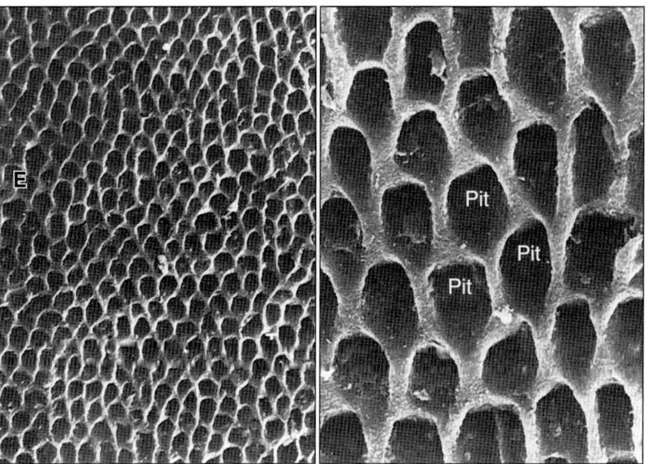

Fig. 7.33 Scanning electron micrograph of the surface of a developing human tooth from which ameloblasts have been removed. The surface consists of a series of pits previously filled by Tomes processes, the walls of which are formed by interrod enamel. (From Warshawsky H, et al.: The development of enamel structure in rat incisors as compared to the teeth of monkey and man, *Anat Rec* 200:371–399, 1981.)

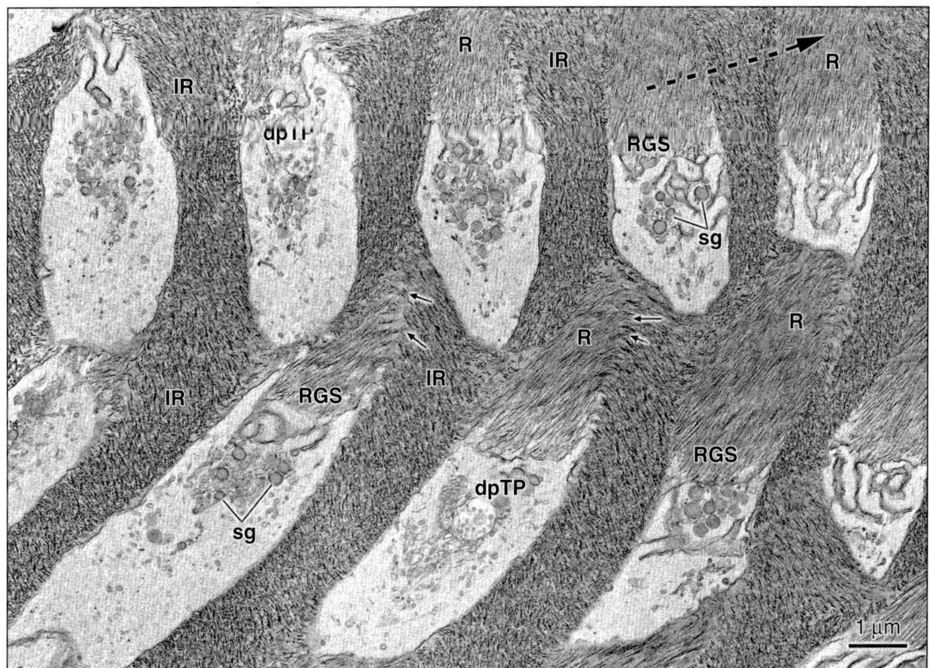

Fig. 7.34 In cross section the distal portions of Tomes processes *(dpTP)* appear as ovoid profiles surrounded by interrod enamel *(IR)*. They decrease in size toward the dentinoenamel junction *(dashed arrow)* as the rod *(R)* grows in diameter. The crystals making up the rod blend in with those of interrod enamel (*small arrows,* zone of confluence) at the point where the rod begins forming. *RGS,* Rod growth sites; *sg,* secretory granule.

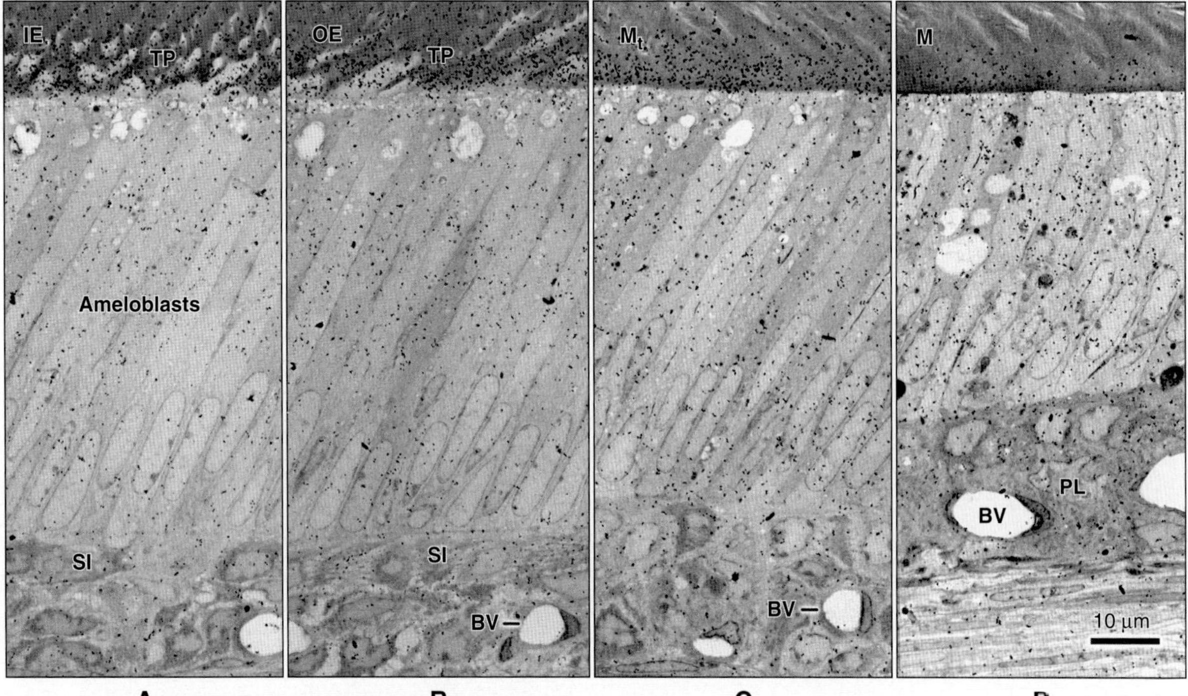

Fig. 7.35 Special scanning electron microscope radioautographic preparations after administration of 3H-methionine to radiolabel secretory products (mainly amelogenins) of ameloblasts. The black silver grains over enamel indicate the presence of newly formed amelogenins. (A, B) As expected, secretory-stage ameloblasts actively secrete proteins during inner *(IE)* and outer *(OE)* enamel formation. (C, D) The presence of grains over the surface enamel during the transition phase *(M_t)* and early maturation *(M)* indicates that ameloblasts still produce some enamel matrix proteins during the early part of the maturation stage. (C) This micrograph is from the beginning of transition; note that the stratum intermedium *(SI)* has started to reorganize to form part of the papillary layer *(PL)*. *BV,* Blood vessel; *TP,* Tomes process.

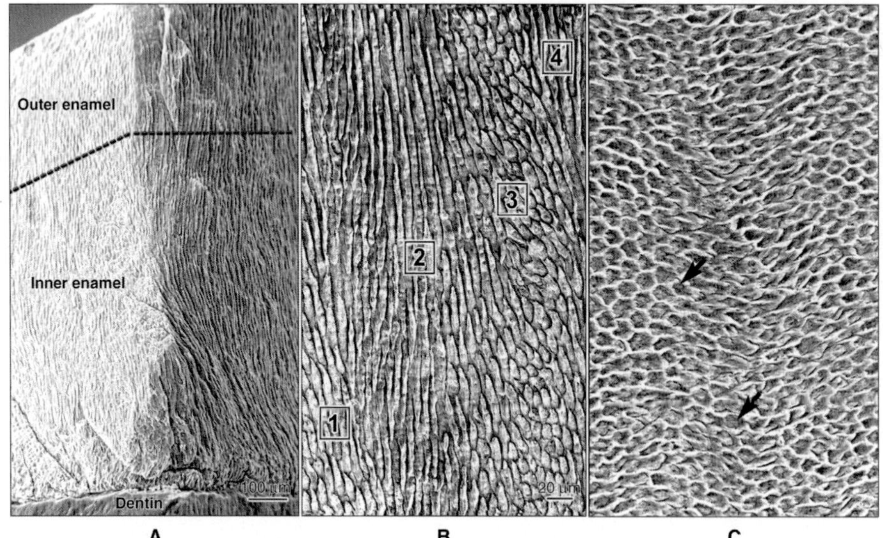

Fig. 7.36 (A, B) Scanning electron microscope images showing the complex trajectory of rods in the inner two-thirds of the enamel layer in human teeth. (B) The rods are organized in groups exhibiting different orientations; this image shows four adjacent groups. (C) In this fractured preparation, rods are seen in the interrod pits *(arrows)*.

During the maturation stage, ameloblasts undergo programmed cell death (apoptosis) (Box 7.1). The particularities of the rat incisor have allowed researchers to obtain a quantitative evaluation of the extent of the process in this tooth; approximately 25% of the cells die during the transitional phase, and another 25% die as enamel maturation proceeds. Whether the magnitude of cell loss is the same in human teeth is not known. However, considering the overall similarities in amelogenesis between teeth of continuous and limited eruption, it can be assumed safely that the initial ameloblast population is significantly reduced in all teeth during the maturation phase. Curiously, apoptosis

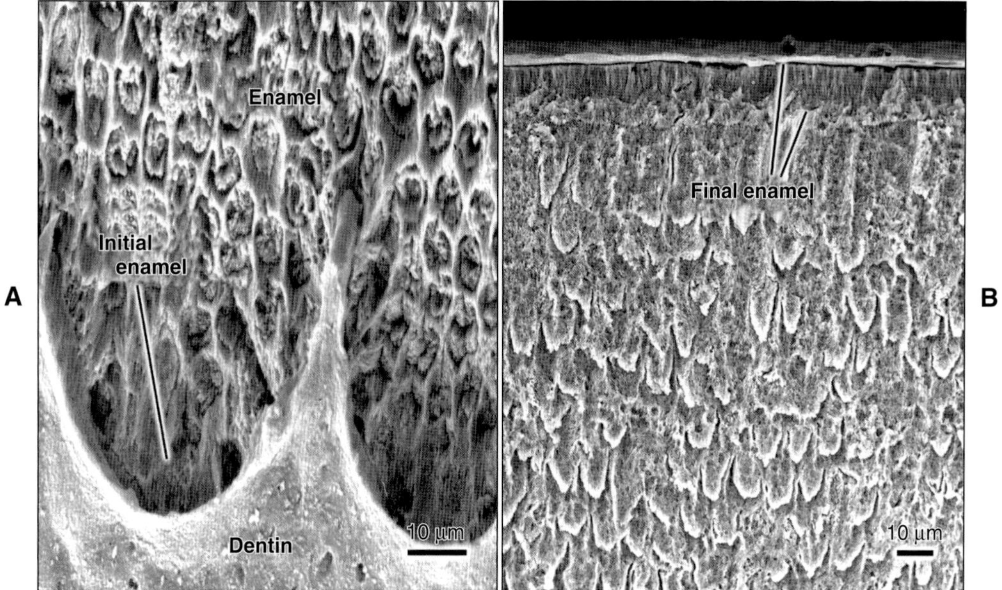

Fig. 7.37 The (A) first (initial) and (B) last (final) enamel layers are aprismatic (i.e., they do not contain rods).

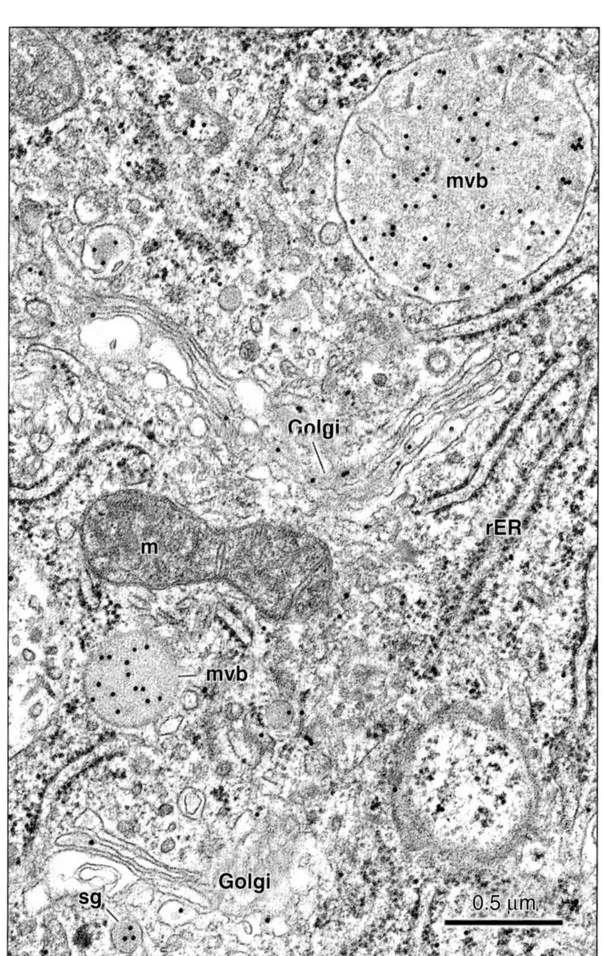

Fig. 7.38 As illustrated in this immunocytochemical preparation *(black dots)*, early maturation-stage ameloblasts contain amelogenin in their Golgi apparatus, indicating that they still synthesize enamel proteins. Elements of the lysosomal system, such as multivesicular bodies *(mvbs)*, are also immunoreactive. *m,* Mitochondria; *rER,* rough endoplasmic reticulum; *sg,* secretory granule.

BOX 7.1 Key Features of Cell Death

Necrosis (Accidental Cell Death)

Cell death that results from irreversible injury to the cell. Cell membranes swell and become permeable. Lytic enzymes destroy the cellular contents, which then leak into the intercellular space, leading to the mounting of an inflammatory response.

Programmed Cell Death

An active cellular process that culminates in cell death. This process may occur in response to developmental or environmental cues or as a response to physiologic damage detected by the internal surveillance networks of the cell.

Apoptosis

One type of programmed cell death characterized by a particular pattern of morphologic changes. The name comes from the ancient Greek, referring to shedding of the petals from flowers or leaves from trees. Apoptosis is observed in all metazoans, including plants and animals, but the genes encoding proteins involved in apoptosis have yet to be detected in single-celled organisms, such as yeasts.

Apoptotic death occurs in two phases. During the latent phase, the cell looks morphologically normal but is actively making preparations for death. The execution phase is characterized by a series of dramatic structural and biochemical changes that culminate in the fragmentation of the cell into membrane-enclosed apoptotic bodies. Activities that cause cells to undergo apoptosis are said to be proapoptotic. Activities that protect cells from apoptosis are said to be antiapoptotic.

From Pollard TD, Earnshaw WC: *Cell biology*, Philadelphia, PA, 2004, Saunders.

also takes place in the enamel knots (see Chapter 5) as part of the morphogenetic events.

Cell death is a fundamental mechanism during embryonic development and throughout the life of an organism. In embryogenesis, cells die at specific times during development to permit orderly morphogenesis. Two major ways by which cell death can occur are accidental (induced) cell death (necrosis) and programmed cell death (apoptosis). Also now recognized is that programmed cell death can occur without exhibiting the dramatic structural changes typical of apoptosis. The main features of necrosis and apoptosis are summarized in Box 7.1, and the corresponding cellular changes are schematically illustrated in Fig. 7.39 (apoptosis) and Fig. 7.40 (necrosis). The Bcl-2 (B-cell lymphoma 2) gene family is a major regulator of apoptosis and comprises protector, killer, and regulator proteins (Fig. 7.41). Specialized proteinases (caspases) also inactivate cellular survival pathways and activate factors that promote death.

Maturation Proper

Next, the principal activity of ameloblasts is the bulk removal of water and organic material from the enamel to allow introduction of additional inorganic material. The most visually dramatic activity of these cells is modulation—the cyclic creation, loss, and recreation of a highly invaginated ruffle-ended apical surface (the cells alternate between possessing a ruffled border [ruffle ended] and a smooth border [smooth ended]) (Fig. 7.42; see also Figs. 7.13, 7.14, and 7.15). Modulation can be visualized by special stains (Fig. 7.43) and occurs in waves traveling across the crown of a developing tooth from least mature regions to most mature regions of the enamel (e.g., in an apical-incisal direction in continuously erupting teeth and cervical-incisal [occlusal] direction in teeth of limited eruption). Available evidence suggests that ameloblasts in some species modulate rapidly—as often as once every 8 hours—thereby yielding three complete modulation cycles per day. The significance of the modulations is not yet fully understood, but they appear to be related to maintaining an environment that allows accretion of mineral content and loss of organic matrix, in part through alterations in permeability of the enamel organ. One proposal is that the acidification associated with ongoing mineral accretion during maturation causes ruffle-ended ameloblasts to produce bicarbonate ions. This process continuously alkalizes the enamel fluid to prevent reverse demineralization of the growing crystallites and maintain pH conditions optimized for functioning of the matrix-degrading enzymes, which prefer slightly acidic to near-neutral conditions. Interstitial fluids that may leak into the maturing enamel during the smooth-ended phase also may contribute to neutralizing the pH of the enamel fluid. Ruffle-ended ameloblasts possess proximal junctions that are leaky and distal junctions that are tight, whereas most smooth-ended ameloblasts have distal junctions that are leaky and proximal ones that are tight (Fig. 7.44). Ruffle-ended ameloblasts show considerable endocytotic activity and contain numerous lysosomes, calcium-binding proteins, and membrane-associated calcium–adenosine triphosphatases (ATPases) that appear to promote the pumping of calcium ions into the maturing enamel. Smooth-ended ameloblasts, however, leak small proteins and other molecules, show little endocytotic activity, and have almost no membrane calcium-ATPase activity.

Data available to date suggest the calcium ions required for active crystal growth pass through the ruffle-ended ameloblasts (because their distal junctions are tight) but along the sides of the more leaky smooth-ended ameloblasts. Active incorporation of mineral ions into crystals occurs mainly in relation to the ruffle-ended cells. Regarding the withdrawal of organic matrix from maturing enamel, sufficient evidence is now available to indicate that active resorption of intact proteins by ameloblasts is not the main mechanism for the loss of organic matrix observed during enamel maturation. This is attributed largely to the action of bulk-degrading enzymes that act extracellularly to digest the various matrix proteins into fragments small enough to leave the enamel layer. Polypeptide fragments leaving the enamel likely pass between the leaky distal junctions of smooth-ended cells and diffuse laterally among the ameloblasts to be taken up along their basolateral surfaces. When cells become ruffle ended because the proximal junctional complex now in turn becomes leaky, some of the laterally

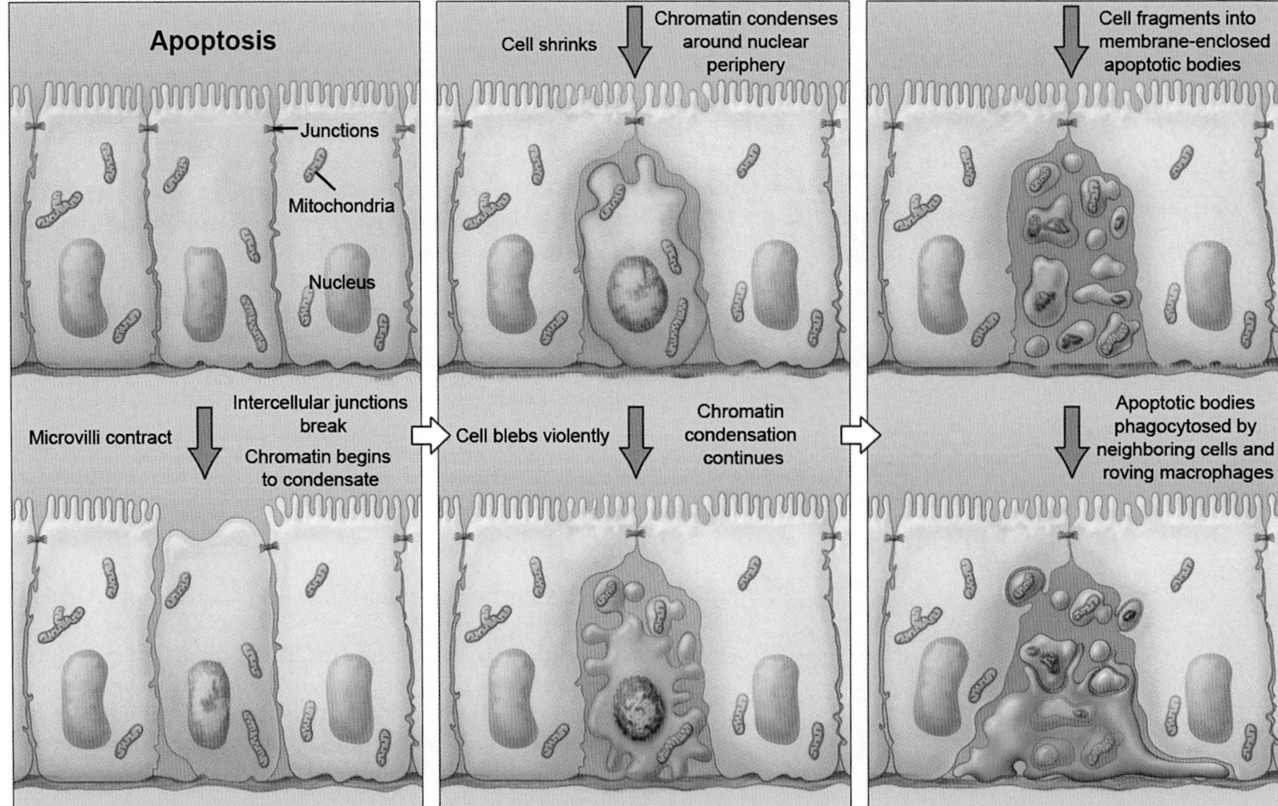

Fig. 7.39 Cascade of events that occur in apoptosis. (From Pollard TD, et al.: *Cell biology,* ed 4, Elsevier, 2022.)

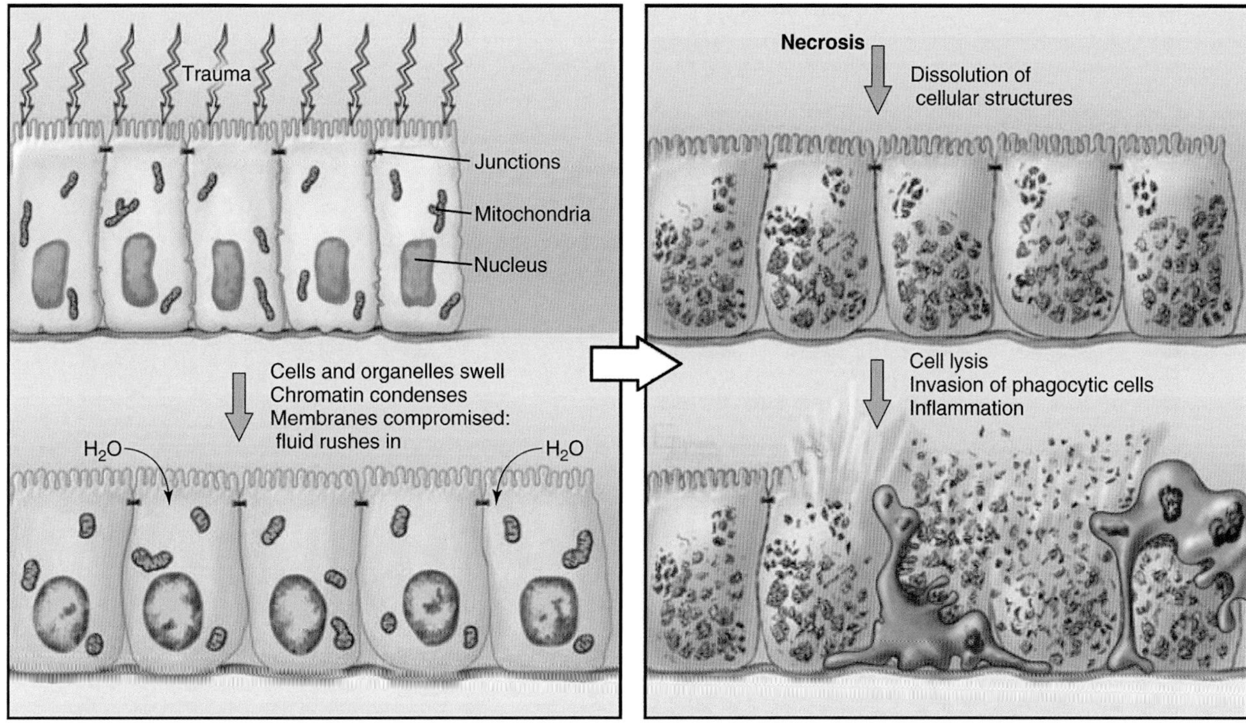

Fig. 7.40 Cascade of events that occur in necrosis. (From Pollard TD, et al.: *Cell biology,* ed 4, Elsevier, 2022.)

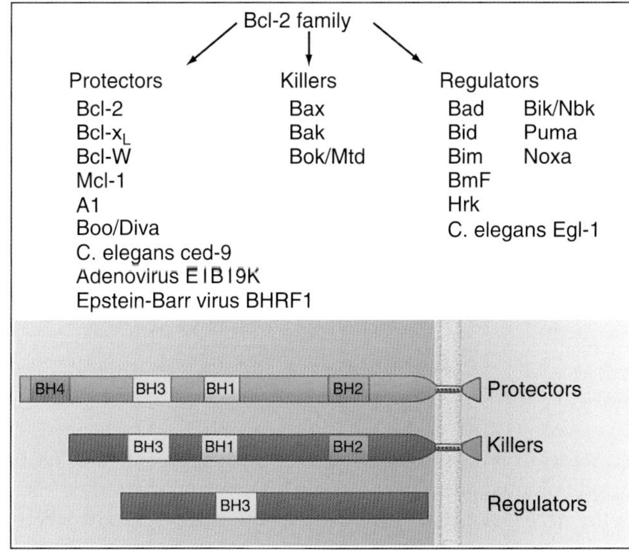

Fig. 7.41 The Bcl-2 family of apoptosis-regulating proteins. (From Pollard TD, et al.: *Cell biology,* ed 4, Elsevier, 2022.)

diffusing peptides could disperse throughout the papillary layer and perhaps beyond. Some protein fragments from the enamel layer also may be taken up by endocytosis across the membrane infoldings of the ruffled border. Just as ameloblasts complete the transitional phase and begin the first series of modulation cycles, they deposit an atypical basal lamina at their now-flattened apex (no part of Tomes process is recognizable at this stage). This interfacial layer adheres to the enamel surface, and the ameloblasts attach to it by means of hemidesmosomes (Fig. 7.45). Typical basal lamina constituents, such as types IV and VII collagen, have not been demonstrated in it; however, the layer has been shown to contain laminin-332 (previously known as *laminin-5*), a bridging heterotrimer molecule that is essential for hemidesmosomal attachment to organic extracellular matrix components. Patients with laminin-332 deficiency show focal enamel hypoplasia, and targeted disruption of laminin-332 function in mice affects the appearance of ameloblasts and enamel formation.

Interestingly, during postsecretory transition and leading into early maturation, ameloblasts secrete an acidic phosphoprotein called *odontogenesis-associated phosphoprotein (ODAPH).* Mutations in the gene encoding for this protein are associated with recessive hypomineralized amelogenesis imperfecta. In a mouse model expressing a truncated form of ODAPH, ameloblasts detach from the enamel layer forming a cyst, and modulation does not take place, causing complete failure of enamel maturation. It is important to reiterate here that there are two major events during postsecretory transition that usher in maturation. One is cell death, without which the excess of cells would likely cause buckling of the enamel organ. The other is structuring of the atypical basal lamina, which is needed to keep the enamel organ adherent to the tooth surface, creating a secluded environment for controlling enamel maturation.

The atypical basal lamina is known to be rich in glycoconjugates and to contain some unique proteins (Fig. 7.46) whose nature and role are only just now beginning to be elucidated (see the following discussion). Thus it likely represents a unique structure both in composition and function; in addition to an adhesive role, the presence of highly glycosylated molecules may confer to this lamina charge-selective property, which could help regulate the movement of material into and out of the enamel layer. Also, it is situated such that it could relay to the ameloblasts information about the status of the dynamic enamel compartment.

At this point, recapitulating the many functions that cells of the inner enamel epithelium exhibit during their life cycle is worthwhile. Initially, the cells undergo frequent mitoses and are involved in establishing the crown pattern of the tooth (morphogenesis). Then, the

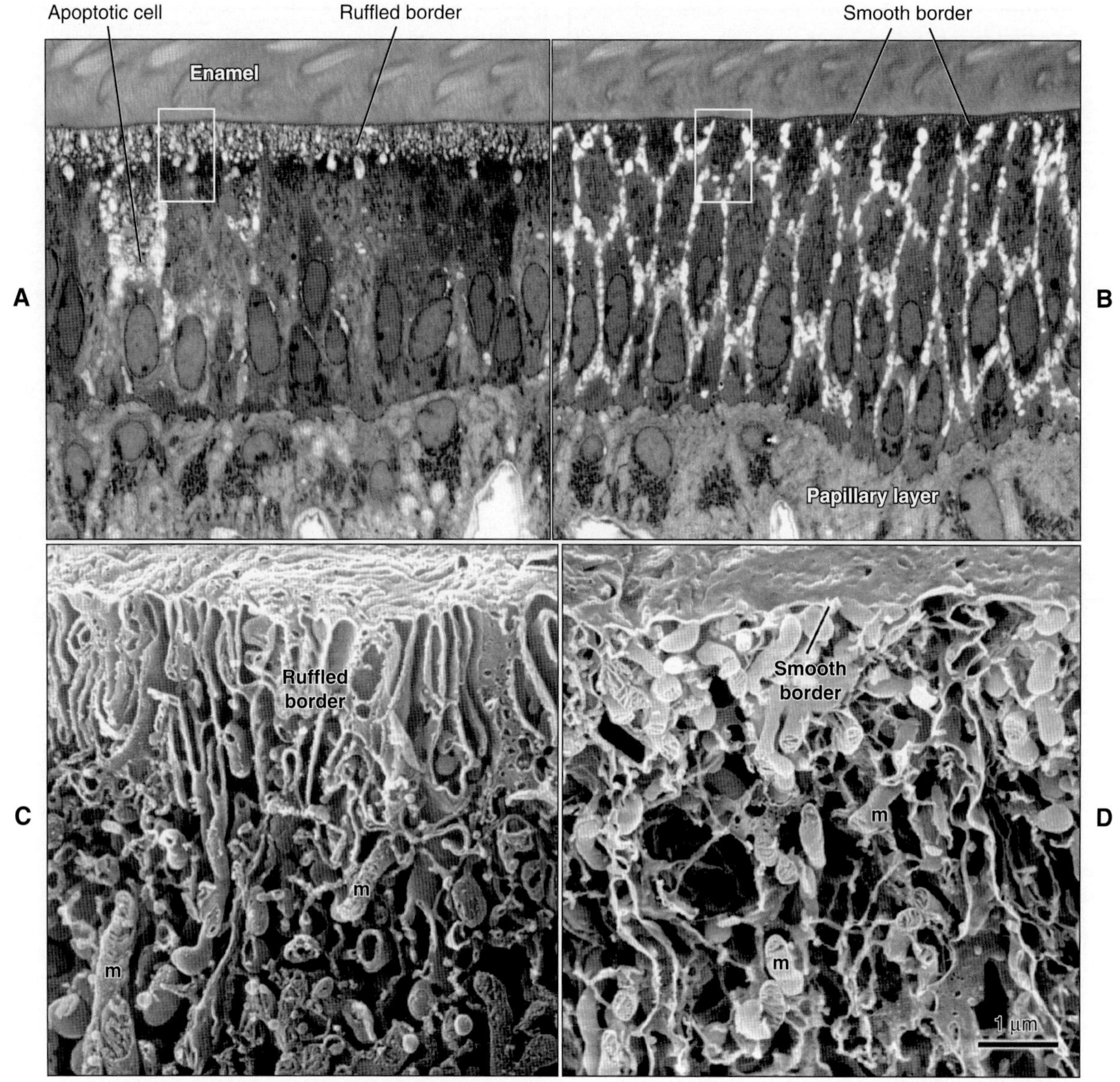

Fig. 7.42 Scanning electron micrographs of (A, B) tissue sections and (C, D) fractured samples showing the (A, C) ruffle-ended and (B, D) smooth-ended apices of maturation-stage ameloblasts. (C, D) are from areas similar to the boxed area in (A, B), respectively. *m,* Mitochondria.

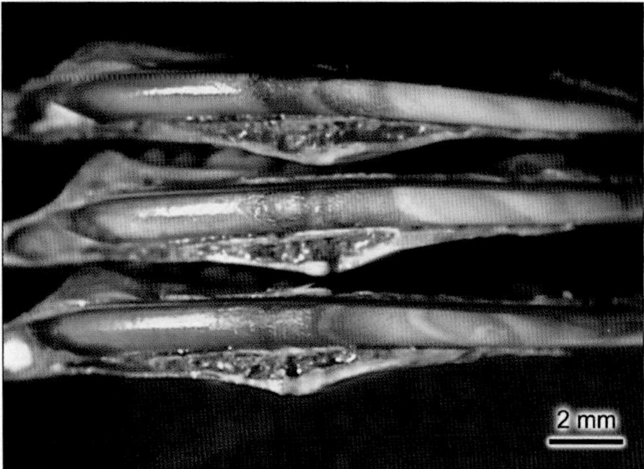

Fig. 7.43 The modulation cycle of ameloblasts can be visualized by special stains. Indicator dyes were used to detect regional variations in pH along the maturing enamel of rat incisors. The large bands correspond to regions overlaid by ruffle-ended ameloblasts, whereas smaller ones correspond to those associated with smooth-ended cells. (Courtesy C.E. Smith.)

cells undergo morphologic changes, and they become ameloblasts (histodifferentiation). These changes are preparatory to their entering the next phase, active secretion of the enamel matrix, wherein they develop the Tomes process. The secretory stage is followed by a short transitional phase of cell restructuring leading to enamel maturation proper, wherein the ameloblasts exhibit cyclic variations with ruffle- and smooth-ended borders against the enamel surface, the ruffle-ended cells allowing incorporation of inorganic material and the smooth-ended cells permitting exit of protein fragments and water.

Ameloblast Secretory Products

The organic matrix of enamel is made from noncollagenous proteins consisting only of several enamel proteins and enzymes (Table 7.2). Of the enamel proteins, 90% are a heterogeneous group of low-molecular-weight proteins known as *amelogenins.* The remaining 10% consists of nonamelogenins, such as enamelin and ameloblastin. The electrophoretic profile of whole enamel homogenates from immature enamel is

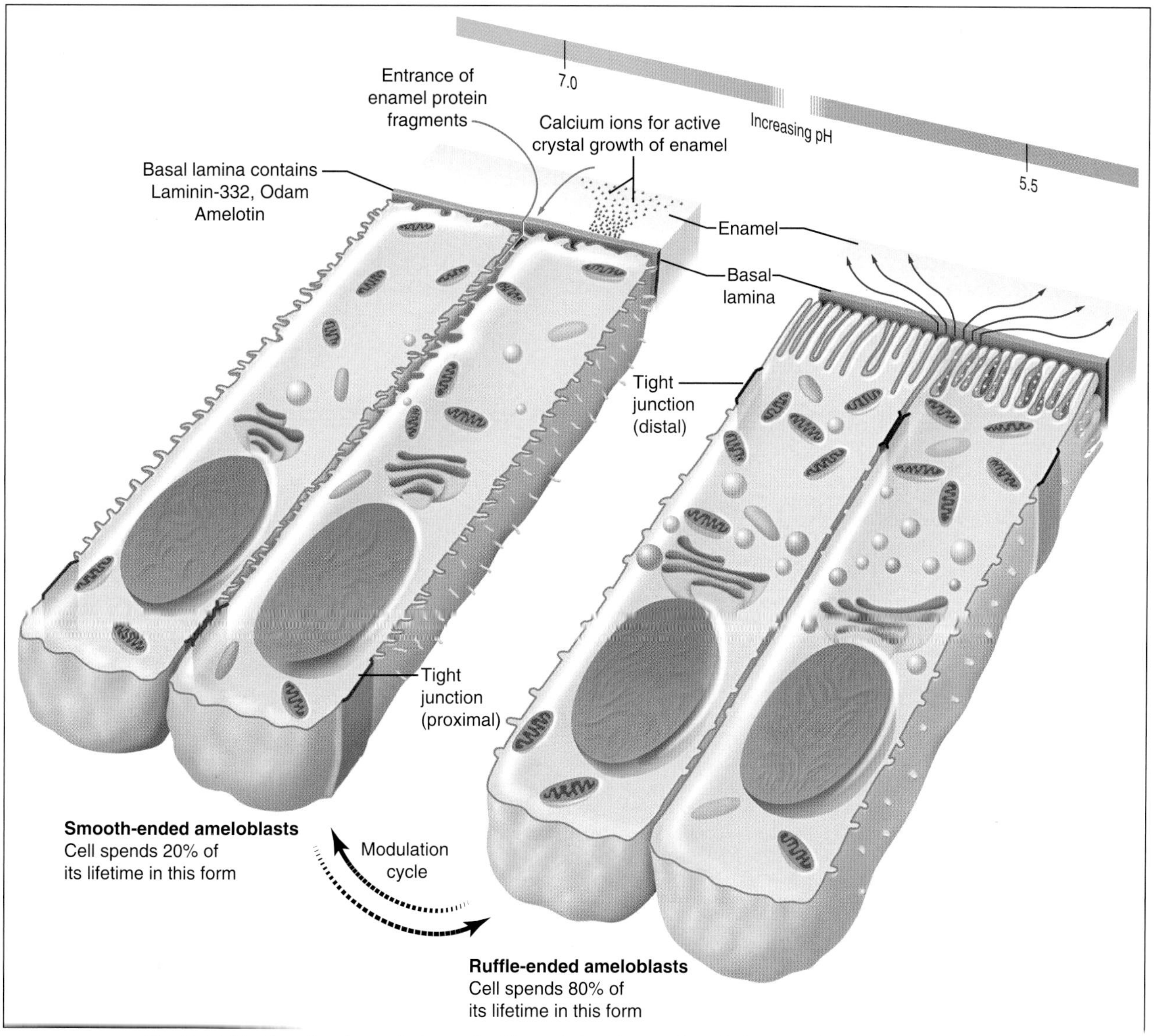

Fig. 7.44 The functional morphology of ruffle-ended and smooth-ended maturation stage ameloblasts.

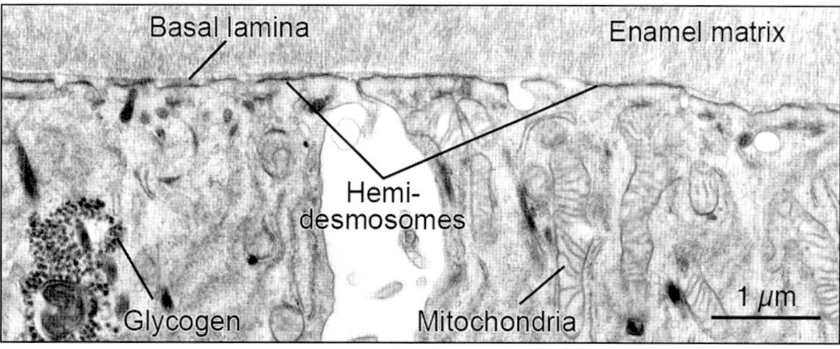

Fig. 7.45 There is a basal lamina at the interface between ameloblasts and maturing enamel. The cells attach to the basal lamina by hemidesmosomes.

complex and represents a composite image of newly secreted and partially degraded forms of both categories of proteins. Amelogenins are hydrophobic proteins rich in proline, histidine, and glutamine, showing little posttranslational modifications (single phosphorylation site) and with reported molecular weights ranging between 5 and 45 kDa. Their heterogeneity is brought about in three ways. The genes responsible for transcribing amelogenin are found on X and Y chromosomes; because these two genes are not 100% homologous, a sexual heterogeneity exists at the outset. The functional significance of this sexual dimorphism is not known. Second, the amelogenin gene contains several exons, which can be spliced in numerous ways to produce mature mRNAs that may include all exons or lack some of them, producing as many as nine isoforms. The functional significance of alternatively spliced forms of amelogenins has not yet been fully determined. Third,

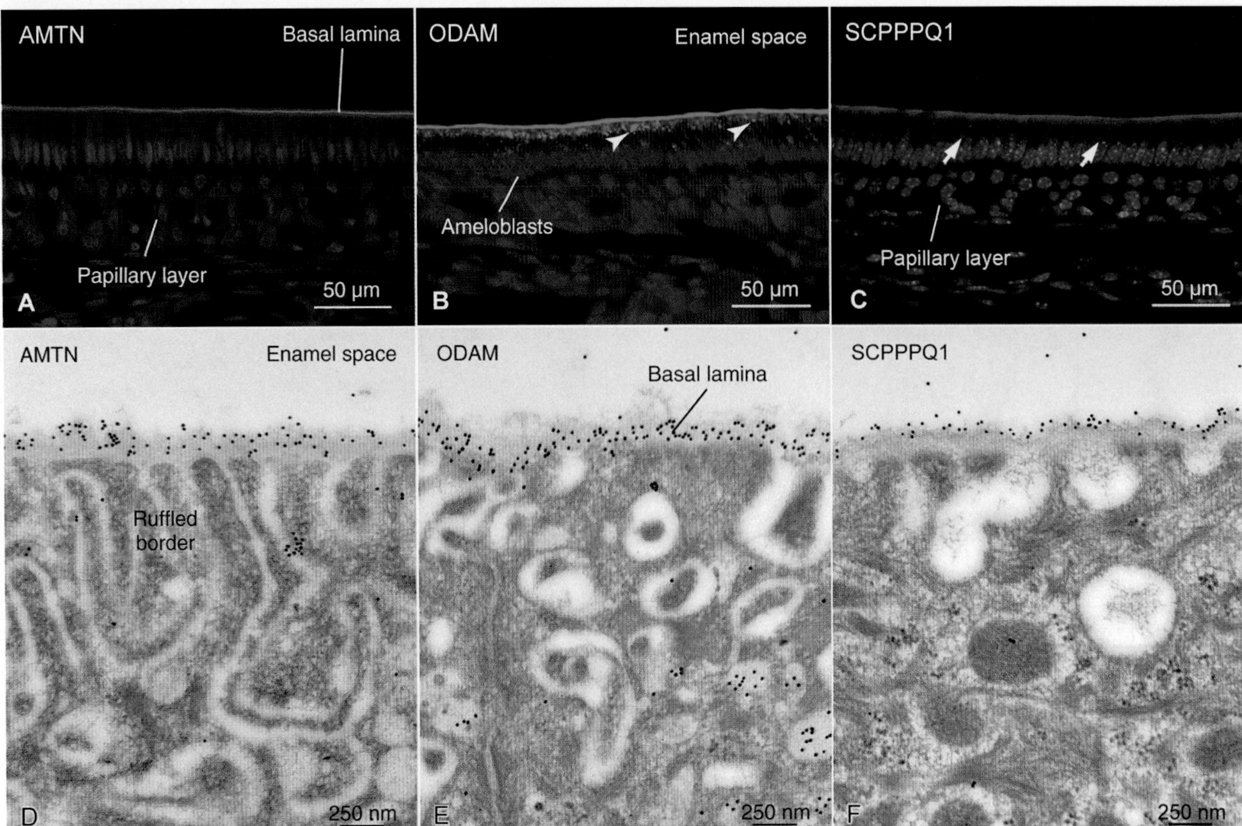

Fig. 7.46 At the start of the maturation stage, ameloblasts deposit an atypical basal lamina against the enamel surface, to which it adheres firmly. (A–C) Immunofluorescence images showing that amelotin (A, *AMTN*), odontogenic ameloblast-associated (B, *ODAM*), and secretory calcium-binding phosphoprotein-proline-glutamine-rich 1 (C, *SCPPPQ1*) are present at the interface between ameloblasts and enamel. Note also the distinctive presence of ODAM but not AMTN in the apical portion of the ameloblasts *(arrowheads)*, and the Golgi region labeling for SCPPPQ1 in late maturation stage ameloblasts *(arrows)*. (C–E) Transmission electron micrographs of immunogold preparations of ruffle-ended ameloblasts and illustrating the presence of AMTN (D), ODAM (E) and SCPPPQ1 (F) in the basal lamina at their apical surface.

amelogenins undergo short-term (minor) and long-term (extensive) extracellular processing by proteolytic enzymes into low-molecular-weight fragments, of which tyrosine-rich amelogenin polypeptide and leucine-rich amelogenin polypeptide are significant because they constitute the bulk of the residual organic matrix in maturing enamel.

Ameloblastin and enamelin are the best-studied members of the nonamelogenin family. A 65-kDa sulfated protein also has been described. Nonamelogenins are believed to undergo rapid extracellular processing, and intact molecules do not accumulate in enamel for long periods. Another nonamelogenin called *tuftelin* has been reported, but its role as an enamel matrix protein is questionable because it is present in several tissues and lacks a signal peptide for secretion. The fact that nonamelogenins represent minor components of forming enamel does necessarily imply that they are produced in small amounts but is likely a reflection of their short half-life (i.e., they do not accumulate over time and undergo rapid degradation).

Members of at least two general families of proteinases are involved in the extracellular processing and degradation of enamel proteins (see Table 7.2). Enamelysin (Mmp20), an enzyme from the matrix metalloproteinase (MMP) family, is involved in the short-term processing of newly secreted matrix proteins. Another enzyme from the serine proteinase family, originally termed *enamel matrix serine protease 1* and now called *kallikrein 4 (Klk4)*, functions as a bulk digestive enzyme during the maturation stage. Both proteinases are secreted in a latent proenzyme form.

There has been considerable effort in identifying ameloblast products that are secreted into the enamel layer where they would be in a position to affect crystal formation and growth and structuring of the layer. Efforts to better define the secretome of ameloblasts, in general, have led to the identification of three novel secreted proteins produced by maturation-stage ameloblasts. (These do not represent enamel matrix constituents in the sense that they do not have an active role in structuring the enamel layer.) They are amelotin (AMTN), odontogenic ameloblast–associated (ODAM) (a fragment of ODAM was originally isolated from the amyloid of calcifying odontogenic epithelial tumors), and secretory calcium-binding phosphoprotein proline-glutamine rich 1 (SCPPPQ1) (see Table 7.2). All three proteins have been immunolocalized to the atypical basal lamina at the interface between ameloblasts and maturing enamel (see Fig. 7.46). They therefore represent novel components of the atypical basal lamina, and thus they may participate in its supramolecular organization and in the molecular mechanism that mediates adhesion of the enamel organ to the maturing enamel surface. Using light microscopy, ODAPH was detected at the interface between the ameloblasts and the enamel surface and proposed to play role in "maintaining the integrity of the atypical basal lamina."[1] However, the association of ODAPH with the basal lamina awaits high-resolution immunolocalization. These proteins may also have other functions related to cell or matrix events taking place

[1]Ji Y, et al.: Maturation stage enamel defects in Odontogenesis-associated phosphoprotein (*Odaph*) deficient mice, *Dev Dyn* 250:1505–1517, 2021, https://doi.org/10.1002/dvdy.336. First published: 26 March 2021.

TABLE 7.2 Summary of Secreted Proteins Associated With Enamel Formation[a]

	Name	Symbol/ Gene Location	Features
Proteins Contributing to Appositional Growth in Thickness of the Enamel Layer			
	Amelogenin	AMELX; AMELY Xp22.3; Yp11.2	• Represents the main protein present in forming enamel; expression stops when enamel reaches full thickness. • Has a relatively low molecular weight (~25 kDa) with few posttranslational modifications. • Ameloblasts secrete several versions (isoforms) of the protein arising from active transcription of X and Y chromosomes and from alternative splicing of its mRNA; most secreted isoforms are truncated relative to hypothetical full-length transcript. • The N-terminal end of the secreted protein characteristically begins with the amino acid sequence MPLPP–, and the C-terminal end usually finishes with –KREEVD • Has unusual solubility properties relative to temperature, pH, and calcium ion concentrations; solutions of the protein are capable of transforming into a jelly under physiologic conditions. • Shows a marked tendency for self-aggregation; it creates unit structures called *nanospheres* (~20 nm) that themselves aggregate into larger quaternary arrangements, including chains and ribbons. • Inhibits lateral growth (volumetric expansion) of hydroxyapatite crystals. *Loss of function:* A thin hypoplastic enamel layer is formed that lacks enamel rods.
Nonamelogenins	Ameloblastin	AMBN 4q13.3	• Present in much smaller amounts compared with amelogenin (~10% of matrix); it is found mostly in newly formed (secretory stage) enamel and more so at the outer surface than in deeper areas closest to the dentinoenamel junction. • Roughly 2.5 times larger in molecular weight than amelogenin (~65 kDa); it has sulfated O-linked sugars. • Cleaved rapidly into several fragments soon after it is secreted from ameloblasts; one fragment has calcium-binding properties. • Ameloblasts continue to express ameloblastin throughout the maturation stage, although ameloblastin does not appear to cross the basal lamina and enter into the maturing enamel layer. • Believed to assist ameloblasts in adhering to the forming enamel surface during the secretory stage. *Mutant protein:* Terminal differentiating ameloblasts detach from the dentin, and enamel formation aborts. Enamel organ regresses and becomes cystic.
	Enamelin	ENAM 4q13.3	• Largest (~186 kDa) and least abundant (>5%) of the enamel matrix proteins. • Believed to undergo extensive posttranslational modifications; it has N-linked sugars and is phosphorylated. • The full-length protein and its largest derivative fragments (to ~89 kDa), created as soon as the protein is secreted, are not detected inside forming (secretory stage) enamel; these are present only at the growing enamel surface. • Small fragments from enamelin, however, do linger within enamel (e.g., 32 kDa and 25 kDa); these bind strongly to mineral and are inhibitory to crystal growth. • Believed to function in part as a modulator for de novo formation of mineral and to promote crystal elongation. *Loss of function and mutant protein:* No defined enamel layer
Proteins Involved in Postsecretory Processing and Degradation of Amelogenins and Nonamelogenins			
	Enamelysin	MMP20 11q22.3	• Calcium-dependent metalloproteinase of the matrix metalloprotease subfamily; it has some unique structural features. • Found primarily in newly formed (secretory stage) enamel. • Believed to cleave the hydrophilic C-terminal ends of amelogenins and other internal sites; it is suspected to be responsible for cleaving ameloblastin and enamelin into certain large fragments. *Loss of function:* Results in formation of a thin hypomatured enamel layer.
	Enamel matrix serine protease (now called *kallikrein4*)	KLK4 19q13.4	• Serine proteinase of the tissue kallikrein subfamily (kallikrein-related peptidase 4); it also is expressed in prostate. • Believed to be secreted into enamel that has achieved full thickness when ameloblasts lose their Tomes processes and start their modulation cycles along the enamel surface. • Slowly degrades residual amelogenins and fragments from nonamelogenins into small polypeptides. *Loss of function:* Hypomaturation of enamel.
Proteins Related to Basal Lamina Covering Maturing and Mature Preeruptive Enamel			
	Amelotin	AMTN 4q13.3	• Secreted by ameloblasts during and shortly after transition to the maturation stage. • Resides in the surface basal lamina along with laminin-332 throughout maturation and is found at the interface between the junctional epithelium and the tooth. • Precise function to be determined.

Continued

TABLE 7.2 Summary of Secreted Proteins Associated With Enamel Formation[a]—cont'd

	Name	Symbol/ Gene Location	Features
			Putative surface mineralization function *Loss of function:* • Mild and selective enamel phenotype • No junctional epithelium phenotype
	Odontogenic ameloblast–associated	ODAM 4q13.3	• Secreted by ameloblasts during and shortly after transition to the maturation stage. • Located in the surface basal lamina throughout maturation and is found in the basal lamina located at the surface of junctional epithelium and among the incompletely differentiated cells of the junctional epithelium. • Disruption of periodontal integrity induces expression of the protein by epithelial cell rests of Malassez. • Precise function to be determined. *Loss of function:* • No enamel phenotype • Junctional epithelium defects
	Secretory calcium-binding phosphoprotein-proline-glutamine-rich 1	SCPPPQ1	• Secreted by ameloblasts from mid- to late maturation • Produced by the junctional epithelium
	Odontogenesis-associated phosphoprotein	4q21.1 ODAPH	• Secreted by ameloblasts from postsecretory transition to early maturation • Presumably associated with the forming atypical basal lamina. • Precise localization and role remain to be determined. *Mutation, loss of function:* • Detachment/cyst of enamel organ • Complete failure of enamel maturation • Recessive hypomineralized amelogenesis imperfecta
Legacy Proteins			
	First described enamelin		• The EDTA-soluble protein described in older literature as "enamelin" turned out to be albumin derived from blood contamination.
	Tuftelin		• Described in older literature; has no signal peptide and therefore does not represent a protein intentionally secreted extracellularly.
	Amelin/sheathlin		• These are older terms for the protein now referred to as *ameloblastin.*

[a]Modified from a table prepared by C.E. Smith.
EDTA, Ethylenediaminetetraacetic acid.

during enamel maturation (e.g., there is some evidence that AMTN may also participate in mineralization of the final enamel layer). As discussed in Chapter 12, AMTN, ODAM, and SCPPPQ1 also are expressed in the junctional epithelium where cell adhesion via hemidesmosomes to the tooth surface plays an important role in maintaining periodontal integrity and health.

The extracellular matrix of developing dental enamel is now reasonably well defined in terms of its major protein components. Forming enamel does not exhibit a distinct, unmineralized preenamel layer (such as osteoid or predentin) that accumulates and gradually transforms into a mineralized layer at an interfacial region, referred to as a *mineralization front.* Instead, as indicated previously, the enamel matrix proteins participate in mineralization as soon as they are released by the ameloblasts, and crystals grow directly against the secretory surfaces (Fig. 7.47). At these growth sites, the interface between the membrane and the lengthening extremity of crystals can in fact be regarded as a mineralization front. Although the background matrix formed by the marginally soluble amelogenins may provide some physical support, because of their transient nature enamel proteins likely do not play any major structuring and support function as collagen does in bone, dentin, and cellular cementum.

Morphologically, the organic matrix of young, forming enamel appears uniform in decalcified histologic preparations; however, immunocytochemical analyses reveal that enamel proteins are differentially distributed across the enamel layer (Fig. 7.48). Intact or relatively intact nonamelogenin molecules, such as ameloblastin and enamelin, are concentrated near the cell surface at sites where they are secreted, whereas mostly degradation fragments are found in deeper (older) enamel. The areas where there is concentration of intact molecules correspond to the position in enamel where rod/interrod crystals grow in length by the addition of increments of amorphous calcium phosphate (ACP) at their tip (enamel growth sites). These nonamelogenins create by themselves and/or through interactions with cell membrane–associated molecules conditions favorable for crystal elongation. The critical molecular participants proposed to be implicated in the tethering of elongating crystallites to the cell membrane include among others the basal lamina protein laminin-332 and a complex of ameloblastin (AMTN)/enamelin (ENAM) that shapes ACP into crystallites (Box 7.2). While genetic manipulations are certainly a major asset, the high-resolution localization of laminin-332 at this critical interface would provide visual demonstration for this exquisite concept that guides and shapes crystal elongation. It will also be interesting to see how the concept ties in with the "crystal ghosts" proposed many years ago by the pioneering work of Bonucci and Warshawsky.

On the other hand, intact and fragmented forms of amelogenin are least concentrated at growth sites and are found abundantly throughout

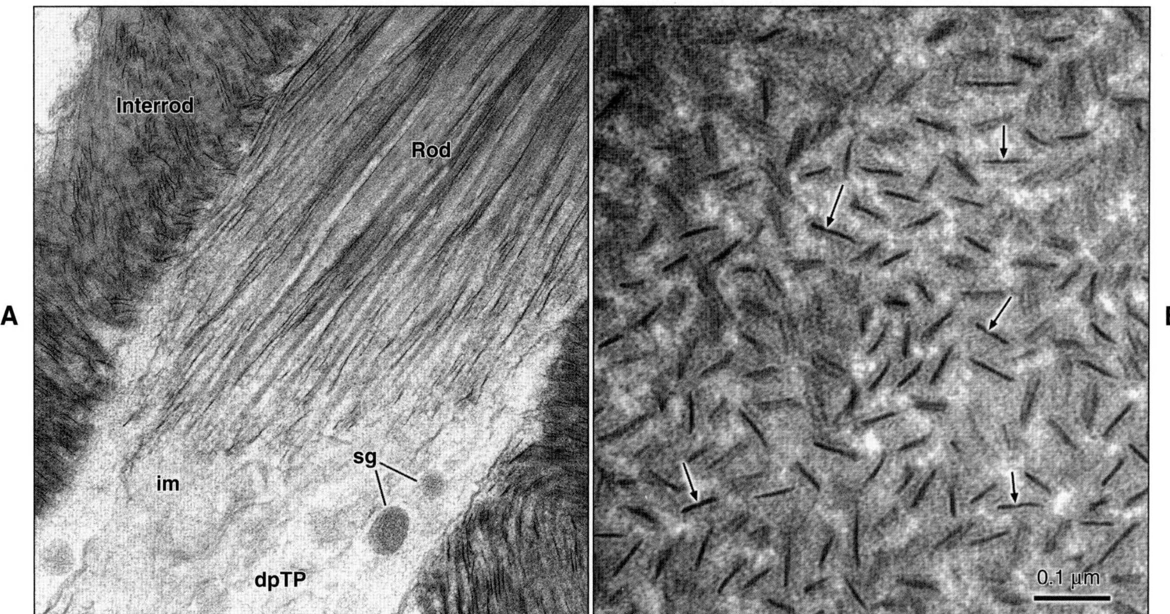

Fig. 7.47 (A) Transmission electron microscope image illustrating the relationship of rod enamel crystals to a distal portion of Tomes process *(dpTP)* and surrounding interrod enamel. The elongating extremity of the rod crystals abut the infolded membrane *(im)* at the secretory surface, an area that can be regarded as a mineralization front. (B) In cross section, newly formed crystals appear as small, needlelike structures *(arrows)* surrounded by granular organic matrix. *sg,* Secretory granules.

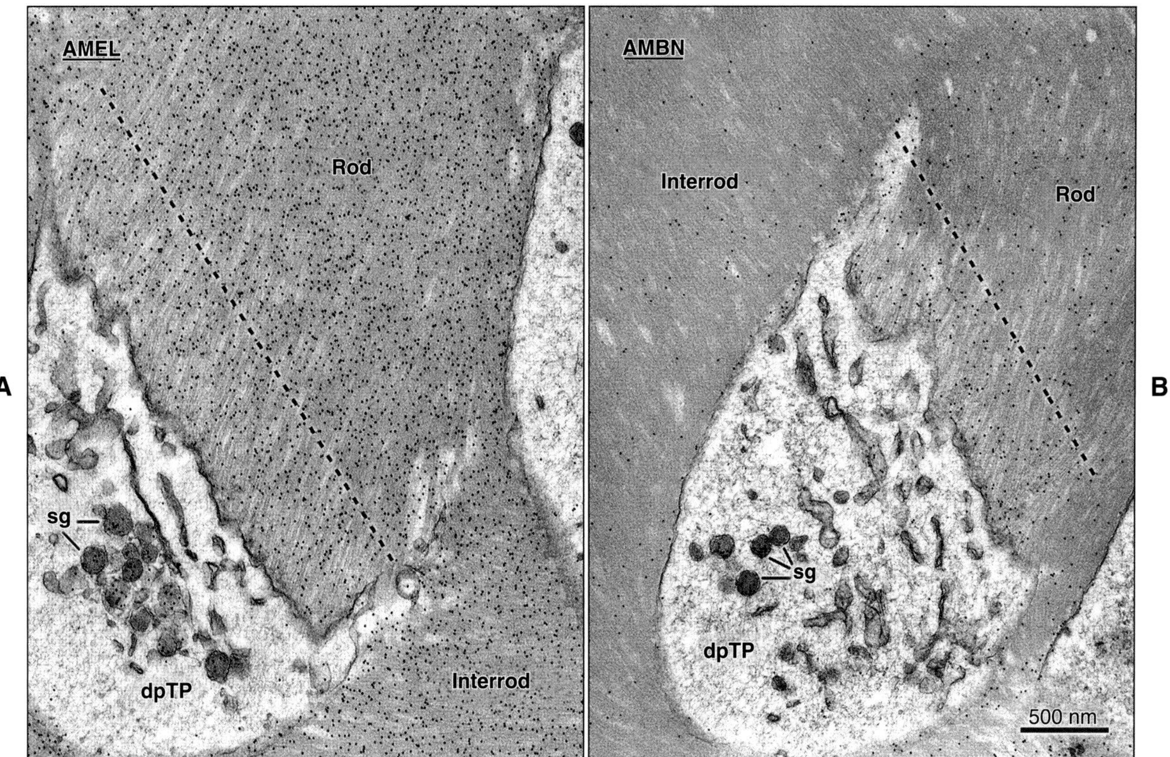

Fig. 7.48 Comparative immunocytochemical preparations illustrating the differential distribution of (A) amelogenin *(AMEL)* and (B) ameloblastin *(AMBN),* here in relation to a distal portion of Tomes process *(dpTP).* Amelogenins are less concentrated in a narrow region near the secretory surface on the process (fewer *black dots* occur between the cell and the *dashed line* than beyond), whereas most of the ameloblastin is found in this border region where enamel crystals elongate. *sg,* Secretory granule.

the enamel layer. Amelogenins and ameloblastin (and likely also enamelin) are synthesized together and are contained within the same secretory granule (see Fig. 7.28). Given that they are cosecreted, their segregation at growth sites is intriguing and may result from microenvironmental conditions, the physicochemical properties of the proteins, or some special attribute of the secretory granule populations. Amelogenins are believed to form supramolecular aggregates (nanospheres) that surround crystals along their long axis and are visible on sections of enamel examined under the electron microscope as a granular background material between crystals (see Fig. 7.47B). Recent analyses showed that amelogenins can also assemble as nanoribbon structures that sustain the uniaxial growth of apatite nanofibers. Radiolabeling studies indicate that newly formed amelogenins diffuse away from secreted surfaces and eventually randomize throughout the enamel layer. As such they may add volume into the enamel layer into which the crystal can elongate and assemble. This possibility has received further support by a recent three-dimensional analysis of the forming enamel layer in amelogenin knockout mice, in which it was concluded that "amelogenin does not directly nucleate, shape, or orient enamel ribbons, but separates and supports the enamel ribbons, and expands the enamel matrix to accommodate continued ribbon elongation."[2]

[2]Smith CE, et al.: Ultrastructure of early amelogenesis in wild-type, Amelx-/-, and Enam-/- mice: enamel ribbon initiation on dentin mineral and ribbon orientation by ameloblasts, *Mol Genet Genomic Med* 4(6):662–683, 2016, https://doi.org/10.1002/mgg3.253.

Based on the biochemical characteristics and differential distribution of the various enamel proteins, members of the nonamelogenin family are believed to broadly promote and guide the formation of enamel crystals. Amelogenins regulate growth in thickness and width of crystals, thereby preventing crystals from fusing during their formation, and must be removed to permit subsequent enlarging of crystals during maturation.

The expression of matrix proteins at early stages by cells that are not fully differentiated, including the inverted expression of matrix proteins by epithelial and ectomesenchymal cells, may be part of the reciprocal epithelial-mesenchymal signaling during tooth morphogenesis and histodifferentiation. The early secretion of amelogenin at a time when odontoblasts have not yet differentiated fully, mantle predentin is not yet discernible, and enamel mineralization has not yet started suggests that this protein is multifunctional. Initially, amelogenins may participate in epithelial-mesenchymal events. Because no overt sign of mineral deposition exists among the initial patches of enamel proteins, any role amelogenin may have in crystal nucleation likely is associated with the temporal expression of specific isoforms, extracellular processing of major isoforms, or the arrival of other proteins such as ameloblastin. When enamel mineralization is ongoing, amelogenin then may function to regulate the environment into which crystals form.

Studies using knockout mice (which do not express a given protein), transgenic mice (which overexpress a selected protein or have point mutations), and mutant mice (which express altered or defective proteins) are providing invaluable information on the function of the various ameloblast products. Transgenic mice express mutated

BOX 7.2 Understanding Enamel Formation Through Human and Mouse Genetics

Until recently, we had little insight into how dental enamel forms at the molecular level. Human and mouse genetic studies are changing that. There are dozens of human hereditary conditions that include enamel malformations as a phenotype, and many of the mutated genes causing these conditions have been identified. These include ameloblast membrane proteins and extracellular matrix molecules that are critical for the attachment and elongation of enamel mineral ribbons. The most important of these for understanding the attachment and elongation enamel ribbons are *COL17A1, ITGAV, ITGB6, ITGA6, ITGB4, LAMA3, LAMB3, LAMC2, ENAM, AMBN, AMELX, MMP20,* and *SLC13A5.*

Collagen 17 is a homotrimeric transmembrane protein that mediates adhesion of the cell to the underlying extracellular matrix. It contains an extracellular collagen triple-helical domain that in some tissues is cleaved by proteinases of the ADAMs family. Type XVII collagen can bind to integrins and laminins. Integrins are cell adhesion receptors that bind to both intracellular and extracellular matrix proteins, thereby functionally linking the cell cytoskeleton to the extracellular matrix (ECM). Integrins are comprised of transmembrane αβ heterodimers that anchor the membrane to the ECM, while transferring extracellular information into the cell. Secretory ameloblasts express two integrin heterodimers that are necessary for proper enamel ribbon formation: α6ß4 and αVß6. *Itgb6* knockout mice upregulated the expression of *Amelx* by 21-fold and *Enam* by 7.6 fold.

Laminins are a family of heterotrimeric-secreted glycoproteins, each containing an alpha chain, beta chain, and gamma chain. Laminin-332, encoded by *LAMA3, LAMB3,* and *LAMC2,* is secreted throughout the secretory stage, although the secreted laminin does not disperse throughout the matrix. Laminin-332 binds to selected integrins and is known to bind to the integrin β4 subunit of the α6β4 integrin. In skin, laminin-332 is an essential component of the basement membrane that attaches the epidermis to the dermis and is essential for skin integrity. In developing teeth, laminin-332 is essential for the adhesion of ameloblasts to the surface of the forming enamel. Ameloblasts in *Lama3* null mice detach from the underlying enamel matrix immediately following the onset of enamel mineral deposition. Laminin-332 is unlikely to extend the full distance to the tips of the enamel ribbons (250-300Å from the plasma membrane). It must bind to secreted enamel proteins that, in turn, bind to the mineral ribbons.

The secreted enamel proteins are enamelin (ENAM), ameloblastin (AMBN), and amelogenin (AMELX). These proteins belong to the secretory calcium-binding phosphoprotein gene family that arose by tandem duplications of *SPARC-L1.* ENAM, AMBN, and AMELX are proline-rich intrinsically disordered proteins, meaning they are unable to fold into a unique and stable tertiary structure. They adopt a functional fold when they bind to a partner molecule or a mineral surface. Matrix metallopeptidase 20 (MMP20) is a secreted protease that cleaves these enamel proteins. ENAM, AMBN, AMEL, and MMP20 are functionally tooth specific, as the genes encoding them are pseudogenized (disrupted) in vertebrates that have lost the ability to make teeth during evolution.

Immunogold transmission electron microscopy has shown that uncleaved enamelin is found only along the mineralization front. AMBN also localizes along the mineralization front and accumulates in the matrix (especially in the sheath space between rod and interrod enamel). Although AMELX is abundant throughout the enamel matrix, where it comprises perhaps 90% of total protein, it is particularly scarce at the mineralization front. No enamel mineral ribbons form in *Enam* or *Ambn* null mice. *Amelx* null mice form an initial enamel comprised of characteristic, oriented enamel mineral ribbons, but mineral deposition becomes increasingly pathologic, and fanlike structures of octacalcium phosphate (OCP) form, rather than rod/interrod structures comprised of calcium hydroxyapatite (HAP). Similar fan-shaped OCP structures form in *Mmp20* null mice, identifying AMELX cleavage products as necessary regulators of the transition of the initially amorphous calcium phosphate (ACP) mineral ribbons into HAP.

Enamel crystallites get their characteristic ribbonlike shape before they become crystalline HAP. Being comprised of ACP, the newly elongated portion of the ribbons do not have crystalline faces that can be shaped by proteins binding to and selectively inhibiting ion absorption onto specific crystal faces. Not having in intrinsic shape of their own, ACP mineral ribbons require a mold to obtain their uniformly thin cross-sectional shapes at the mineralization front. This mold is presumed to bind laminin-332 and is most likely comprised of ENAM and AMBN. AMELX and its cleavage products fill the space between enamel mineral ribbons and regulate their transition from ACP to HAP. MMP20 cleavages degrade the ENAM/AMBN molds, which disappear with increasing distance from the mineralization front,

Continued

BOX 7.2 Understanding Enamel Formation Through Human and Mouse Genetics—cont'd

allowing for a smooth increase in the cross-sectional dimensions of the crystallites with depth by a steady rate of ions depositing onto the sides of the ribbons.

The current model for the enamel mineralization front is shown in Box 7.2 Fig. 1. This model is consistent with all observations and indicates that the mechanism of enamel mineral ribbon formation is an evolutionary adaptation of the ameloblast basement membrane. This dynamic system accomplishes (a) ameloblast attachment to the underlying mineral, (b) a means for the addition of ions or mineral onto the tips of existing mineral ribbons, (c) orientation of the ribbons in the direction of the retreating membrane, and (d) communication of extracellular information into intracellular reactions through effectors such as plectin (*Plec*) that bind to the integrin cytoplasmic tail.

Genetic studies have identified other critical membrane components expressed by secretory-stage ameloblasts. Solute carrier family 13 member 5 (SLC13A5) channels tribasic citrate ions into the enamel matrix. Citrate binds to and stabilizes the thin mineral ribbons. The membrane-bound acid phosphatase 4 (ACP4) apparently dephosphorylates enamel proteins prior to their endocytosis. RELT is a critical tumor necrosis factor receptor expressed throughout the secretory stage, although the ligand that binds it is unknown. Latent transforming growth factor binding protein 3 is cosecreted with transforming growth factor β (TGF-β) to mediate matrix-cell interactions through a TGF-β receptor.

The molecular mechanisms of dental enamel formation are still poorly understood, but advances in human and mouse genetics have provided us with solid identification of many of the critical molecular participants and the ability to frame hypothetical molecular models that can be tested to refine our understanding of amelogenesis at the molecular level.

James P. Simmer
Department of Biologic and Materials Sciences
University of Michigan School of Dentistry
Ann Arbor, Michigan, United States

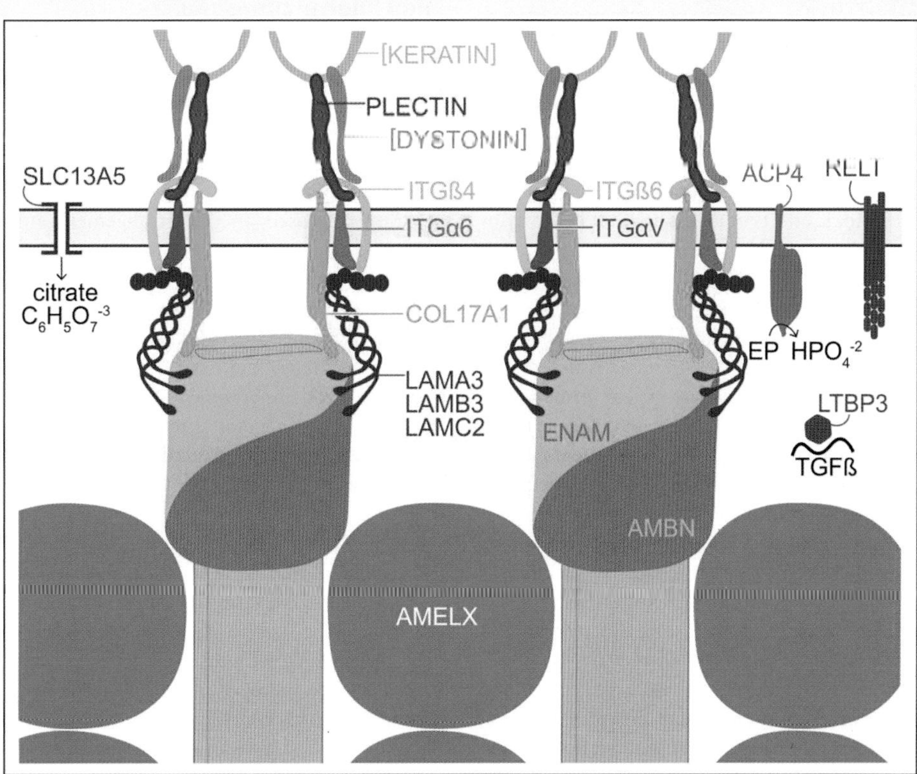

Box 7.2 Fig. 1 Hypothetic molecular model for ameloblast attachment to enamel mineral ribbons while orienting their elongation in the direction of the retrograde movement of the ameloblast membrane. (Courtesy Shelly Zhang, From Simmer JP, et al.: A genetic model for the secretory stage of dental enamel formation, *J Struct Biol* 213(4):107805, 2021.)

forms of amelogenin, and knockout mice exhibit major enamel structural defects that affect overall thickness and enamel rod structure. Consistent with their proposed role in promoting and sustaining mineral formation, no structured enamel layer forms in mice expressing defective ameloblastin or enamelin. This is also the case when expression of enamelin is completely abrogated, attesting to the critical role of nonamelogenins. In animals with defective or absent enamel proteins, tooth induction and formation proceed apparently normally at the histologic level. This raises questions about the proposed signaling functions discussed previously and suggests the possible existence of redundant mechanisms.

Surprisingly, crystals still increase considerably in width and thickness in knockout mice for *Mmp20* and *Klk4*, which exhibit significantly reduced proteolytic activity. The enamel is hypomineralized, rod/interrod organization is disturbed, and enamel proteins persist during maturation. The enamel is thinner in *Mmp20* knockout mice because this enzyme is active during secretion when the full thickness of the enamel layer is created. On the other hand, *Klk4* knockouts show no major thickness problems because this maturation-stage enzyme comes into play only after the full thickness of the enamel is established. Interestingly, the *Klk4* knockout also shows enamel weakness near the dentinoenamel junction, and the enamel layer abrades away when the teeth erupt into the oral cavity, suggesting the maturation process also strengthens the interfacial relationship between enamel and dentin.

As mentioned, ameloblasts produce basal lamina components during presecretion and maturation. Disruption of the production of laminin-332, a heterotrimeric protein composed of alpha 3, beta 3, and gamma 2 chains causes enamel hypoplasia. A mouse model expressing laminin-332 containing human laminin gamma 2 (instead of the mouse form) exhibits severe hypomineralization because the integrity of the atypical basal lamina present during enamel maturation is affected. The ameloblastin knockout only shows a mild and selective phenotype, and there is no histologically apparent enamel phenotype in the ODAM and SCPPPQ1 knockouts.

MINERAL PATHWAY AND MINERALIZATION

The way in which mineral ions are introduced into forming enamel is of interest because it spans the secretory and maturation phases of enamel formation, with the latter demanding a large increase in the influx of mineral. The enamel layer is a secluded environment essentially created and maintained by the enamel organ. The route by which calcium moves from the blood vessels through the enamel organ to reach enamel likely implicates intercellular and transcellular routes. Several years ago, a smooth tubular network, opening onto enamel, was described in secretory stage ameloblasts. It then was speculated that the network might have a role in calcium ion control, similar to the sarcoplasmic reticulum, which it resembles. Transcellular routing can occur across the cell through the action of cytoplasmic buffering and transport proteins (i.e., calbindins) or via high-capacity stores associated with the endoplasmic reticulum. These mechanisms would permit avoidance of the cytotoxic effects of excess calcium in the cytoplasm. The stratum intermedium may also participate in the translocation of calcium, since calcium-ATPase activity has been localized at the cell membrane of the stratum intermedium.

No matrix vesicles are associated with the mineralization of enamel, as is the case for collagen-based calcified tissues. In these tissues, matrix vesicles provide a closed environment to initiate crystal formation in a preformed organic matrix. What is observed instead is formation of crystallites directly against mantle dentin and their subsequent elongation against the ameloblast membrane at sites where enamel proteins are released (see Fig. 7.47A) so that no equivalent of predentin or osteoid is ever created. Because there is an apparent continuity between enamel and dentin crystallites, some believe that the first enamel crystallites are nucleated by apatite crystallites located within the dentin (see Fig. 7.30).

Although amelogenesis is described correctly as a two-step process involving the secretion of partially mineralized enamel and its subsequent maturation, studies involving microradiography of thin ground sections and computer enhancement indicate that the mineralization of enamel may involve several stages. These stages result in the creation of an enamel layer that is most highly mineralized at its surface, with the degree of mineralization decreasing toward the dentinoenamel junction until the innermost layer is reached, where mineralization apparently is increased.

REGULATION OF pH DURING ENAMEL FORMATION

The pH values of forming enamel are maintained near neutral during secretion; however, they show considerable variation during maturation, shifting from acidic to near-neutral values and then rising to higher pH levels in more mature enamel. The pathways known to date to be used by ameloblasts in pH regulation involve carbonic anhydrases (mainly CA2 and CA6) to generate local bicarbonate, chloride ion exchangers and channel to exchange chloride ions across the apical plasma membrane, bicarbonate cotransporters to permit the passage of bicarbonates from external sources across the basal end to the apical pole of ameloblasts, and an exchanger (possibly Na^+/H^+) to remove H^+ ions generated during intracellular production of bicarbonate (Fig. 7.49). These various mechanisms bear resemblance to what takes place in the striated duct cells of salivary glands (see Chapter 11). Based on the abnormal phenotypes resulting from the lack of expression of the genes or proteins associated with these pathways, it has been surmised that the development of enamel requires correct maintenance of pH at all stages of enamel formation. In the case of CAs, given that no abnormal enamel phenotypes have been associated with disruptions in gene expression to date, it is likely that the various isoforms have compensatory capacity.

Readers are referred to a recent review by Bronckers (see Recommended Reading) for a comprehensive view of the complex mechanisms for pH cycling and buffering and ion transport during enamel maturation, the details of which lie beyond this histologic treatise.

STRUCTURAL AND ORGANIZATIONAL FEATURES OF ENAMEL

Rod Interrelationships

In human teeth, rods tend to be maintained in groups arranged circumferentially around the long axis of the tooth. In general, rods run in a perpendicular direction to the surface of the dentin, with a slight inclination toward the cusp as they pass outward. Near the cusp tip they run more vertically, and in cervical enamel they run mainly horizontally.

Superimposed on this arrangement are two other patterns that complicate enamel structure. First, each rod, as it runs to the surface, follows an irregular course, bending to the right and left in the transverse plane of the tooth (except in cervical enamel in which the rods have a straight course) and up and down in the vertical plane. Second, in approximately the inner two-thirds of the enamel layer, adjacent groups of rods intertwine and thus have dissimilar local orientations but a similar general direction. These complex interrelationships produce some of the structural features seen in enamel and must be remembered to interpret enamel structure.

Striae of Retzius

The striae of Retzius generally are identified using ground sections of calcified teeth but can also be seen in forming enamel. In a longitudinal section of the tooth, they are seen as a series of lines extending from the dentinoenamel junction toward the tooth surface (Fig. 7.50); in a cross section, they appear as concentric rings (Fig. 7.51). Although striae of Retzius generally are ascribed to a weekly rhythm in enamel production resulting in a structural alteration of the rod, the basis for their production is still not clear. Another proposal suggests that they reflect appositional or incremental growth of the enamel layer. As the crown becomes bigger, new cohorts of cells are added cervically to compensate for the increase in size. These cells undergo a passive decussation as the enamel layer grows in thickness to assume a more coronal position (Fig. 7.52). The demarcation between the enamel produced by these cohorts may appear as a line of Retzius, according to some investigators. The neonatal line, when present, is an enlarged stria of Retzius that apparently reflects the great physiologic changes occurring at birth. Accentuated incremental lines also are produced by systemic disturbances (e.g., fevers) that affect amelogenesis.

Cross Striations

Human enamel is known to form at a rate of approximately 4 μm/day. Ground sections of enamel reveal what appear to be periodic bands or cross striations at 4-μm intervals across rods. What may seem to be cross striations on longitudinally sectioned rods on ground sections also have been demonstrated to be obliquely sectioned groups of rods.

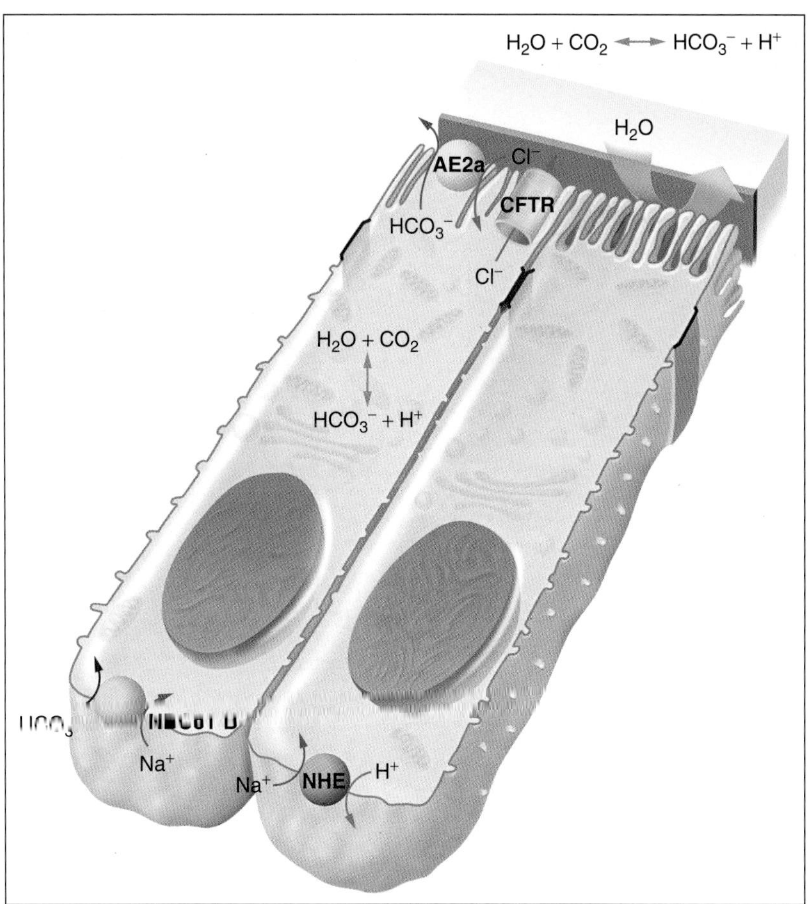

Fig. 7.49 Schematic illustration of selected pathways implicated in pH regulation in enamel. *AE2a*, Cl^-/HCO_3^- anion exchanger 2; *CFTR*, interacting proteins cystic fibrosis transmembrane conductance regulator; *NBCe1-B*, electrogenic sodium bicarbonate cotransporter; *NHE*, sodium/hydrogen exchanger regulatory factor. (From Lacruz RS, et al.: Regulation of pH during amelogenesis, *Calcif Tissue Int* 86:91–103, 2010; Simmer JP, et al.: Regulation of dental shape and hardness, *J Dent Res* 89:1024–1038, 2010.)

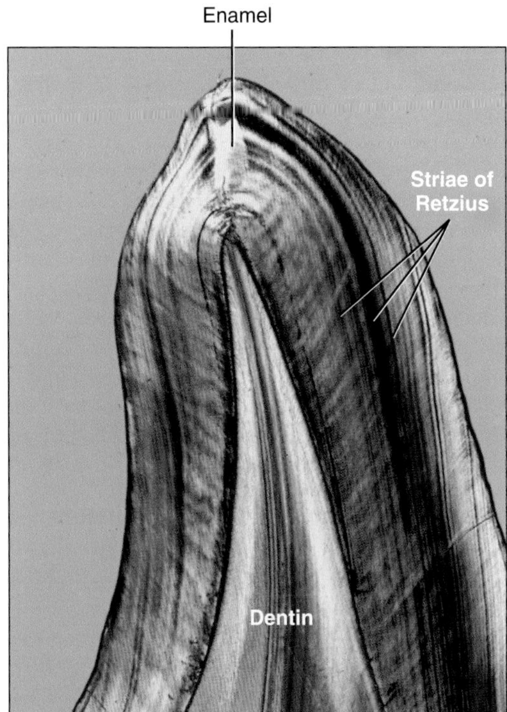

Fig. 7.50 Longitudinal ground section showing disposition of the striae of Retzius using polarized light microscopy. The wider stria corresponds to the neonatal line. (Courtesy P. Tambasco de Oliveira.)

Thus the light microscope may produce an illusion of longitudinally sectioned rods that are really, as demonstrated by electron microscopy, an alignment of obliquely cut rods in horizontal rows. With a scanning electron microscope, alternating constrictions and expansions of the rods sometimes are visible; close examination reveals that the constrictions are gouges in the rod structure (Fig. 7.53). Such a pattern could reflect a diurnal rhythmicity in rod formation, the organization of crystallites within the rod, or structural interrelations between rod and interrod enamel.

Bands of Hunter and Schreger

The bands of Hunter and Schreger are an optical phenomenon produced by changes in direction between adjacent groups of rods. The bands are seen most clearly in longitudinal ground sections viewed by reflected light and are found in the inner two-thirds of the enamel. These bands appear as dark and light alternating zones that can be reversed by altering the direction of incident illumination (Fig. 7.54). Scanning electron microscopy clearly reveals the difference in orientation of groups of rods within these zones (Fig. 7.55; see also Fig. 7.36).

Gnarled Enamel

Over the cusps of teeth, the rods appear twisted around each other in a seemingly complex arrangement known as *gnarled enamel.* Recall that rods are arranged radially in horizontal planes, each plane surrounding the longitudinal axis of the tooth like a washer. The rods undulate back and forth within the planes. This undulation in vertically directed rods around a ring of small circumference readily explains gnarled enamel.

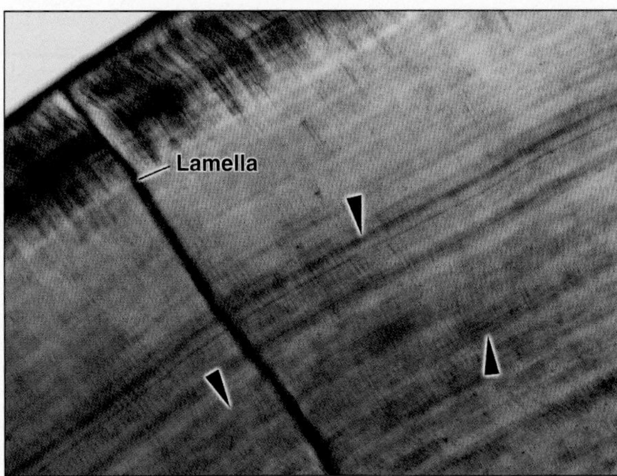

Fig. 7.51 Light microscope view of striae of Retzius in a ground section. In cross section the striae appear as a series of concentric, dark lines *(arrowheads)*. An enamel lamella can be seen running from the outer surface to the dentinoenamel junction.

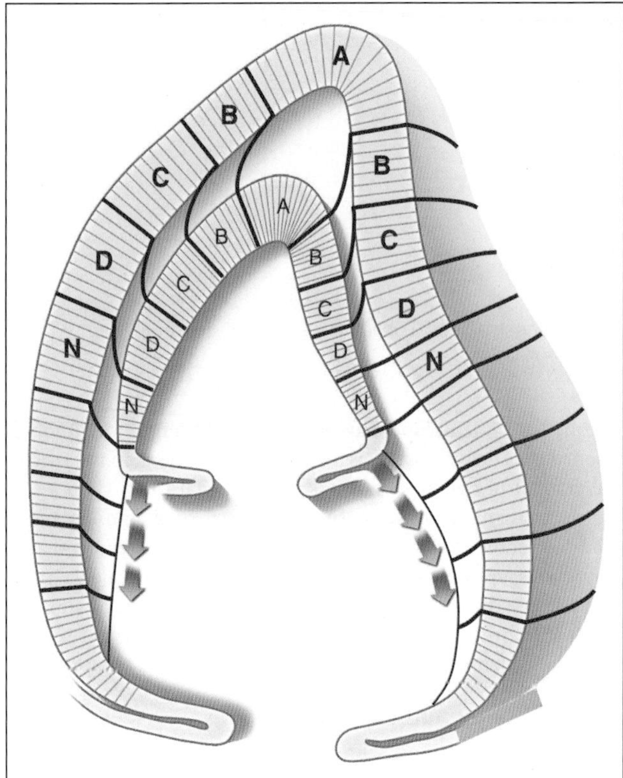

Fig. 7.52 Diagram illustrating the increase in crown size and corresponding growth of the enamel organ in a tooth of limited eruption. The ameloblast cohorts are labeled *A* to *N*. As the crown becomes larger, these cohorts are displaced apically on the enlarged crown by their own production of enamel. The trajectory followed by rods produced by the cohorts is outlined by the dark lines. The junction between the enamel rods produced by the various cohorts is believed to be responsible for the incremental pattern of enamel and to follow the general direction of the striae of Retzius. New ameloblasts differentiate cervically in the direction of the arrows as the crown grows in size. (From Warshawsky H: Ultrastructural studies on amelogenesis. In Butler WT, editor: *The chemistry and biology of mineralized tissues,* Birmingham, AL, 1985, Ebsco Media.)

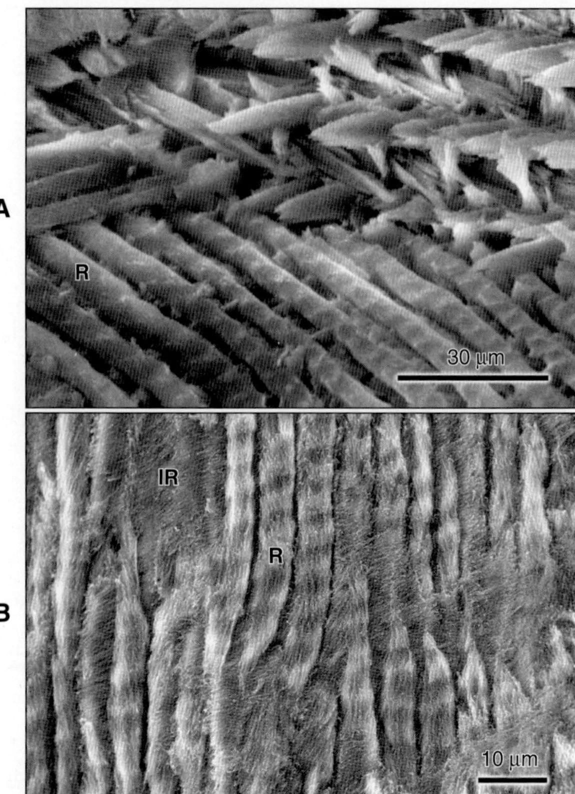

Fig. 7.53 In scanning electron microscopy, periodic varicosities and depressions are seen along enamel rods *(R)* in (A) rodent and (B) human teeth, producing the impression of cross striations along their length. *IR,* Interrod enamel.

Enamel Tufts and Lamellae

Enamel tufts and lamellae may be likened to geologic faults and have no known clinical significance. They are best seen in transverse sections of enamel (Fig. 7.56). Enamel tufts project from the dentinoenamel junction for a short distance into the enamel. They appear to be branched and contain greater concentrations of enamel proteins than the rest of the enamel. Because a special protein (tuft protein) has been reported at these sites, tufts are believed to occur developmentally as a result of abrupt changes in the direction of groups of rods that arise from different regions of the scalloped dentinoenamel junction. Lamellae extend for varying depths from the surface of enamel and consist of linear, longitudinally oriented defects filled with organic material. This organic material may derive from trapped enamel organ components or connective tissue surrounding the developing tooth. Tufts and lamellae are usually best demonstrated in ground sections, but they also can be seen in carefully demineralized sections of human enamel because of their higher protein content. Cracks in the enamel sometimes can be mistaken for lamellae, but they can be distinguished from the latter because they generally do not contain organic material.

Dentinoenamel Junction and Enamel Spindles

The junction between enamel and dentin is established as these two hard tissues begin to form and is seen as a scalloped profile in cross section (Fig. 7.57; see also Figs. 7.23A, 7.37A, and 7.56). Before enamel forms, some developing odontoblast processes extend into the ameloblast layer and, when enamel formation begins, become trapped to form enamel spindles (Fig. 7.58). The electron microscope reveals that crystals of dentin and enamel intermix (Fig. 7.59; see also Fig. 7.30).

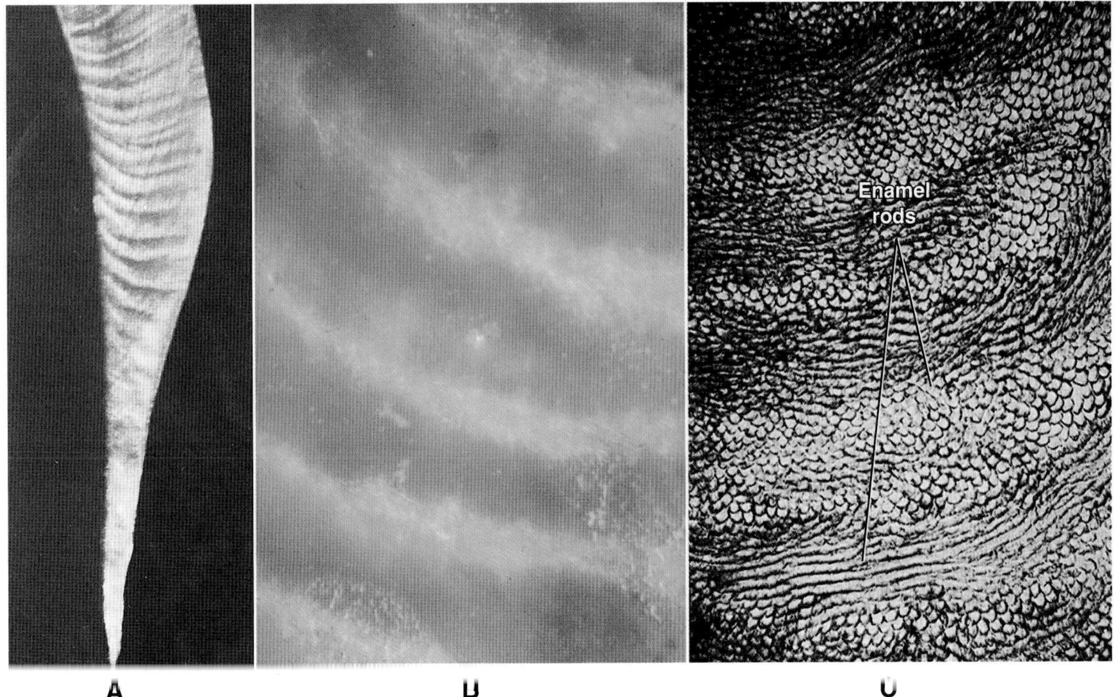

Fig. 7.54 Longitudinal section of enamel viewed by incident light. (A) The series of alternating light and dark bands of Hunter and Schreger are apparent. (B) Higher-power view of a band of Hunter and Schreger as viewed by incident light. (C) Section corresponding to (B) viewed under transmitted light. The differing orientation of enamel rods is clearly evident.

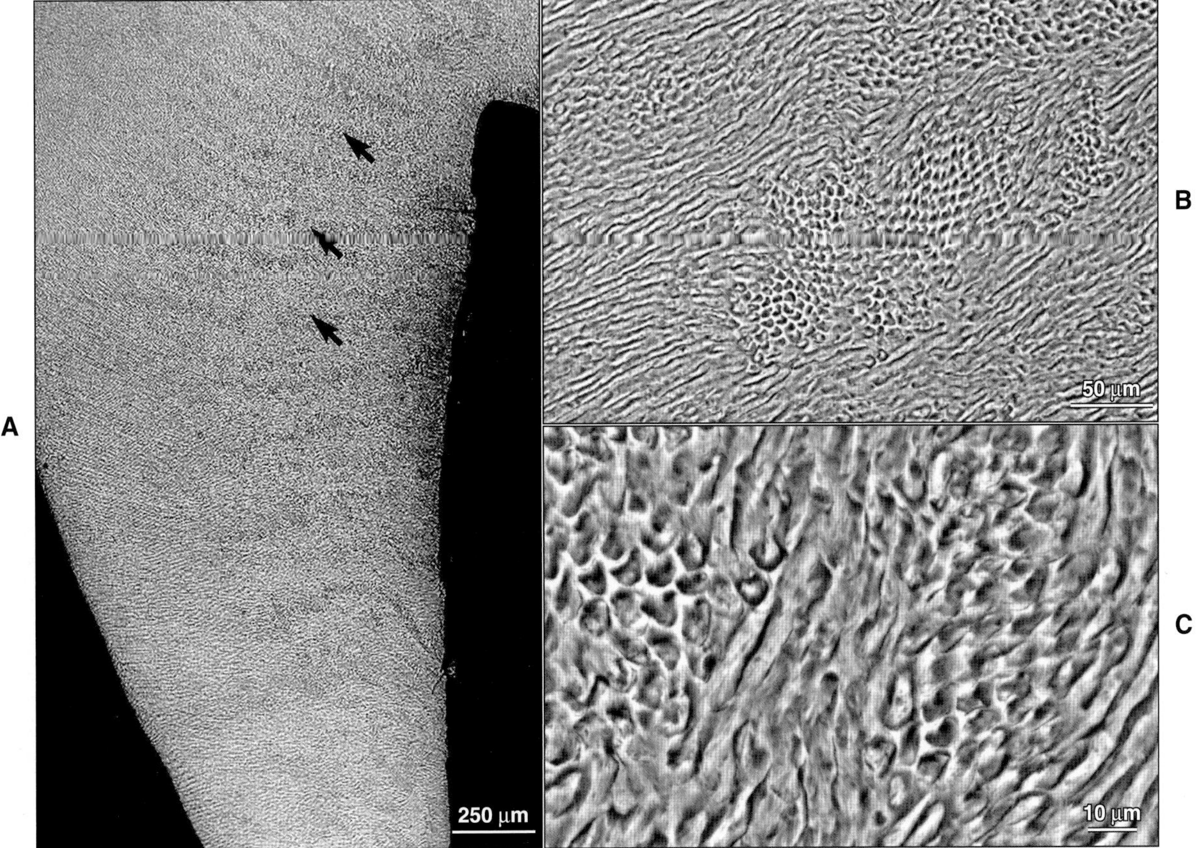

Fig. 7.55 Scanning electron imaging at increasing magnification (A–C) showing alternating changes in groups of rods *(arrows)* in the inner two-thirds of the enamel layer and which corresponds to the Hunter and Schreger bands seen in light microscopy (see Fig. 7.54).

The scanning electron microscope reveals the junction to be a series of ridges rather than spikes, an arrangement that probably increases the adherence between dentin and enamel (see Fig. 7.37A); in this regard, it is worth noting that the ridging is most pronounced in coronal dentin where occlusal stresses are the greatest (Fig. 7.57C). The shape and nature of the junction prevent shearing of the enamel during function.

Enamel Surface

The surface of enamel is characterized by several structures. The striae of Retzius often extend from the dentinoenamel junction to the outer surface of enamel, where they end in shallow furrows known as *perikymata* (Figs. 7.60, 7.61, and 7.62). Perikymata run in circumferentially horizontal lines across the face of the crown. In addition, lamellae or cracks in the enamel appear as jagged lines in various regions of the tooth surface. The surface structure of enamel varies with age. In unerupted teeth, the enamel surface consists of a structureless surface layer (final enamel) that is lost rapidly by abrasion, attrition, and erosion in erupted teeth. As the tooth erupts, it is covered by a pellicle consisting of debris from the enamel organ that is lost rapidly. A salivary pellicle, a nearly ubiquitous organic deposit on the surface of teeth, always reappears shortly after teeth have been polished mechanically. Dental plaque forms readily on the pellicle especially in more protected areas of the dentition.

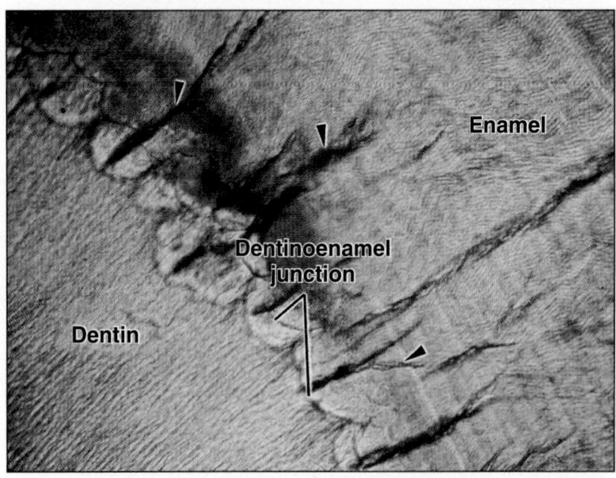

Fig. 7.56 Transverse ground section of enamel. Enamel tufts are the branched structures extending from the dentinoenamel junction into the enamel *(arrowheads)*. The junction is seen as a scalloped profile.

AGE CHANGES

Enamel is a nonvital tissue that is incapable of regeneration. With age, enamel becomes progressively worn in regions of masticatory attrition. Wear facets increasingly are pronounced in older persons, and, in some cases, substantial portions of the crown (enamel and dentin) become eroded. Other characteristics of aging enamel include discoloration, reduced permeability, and modifications in the surface layer. Linked to these changes is an apparent reduction in the incidence of caries.

Teeth darken with age. Whether this darkening is caused by a change in the structure of enamel is debatable. Although darkening could be caused by the addition of organic material to enamel from the environment, darkening also may be caused by a deepening of dentin color (the layer becomes thicker with age) seen through the progressively thinning layer of translucent enamel.

No doubt exists that enamel becomes less permeable with age. Young enamel behaves as a semipermeable membrane, permitting the slow passage of water and substances of small molecular size through pores between the crystals. With age the pores diminish as the crystals acquire more ions and as the surface increases in size.

The surface layer of enamel reflects most prominently the changes within this tissue. During aging, the composition of the surface layer changes as ionic exchange with the oral environment occurs. In particular, a progressive increase in the fluoride content affects the surface layer (and that, incidentally, can be achieved by topical application).

DEFECTS OF AMELOGENESIS

Amelogenesis imperfecta is a group of inherited defects causing disruption to the structure and clinical appearance of tooth enamel (Fig. 7.63). The phenotypic classification of amelogenesis imperfecta reflects the stage of enamel formation during which the problem occurs, giving rise to hypoplastic, hypocalcified, or hypomature defective enamel. An

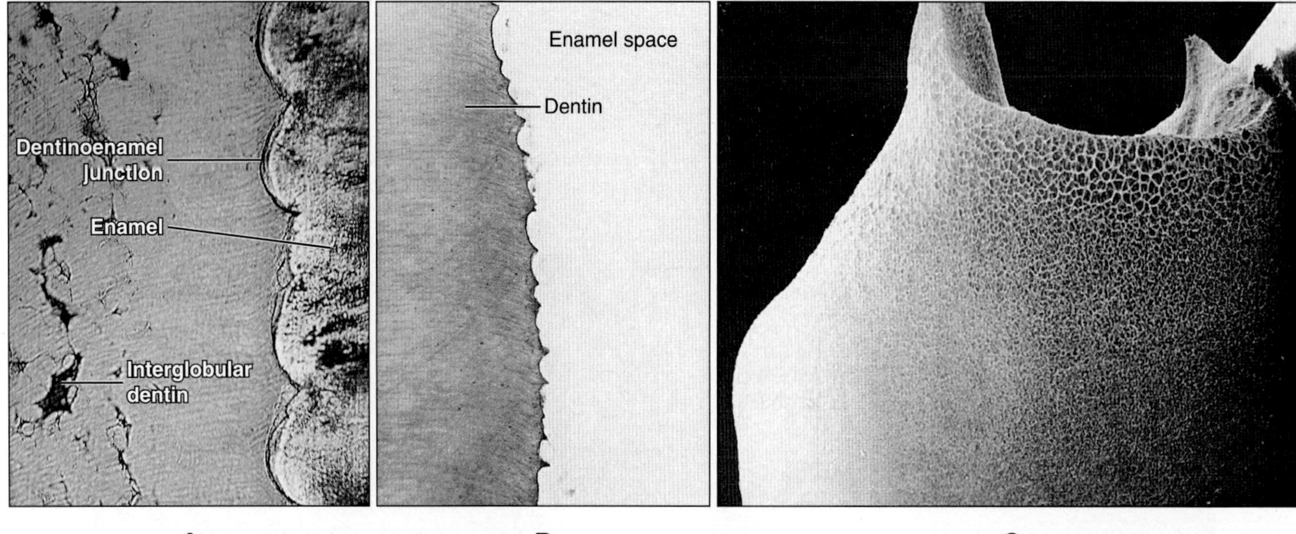

Fig. 7.57 Dentinoenamel junction. (A) Ground section. (B) Demineralized section after the enamel has been lost. The scalloped nature of the junction when seen in one plane is striking. (C) A low-power scanning electron micrograph of a premolar from which the enamel has been removed shows that the scalloping is accentuated where the junction is subjected to most functional stress. (C, Courtesy W.H. Douglas.)

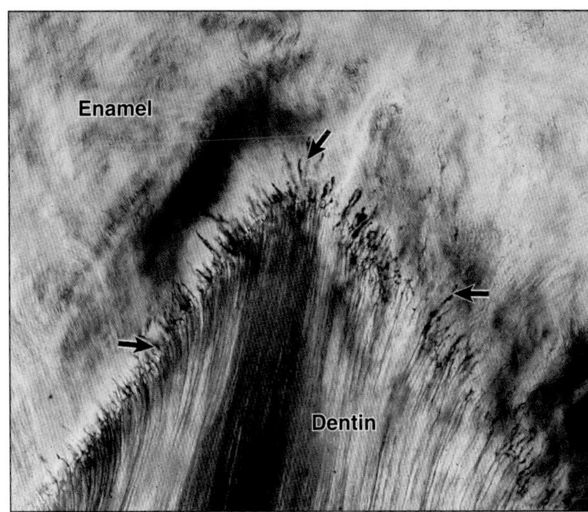

Fig. 7.58 Enamel spindles *(arrows)* in a ground section extend from the dentinoenamel junction into the enamel and most commonly are found at cusp tips.

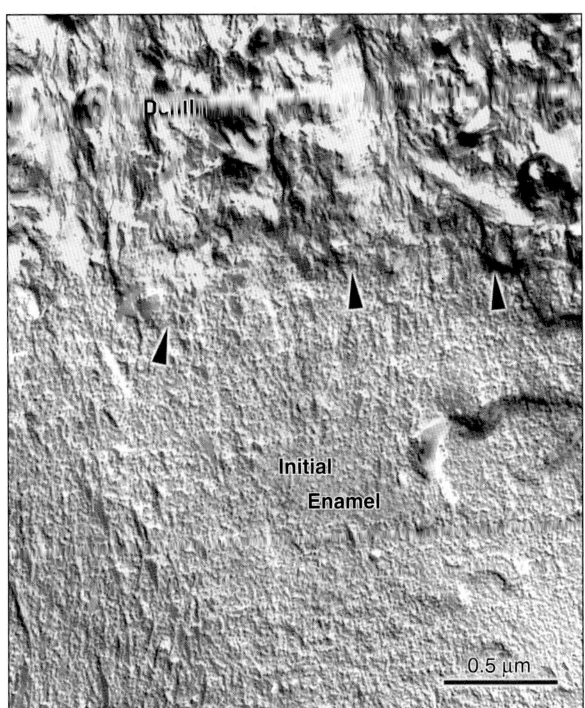

Fig. 7.59 Freeze-fracture preparation at the dentinoenamel junction *(arrowheads)*. The distinctive appearance of the collagenous dentin and noncollagenous (initial) enamel layer is notable.

X-linked, autosomal dominant form (one copy of the gene altered) and an autosomal recessive form (both copies of the gene altered) of the disease have been described. Mutations in various genes, including amelogenin (AMEL) X-linked, enamelin (ENAM), distal-less homeobox 3 (DLX3), family with sequence similarity 83 member H (FAM83H), Mmp20, Klk4, and WD repeat domain 72, have been associated with amelogenesis imperfecta. Not all cases can be accounted by these mutations, suggesting that other genes may contribute to its pathogenesis. Recently it has been shown that deletion of ameloblastin exon 6 and of amelotin exons 3 to 6 cause nonsyndromic human amelogenesis imperfecta.

In addition to this genetic dysplasia, many other conditions produce defects in enamel structure. Such defects occur because ameloblasts are particularly sensitive to changes in their environment. Even minor physiologic changes affect them and elicit changes in enamel structure that can be seen only histologically. More severe insults greatly disturb enamel production or produce death of the ameloblasts, and the resulting defects are easily visible clinically.

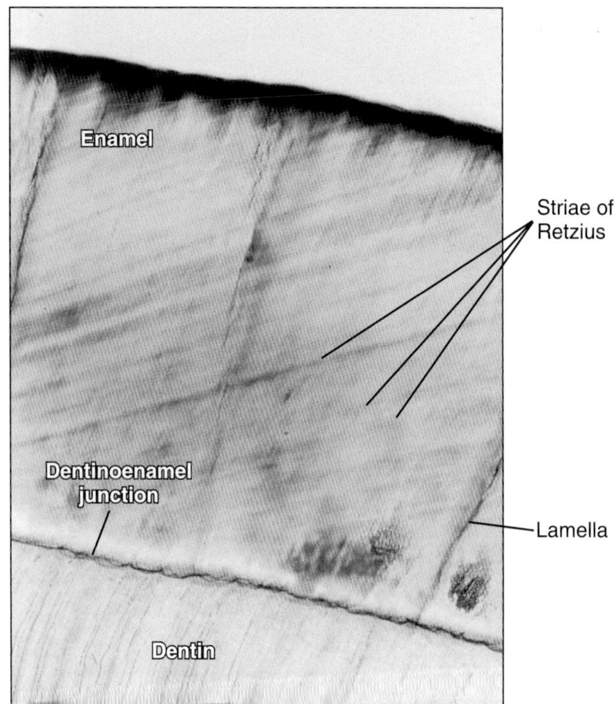

Fig. 7.60 Ground section of enamel showing striae of Retzius and lamellae.

Three conditions affecting enamel formation occur frequently. Defects in enamel can be caused by febrile diseases. During the course of such a disease, enamel formation is disturbed so that all teeth forming at the time become characterized by distinctive bands of malformed enamel. On recovery, normal enamel formation is resumed (Fig. 7.64).

Second, defects can be formed by tetracycline-induced disturbances in teeth. Tetracycline antibiotics are incorporated into mineralizing tissues; in the case of enamel, this incorporation may result in a band of brown pigmentation or even total pigmentation. Hypoplasia or absence of enamel also may occur. The degree of damage is determined by the magnitude and duration of tetracycline therapy.

Finally, the fluoride ion can interfere with amelogenesis (Fig. 7.65). Chronic ingestion of fluoride ion concentrations in excess of 5 ppm (five times the amount in fluoridated water supplies) interferes sufficiently with ameloblast function to produce mottled enamel. Mottled enamel is unsightly and often is seen as white patches of hypomineralized and altered enamel. Such enamel, though unsightly, still resists caries.

CLINICAL IMPLICATIONS

An appreciation of the histology of enamel is important for understanding the principles of fluoridation, acid-etching techniques, and dental caries.

Fluoridation

If the fluoride ion is incorporated into or adsorbed on the hydroxyapatite crystal, the crystal becomes more resistant to acid dissolution. This reaction partly explains the role of fluoride in caries prevention

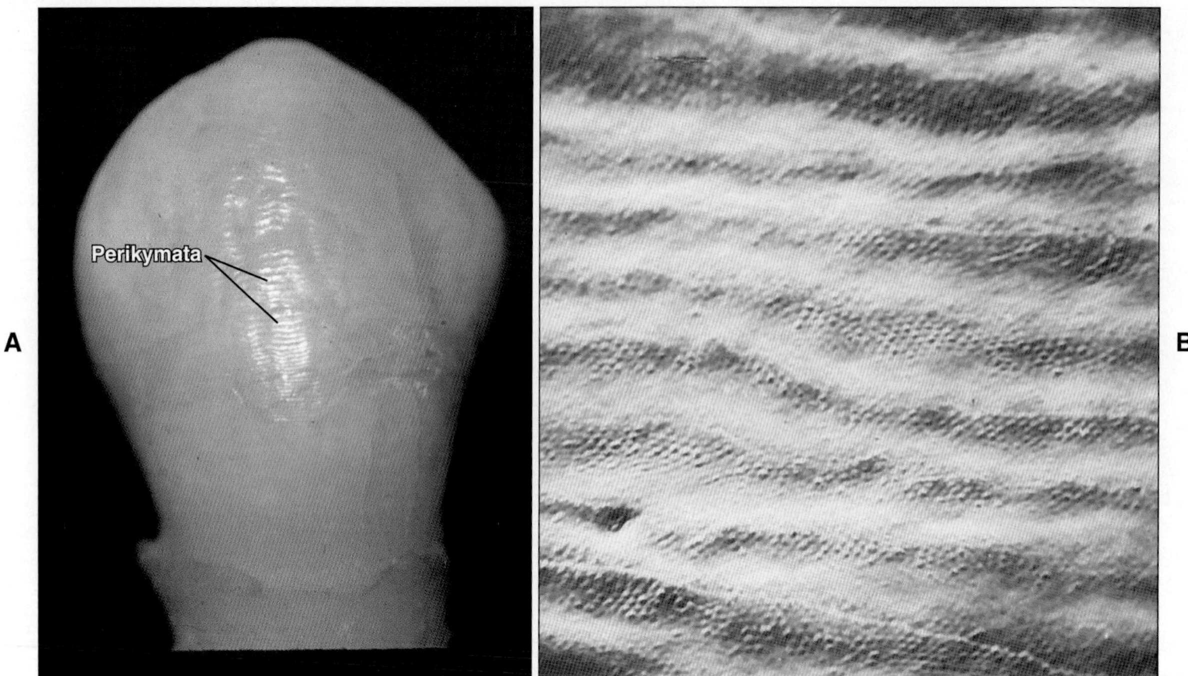

Fig. 7.61 (A) Micrograph illustrating perikymata on the surface of a tooth. (B) Scanning electron micrograph of the labial surface of a tooth, showing the perikymata. (Courtesy D. Weber.)

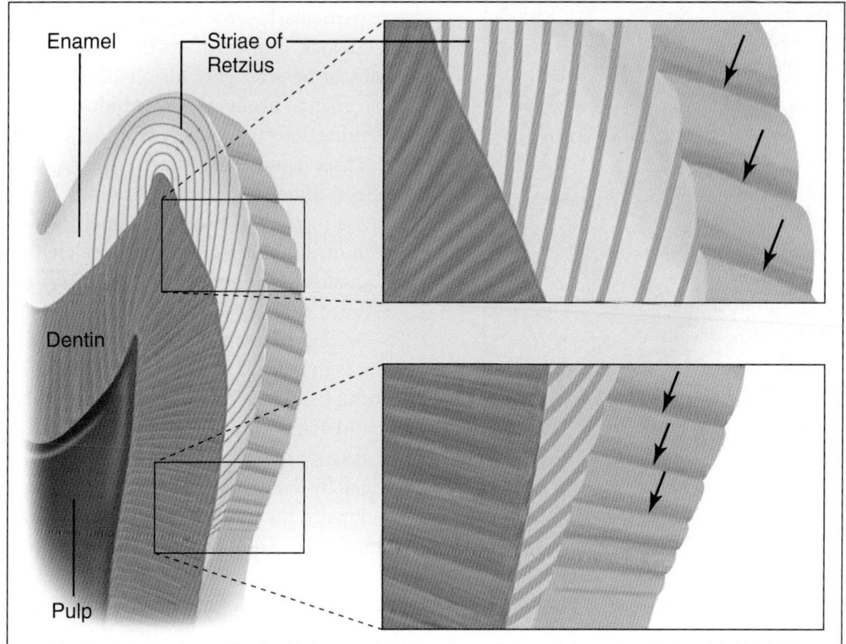

Fig. 7.62 The relationship between the striae of Retzius and surface perikymata *(arrows)*. (From Fejerskov O, Thylstrup A: Dental enamel. In Mjör I, Fejerskov O, editors: *Human oral embryology and histology*, Copenhagen, Denmark, 1986, Munksgaard.)

because the caries process is initiated by demineralization of enamel. Obviously, if fluoride is present as enamel is being formed, all the enamel crystals will be more resistant to acid dissolution. The amount of fluoride must be controlled carefully, however, because of the sensitivity of ameloblasts to the fluoride ion and the possibility of producing unsightly mottling. The semipermeable nature of enamel enables topical application to provide a higher concentration of fluoride in the surface enamel of erupted teeth.

The presence of fluoride enhances chemical reactions that lead to the precipitation of calcium phosphate. An equilibrium exists in the oral cavity between calcium and phosphate ions in the solution phase (saliva) and in the solid phase (enamel), and fluoride shifts this equilibrium to favor the solid phase. Clinically, when a localized region of enamel has lost mineral (e.g., a white spot lesion), the enamel may be remineralized if the destructive agent (dental plaque) is removed. The remineralization reaction is enhanced greatly by fluoride.

A

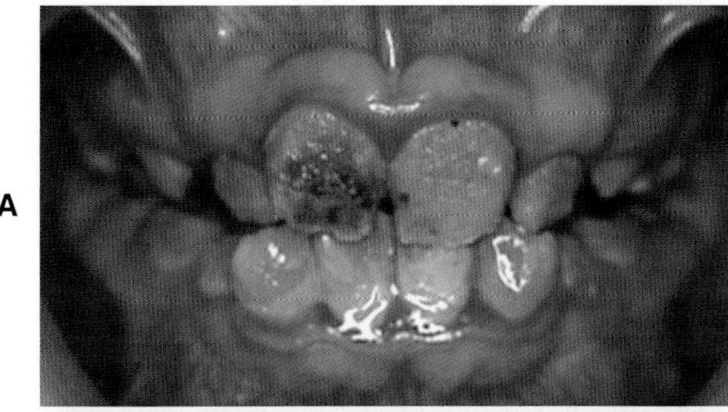

B

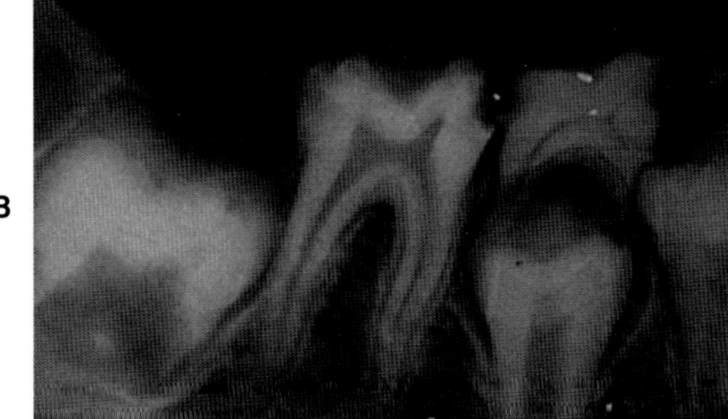

Fig. 7.63 (A) Oral photograph of the appearance of teeth in an individual affected by X-linked amelogenesis imperfecta resulting from amelogenin X-linked mutations. Note the severe hypomineralization with altered color of the enamel. (B) The intraoral x-ray shows the absence or the presence of a very thin enamel layer in erupted teeth. The enamel layer in unerupted teeth shows reduced opacity, making it difficult to distinguish from dentin. (Courtesy M. Schmittbuhl.)

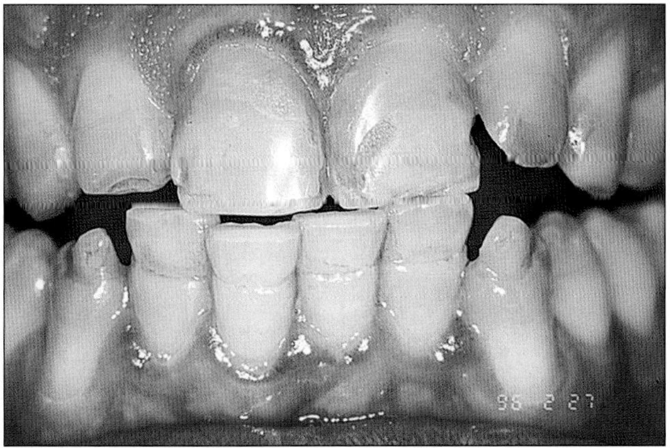

Fig. 7.64 Endogenous developmental stain from a febrile illness. The zone of defective and normal enamel can be readily distinguished. (Courtesy Dr. G. Taybos.)

Acid Etching

Acid etching of the enamel surface (enamel conditioning) has become an important technique in clinical practice. Use of fissure sealants, bonding of restorative materials to enamel, and cementing of orthodontic brackets to tooth surfaces involve acid etching. The process achieves the desired effect in two stages. First, acid etching removes plaque and other debris, along with a thin layer of enamel; second, it increases the porosity of exposed surfaces through selective dissolution of crystals, which provides a better bonding surface for the restorative and adhesive materials.

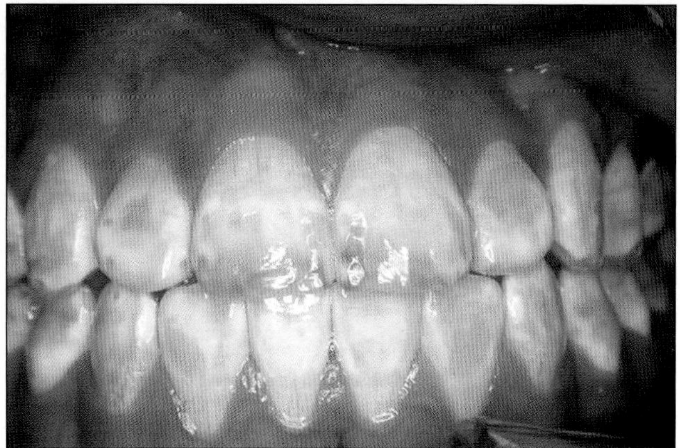

Fig. 7.65 This patient had a moderate level of fluorosis in all teeth, leading to poor aesthetics. (Courtesy Professor E.C. Reynolds.)

Scanning electron microscopy demonstrates the effects of acid etching on enamel surfaces. Three etching patterns predominate (Fig. 7.66) although this can vary substantially with position, age, and degree of surface change such as fluoride incorporation. The most common is type I, characterized by preferential removal of rods. In the reverse, type II, interrod enamel is removed preferentially, and the rod remains intact. Occurring less frequently is type III, which is irregular and indiscriminate. Some debate still occurs as to why acid etchants produce differing surface patterns. The most held view is that the etching pattern depends on crystal orientation. Ultrastructural studies of crystal dissolution indicate that crystals dissolve more readily at their ends than on their sides. Thus crystals lying perpendicular to the enamel surface are the most vulnerable. The type I and II etching patterns can be explained easily by noting that crystals reach the enamel surfaces at differing inclinations in the rods compared with the interrod areas (Fig. 7.67).

Acid conditioning of enamel surfaces is now an accepted procedure for obtaining improved bonding of resins to enamel. Retention depends mainly on a mechanical interlocking. The conditioning agent removes the organic film from the tooth surface and preferentially etches the enamel surface so that firmer contact is established. In areas with rodless enamel, especially in deciduous teeth, slightly more severe etching is required to obtain adequate mechanical retention.

In summary, the process of amelogenesis involves cells that secrete enamel proteins, which immediately participate in mineralizing enamel to approximately 30%. When the entire thickness of enamel has been formed and structured, it then acquires a significant amount of additional mineral coincident with the bulk removal of enamel proteins and water to yield a unique layer consisting of more than 95% mineral. This complicated process is under cellular control, and the associated cells undergo significant morphologic changes throughout amelogenesis, reflecting their evolving physiologic activity. In particular, completion of mineralization is characterized by modulation, a process whereby ameloblasts cyclically alternate their appearance several times so that matrix removal and crystal growth can go on efficiently within the secluded enamel space. One intriguing question is how formation and maturation fields are maintained in a forming tooth until development is advanced enough that these two processes are now temporally separated (i.e., the entire tooth crown is in maturation). A better understanding of the cellular events taking place during amelogenesis, the nanoscale processes involved in creating long enamel crystals, and in structuring them is ultimately expected to lead to the development of biomimetic approaches for the rebuilding of enamel.

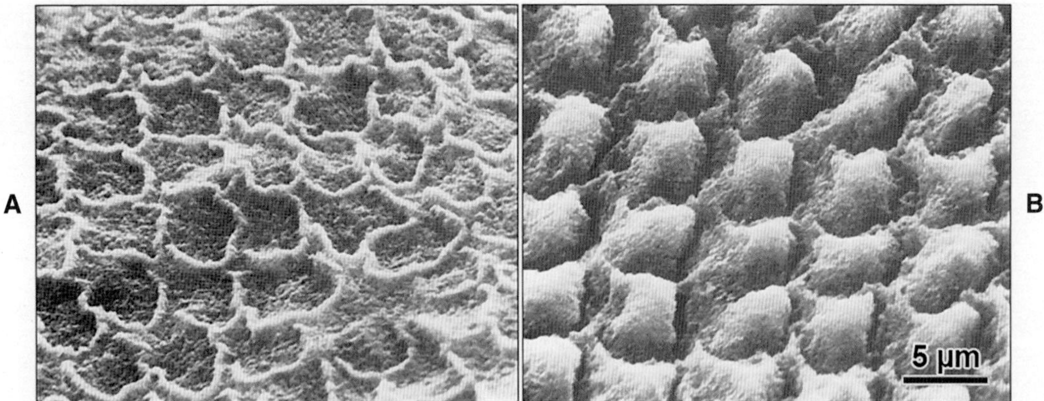

Fig. 7.66 Scanning electron micrographs of etching patterns in enamel. (A) Type I pattern: rod preferentially eroded. (B) Type II pattern: rod boundary (interrod) preferentially eroded. (Courtesy L. Silverstone.)

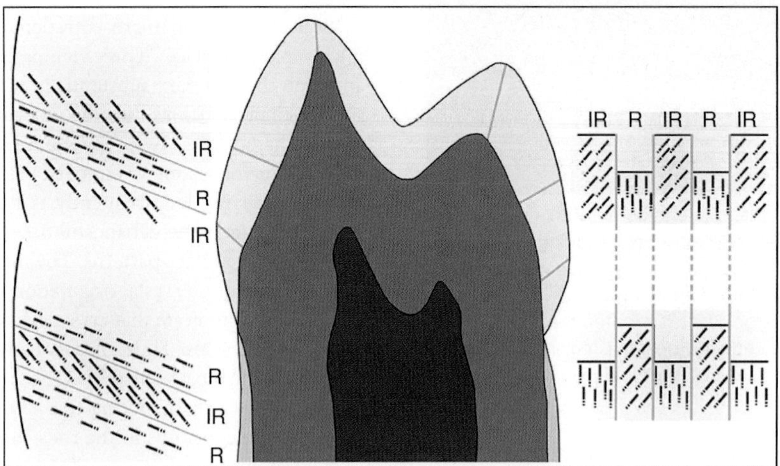

Fig. 7.67 Diagrammatic representation of how the difference in general orientation of rod *(R)* and interrod *(IR)* crystals will result in the different etching topographies illustrated in Fig. 7.66A and B. Crystals are more susceptible to dissolution at their extremities than along their sides, such that the ones arriving perpendicular to the surface will be more affected.

RECOMMENDED READING

Bartlett JD, Simmer JP: New perspectives on amelotin and amelogenesis, *J Dent Res* 94:642–644, 2015.

Bartlett JD, et al.: Protein-protein interactions of the developing enamel matrix, *Curr Top Dev Biol* 74:57–115, 2006.

Bonucci E: Understanding nanocalcification: a role suggested for crystal ghosts, *Mar Drugs* 12(7):4231–4246, 2014, https://doi.org/10.3390/md12074231.

Bronckers ALJJ: Ion transport by ameloblasts during amelogenesis, *J Dent Res* 96:243–253, 2017.

Nanci A, Smith CE: Matrix-mediated mineralization in enamel and the collagen-based hard tissues. In Goldberg M, et al., editors: *Chemistry and biology of mineralized tissues*, Rosemont, IL, 1999, American Academy of Orthopedic Surgeons.

8

Dentin-Pulp Complex

Antonio Nanci

OUTLINE

BASIC STRUCTURE OF DENTIN

Dentin is the hard tissue portion of the pulp-dentin complex and forms the bulk of the tooth (Fig. 8.1). Dentin is a bonelike matrix characterized by multiple closely packed dentinal tubules that traverse its entire thickness and contain the cytoplasmic extensions of odontoblasts that once formed the dentin and thereafter maintained it. The cell bodies of the odontoblasts are aligned along the inner aspect of the dentin, against a layer of predentin, where they also form the peripheral boundary of the dental pulp.

The dental pulp is the soft connective tissue that occupies the central portion of the tooth. The space it occupies is the pulp cavity, which is divided into a coronal portion (or pulp chamber) and a radicular portion (the root canal). The pulp chamber conforms to the general shape of the anatomic crown. Under the cusps the chamber extends into pulp horns, which are especially prominent under the buccal cusp of premolar teeth and the mesiobuccal cusp of molar teeth. Their cusps are particularly significant in dental restoration where care must be taken to prevent exposure of pulp tissue.

The root canal (or *root canal system* as it is called in multirooted teeth) terminates at the apical foramen where the pulp and periodontal ligament meet and the main nerves and vessels enter and leave the tooth. In the developing tooth the apical foramen is wide and centrally located (Fig. 8.2). As the tooth completes its development, the apical foramen becomes smaller in diameter and more eccentric in position. Sizes from 0.3 to 0.6 μm, with the larger diameter occurring in the palatal root of maxillary molars and the distal root of mandibular molars, are typical of the completed foramen. The foramen may be located at the very end (anatomic apex) of the root, but it usually is located slightly more occlusally from the apex. If more than one foramen is present on a root, the largest is designated the apical foramen and the others the accessory foramina.

Connections between the pulp and the periodontal tissues also may occur along the lateral surface of the root through the lateral canals. Such canals, which may contain blood vessels, are not present in all teeth and occur with differing frequencies in different types of teeth. Because the apical foramen and the lateral canals are areas of communication between the pulp space and the periodontium, they can act as avenues for the extension of disease from one tissue to the other. Hence diseases of the dental pulp can produce changes in the periodontal tissues. More rarely do diseases of the periodontium involve the dental pulp.

COMPOSITION, FORMATION, AND STRUCTURE OF DENTIN

Dentin is first deposited as a layer of unmineralized matrix (predentin) that varies in thickness (10–50 μm) and lines its innermost (pulpal) portion. Predentin consists principally of collagen and is similar to osteoid in bone; it is easy to identify in histologic sections because it stains less intensely than mineralized dentin (Fig. 8.3). Predentin gradually mineralizes into dentin as various noncollagenous matrix proteins are incorporated at the mineralization front. The thickness

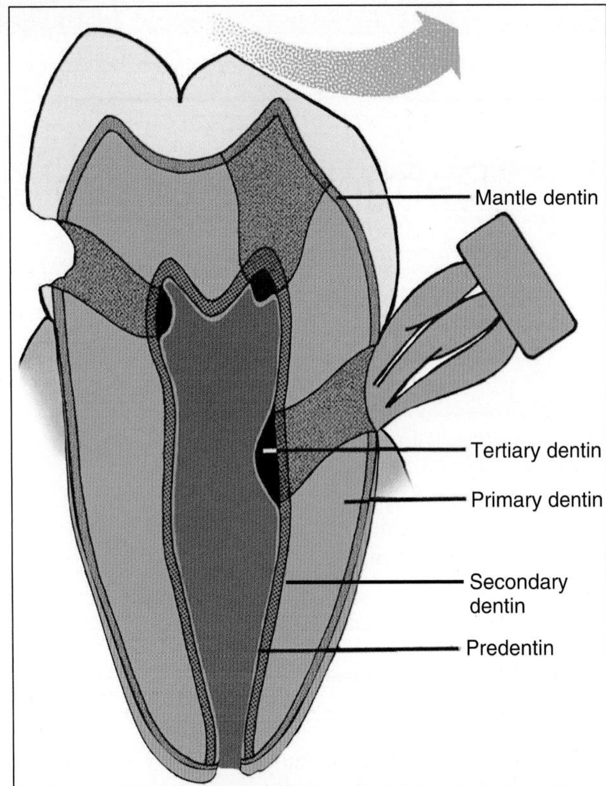

Fig. 8.1 Dentin types and distribution.

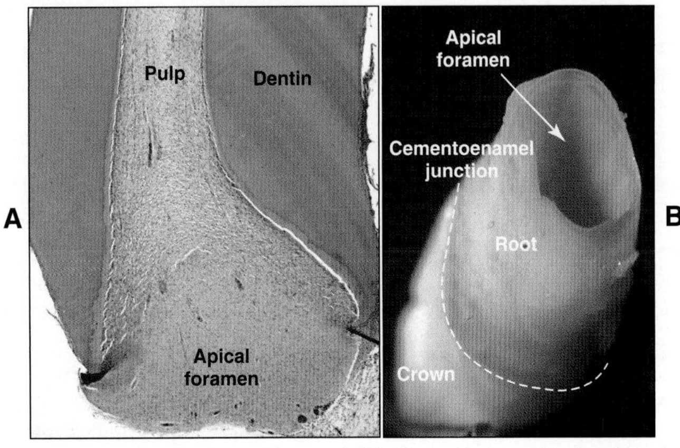

Fig. 8.2 (A) Histologic section and (B) photomicrograph showing the widely open apical foramen in developing teeth.

of predentin remains constant because the amount that calcifies is balanced by the addition of new unmineralized matrix. Predentin is thickest at times when active dentinogenesis is occurring and diminishes in thickness with age.

Mature dentin is made up of approximately 70% inorganic material, 20% organic material, and 10% water. The inorganic component of dentin consists of substituted hydroxyapatite in the form of small plates. The organic phase is about 90% collagen (mainly type I with small amounts of types III and V) with fractional inclusions of various noncollagenous matrix proteins and lipids. Although studies have for a long time focused on identifying proteins specific to bone or dentin, it is now clear that bone matrix proteins can be found in dentin and that dentin matrix proteins also are present in bone (see Table 1.1).

The noncollagenous matrix proteins pack the space between collagen fibrils and accumulate along the periphery of dentinal tubules.

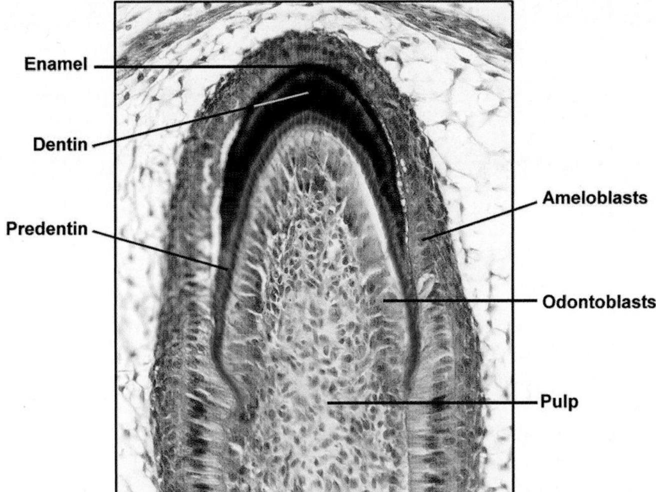

Fig. 8.3 In histologic sections, predentin stains distinctively from dentin.

These proteins comprise the following: dentin phosphoprotein/phosphophorin (DPP), dentin sialoprotein (DSP), dentin glycoprotein (DGP), dentin matrix protein 1 (DMP1), osteonectin (also known as *secreted protein acidic and rich in cysteine [SPARC]* osteocalcin, bone sialoprotein (BSP), osteopontin, matrix extracellular phosphoglycoprotein, proteoglycans, and some serum proteins. DPP, DSP, and DGP are expressed at the gene level as a single molecule called *dentin sialophosphoprotein (DSPP)* that is then processed into individual components with distinct physicochemical properties. DSPP-derived proteins are highly modified after their translation. DPP and DSP represent the major noncollagenous matrix proteins in dentin. DPP is the C-terminal proteolytic cleavage product of DSPP, DSP is the N-terminal one, and DGP lies in the middle of the molecule. As stated in Chapter 7, differentiating odontoblasts also appear to produce, for a short period, enamel proteins such as amelogenin. Reciprocally, differentiating ameloblasts also are believed to transiently produce some dentin proteins.

Collagen type I acts as a scaffold that accommodates a large proportion (estimated at 56%) of the mineral in the holes and pores of fibrils. See Chapter 1 for the participation of noncollagenous matrix proteins in mineralization of collagen fibrils. The noncollagenous matrix proteins regulate mineral deposition and can act as inhibitors, promoters, and/or stabilizers; their distribution is suggestive of their role. For instance, intact proteoglycans appear to be more concentrated in predentin and thus are believed to prevent the premature mineralization of the organic matrix whereas collagen fibrils mature and attain the correct dimension. DPP is an unusual phosphoprotein. It has an isoelectric point of 1 and has numerous aspartic acid-serine-serine residues, and many of its serine residues are phosphorylated. Having a high negative charge, DPP binds large amounts of calcium. In vitro studies show that DPP binds to collagen and is able to initiate hydroxyapatite formation. DSP and DMP1 are predominantly immunodetected in peritubular dentin (see later) where they may inhibit its growth and thus prevent occlusion of the tubule. In addition to their codistribution, DSP and DMP1 exhibit similarities in biochemical features, they thus may have redundant or synergistic functions. DSPP mutations result in a variety of dental phenotypes, including dentin dysplasia and dentinogenesis imperfecta, that affect both the primary and permanent dentition. There are three types of dentinogenesis imperfecta; type I is also associated with osteogenesis imperfecta. In both types I and II, the pulp chamber is no longer visible because of abnormal dentin deposits (Fig. 8.4). Mice that do not express DSPP or DMP1 show enlarged pulp

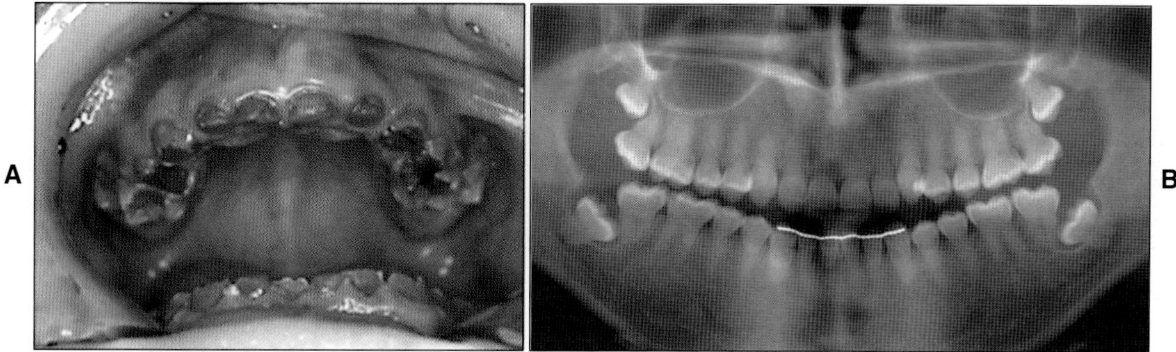

Fig. 8.4 Intraoral photograph (A) and panoramic x-ray (B) of a dentition with dentinogenesis imperfecta type II, an autosomal-dominant genetic defect. Note that the pulp chamber appears opalescent because it has been filled with defective dentin. (Courtesy M. Schmittbuhl.)

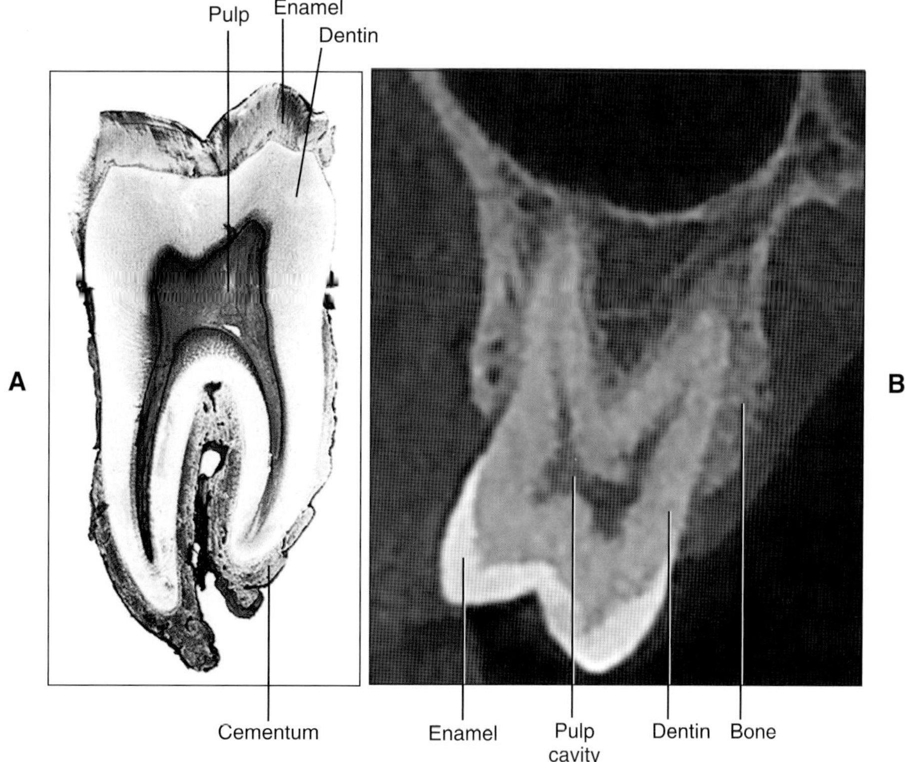

Fig. 8.5 Differential deposition of dentin results in an asymmetric reduction of the pulp chamber, referred to as *pulp recession*, as seen in (A), a specially prepared thick (100-μm) section in which both the hard and soft tissue have been retained and (B) x-ray radiograph.

chambers (as seen in type III dentinogenesis imperfecta), an increase in the thickness of predentin, and hypomineralization, indicating additional functions to the control of peritubular dentin. Noteworthy, DSPP and DMP1 are present in bone and dentin as processed fragments and absence of DMP1 has profound effects on bone.

Dentin is slightly harder than bone and softer than enamel. This difference can be distinguished readily on radiographs on which the dentin appears more radiolucent (darker) than enamel and slightly more radiopaque (lighter) than bone (Fig. 8.5B). Because light can pass readily through the thin, highly mineralized enamel and can be reflected by the underlying yellowish dentin, the crown of a tooth also assumes such coloration. The thicker enamel does not permit light to pass through as readily, and in such teeth the crown appears whiter. Teeth with pulp disease or without a dental pulp often show discoloration of the dentin, which causes a darkening of the clinical crown.

Physically, dentin has an elastic quality that is important for the proper functioning of the tooth because the elasticity provides flexibility and prevents fracture of the overlying brittle enamel. Dentin and enamel are bound firmly at the dentinoenamel junction that appears microscopically, as seen in the previous chapter, as a well-defined scalloped border (see Fig. 7.57). In the root of the tooth, the dentin is covered by cementum, and the junction between these two tissues is less distinct because, in humans, they intermingle.

TYPES OF DENTIN

Primary Dentin

Most of the tooth is formed by primary dentin, which outlines the pulp chamber and is referred to as *circumpulpal dentin* (see Fig. 8.1). The outer layer, near enamel or cementum, differs from the

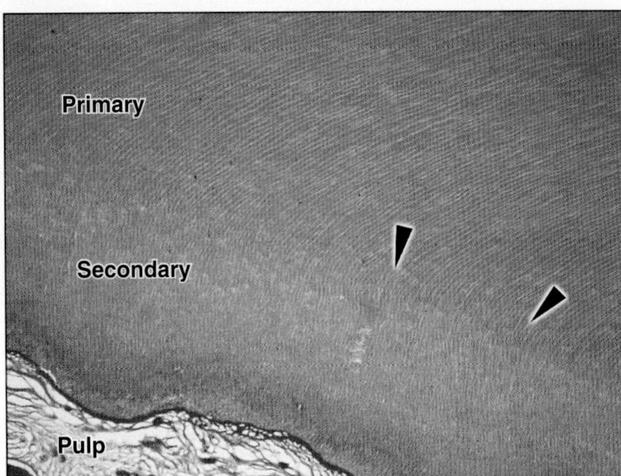

Fig. 8.6 Section of dentin. The region where dentinal tubules change direction *(arrowheads)* delimits the junction between primary and secondary dentin.

rest of the primary dentin in the way it is mineralized and in the structural interrelation between the collagenous and noncollagenous matrix components. This outer layer is generally referred to as *mantle dentin* in coronal dentin.

Secondary Dentin

Secondary dentin develops after root formation has been completed and represents the continuing but much slower deposition of dentin by odontoblasts (Fig. 8.6). Secondary dentin has a tubular structure that, although less regular, is mostly continuous with that of the primary dentin. The ratio of mineral to organic material is the same as for primary dentin. Secondary dentin is not deposited evenly around the periphery of the pulp chamber, especially in the molar teeth. The greater deposition of secondary dentin on the roof and floor of the chamber leads to an asymmetric reduction in its size and shape (see Fig. 8.5A). These changes in the pulp space, clinically referred to as *pulp recession*, can be detected readily on histologic sections and radiographs (see Fig. 8.5B) and are important in determining the form of cavity preparation for certain dental restorative procedures. For example, preparation of the tooth for a full crown in a young patient presents a substantial risk of involving the dental pulp by mechanically exposing a pulp horn. In an older patient, the pulp horn has receded and presents less danger. Some evidence suggests that the tubules of secondary dentin sclerose (fill with calcified material) more readily than those of primary dentin. This process tends to reduce the overall permeability of the dentin, thereby protecting the pulp.

Tertiary Dentin

Tertiary dentin (also referred to as *reactive* or *reparative dentin*) is produced in reaction to various stimuli, such as attrition, caries, or a restorative dental procedure. Unlike primary or secondary dentin that forms along the entire pulp-dentin border, tertiary dentin is produced only by those cells directly affected by the stimulus. The quality (or architecture) and the quantity of tertiary dentin produced are related to the cellular response initiated, which depends on the intensity and duration of the stimulus. Tertiary dentin may have tubules continuous with those of secondary dentin (Fig. 8.7), tubules sparse in number and irregularly arranged (Fig. 8.8), or no tubules at all. The cells forming tertiary dentin line its surface or may become included in the dentin; the latter case is referred to as *osteodentin* (Fig. 8.8). Tertiary dentin is subclassified as reactionary dentin

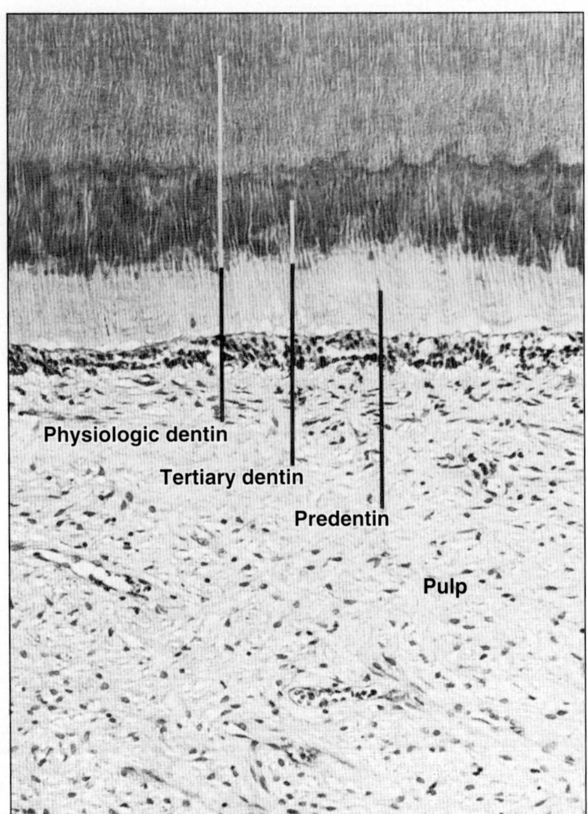

Fig. 8.7 Tertiary dentin with a regular tubular pattern and no cellular inclusions. This dentin probably was deposited slowly in response to a mild stimulus.

deposited by preexisting odontoblasts or reparative dentin formed by newly differentiated odontoblast-like cells.

PATTERN OF DENTIN FORMATION

Dentin formation begins at the bell stage of tooth development in the papillary tissue adjacent to the concave tip of the folded inner enamel epithelium (Fig. 8.9), the site where cuspal development begins. From that point, dentin formation spreads down the cusp slope as far as the cervical loop of the enamel organ, and the dentin thickens until all the coronal dentin is formed. In multicusped teeth, dentin formation begins independently at the sites of each future cusp tip and again spreads down the flanks of the cusp slopes until fusion with adjacent formative centers occurs. Dentin thus formed constitutes the dentin of the crown of the tooth (coronal dentin).

Root dentin forms at a slightly later stage of development and requires the proliferation of epithelial cells (Hertwig epithelial root sheath) from the cervical loop of the enamel organ around the growing pulp to initiate the differentiation of root odontoblasts (see Chapter 5). The onset of root formation precedes the onset of tooth eruption, and by the time the tooth reaches its functional position, about two-thirds of the root dentin will have been formed. Completion of root dentin formation does not occur in the deciduous tooth until about 18 months after it erupts and in the permanent tooth until 2 to 3 years after it erupts. During this period the tooth is said to have an open apex (see Fig. 8.2).

Rates of dentin deposition vary not only within a single tooth but also among different teeth. Dentin formation continues throughout the life of the tooth, and its formation results in a gradual but progressive reduction in the size of the pulp cavity.

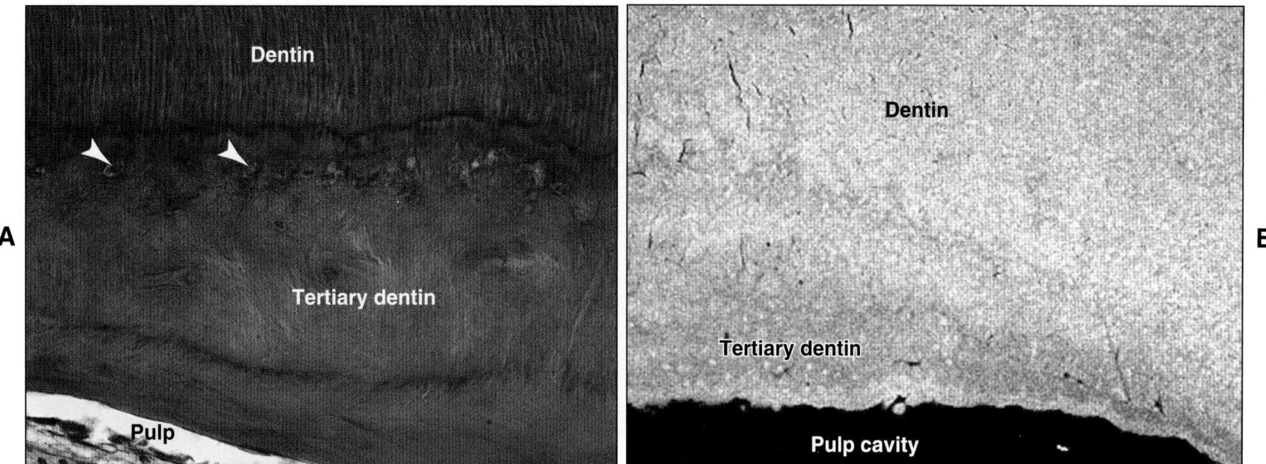

Fig. 8.8 Light (A) and scanning electron (B) micrographs of tertiary (reparative) dentin containing only a few sparse irregular tubules and some cellular inclusions *(arrowheads)*.

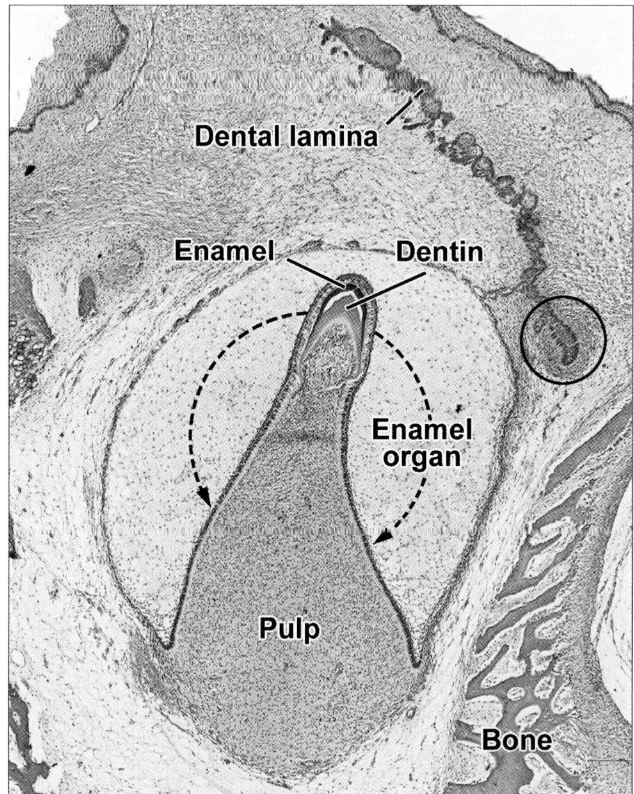

Fig. 8.9 Initial dentin formation during the early bell stage of tooth development. From the apex of the tooth, dentin formation spreads down the slopes of the cusp. The circled structure represents a permanent tooth bud.

DENTINOGENESIS

Dentin is formed by cells called *odontoblasts* that differentiate from ectomesenchymal cells of the dental papilla after an organizing influence that emanates from the inner enamel epithelium. Thus the dental papilla is the formative organ of dentin and eventually becomes the pulp of the tooth, a change in terminology generally associated with the moment dentin formation begins.

Odontoblast Differentiation

A detailed understanding of how odontoblasts differentiate from ectomesenchymal cells is necessary not only to understand normal development, but also to explain and eventually be able to influence their recruitment when required to initiate repair of dentin.

The differentiation of odontoblasts from the dental papilla in normal development is brought about by the expression of signaling molecules and growth factors in the cells of the inner enamel epithelium (see Chapter 5). Their differentiation sequence is illustrated in Figs. 8.10 and 8.11. The dental papilla cells are small and undifferentiated, and they exhibit a central nucleus and few organelles. At this time they are separated from the inner enamel epithelium by an acellular zone that contains some fine collagen fibrils. Almost immediately after cells of the inner enamel epithelium reverse polarity, changes also occur in the adjacent dental papilla. The ectomesenchymal cells adjoining the acellular zone rapidly enlarge and elongate to become preodontoblasts first and then odontoblasts as their cytoplasm increases in volume to contain increasing amounts of protein-synthesizing organelles. The acellular zone between the dental papilla and the inner enamel epithelium is gradually eliminated as the odontoblasts differentiate and increase in size and occupy this zone. These newly differentiated cells are characterized by being highly polarized, with their nuclei positioned away from the inner enamel epithelium.

Formation of Mantle Dentin

After the differentiation of odontoblasts, the next step in the production of dentin is formation of its organic matrix. The first sign of dentin formation is the appearance of distinct, large-diameter collagen fibrils (0.1–0.2 μm in diameter) called von Korff fibers (Figs. 8.12–8.15). These fibers consist of collagen type III associated, at least initially, with fibronectin. These fibers originate deep among the odontoblasts, extend toward the inner enamel epithelium, and fan out in the structureless ground substance immediately below the epithelium. As the odontoblasts continue to increase in size, they also produce smaller collagen type I fibrils that orient themselves parallel to the future dentinoenamel junction (Fig. 8.16). In this way, a layer of mantle predentin appears.

Coincident with this deposition of collagen, the plasma membrane of odontoblasts adjacent to the differentiating ameloblasts extends stubby processes into the forming extracellular matrix (Fig. 8.17). On occasion, one of these processes may penetrate the basal lamina and interpose itself between the cells of the inner enamel epithelium to form what later becomes an enamel spindle (see Chapter 7). As the odontoblast forms these processes, it also buds off a number of small, membrane-bound vesicles known as matrix vesicles, which come to lie superficially near the basal lamina (Fig. 8.17; see also Figs. 8.12 and 8.16). The odontoblast then develops a cell process, the odontoblast process (Tomes fiber), which is left behind in the forming dentin matrix as the odontoblast moves away toward the pulp (see Fig. 8.15). The mineral phase is believed to first appear within the matrix vesicles as single crystals seeded by phospholipids present in the vesicle

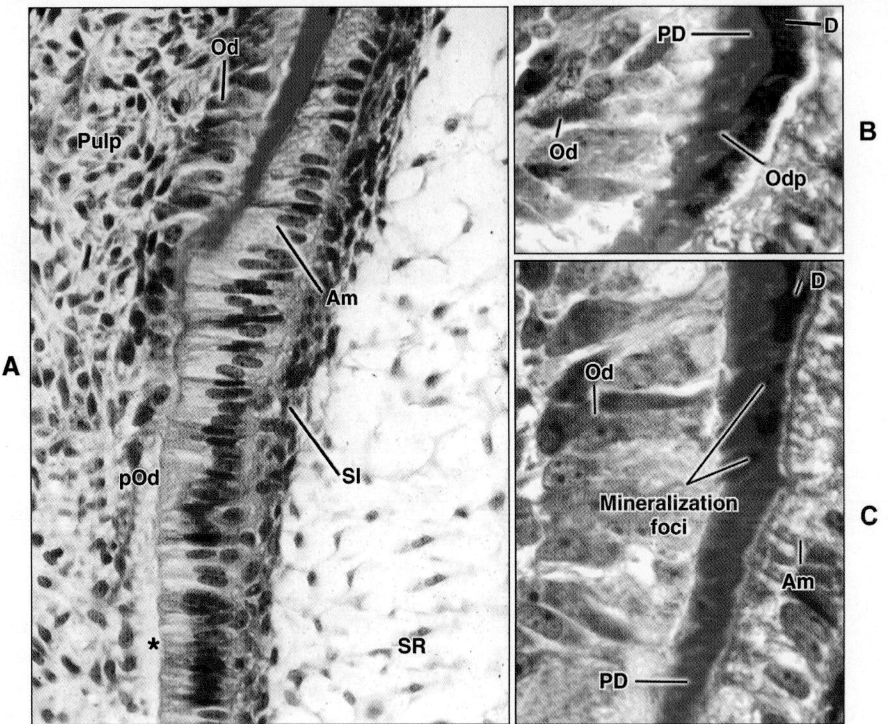

Fig. 8.10 Changes in the dental papilla associated with initiation of dentin formation. (A) An acellular zone *(*)* separates the undifferentiated cells of the dental papilla (preodontoblasts *[pOd]*) from the differentiating inner enamel epithelium (ameloblasts *[Am]*). Preodontoblasts develop into tall and polarized odontoblasts (Od) that will deposit matrix at the interface with ameloblasts. B and C. The matrix first accumulates as an unmineralized layer, predentin *(PD)*, which gradually mineralizes to form mantle dentin *(D)*. *Odp*, Odontoblast process; *SI*, stratum intermedium; *SR*, stellate reticulum.

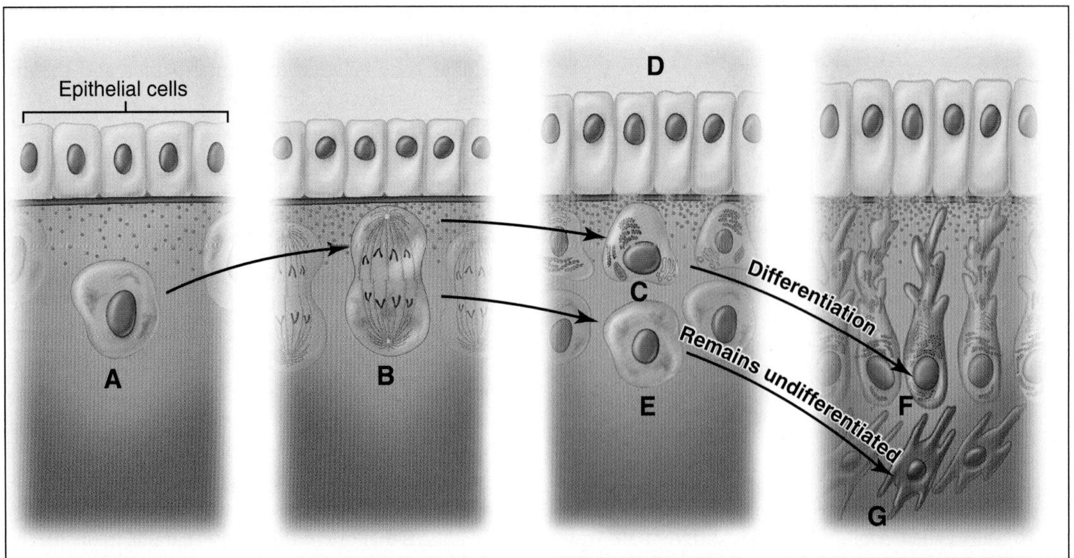

Fig. 8.11 Odontoblast differentiation. The undifferentiated ectomesenchymal cell *(A)* of the dental papilla divides *(B)* with its mitotic spindle perpendicular to the basal lamina *(pink line)*. A daughter cell *(C)*, influenced by the epithelial cells and molecules they produce *(D)*, differentiates into an odontoblast *(F)*. Another daughter cell *(E)*, not exposed to this epithelial influence, persists as a subodontoblast cell *(G)*. This cell has been exposed to all the determinants necessary for odontoblast formation except the last.

membrane (see Fig. 8.16). These crystals grow rapidly and rupture from the confines of the vesicle to spread as a cluster of crystallites that fuse with adjacent clusters to form a continuous layer of mineralized matrix. Matrix vesicles are discussed in more detail in Chapter 1. The deposition of mineral lags behind the formation of the organic matrix so that a layer of organic matrix (predentin) always is found between the odontoblasts and the mineralization front. After mineral seeding, noncollagenous matrix proteins produced by odontoblasts come into play to regulate mineral deposition. In this way coronal mantle dentin is formed in a layer approximately 15 to 20 µm thick onto which then is added the primary (circumpulpal) dentin.

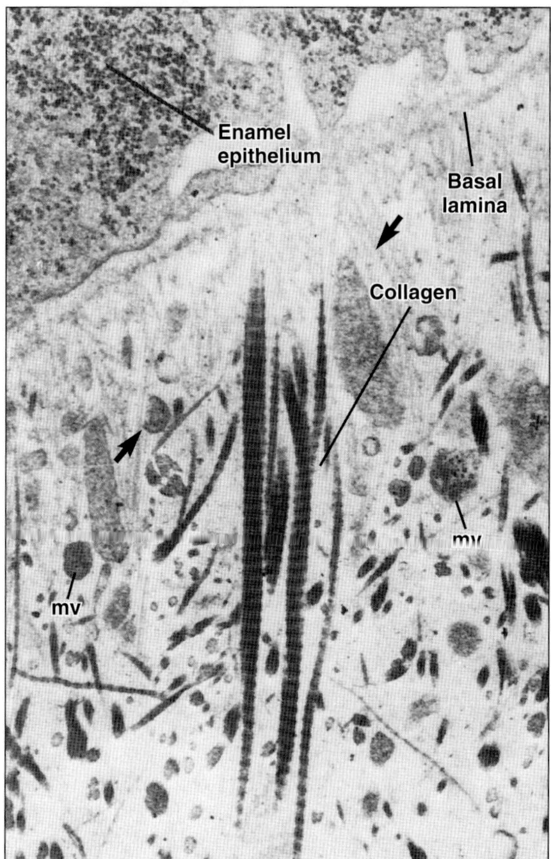

Fig. 8.12 Electron micrograph showing the characteristic deposition of first collagen fibers to form coronal mantle predentin. Large-diameter collagen fibers *(Collagen)* intermingle with aperiodic fibrils *(arrows)* associated with the basal lamina supporting the enamel epithelium. *mv,* Matrix vesicle. (From Ten Cate AR: A fine structural study of coronal and root dentinogenesis in the mouse: observations on the so-called von Korff fibres and their contribution to mantle dentine, *J Anat* 125: 183–197, 1978.)

Vascular Supply

Chapter 1 stated the requirements for good blood supply during the formative phase of hard tissue formation. During dentinogenesis, interesting changes have been observed in rat molars in the distribution and nature of the capillaries associated with the odontoblasts. When mantle dentin formation begins, capillaries are found beneath the newly differentiated odontoblasts. As circumpulpal dentinogenesis is initiated, some of these capillaries migrate between the odontoblasts (Fig. 8.18), and at the same time their endothelium fenestrates to permit increased exchange. With the completion of dentinogenesis, they retreat from the odontoblast layer, and their endothelial lining once again becomes continuous.

Control of Mineralization

A widely-accepted view is that mineralization is achieved by continuous creation of mineral, initially in the matrix vesicle and then at the mineralization front without implication of these vesicles. The question is

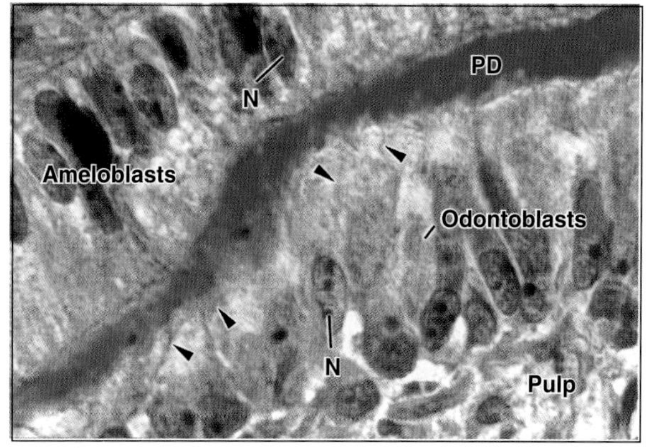

Fig. 8.14 Light micrograph of a paraffin section specially stained for collagen; von Korff fibers appear as convoluted, bluish threadlike structures *(arrowheads)* that originate deep between odontoblasts. *N,* Nucleus; *PD,* predentin.

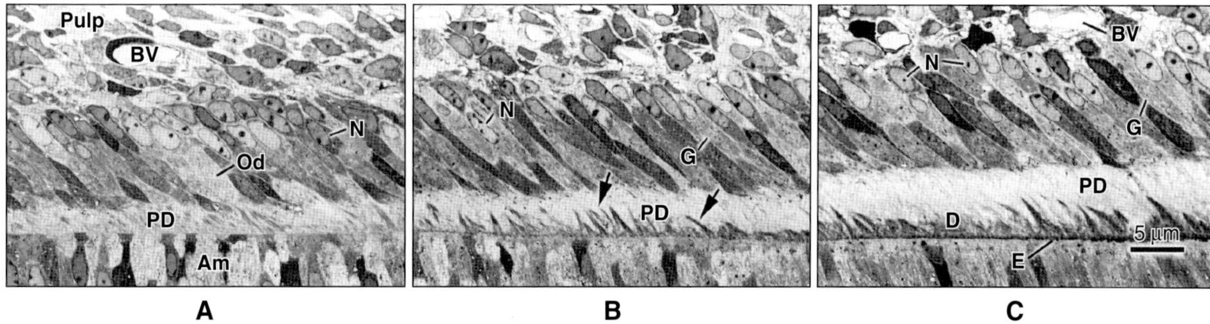

Fig. 8.13 (A–C) Scanning electron micrographs of tissue sections illustrating the formation of the first layer of (mantle) dentin *(D)* in a rat incisor. Differentiated odontoblasts are tall columnar cells tightly grouped in a palisade arrangement. Their nucleus *(N)* is situated basally, the Golgi complex *(G)* occupies much of the supranuclear compartment, and their body is inclined with respect to that of the ameloblasts *(Am)*. (B) A concentration of large-diameter collagen fibrils *(arrows)* can be seen in the forming predentin *(PD)* matrix near the surface of the ameloblasts. (C) As this matrix mineralizes, the fibrils become incorporated in the mantle dentin. *BV,* Blood vessel; *E,* enamel; *Od,* odontoblasts.

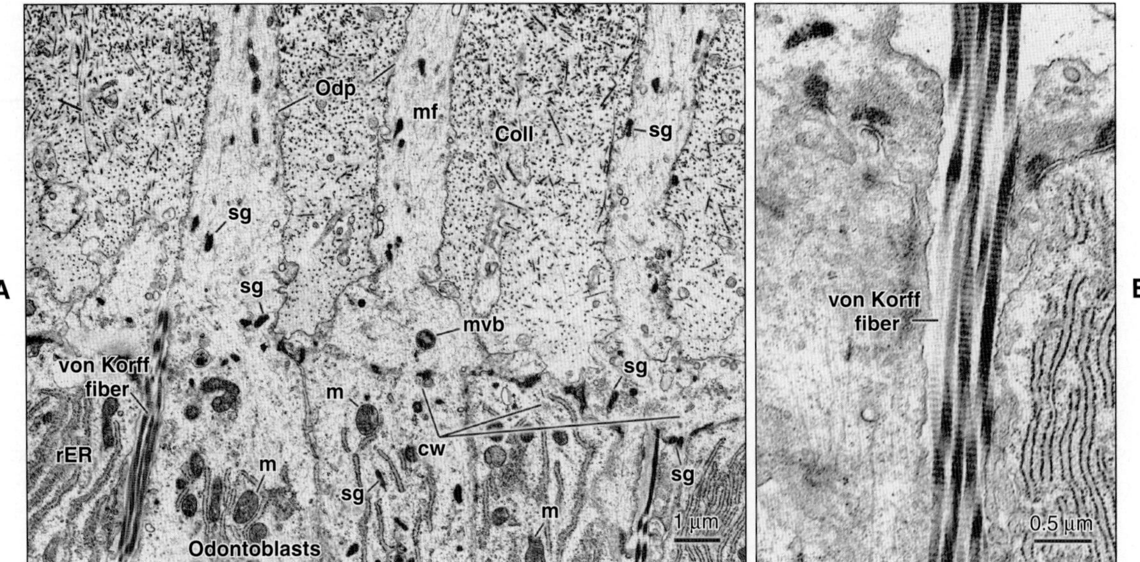

Fig. 8.15 Transmission electron microscope images. (A) The odontoblast process *(Odp)* is the portion of the cell that extends above the cell web *(cw)*. Numerous typical, elongated secretory granules *(sg)*, occasional multivesicular bodies *(mvb)*, and microfilaments *(mf)* are found in the process. The small collagen *(Coll)* fibrils making the bulk of predentin run perpendicularly to the processes and, therefore, appear as dotlike structures in a plane passing longitudinally along odontoblasts. Bundles of larger diameter collagen fibrils (von Korff fibers) run parallel to the odontoblast processes and extend deep between the cell bodies. (B) At higher magnification, a von Korff fiber extending between two odontoblasts shows the typical fibrillar collagen periodicity. *m,* Mitochondria; *rER,* rough endoplasmic reticulum.

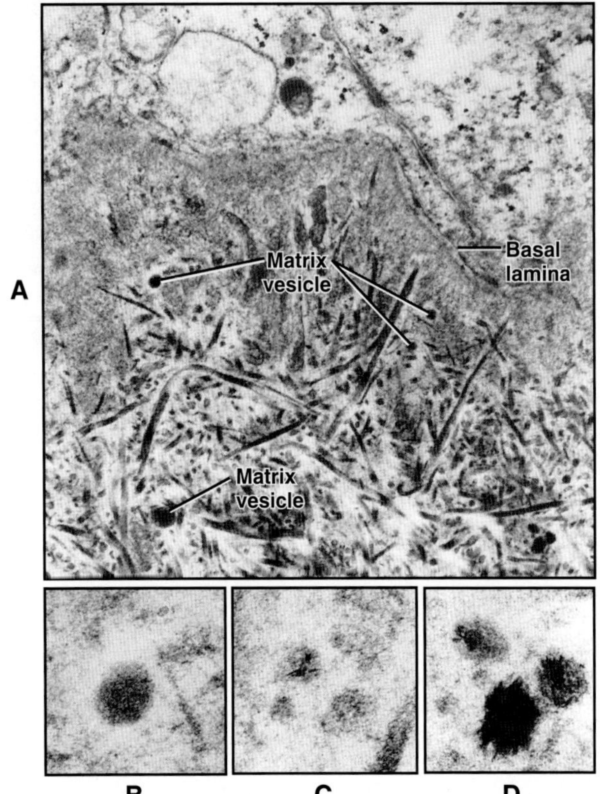

Fig. 8.16 Electron micrograph of initial dentin formation in a human tooth germ at the early bell stage. (A) Collagen fibrils of the first-formed dentin matrix can be seen along with the basal lamina supporting ameloblasts. Intermingled between the collagen fibrils are matrix vesicles in which initial mineralization of the dentin matrix occurs. (B–D) The occurrence and growth of apatite crystals in these vesicles. (From Sisca RF, Provenza DV: Initial dentin formation in human deciduous teeth. An electron microscope study, *Calcif Tissue Res* 9:1–16, 1972.)

whether the odontoblast brings about and controls this mineralization. Clearly the cell exerts control in initiating mineralization by producing matrix vesicles and proteins that can regulate mineral deposition and by adapting the organic matrix at the mineralization front so that it can accommodate the mineral deposits.

The question of how mineral ions reach mineralization sites was reviewed in Chapter 1. In the case of dentinogenesis, some dispute exists because the junctions holding the odontoblasts together in a palisade arrangement are incomplete and thus leaky. Conceptually, simple percolation of tissue fluid supersaturated with calcium and phosphate ions could take place. However, calcium channels of the L type have been demonstrated in the basal plasma membrane of the odontoblast; significantly, when these are blocked, mineralization of the dentin is affected. The presence of alkaline phosphatase activity and calcium adenosine triphosphatase activity at the distal end of the cell is also consistent with a cellular implication in the transport and release of mineral ions into the forming dentin layer.

Pattern of Mineralization

Histologically, two patterns of dentin mineralization can be observed—globular and linear calcification (Figs. 8.19 and 8.20)—that seem to depend on the rate of dentin formation. Globular (calcospheric) calcification involves the deposition of crystals in several discrete areas of matrix by heterogeneous capture in collagen. With continued crystal growth, globular masses are formed that continue to enlarge and eventually fuse to form a single calcified mass. This pattern of mineralization is best seen in the mantle dentin region where matrix vesicles give rise to mineralization foci that grow and coalesce. In circumpulpal dentin, the mineralization front can progress in a globular or linear pattern. The size of the globules seems to depend on the rate of dentin deposition, with the largest globules occurring where dentin deposition is fastest. When the rate of formation progresses slowly, the mineralization front appears more uniform, and the process is said to be linear.

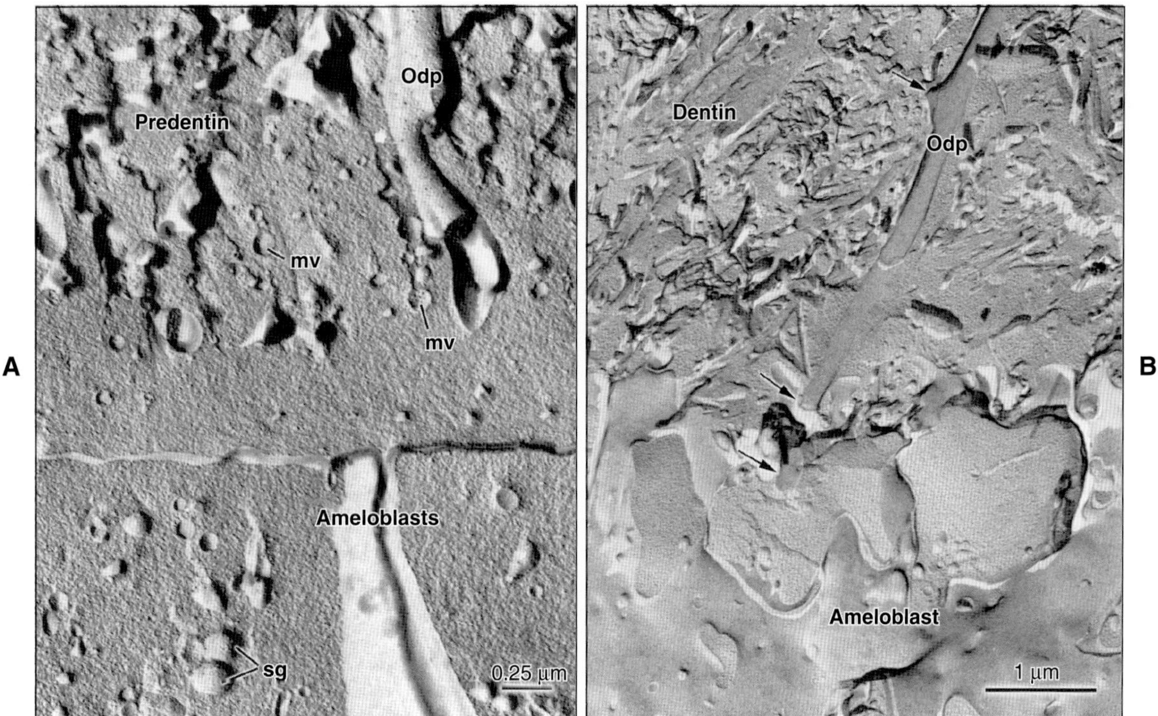

Fig. 8.17 Freeze fracture preparations showing the interface between forming mantle (A) predentin and (B) dentin and ameloblasts at an early time during tooth formation. (A) The presence of abundant, well-defined matrix vesicles *(mv)* in the extracellular matrix indicates that mineralization has not yet started. (B) Odontoblast processes *(Odp)* can establish contact *(arrows)* with ameloblasts, an event believed to be one of the various mechanisms of epithelial-mesenchymal interaction during tooth development. *sg,* Secretory granule.

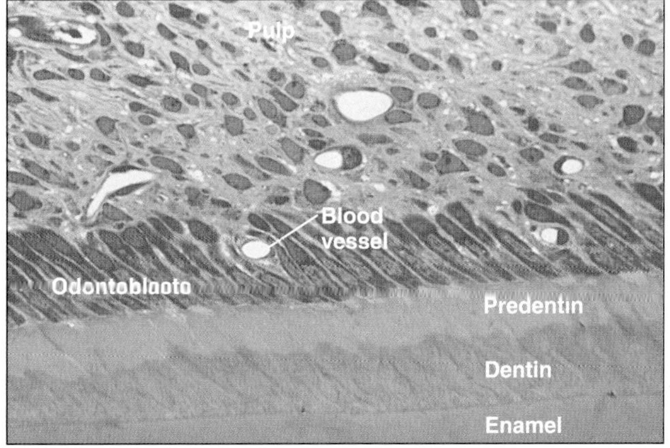

Fig. 8.18 Light photomicrograph of the odontoblast layer. This specimen was fixed by perfusion, which forced blood vessels open, thereby better revealing their distribution in the layer.

Formation of Root Dentin

The epithelial cells of Hertwig root sheath initiate the differentiation of odontoblasts that form root dentin (Fig. 8.21; see also Chapter 9). Root dentin forms similarly to coronal dentin, but some differences have been reported. The outermost layer of root dentin, the equivalent of mantle dentin in the crown, shows differences in collagen fiber orientation and organization in part because the collagen fibers from cementum blend with those of dentin (see Chapter 9). Some reports also indicate that the phosphoprotein content of root dentin differs, that it forms at a slower speed, and that its degree of mineralization differs from that of coronal dentin. These possible differences, however, need to be ascertained and simply may reflect the anatomic context of root dentin rather than fundamental differences.

Secondary and Tertiary Dentinogenesis

Secondary dentin is deposited after root formation is completed, is formed by the same odontoblasts that formed primary dentin, and is laid down as a continuation of the primary dentin. Secondary dentin formation is achieved in essentially the same way as primary dentin formation although at a much slower pace. Secondary dentin can be distinguished histologically from primary dentin by a subtle demarcation line, a slight differential in staining, and a less regular organization of dentinal tubules (see Fig. 8.6). Indeed, in some regions tubules may be altogether absent; as the dentin layer becomes thicker, its inner surface is reduced, resulting in the crowding of odontoblasts and the death of some.

Tertiary dentin is deposited at specific sites in response to injury by damaged odontoblasts or replacement cells from pulp. The rate of deposition depends on the degree of injury; the more severe the injury, the more rapid the rate of dentin deposition. As a result of this rapid deposition, cells often become trapped in the newly formed matrix, and the tubular pattern becomes grossly distorted (Fig. 8.22). In addition to its particular structural organization, the composition of tertiary dentin is also distinctive; during its formation, production of collagen, DSP, and DMP1 appears to be downregulated, whereas that of BSP and osteopontin is upregulated (Fig. 8.23).

HISTOLOGY OF DENTIN

When the dentin is viewed microscopically, several structural features can be identified: dentinal tubules, peritubular and intertubular

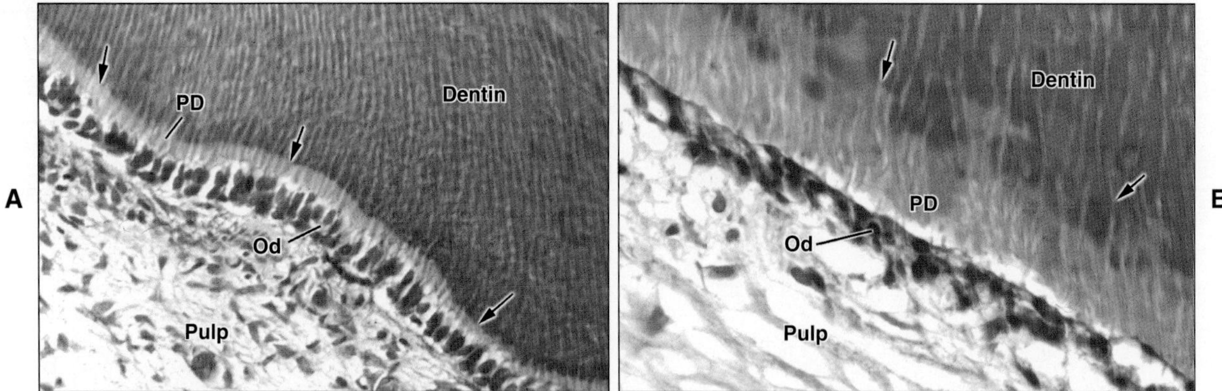

Fig. 8.19 Light photomicrographs of the predentin-dentin interface illustrating (A) linear and (B) globular mineralization fronts *(arrows)*. *Od*, Odontoblasts; *PD*, predentin.

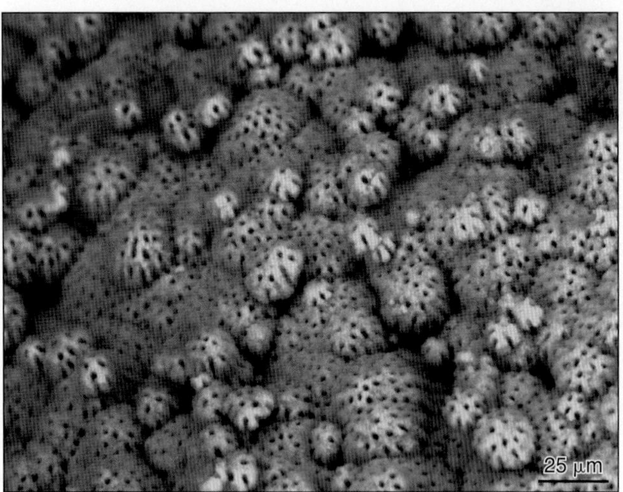

Fig. 8.20 Scanning electron micrograph of globular dentin.

dentin, areas of deficient calcification (interglobular dentin), incremental growth lines, and an area seen solely in the root portion of the tooth known as the *granular layer of Tomes*.

Dentinal Tubules

Odontoblast processes, similar to osteocyte processes, run in canaliculi that traverse the dentin layer and are referred to as *dentinal tubules* (Figs. 8.24 and 8.25). Dentinal tubules extend through the entire thickness of the dentin from the dentinoenamel junction to the mineralization front and form a network for the diffusion of nutrients throughout dentin. The tubules follow an S-shaped path from the outer surface of the dentin to the perimeter of the pulp in coronal dentin. This S-shaped curvature is least pronounced beneath the incisal edges and cusps where the tubules may run an almost straight course (Fig. 8.26). These curvatures result from the crowding of and path followed by odontoblasts as they move toward the center of the pulp. Evidence also indicates that some odontoblasts are deleted selectively by apoptosis as they become crowded. In root dentin, little or no crowding results from decrease in surface area, and tubules run a straight course. In predentin, odontoblast processes run in a compartment delimited by unmineralized collagen fibers (see Fig. 8.25A and B).

The dentinal tubules are tapered structures that are larger near the pulp and thinnest at the dentinoenamel junction. It has been estimated that, in the coronal parts of young premolar and molar teeth, the numbers of tubules range from 59,000 to 76,000/mm^2 at the pulpal surface with approximately half as many per square millimeter near the enamel. This increase per unit volume is associated with crowding of the odontoblasts as the pulp space becomes smaller. A significant reduction in the average density of tubules also occurs in radicular dentin compared with cervical dentin.

Dentinal tubules branch to the extent that dentin is permeated by a profuse anastomosing canalicular system (Fig. 8.27). Major branches occur more frequently in root dentin than in coronal dentin (Fig. 8.28). The tubular nature of dentin bestows an unusual degree of permeability on this hard tissue that can enhance a carious process (Fig. 8.29) and accentuate the response of the pulp to dental restorative procedures. Tubules in carious lesions may fill with bacteria and appear darkly stained in histologic sections (Fig. 8.30; see also Fig. 8.29). The processes in these tubules may disintegrate or retract, leaving behind an empty tubule (dead tract). Reparative dentin seals off such dead tracts at their pulpal extremity, thereby protecting the pulp from infection. Such tracts may also occur normally as a result of the death of odontoblasts from cell crowding, particularly in pulpal horns. In ground sections, empty tubules appear by transmitted light as black because they entrap air.

Peritubular Dentin

Tubules are delimited by a collar of more highly calcified matrix called peritubular dentin (see Fig. 8.25D), which starts at the mineralization front (see Fig. 8.24C). The mechanism by which peritubular dentin forms and its precise composition are still not known; peritubular dentin has been shown to be hypermineralized compared with intertubular dentin. Also, peritubular dentin contains little collagen, and in rodent teeth it appears to be enriched in noncollagenous matrix proteins, such as DSP (Fig. 8.31) and DMP1. This hypermineralized ring of dentin is readily apparent in human teeth when nondemineralized ground sections cut at right angles to the tubules are examined under the light microscope or by scanning electron microscopy (Fig. 8.32).

Sclerotic Dentin

Sclerotic dentin describes dentinal tubules that have become occluded with calcified material. When this occurs in several tubules in the same area, the dentin assumes a glassy appearance and becomes translucent (Fig. 8.33). The amount of sclerotic dentin increases with age and is most common in the apical third of the root and in the crown midway between the dentinoenamel junction and the surface of the pulp. The occlusion of dentinal tubules with mineral begins in root dentin of 18-year-old premolars without any identifiable external influence—hence the assumptions that sclerotic dentin is a physiologic response and that occlusion is achieved by continued

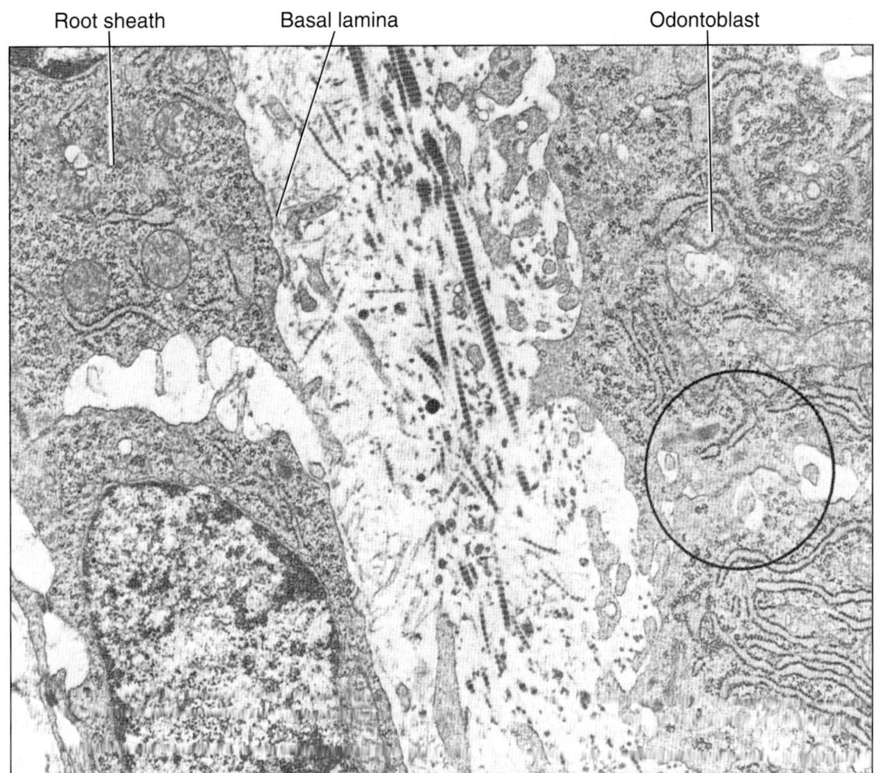

Fig. 8.21 Electron micrograph illustrating initial root dentinogenesis. Cells of Hertwig epithelial root sheath have initiated differentiation of odontoblasts that are about to begin the formation of root dentin. The first collagen fibers of the matrix are aligned parallel to the basal lamina, which supports the root sheath cells and which, at this stage, is becoming discontinuous. The circled area outlines a junctional complex between two odontoblasts. (From Ten Cate AR: A fine structural study of coronal and root dentinogenesis in the mouse: observations on the so-called von Korff fibres and their contribution to mantle dentine, *J Anat* 125:183–197, 1978.)

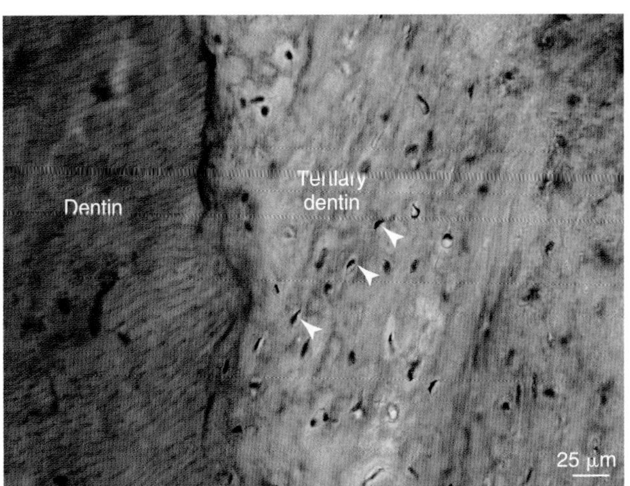

Fig. 8.22 Light micrograph of tertiary dentin containing cellular inclusions *(arrowheads)*.

deposition of peritubular dentin (Fig. 8.34A). However, occlusion of the tubules may occur in several other ways: deposition of mineral within the tubule without any dentin formation (see Fig. 8.34B), a diffuse mineralization that occurs with a viable odontoblast process still present (see Fig. 8.34C), and mineralization of the process itself and tubular contents, including intratubular collagen fibrils (see Fig. 8.34D). Because sclerosis reduces the permeability of dentin, it may help to prolong pulp vitality.

Intertubular Dentin

Dentin located between the dentinal tubules is called *intertubular dentin* (see Figs. 8.25D and 8.32). Intertubular dentin represents the primary formative product of the odontoblasts and consists of a tightly interwoven network of type I collagen fibrils (50–200 nm in diameter) in and around which apatite crystals are deposited. The fibrils are arranged randomly in a plane at roughly right angles to the dentinal tubules. The ground substance consists of noncollagenous matrix proteins and some plasma proteins.

Interglobular Dentin

Interglobular dentin describes areas of unmineralized or hypomineralized dentin where globular zones of mineralization (calcospherites) have failed to fuse into a homogeneous mass within mature dentin (Fig. 8.35). These areas are especially prevalent in human teeth in which the person has had a deficiency in vitamin D or exposure to high levels of fluoride at the time of dentin formation. Interglobular dentin is most common in the circumpulpal dentin just below the mantle dentin, where the pattern of mineralization is largely globular. Because this irregularity of dentin is a particularity of mineralization and not of matrix formation, the normal architectural pattern of the tubules remains unchanged, and they run uninterrupted through the interglobular areas. However, no peritubular dentin exists where the tubules pass through the unmineralized areas.

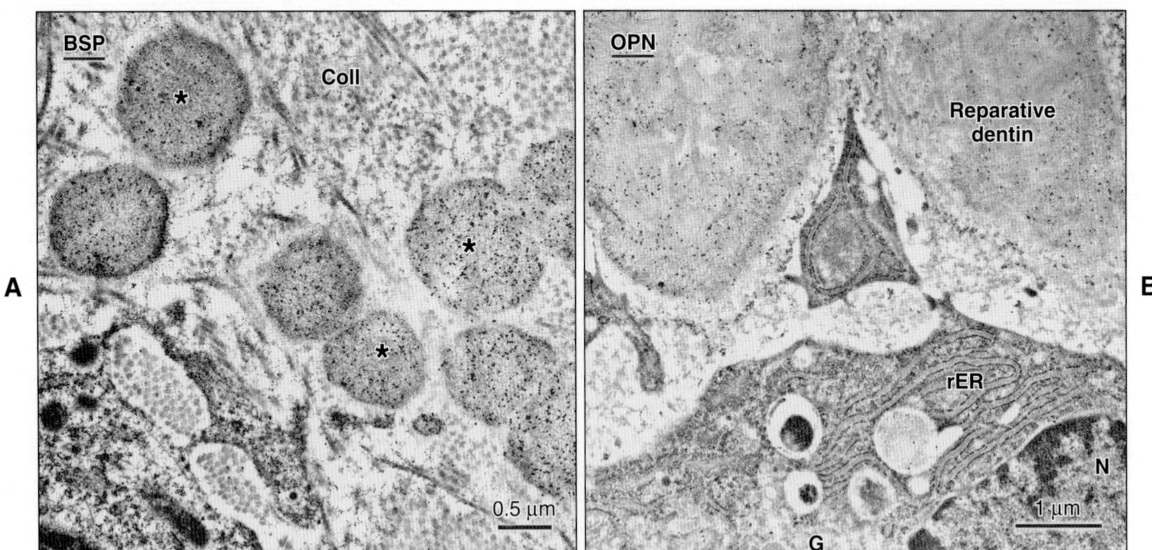

Fig. 8.23 As illustrated by these immunogold preparations, reparative dentin is poor in collagen and enriched in noncollagenous matrix proteins, such as bone sialoprotein *(BSP)* and osteopontin *(OPN)*. (A) In this situation, reparative dentin began formation as globular masses *(*)* among collagen fibrils *(Coll)*. (B) The globules grew and fused to form larger masses of mineralized matrix. *G,* Golgi complex; *N,* nucleus; *rER,* rough endoplasmic reticulum.

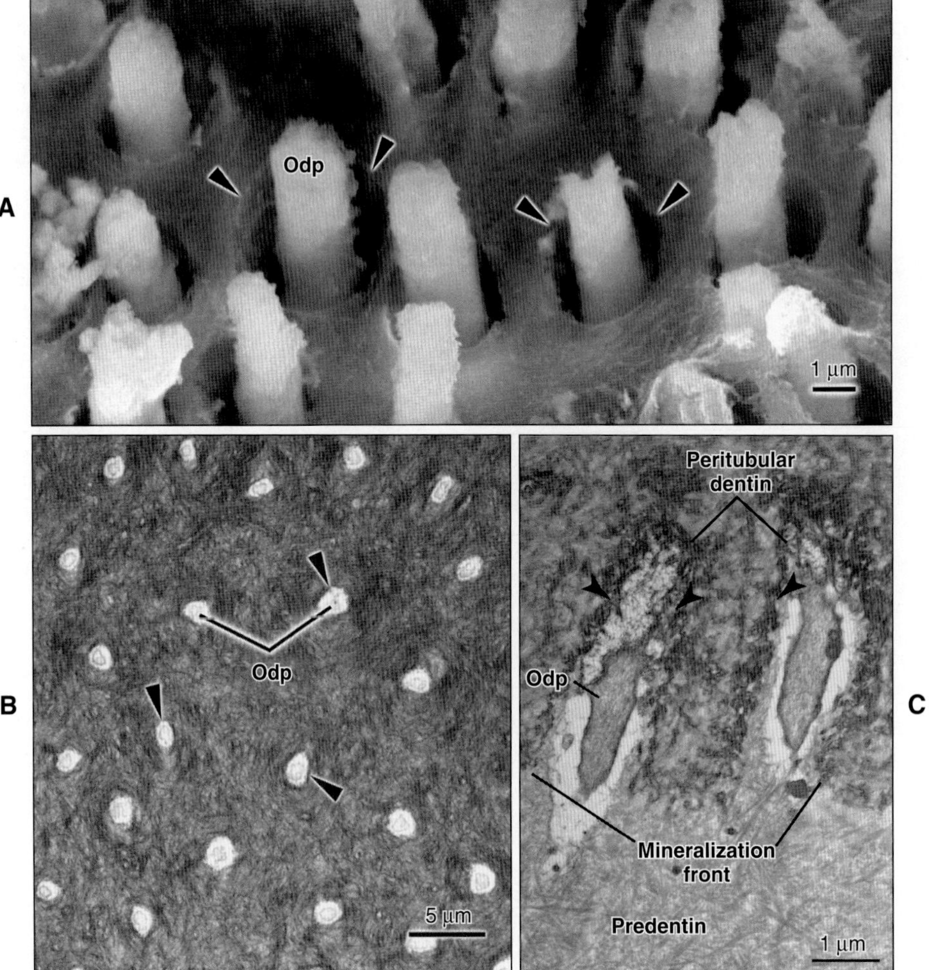

Fig. 8.24 Images from (A) scanning electron microscope and (B) light microscope. Odontoblast processes *(Odp)* run in canaliculi called *dentinal tubules (arrowheads)*. (C) A transmission electron micrograph showing that dentinal tubules are lined by peritubular dentin starting at the mineralization front and extending to dentin.

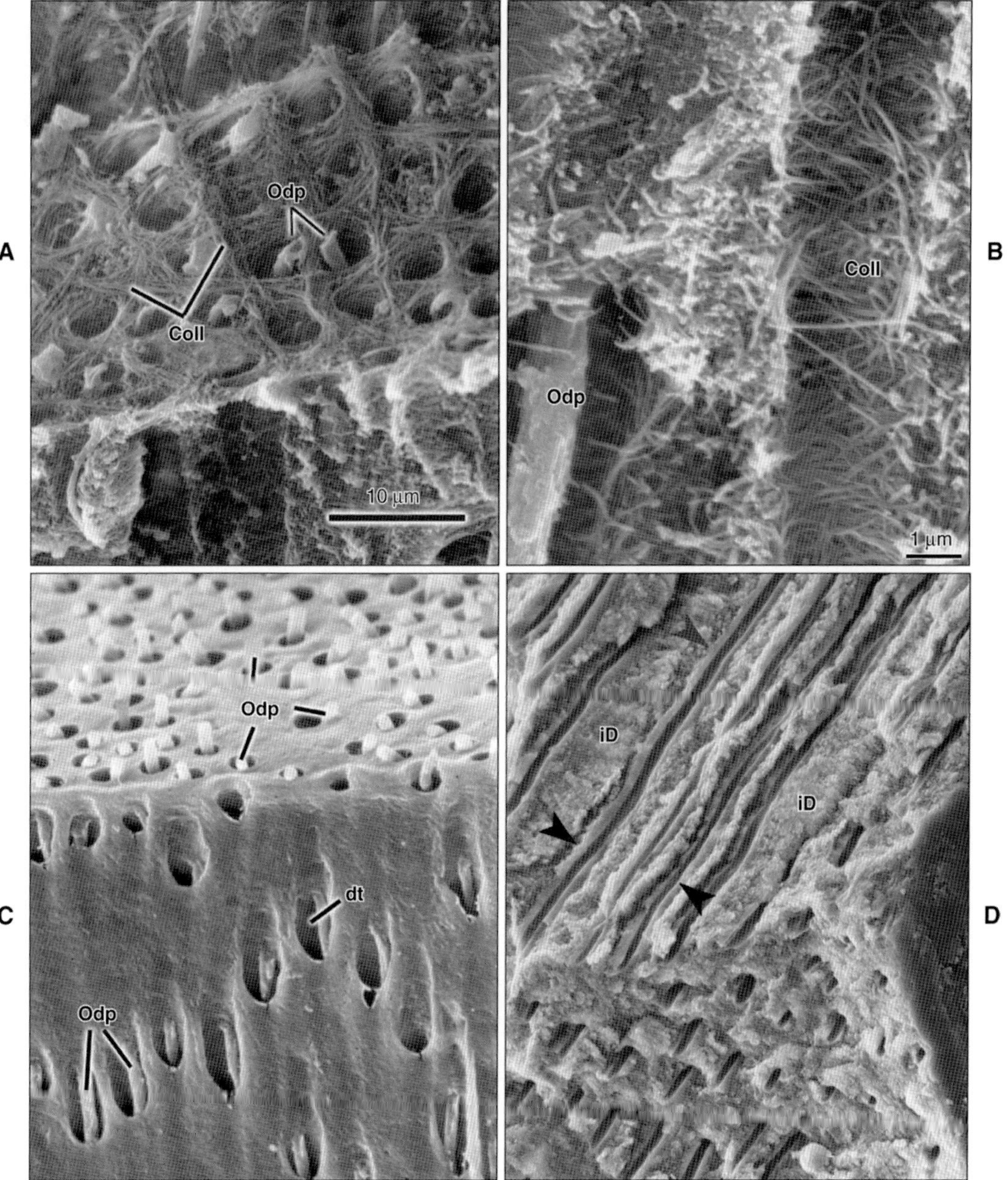

Fig. 8.25 Scanning electron microscope preparations of predentin (A, B) and dentin (C, D). (A, B) Although no dentinal tubules *(dt)* occur in predentin, each odontoblast process *(Odp)* is surrounded by a meshwork of intertwined collagen *(Coll)* fibrils that outline the future dentinal tubule. As visible in cross-sectional (A) and longitudinal (B) profile, the fibrils run circumferentially and perpendicular to the process. (C) In healthy dentin, each tubule is occupied by a process or its ramifications. (D) The dentinal tubule is delimited by a layer of peritubular dentin *(arrowheads)* that is poor in collagen and more mineralized than the rest of the dentin. The dentin between tubules is referred to as *intertubular dentin (iD)*.

Incremental Growth Lines

The organic matrix of primary dentin is deposited incrementally at a daily rate of approximately 4 µm; at the boundary between each daily increment, minute changes in collagen fiber orientation can be demonstrated by means of special staining techniques. Superimposed on this daily increment is a 5-day cycle in which the changes in collagen fiber orientation are more exaggerated. These incremental lines run at right angles to the dentinal tubules and generally mark the normal rhythmic, linear pattern of dentin deposition in an inward and rootward direction (Fig. 8.36). The 5-day increment can be seen readily in conventional and ground sections as the incremental lines of von Ebner (situated ~20 µm apart). Close examination of globular mineralization shows that the rate in organic matrix is approximately 2 µm every 12 hours. Thus the organic matrix of dentin is deposited rhythmically at a daily rate of about 4 µm a day and is mineralized in a 12-hour cycle. As mentioned, the rate of deposition of secondary dentin is slower and asymmetric.

Another type of incremental pattern found in dentin is the contour lines of Owen. Some confusion exists about the exact connotation of this term. As originally described by Owen, the contour lines result from a coincidence of the secondary curvatures between neighboring dentinal tubules. Other lines, however, that have the same disposition

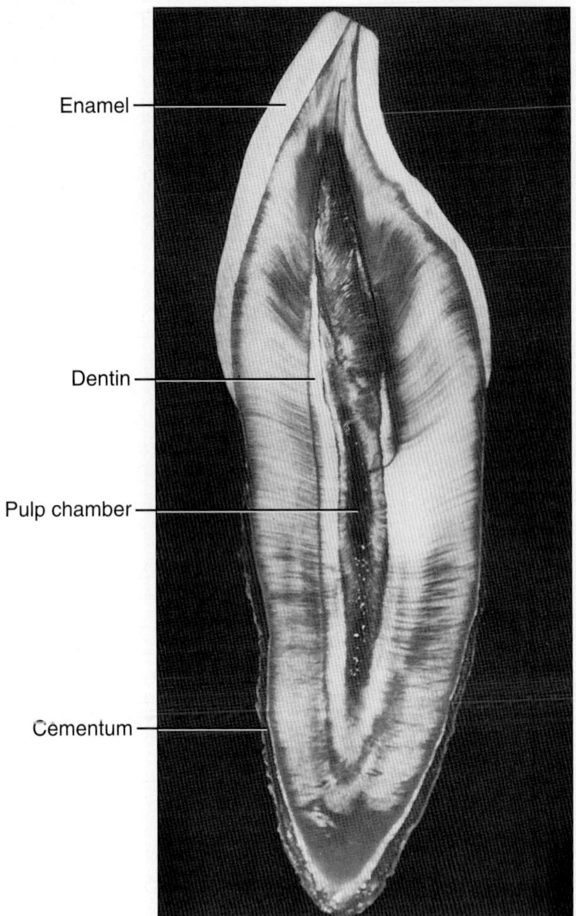

Fig. 8.26 Ground section showing the S-shaped primary curvature of the dentinal tubules in the crown and their straight course in the root.

but caused by accentuated deficiencies in mineralization now are known more generally as *contour lines of Owen*. These are recognized easily in longitudinal ground sections. An exceptionally wide contour line is the neonatal line found in those teeth that mineralize at birth and reflects the disturbance in mineralization created by the physiologic trauma of birth. Periods of illness or inadequate nutrition also are marked by accentuated contour lines within the dentin.

Granular Layer of Tomes

When root dentin is viewed under transmitted light in ground sections (and only in ground sections), a granular-appearing area, the granular layer of Tomes, can be seen just below the surface of the dentin where the root is covered by cementum (Figs. 8.37 and 8.38). A progressive increase in granularity occurs from the cementoenamel junction to the apex of the tooth. A number of interpretations have been proposed for these structures. This granular appearance was once believed to be associated with minute hypomineralized areas of interglobular dentin. They also were proposed to be true spaces; however, these cannot be seen in hematoxylin-eosin–stained sections or on electron micrographs. Finally, the spaces have been suggested to represent sections made through the looped terminal portions of dentinal tubules found only in root dentin and seen only because of light refraction in thick ground sections. More recent interpretation relates this layer to a special arrangement of collagen and noncollagenous matrix proteins at the interface between dentin and cementum (see Chapter 9).

PULP

The dental pulp is the soft connective tissue that supports the dentin. When its histologic appearance is examined, four distinct zones can be distinguished: (1) the odontoblastic zone at the pulp periphery; (2) a cell-free zone of Weil beneath the odontoblasts, which is prominent in the coronal pulp; (3) a cell-rich zone, where cell density is high, which, again, is seen easily in coronal pulp adjacent to the cell-free zone; and

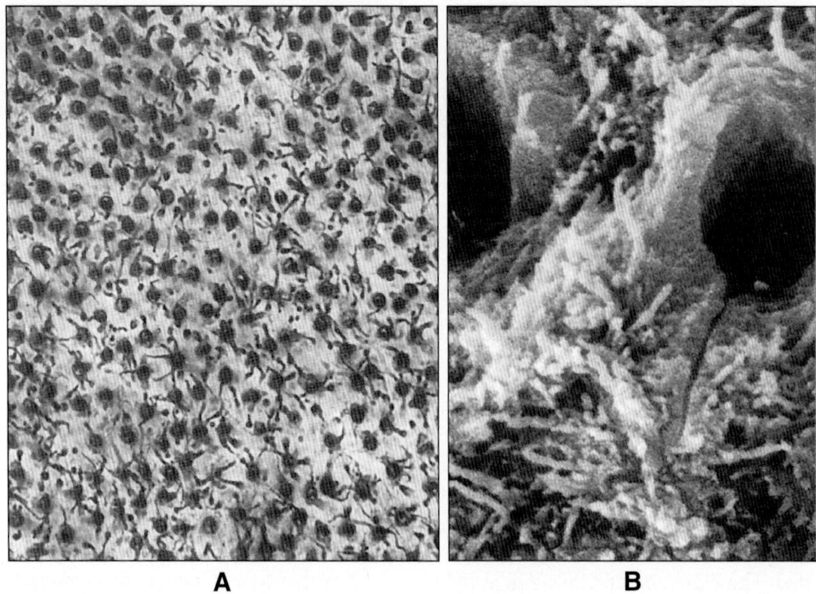

Fig. 8.27 Dentinal tubule branching. (A) Light microscope cross section of dentin stained with silver nitrate, showing the extensive fine branching network of the tubular compartment. (B) Scanning electron micrograph showing microbranch extends from a larger dentinal tubule through the peritubular dentin. A thin layer of peritubular dentin also borders the microbranch.

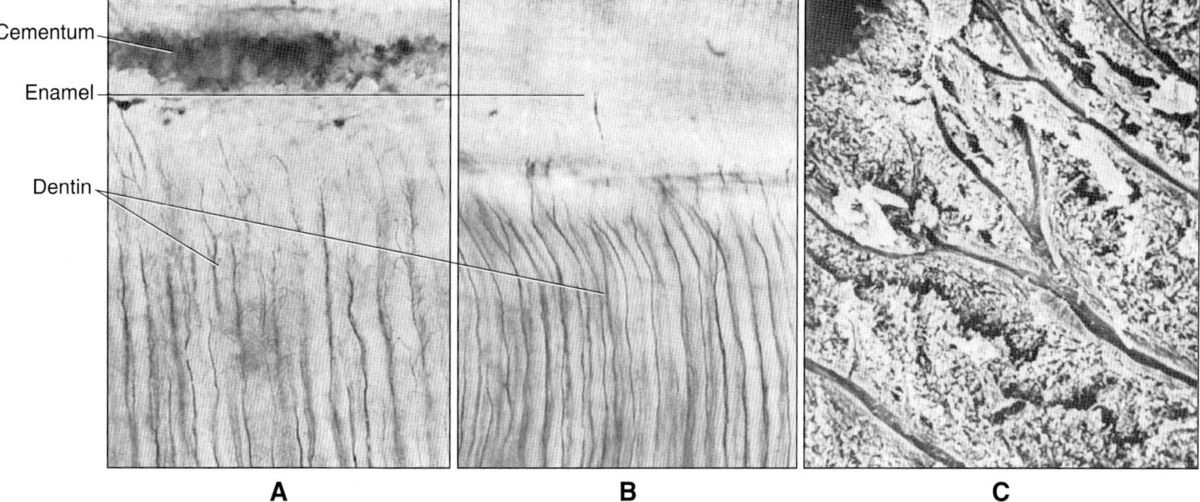

Fig. 8.28 Terminal branching of dentinal tubules is more profuse in root dentin (A) than in coronal dentin (B). (C) Scanning electron micrograph showing branching.

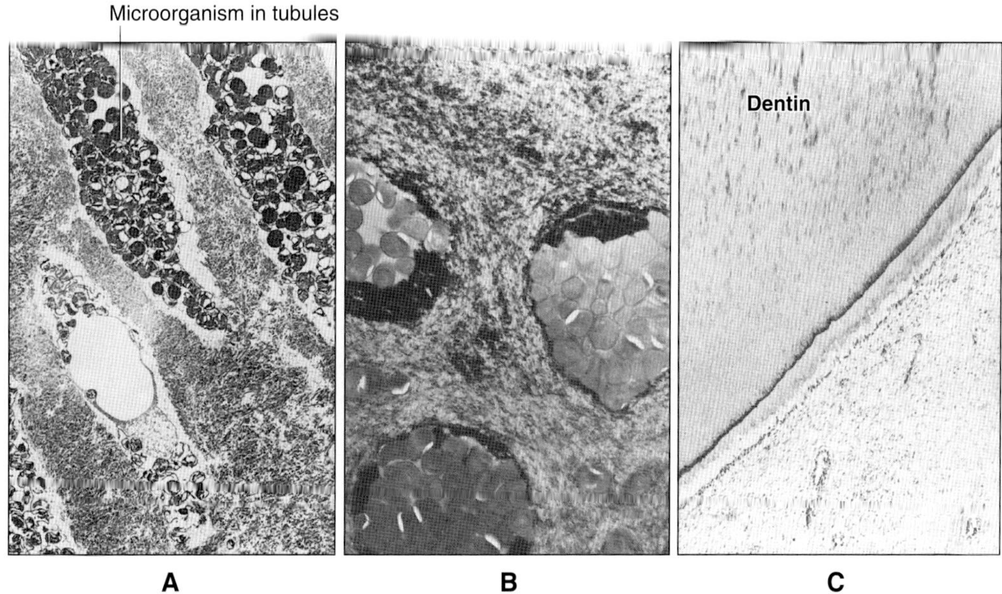

Fig. 8.29 Caries of dentin. Transmission electron micrographs show the natural pathway created for microorganisms by the dentinal tubules in longitudinal section (A) and in cross section (B). (C) The microorganisms absorb stain; in light microscope sections, the tubules of carious dentin are seen as dark streaks. (B, Courtesy N.W. Johnson.)

(4) the pulp core, which is characterized by the major vessels and nerves of the pulp (Figs. 8.39 and 8.40). The principal cells of the pulp are the odontoblasts, fibroblasts, undifferentiated ectomesenchymal cells, macrophages, and other immunocompetent cells. Interestingly, the tooth pulp has been shown to be a convenient source of multipotent stem cells.

Odontoblasts

The most distinctive cells of the dental pulp, and therefore the most easily recognized, are the odontoblasts. Odontoblasts form a layer lining the periphery of the pulp and have a process extending into the dentin (Fig. 8.41A). In the crown of the mature tooth, odontoblasts often appear to be arranged in a palisade pattern three to five cells deep. This appearance is an artifact caused by crowding of the odontoblasts as they migrate centripetally and by a tangential plane of section. The number of odontoblasts corresponds to the number of dentinal tubules and, as mentioned, varies with tooth type and location within the pulp space. The odontoblasts in the crown are larger than odontoblasts in the root. In the crown of the fully developed tooth, the cell bodies of odontoblasts are columnar and measure approximately 50 µm in height, whereas in the midportion of the pulp they are more cuboid and in the apical part more flattened.

The morphology of odontoblasts reflects their functional activity and ranges from an active synthetic phase to a quiescent phase

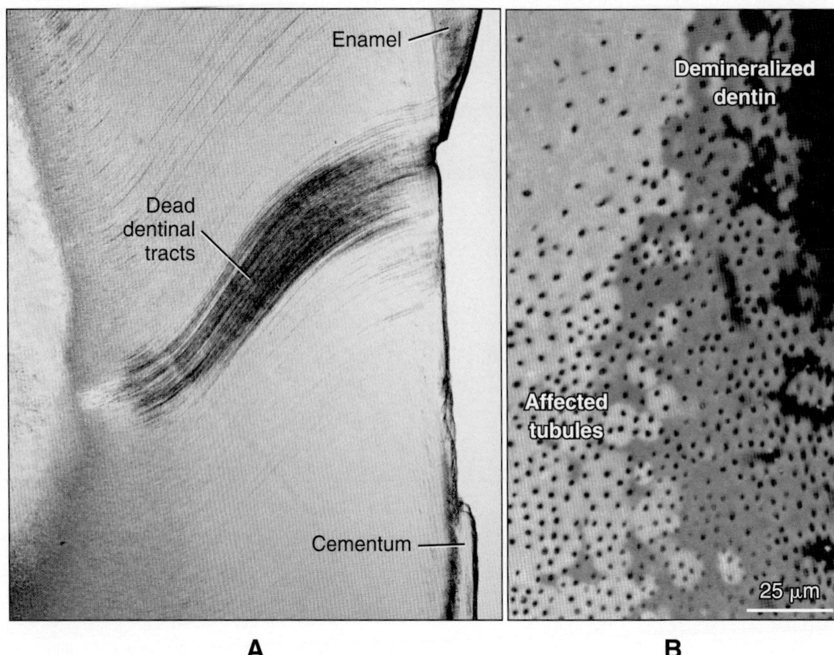

Fig. 8.30 (A) Light micrograph showing dead tracts on the radicular carious lesion, which appear dark under transmitted light. (B) Scanning electron micrograph showing empty tubules under a carious lesion.

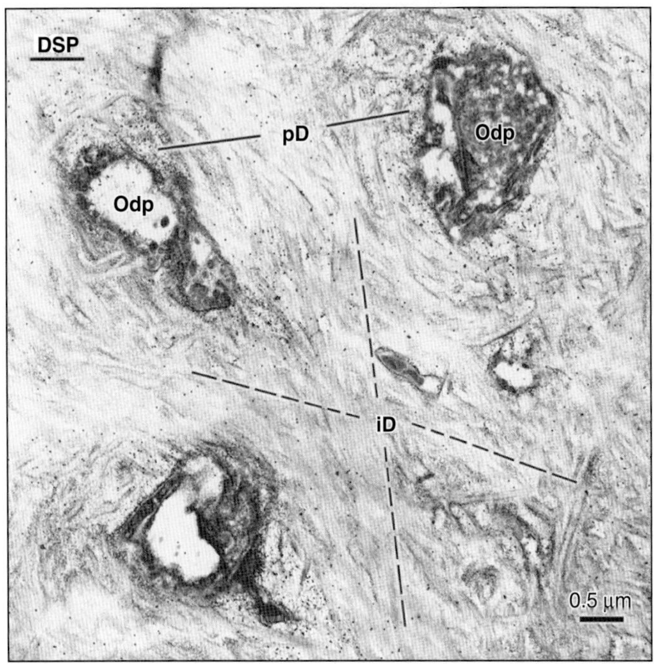

Fig. 8.31 Immunogold preparation illustrating an accumulation of dentin sialoprotein *(DSP; black particles)* around odontoblast processes *(Odp)* in certain regions of a rat incisor. Less collagen is present in these areas corresponding to the position of peritubular dentin *(pD)*. The matrix between these areas is the intertubular dentin *(iD)* and constitutes the bulk of the dentin.

(Fig. 8.42). By light microscopy, an active cell appears elongated and can be seen to possess a basal nucleus, much basophilic cytoplasm, and a prominent Golgi zone. A resting cell, by contrast, is stubby with little cytoplasm and has a more hematoxophilic nucleus. By electron microscopy, another stage in the life cycle of odontoblasts can be discerned. In addition to the secretory and resting (or aged) states recognizable by light microscopy, defining a transitional stage intermediate between the secretory and resting states is also possible. The organelles of an active odontoblast are prominent, consisting of numerous vesicles, much endoplasmic reticulum, a well-developed Golgi complex located on the dentinal side of the nucleus, and numerous mitochondria scattered throughout the cell body (Figs. 8.43 and 8.44; see also Fig. 8.41B). The nucleus contains an abundance of peripherally dispersed chromatin and several nucleoli. The pathway for collagen synthesis within the odontoblast and its intracellular and extracellular assembly is similar to that described for the fibroblast (summarized in Fig. 4.12). Spheric and cylindric distentions are implicated in the processing of the procollagen molecule (Fig. 8.45; see also Fig. 8.44B). The cylindric distentions bud off as secretory granules that exhibit a characteristic elongated shape and electron density. The secretory granules then are transported toward the odontoblast process where their content is released (Fig. 8.46A). Debate continues as to whether the noncollagenous matrix proteins produced by odontoblasts are packaged within the same secretory granule with collagen or in a distinct granule population. Indeed, immunolabeling for BSP and osteocalcin can be found in round granules (Fig. 8.47), whereas their presence in the elongated, collagen-containing ones has not yet been convincingly demonstrated. Other membrane-bound granules, similar in appearance to lysosomes, are present in the cytoplasm as are numerous filaments and microtubules. Decreasing amounts of intracellular organelles reflect decreased functional activity of the odontoblast. Thus the transitional odontoblast is a narrower cell with its nucleus displaced from the basal extremity and exhibiting condensed chromatin. The amount of endoplasmic reticulum is reduced, and autophagic vacuoles are present and are associated with the reorganization of cytoplasm. Resting, or aged, odontoblasts are smaller cells crowded together. The nucleus of such a cell is situated more apically, creating a prominent infranuclear region in which fewer cytoplasmic organelles are clustered. The supranuclear region is devoid of organelles, except for large, lipid-filled vacuoles in a cytoplasm containing tubular and filamentous structures. Secretory granules are scarce or even absent.

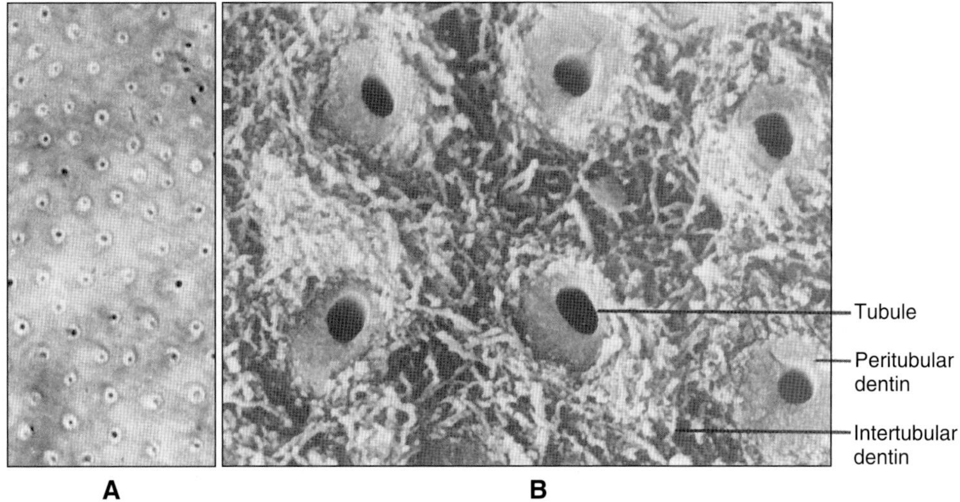

Fig. 8.32 Peritubular dentin seen in ground section by (A) light microscopy and (B) scanning electron microscopy. The dark central spots are empty dentinal tubules surrounded by a well-defined collar of peritubular dentin.

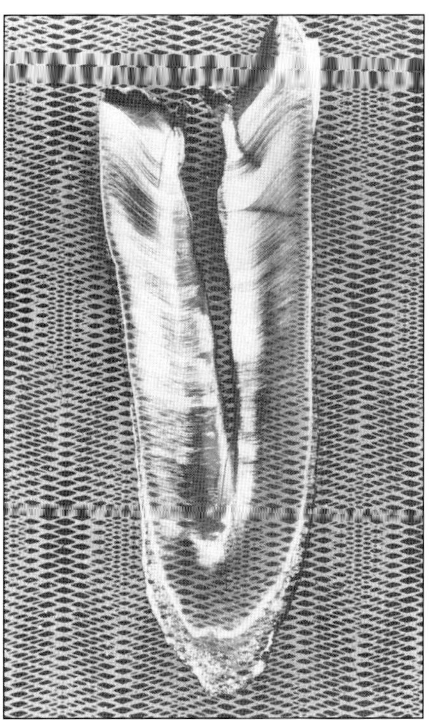

Fig. 8.33 Ground section, approximately 100 μm thick, of an old tooth. The section has been placed over a pattern, which can be seen through the apical translucent sclerotic dentin but not through normal dentin.

The odontoblast process begins at the neck of the cells just above the apical junctional complex where the cell gradually begins to narrow as it enters predentin (Fig. 8.48; see also Figs. 8.15A, 8.41A, 8.46A). A major change in the cytologic condition of odontoblasts occurs at the junction between the cell body and the process. The process is devoid of major organelles but displays an abundance of microtubules and filaments arranged in a linear pattern along its length (see Figs. 8.15A and 8.46). Coated vesicles and pits that reflect pinocytotic activity along the process membrane also are present (Fig. 8.49).

Junctions occur between adjacent odontoblasts involving gap junctions, occluding zones (tight junctions) and desmosomes. Distally, where the cell body [illegible] the process the junctions take the form of a junctional complex (see Fig. 8.46A) consisting mostly of adherent junctions interspersed with areas of tight junctions. The actin filaments inserting into the adherent junction are prominent and form a terminal cell web (see Figs. 8.15A, 8.41A, and 8.46A). This junctional complex does not form a zonula that completely encircles the cell, as occurs in epithelia; it is focal, and there is some debate whether it can restrict the passage of molecules and ions from the pulp into the dentin layer. For instance, some molecular tracers have been shown to reach the predentin via the interodontoblastic space, but others are unable to do so. Serum proteins seem to pass freely between odontoblasts and are found in dentin.

Gap junctions occur frequently on the lateral surfaces of odontoblasts and are found at the base of the cell where junctions are established with pulpal fibroblasts. The number and location of gap junctions are variable, however, because they can form, dissolve, and reform rapidly as function dictates (Fig. 8.50).

The lifespan of the odontoblasts generally is believed to equal that of the viable tooth because the odontoblasts are end cells, which means that, when differentiated, they cannot undergo further cell division. This fact poses an interesting problem. On occasion, when the pulp tissue is exposed, repair can take place by the formation of new dentin. This means that new odontoblasts must have differentiated and migrated to the exposure site from pulp tissue, most likely from the cell-rich subodontoblast zone. The differentiation of odontoblasts during tooth development requires a cascade of determinants, including cells of the inner enamel epithelium (Hertwig root sheath). Epithelial cells, however, are no longer present in the developed tooth, and the stimulus for differentiation of new odontoblasts under these circumstances is thus different and not yet understood.

The dentinal tubule and its contents bestow on dentin its vitality and ability to respond to various stimuli. The tubular compartment therefore assumes significance in any analysis of dentinal response to clinical procedures such as cavity preparation or the bonding of materials to dentin.

The account given of the tubule and the odontoblast process so far has been fairly uncontroversial; dentin is tubular, each tubule is (or

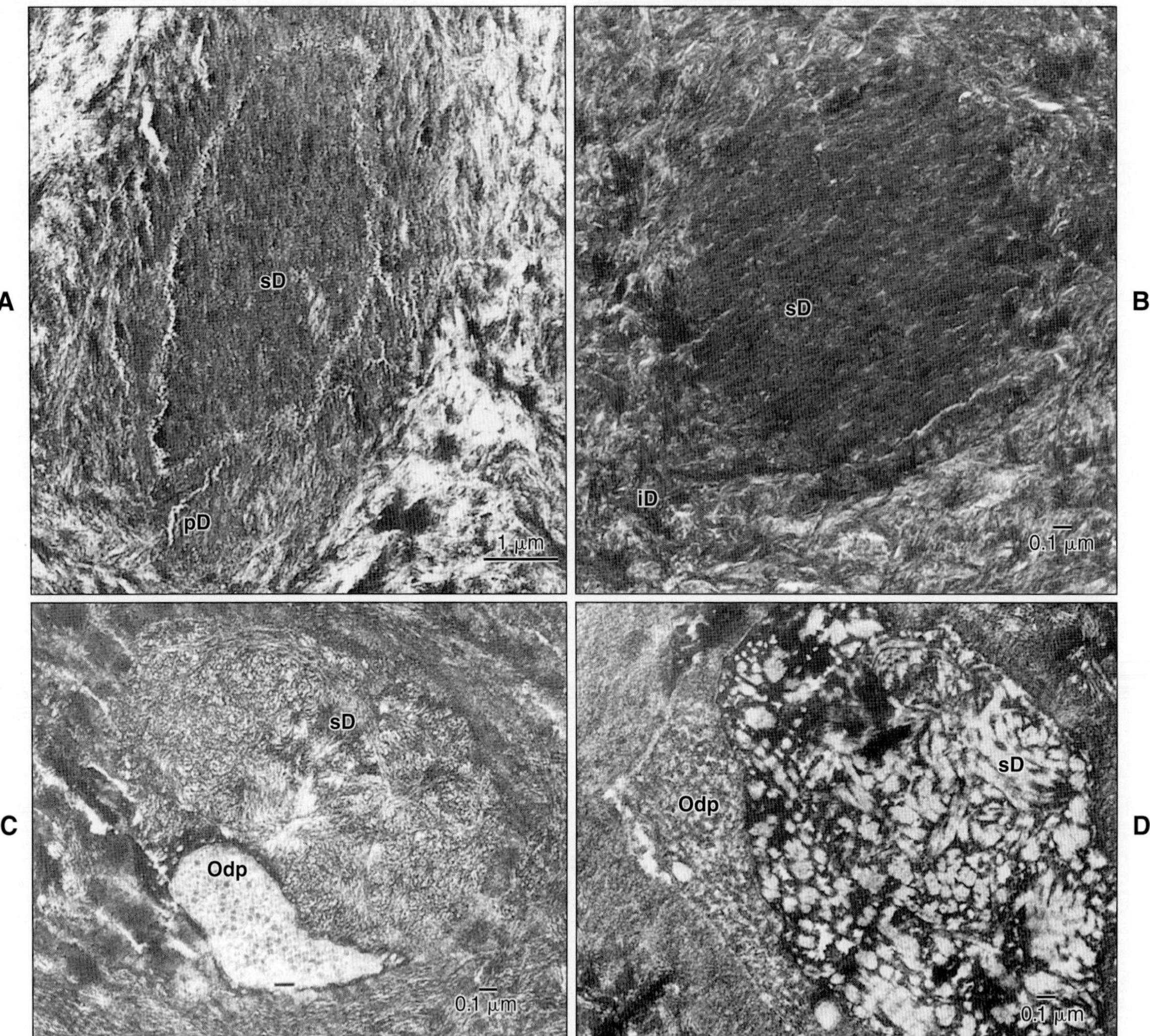

Fig. 8.34 Sclerosis of the dentinal tubule, which occurs in different ways. (A) The tubule is filled with an even deposition of mineral, which has been interpreted as a spread of peritubular dentin. However, at (B), tubular occlusion has occurred in a similar way, although no peritubular dentin is recognizable. (C) Diffuse mineralization is occurring in the presence of a viable odontoblast process *(Odp)*. (D) Mineralization occurs within the odontoblast process and around collagen fibrils deposited within the tubule as a reactionary response. *iD,* Intertubular dentin; *pD,* peritubular dentin; *sD,* sclerotic dentin. (A, D, From Tsatsas BG, Frank RM: Ultrastructure of dentinal tubular substances near the dentino-enamel junction, *Calcif Tissue Res* 9:238–242, 1972; B, from Frank RM, Nalbandian H: Teeth. In *Handbook of microscopic anatomy*, vol 6, New York, NY, 1989, Springer Verlag; C, from Frank RM, Voegel JC: Ultrastructure of human odontoblast process and its mineralization during dental caries, *Caries Res* 14:367–380, 1980.)

was once) occupied by an odontoblast process, the tubule is delimited by a layer of peritubular dentin, and fluid circulates between dentin and the process. This explanation is simplistic, however, and a number of debatable issues require amplification, especially because the dentin-pulp complex is so crucial to the everyday practice of dentistry. Perhaps the most important issue is the extent of the odontoblast process within the dentinal tubule. Using labeled antibodies against proteins making up the cytoskeleton (actin, vimentin, and tubulin), researchers have shown that the majority of dentinal tubules exhibit these components along their entire extent, up to the dentinoenamel junction. Because these proteins are exclusively intracellular, the presence of a process can be inferred.

Another question concerns the contents of the space between the odontoblast process and the tubule wall, the so-called *dentinal fluid.* The assumption has been made that the space is filled with fluid (equivalent to tissue fluid), but this is difficult to prove because the demonstration of fluid is achieved only after cavity preparation, which causes the fluid to leak out. What information exists concerning tubule content indicates that proteoglycans, tenascin, fibronectin, and the serum proteins (albumin, HS glycoprotein, transferrin [in ratios differing from those found in serum]) may be present; this is clearly a complex mixture about which much more needs to be learned.

Fibroblasts

The cells occurring in greatest numbers in the pulp are fibroblasts (Figs. 8.51 and 8.52). Fibroblasts are particularly numerous in the coronal portion of the pulp where they form the cell-rich zone. The function of fibroblasts is to form and maintain the pulp matrix,

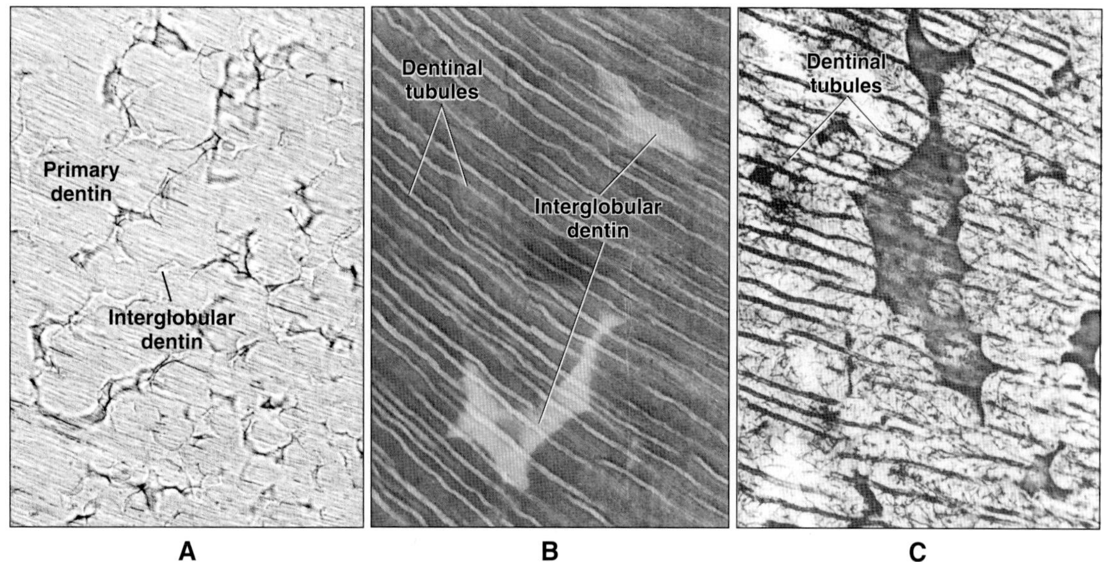

Fig. 8.35 Interglobular dentin. (A) Ground section. (B) Demineralized section stained with hematoxylin-eosin. (C) Demineralized section stained with silver nitrate. The spheric borders of the interglobular areas indicate the failure of calcospherite fusion. (B) Staining of nonmineralized matrix is lighter; in (C) it is darker. Dentinal tubules pass through the interglobular dentin, but no peritubular dentin is present in these areas. Silver nitrate staining reveals numerous smaller tubules into which run the branches of the odontoblast process. (C, Courtesy Dr. Alexanian.)

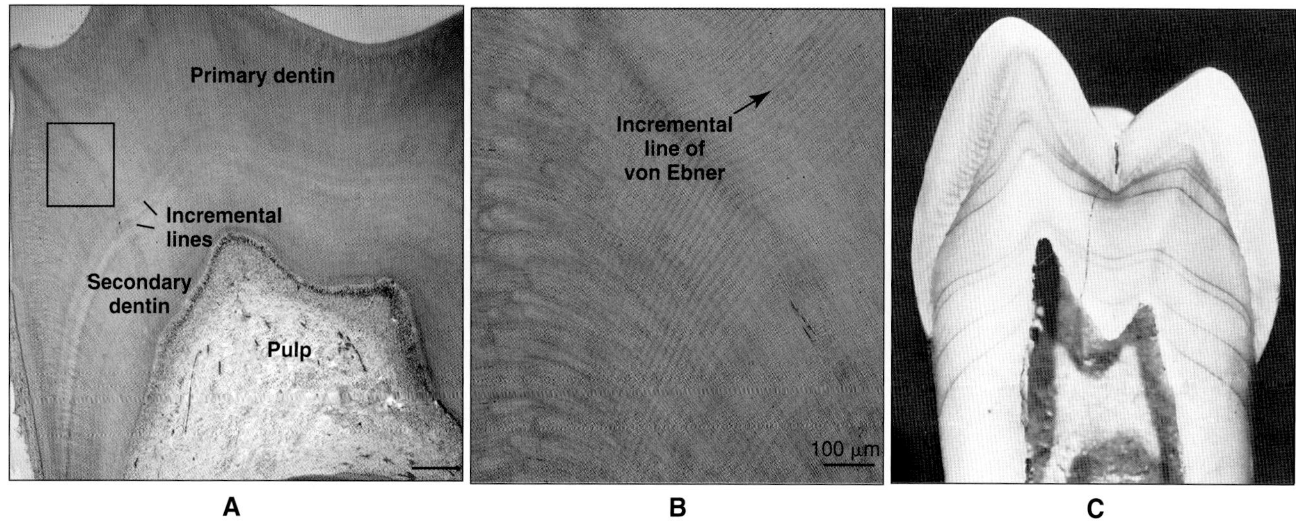

Fig. 8.36 (A) Histologic section showing fine incremental deposition of von Ebner lines in dentin. (B) A higher magnification of the boxed area in (A). (C) Tooth section of a person who received tetracycline intermittently. The drug has been incorporated at successive dentin-forming fronts, mimicking incremental line patterns in both coronal and radicular dentin.

which consists of collagen and ground substance. The histologic appearance of these fibroblasts reflects their functional state. In young pulps the fibroblasts are actively synthesizing matrix and therefore have a plump cytoplasm and extensive amounts of all the usual organelles associated with synthesis and secretion. With age, the need for synthesis diminishes, and the fibroblasts appear as flattened spindle-shaped cells with dense nuclei. Fibroblasts of the pulp also have the capability of ingesting and degrading collagen when appropriately stimulated (see Chapter 4). Apoptotic cell death (see Chapter 7) of pulpal fibroblasts, especially in the cell-rich zone, indicates that some turnover of these cells is occurring. The fine structure of a young pulp is shown in Fig. 8.52. Desmosomes are often present between these cells.

Undifferentiated Ectomesenchymal Cells

Undifferentiated mesenchymal cells represent the pool from which connective tissue cells of the pulp are derived. Depending on the stimulus, these cells may give rise to odontoblasts and fibroblasts. These cells are found throughout the cell-rich area and the pulp core and often are related to blood vessels. Under the light microscope, undifferentiated mesenchymal cells appear as large polyhedral cells possessing a large, lightly stained, centrally placed nucleus. These cells display

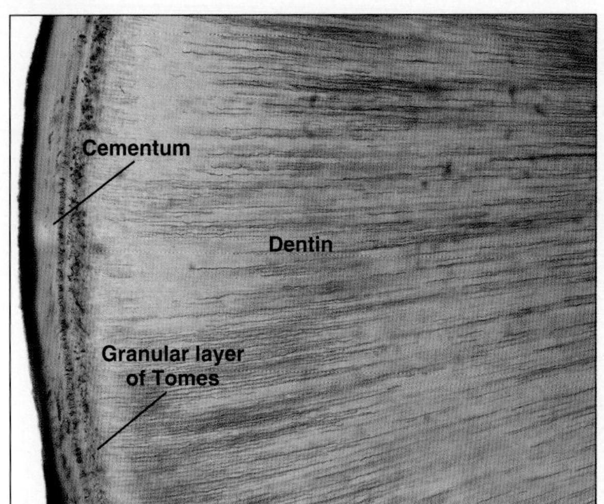

Fig. 8.37 Transverse ground section across the root of a tooth. The granular layer of Tomes is visible just beneath the cementum.

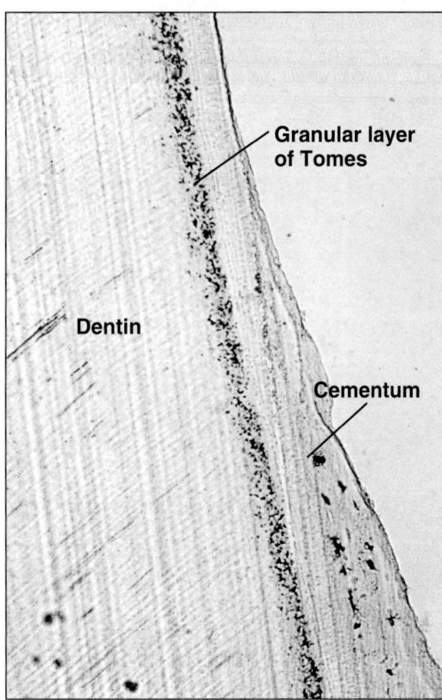

Fig. 8.38 Longitudinal ground section of the granular layer of Tomes.

abundant cytoplasm and peripheral cytoplasmic extensions. In older pulps the number of undifferentiated mesenchymal cells diminishes along with the number of other cells in the pulp core. This reduction, along with other aging factors, reduces the regenerative potential of the pulp.

Dental Pulp Stem Cells

Mesenchymal stem cells have been isolated from the dental pulp of adult and deciduous teeth. These postnatal dental pulp stem cells have a self-renewal capability and, under appropriate environmental conditions, can differentiate into odontoblasts, chondrocytes, adipocytes, and neurons. It has also been shown that these cells have the capacity to give rise to osteoblasts and may therefore be a promising tool for bone regeneration.

Inflammatory Cells

Macrophages tend to be located throughout the pulp center. Macrophages appear as large oval or sometimes elongated cells that, under the light microscope, exhibit a dark-stained nucleus. Pulp macrophages, as at other sites derived from blood, are involved in the elimination of dead cells, the presence of which further indicates that turnover of dental pulp fibroblasts occurs.

In normal pulps, T lymphocytes are found, but B lymphocytes are scarce. There are also some leukocytes (neutrophils and eosinophils), which increase substantially during infection.

Bone marrow–derived, antigen-presenting dendritic cells (Fig. 8.53) are found in and around the odontoblast layer in nonerupted teeth and in erupted teeth beneath the odontoblast layer. They have a close relationship to vascular and neural elements, and their function is similar to that of the Langerhans cells found in epithelium (see Chapter 12) in that they capture and present foreign antigen to the T cells. These cells participate in immunosurveillance and increase in number in carious teeth where they infiltrate the odontoblast layer and can project their processes into the tubules.

Matrix and Ground Substance

The extracellular compartment of the pulp (matrix) consists of collagen fibers and ground substance. The fibers are principally types I and III collagen. In young pulps, single fibrils of collagen are found scattered between the pulp cells. Whereas the overall collagen content of the pulp increases with age, the ratio between types I and III remains stable, and the increased amount of extracellular collagen organizes into fiber bundles (Fig. 8.54). The greatest concentration of collagen generally occurs in the most apical portion of the pulp. This fact is of practical significance when a pulpectomy is performed during the course of endodontic treatment. Engaging the pulp with a barbed broach in the region of the apex affords a better opportunity to remove the tissue intact than does engaging the broach more coronally, where the pulp is more gelatinous and liable to tear.

The ground substance of these tissues resembles that of any other loose connective tissue. Composed principally of glycosaminoglycans, glycoproteins, and water, the ground substance supports the cells and acts as the medium for transport of nutrients from the vasculature to the cells and of metabolites from the cells to the vasculature. Alterations in composition of the ground substance caused by age or disease interfere with this function, producing metabolic changes, reduced cellular function, and irregularities in mineral deposition.

VASCULATURE AND LYMPHATIC SUPPLY

The circulation establishes the tissue fluid pressure found in the extracellular compartment of the pulp. Blood vessels enter and exit the dental pulp by way of the apical and accessory foramina. One or sometimes two vessels of arteriolar size (~150 μm) enter the apical foramen with the sensory and sympathetic nerve bundles. Smaller vessels enter the pulp through the minor foramina. Vessels leaving the dental pulp are associated closely with the arterioles and nerve bundles entering the apical foramen. Once the arterioles enter the pulp, an increase in the caliber of the lumen occurs with a reduction in thickness of the vessel wall. The arterioles occupy a central position within the pulp and, as they pass through the radicular portion of pulp, give off smaller lateral branches that extend toward and branch into the subodontoblastic area. The number of branches given off in this manner increases as the arterioles pass coronally so that, in the coronal region of the pulp, they divide and subdivide to form an extensive vascular capillary network. Occasionally, U-looping of pulpal arterioles is seen, and this anatomic configuration is believed to be related to the regulation of blood flow.

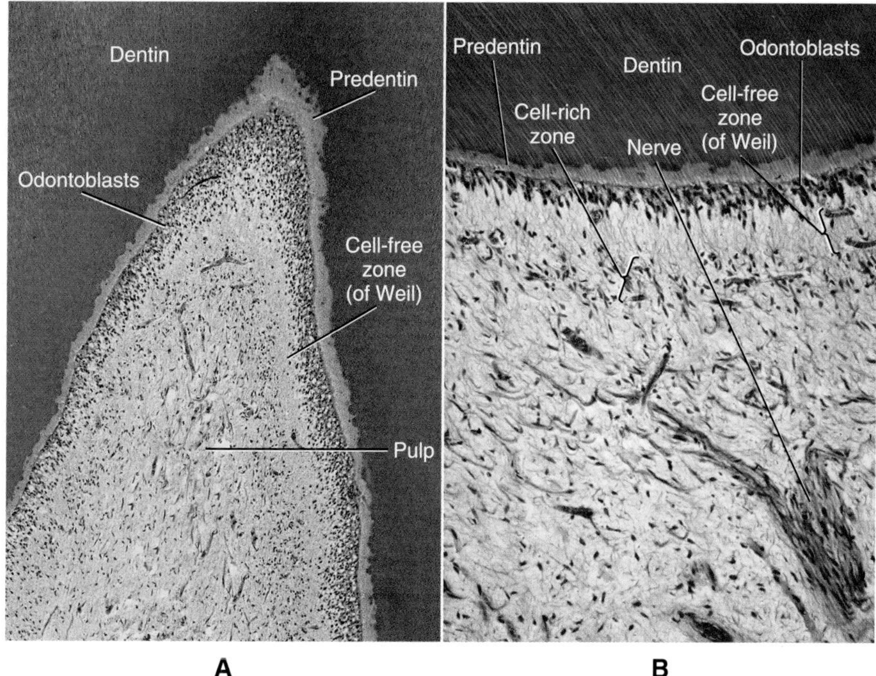

[illegible] (A) [illegible] power photomicrograph of the dentin-pulp complex. (B) At higher power, the cell-free zone (of Weil) beneath the odontoblast layer is clearly visible as is the [illegible]

The extensive vascular network in the coronal portion of pulp can be demonstrated by scanning electron microscopy of vascular casts (Fig. 8.55). The main portion of the capillary bed is located in the subodontoblastic area. Some terminal capillary loops extend upward between the odontoblasts to abut the predentin if dentinogenesis is occurring (see Figs. 8.18 and 8.41A). Located on the periphery of the capillaries at random intervals are pericytes, which form a partial circumferential sheath about the endothelial wall. These cells are believed to be contractile cells capable of reducing the size of the vessel lumen. Arteriovenous anastomoses also have been identified in the dental pulp (Fig. 8.56). The anastomosis is of arteriolar size, with an endothelium whose cells bulge out into the lumen. Anastomoses are points of direct communication between the arterial and venous sides of the circulation.

The efferent (drainage) side of the circulation is composed of an extensive system of venules, the diameters of which are comparable to those of arterioles, but their walls are much thinner, making their lumina comparatively larger. The muscle layer in the venule walls is intermittent and thin.

Lymphatic vessels also occur in pulp tissue; they arise as small, blind, thin-walled vessels in the coronal region of the pulp (Fig. 8.57) and pass apically through the middle and radicular regions of the pulp to exit via one or two larger vessels through the apical foramen. The lymphatic vessels are differentiated from small venules by the presence of discontinuities in their vessel walls and the absence of red blood cells in their lumina.

Sympathetic adrenergic nerves terminate in relation to the smooth muscle cells of the arteriolar walls (Fig. 8.58A). Afferent free nerve endings terminate in relation to arterioles, capillaries, and veins (see Fig. 8.58B); they serve as effectors by releasing various neuropeptides that exert an effect on the vascular system.

INNERVATION OF THE DENTIN-PULP COMPLEX

The dental pulp is innervated richly. Nerves enter the pulp through the apical foramen, along with afferent blood vessels, and, together, form the neurovascular bundle. Depending on the size of the foramina, nerves can also accompany blood vessels through accessory foramina. In the pulp chamber the nerves generally follow the same course as the afferent vessels, beginning as large nerve bundles that arborize peripherally as they extend occlusally through the pulp core (Fig. 8.59). These branches ultimately contribute to an extensive plexus of nerves in the cell-free zone of Weil just below the cell bodies of the odontoblasts in the crown portion of the tooth. This plexus of nerves, called the *subodontoblastic plexus of Raschkow*, can be demonstrated in silver nitrate–stained sections under light microscope (Fig. 8.60) or by immunocytochemical techniques to detect various proteins associated with nerves (Fig. 8.61A). In the root, no corresponding plexus exists. Instead, branches are given off from the ascending trunks at intervals that further arborize, with each branch supplying its own territory (see Fig. 8.61B).

The nerve bundles that enter the tooth pulp consist principally of sensory afferent nerves of the trigeminal (fifth cranial) nerve and sympathetic branches from the superior cervical ganglion. Each bundle contains myelinated and unmyelinated axons (Fig. 8.62). Fine structural investigations of animal tooth pulp have shown increased discontinuities in the investing perineurium as nerves ascend coronally. Furthermore, as the nerve bundles ascend coronally, the myelinated axons gradually lose their myelin coating so that a proportional increase in the number of unmyelinated axons occurs in the more coronal aspect of the tooth.

Although most of the nerve bundles terminate in the subodontoblastic plexus as free, unmyelinated nerve endings, a small number of axons pass between the odontoblasts (see Fig. 8.60A) and sometimes extend into dentinal tubules (Fig. 8.63). No organized junction or synaptic relationship has been noted between axons and the odontoblast process. Occasionally, some nerves enter the dentinal tubules; however, the number of tubules containing nerve fibers in relation to the overall number of tubules is small. The literature also contains reports of nerves running within predentin at right angles to the tubules, and such loops generally are assumed to represent isolated nerve fibrils

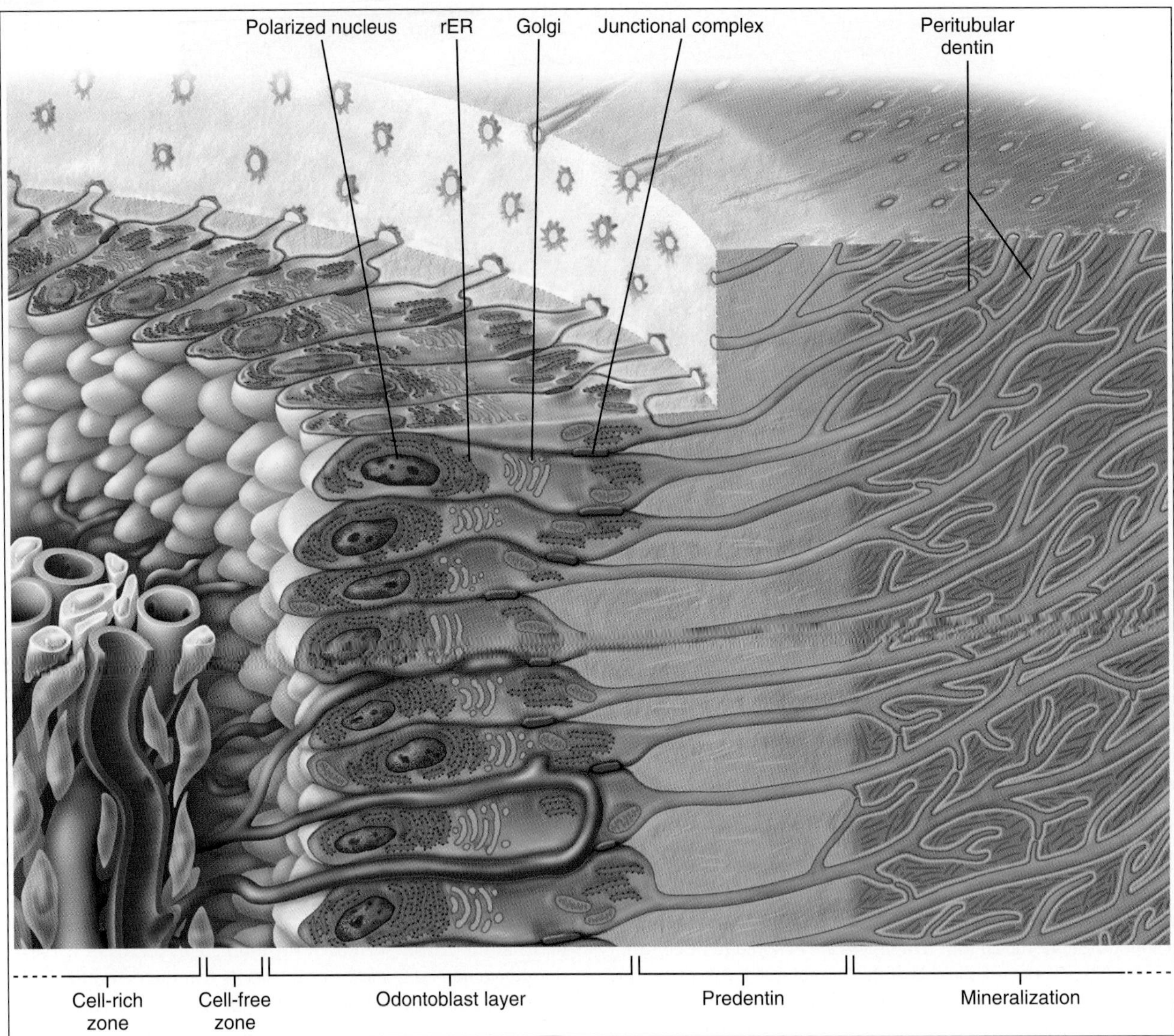

Fig. 8.40 Schematic representation of the cells bordering the pulp. *rER,* Rough endoplasmic reticulum.

from the plexus of Raschkow that are caught up by the advancing process of dentinogenesis (Fig. 8.64). However, this description may be too simplified; recent studies examining tangential sections of predentin have indicated that some of these fibers undergo dendritic ramification (Fig. 8.65). The functional significance, if any, of this pattern of innervation within the predentin has not been determined.

DENTIN SENSITIVITY

One of the most unusual features of the pulp-dentin complex is its sensitivity. The extreme sensitivity of this complex is difficult to explain because this characteristic provides no apparent evolutionary benefit. The overwhelming sensation appreciated by this complex is pain, although evidence now indicates that pulpal afferent nerves can distinguish mechanical, thermal, and tactile stimuli as well (but always as some form of discomfort). Convergence of pulpal afferent nerves with other pulpal afferent nerves and afferent nerves from other orofacial structures in the central nervous system often makes pulpal pain difficult to localize.

Among the numerous stimuli that can evoke a painful response when applied to dentin are many that are related to clinical dental practice such as cold air or water, mechanical contact by a probe or bur, and dehydration with cotton wool or a stream of air. Of interest is the observation that some products such as histamine and bradykinin, known to produce pain in other tissues, do not produce pain in dentin.

Three mechanisms, all involving an understanding of the structure of dentin and pulp, have been proposed to explain dentin sensitivity: (1) The dentin contains nerve endings that respond when it is stimulated; (2) the odontoblasts serve as receptors and are coupled to nerves in the pulp; and (3) the tubular nature of dentin permits fluid movement to occur within the tubule when a stimulus is applied, a movement registered by pulpal free nerve endings close to the odontoblasts (Fig. 8.66). Regarding the first possibility, all that can be stated is that some nerves occur within some tubules in the inner dentin, but dentin sensitivity does not depend solely, if at all, on the stimulation of such nerve endings.

The second possible mechanism to explain dentin sensitivity considers the odontoblast to be a receptor cell. This attractive concept has been considered, abandoned, and reconsidered for many reasons. The point once was argued that because the odontoblast is of neural crest origin, it retains an ability to transduce and propagate an impulse. What was missing was the demonstration of a synaptic relationship between the odontoblast and pulpal nerves. That the membrane potential of odontoblasts measured in vitro is too low to permit transduction and

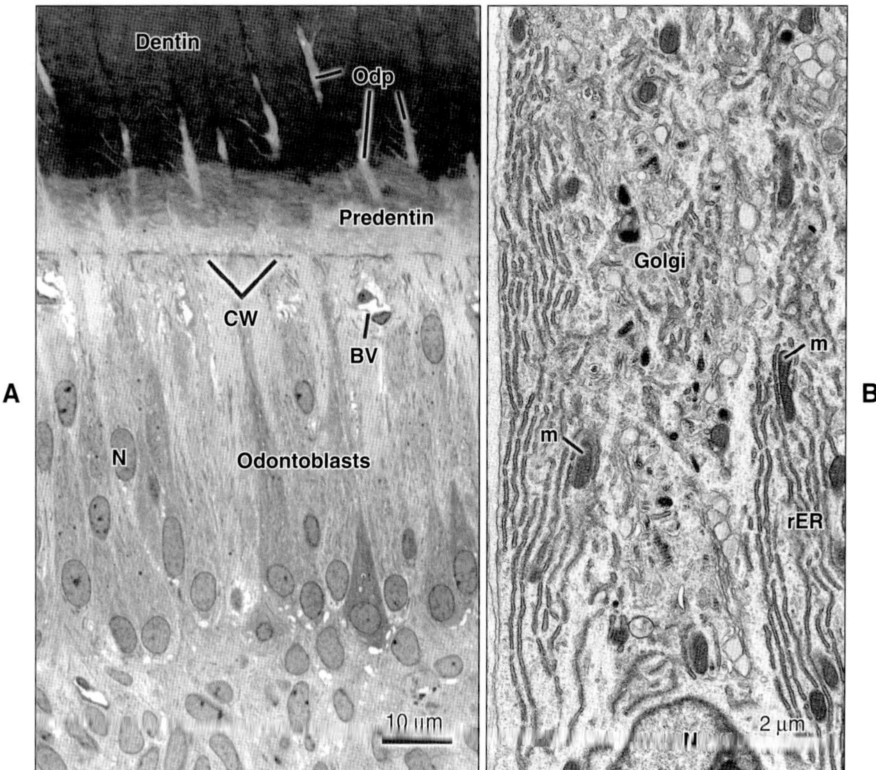

Fig. 8.41 (A) Low-magnification view of odontoblasts taken by examining the section in the scanning electron microscope. These tall, bowling pin–shaped cells border the pulp and form a tight layer against predentin. Despite the presence of nuclei *(N)* at different levels, there is only one layer of odontoblasts that extend cell processes *(Odp)* across predentin into dentin. Note the fine branches on these processes. Blood vessels *(BV)* are present among the cells. (B) Transmission electron micrograph; a large portion of the supranuclear compartment of odontoblasts is occupied by an extensive Golgi complex *(Golgi)* surrounded by abundant rough endoplasmic reticulum *(rER)* profiles. *CW,* Cell web; *m,* mitochondria.

that local anesthetics and protein precipitants do not abolish sensitivity also militated against this concept. The fact that odontoblast processes extend to the dentinoenamel junction and the demonstration of gap junctions between odontoblasts (and possibly between odontoblasts and pulpal nerves) are consistent with the direct role of the odontoblast in dentin sensitivity.

The third mechanism proposed to explain dentin sensitivity involves movement of fluid through the dentinal tubules. This hydrodynamic theory, which fits much of the experimental and morphologic data, proposes that fluid movement through the tubule distorts the local pulpal environment and is sensed by the free nerve endings in the plexus of Raschkow. Thus when dentin is first exposed, small blebs of fluid can be seen on the cavity floor. When the cavity is dried with air or cotton wool, a greater loss of fluid is induced, leading to more movement and more pain. The increased sensitivity at the dentinoenamel junction is explained by the profuse branching of the tubules in this region. The hydrodynamic hypothesis also explains why local anesthetics applied to exposed dentin fail to block sensitivity and why pain is produced by thermal change, mechanical probing, hypertonic solutions, and dehydration.

Attention must be drawn, however, to the fact that dentin sensitivity bestows no benefit on the organism and to the possibility that this sensitivity results from more important functional requirements of the innervated dentin-pulp complex. Increasingly, appreciation is given to the fact that pulpal innervation has a significant role to play in pulpal homeostasis and its defense mechanisms and that this role involves interplay between nerves, blood vessels, and immunocompetent cells, which have been shown to contact the vascular and neural elements of the pulp. Immunocompetent cells contact vascular endothelium and have close association with free nerve endings (Fig. 8.67). Furthermore, immunocompetent cells express receptors for various neuropeptides. This common biochemical language between the immune, nervous, and vascular systems suggests a functional unit of importance in pulp biology.

PULP STONES

Pulp stones, or denticles, frequently are found in pulp tissue (Fig. 8.68). As their name implies, they are discrete calcified masses with calcium-phosphorus ratios comparable to that of dentin. They may be singular or multiple in any tooth and are more common at the orifice of the pulp chamber or within the root canal. Histologically they usually consist of concentric layers of mineralized tissue formed by surface accretion around blood thrombi, dying or dead cells, or collagen fibers. Occasionally a pulp stone may contain tubules and be surrounded by cells resembling odontoblasts. Such stones are rare and, if seen, occur close to the apex of the tooth. Such stones are referred to as true pulp stones as opposed to stones having no cells associated with them.

Pulp stones may form in several teeth and, indeed, in every tooth in some individuals. If, during the formation of a pulp stone, union occurs between it and the dentin wall or if secondary dentin deposition surrounds the stone, the pulp stone is said to be attached, as distinguished from a free stone (which is completely surrounded by soft tissue). The presence of pulp stones is significant in that they reduce

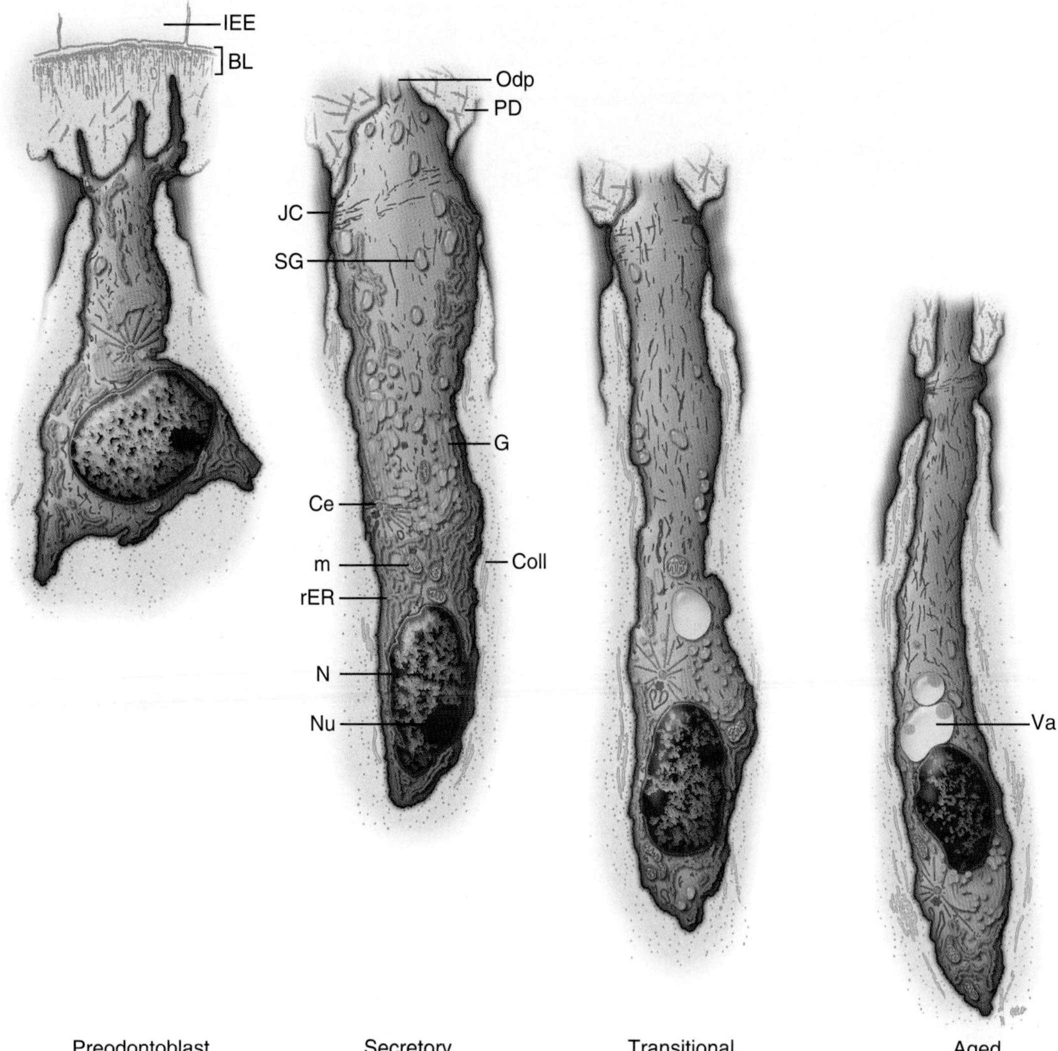

Fig. 8.42 Diagrammatic representation of the various functional stages of the odontoblast. *BL,* Basal lamina; *Ce,* centriole; *Coll,* collagen; *G,* Golgi complex; *IEE,* inner enamel epithelium; *JC,* junctional complex; *m,* mitochondria; *N,* nucleus; *Nu,* nucleolus; *Odp,* odontoblast process; *PD,* predentin; *rER,* rough endoplasmic reticulum; *SG,* secretory granule; *Va,* vacuole. (From Couve E: Ultrastructural changes during the life cycle of human odontoblast, *Arch Oral Biol* 31:643–651, 1986.)

the overall number of cells within the pulp and act as an impediment to debridement and enlargement of the root canal system during endodontic treatment.

AGE CHANGES

The dentin-pulp complex, like all body tissues, undergoes change with time. The most conspicuous change is the decreasing volume of the pulp chamber and root canal brought about by continued dentin deposition (Fig. 8.69). In old teeth the root canal is often no more than a thin channel (Fig. 8.70); indeed, the root canal on occasion can appear to be obliterated almost completely. Such continued restriction in pulp volume probably brings about a reduction in the vascular supply to the pulp and initiates many of the other age changes found in this tissue.

From about the age of 20 years, cells gradually decrease in number until age 70, when the cell density has decreased by about half. The distribution of collagen fibrils may change with age, leading to the appearance of fibrous bundles.

With age come a loss and a degeneration of myelinated and unmyelinated axons that correlate with an age-related reduction in sensitivity. There is also an increase in dead tracts and sclerotic dentin, which, together with the presence of reparative dentin, contributes to reducing sensitivity.

Another age change is the occurrence of irregular areas of dystrophic calcification, especially in the central pulp (Fig. 8.71). Dystrophic calcifications generally originate in relation to blood vessels or as diffuse mineral deposits along collagen bundles.

That the pulp supports the dentin and that age changes within the pulp are reflected in the dentin have been emphasized. Within dentin the deposition of intratubular dentin continues, resulting in a gradual reduction of the tubule diameter. This continued deposition often leads to complete closure of the tubule, as can be seen readily in a ground section of dentin because the dentin becomes translucent (or sclerotic). Sclerotic dentin is common near the root apex in teeth from middle-aged individuals (see Fig. 8.33). Associated with sclerotic dentin are an increased brittleness and a decreased permeability of the

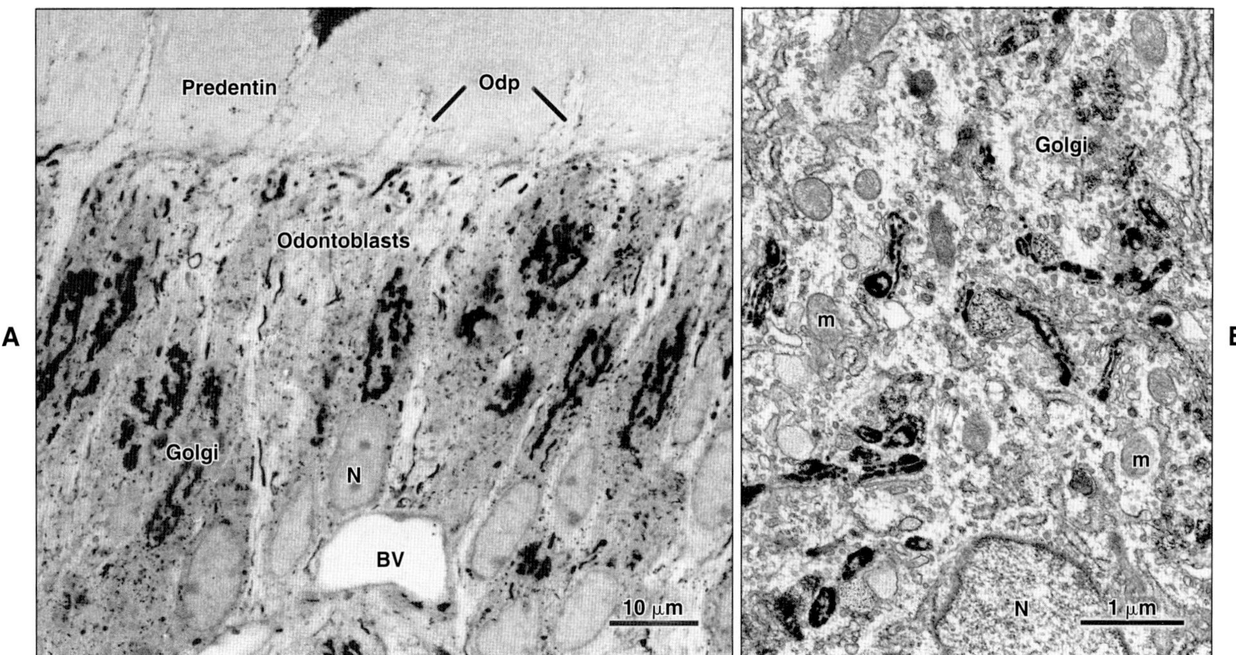

Fig. 8.43 Cytochemical preparations for a Golgi-associated phosphatase visualized using scanning (A) and transmission (B) electron microscopes, illustrating the position and extent of this protein-synthesizing organelle in the supranuclear compartment. Reaction product is found selectively in the intermediate saccules of the Golgi complex. *BV,* Blood vessel; *m,* mitochondria; *N,* nucleus; *Odp,* odontoblast process.

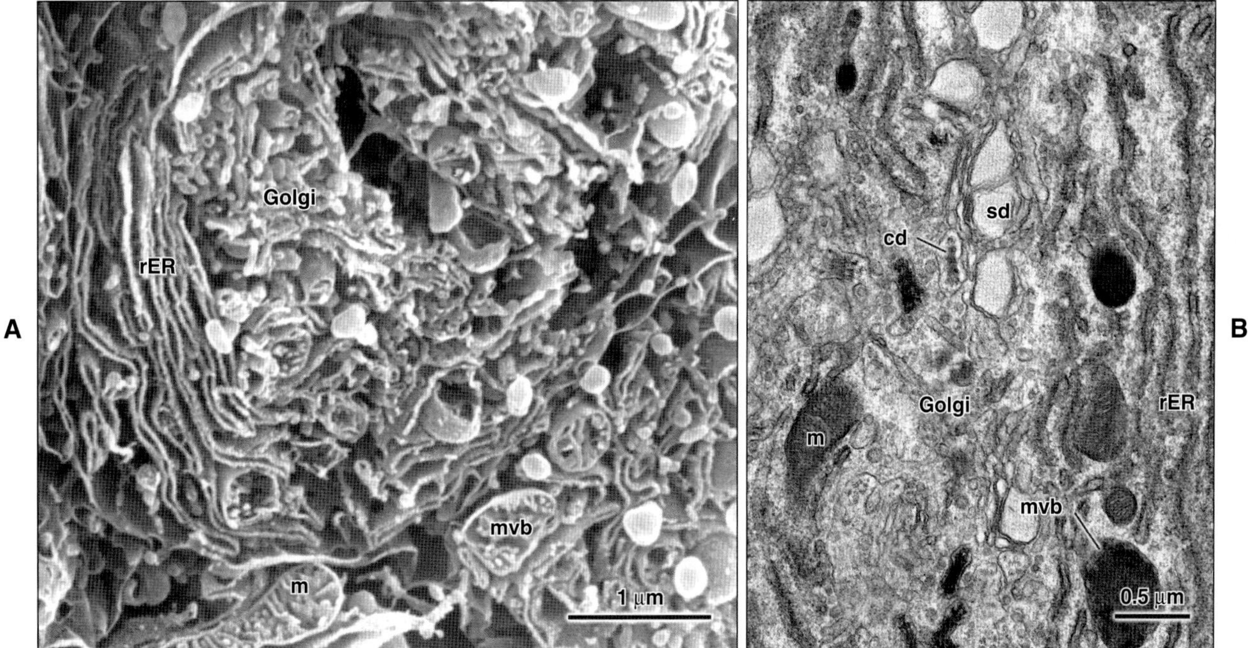

Fig. 8.44 (A) Scanning electron micrograph of a cross-fractured odontoblast at the level of the Golgi *(Golgi)* complex. Rough endoplasmic reticulum *(rER)* surrounds the Golgi complex. (B) Transmission electron micrograph; Golgi saccules exhibit cylindric *(cd)* and spheric *(sd)* distentions in which the collagen molecule is processed. *m,* Mitochondria; *mvb,* multivesicular body.

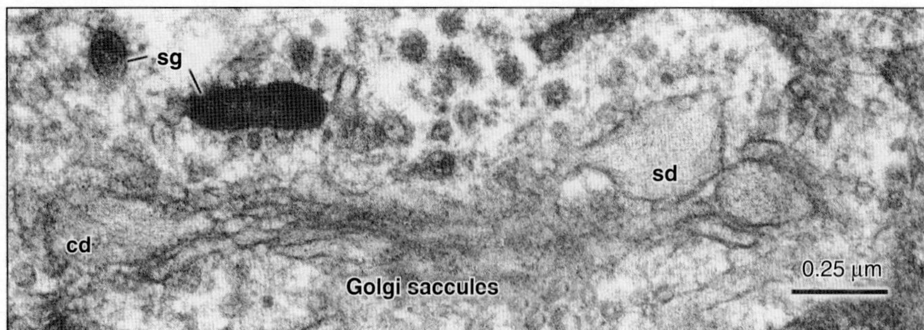

Fig. 8.45 Transmission electron micrograph of a Golgi stack. Cylindric *(cd)* and spheric *(sd)* distentions can be seen at the extremities of the saccules. Cds, when mature, bud off as atypical elongated and electron-dense collagen-containing secretory granules *(sg)*.

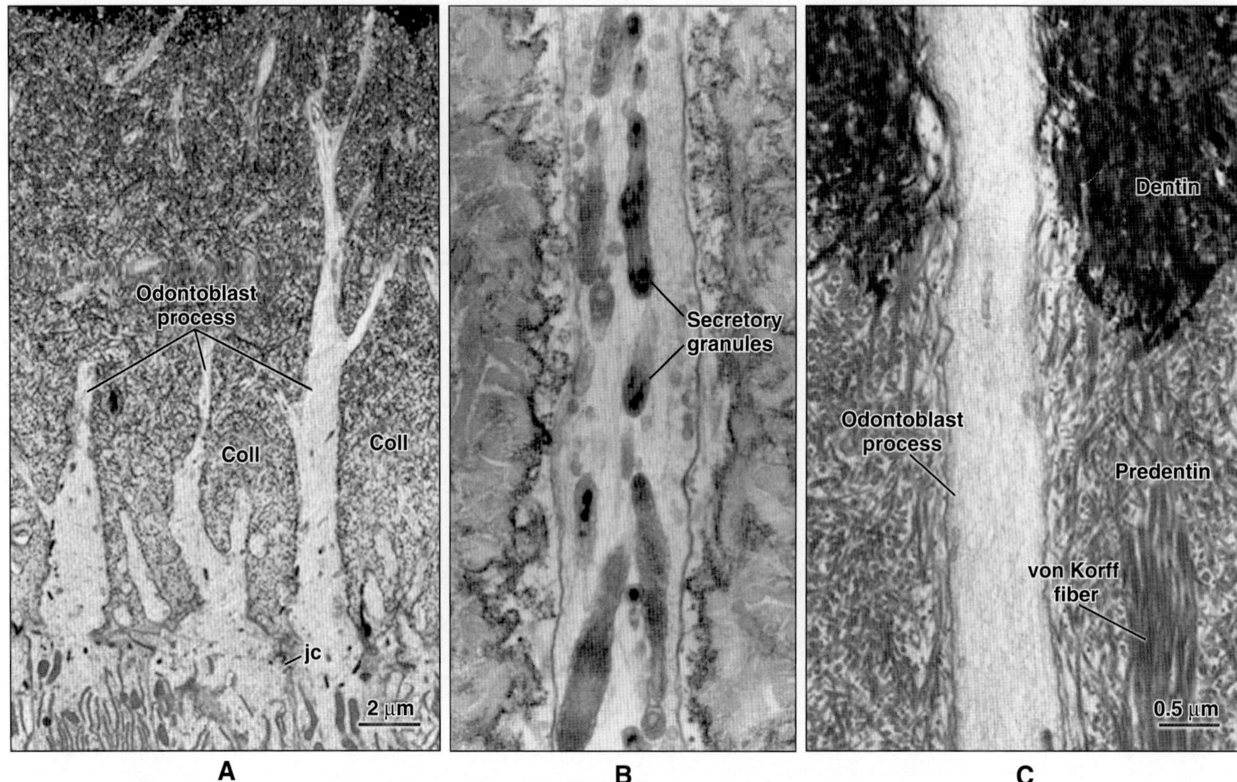

Fig. 8.46 Electron micrographs of the odontoblast process. (A) The process is an arborizing cell extension that extends above the apical junctional complex *(jc)* into predentin and dentin. The fibrils become thicker and more compact toward the dentin. (B) Numerous collagen-containing secretory granules are found in the process, particularly near its base where the surrounding collagen fibrils *(Coll)* are packed less densely. (C) Process at the predentin-dentin junction. A bundle of larger collagen fibrils, von Korff fibers, runs parallel to the process. Note the paucity of elongated, collagen-containing secretory granules at this level.

dentin. Another age change found within dentin is an increase in dead tracts (Fig. 8.72).

RESPONSE TO ENVIRONMENTAL STIMULI

Many of the age changes in the pulp-dentin complex render it more resistant to environmental injury. For example, the spread of caries is slowed by tubule occlusion. Age changes also accelerate in response to environmental stimuli, such as caries or attrition of enamel. The response of the complex to gradual attrition is to produce more sclerotic dentin and deposit secondary dentin at an increased rate. If the stimulus is more severe, tertiary dentin is formed at the ends of the tubules affected by the injury.

Age change, however, also lessens the ability of the pulp-dentin complex to repair itself. Injury has been defined as the interference of a stimulus with cellular metabolism. If pulpal injury occurs, the age of the pulp determines its ability to repair the damage. Because cell metabolism is high in young pulps, their cells are prone to injury, which manifests as altered cell function, but recovery occurs rapidly. If injury is such that the odontoblasts are destroyed, the possibility exists in young pulps for the differentiation of new odontoblasts from the mesenchymal cells of the pulp and the formation of repair dentin. This potential is reduced considerably with age.

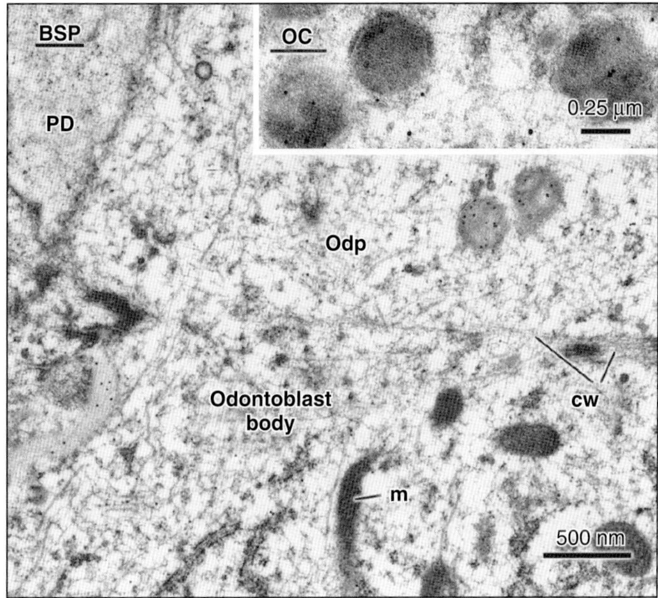

Fig. 8.47 Immunogold preparations for bone sialoprotein *(BSP)* and osteocalcin *(OC, inset)*. Round granules are immunoreactive *(black dots)* for these two matrix proteins, suggesting that a secretory granule population may exist, distinct from the elongated collagen-containing ones that may be responsible for the transport and secretion of noncollagenous dentin matrix proteins. A cell web *(cw)* is associated with the apical junctions and separates the odontoblast body from the process *(Odp)*. *m*, Mitochondria; *PD*, predentin.

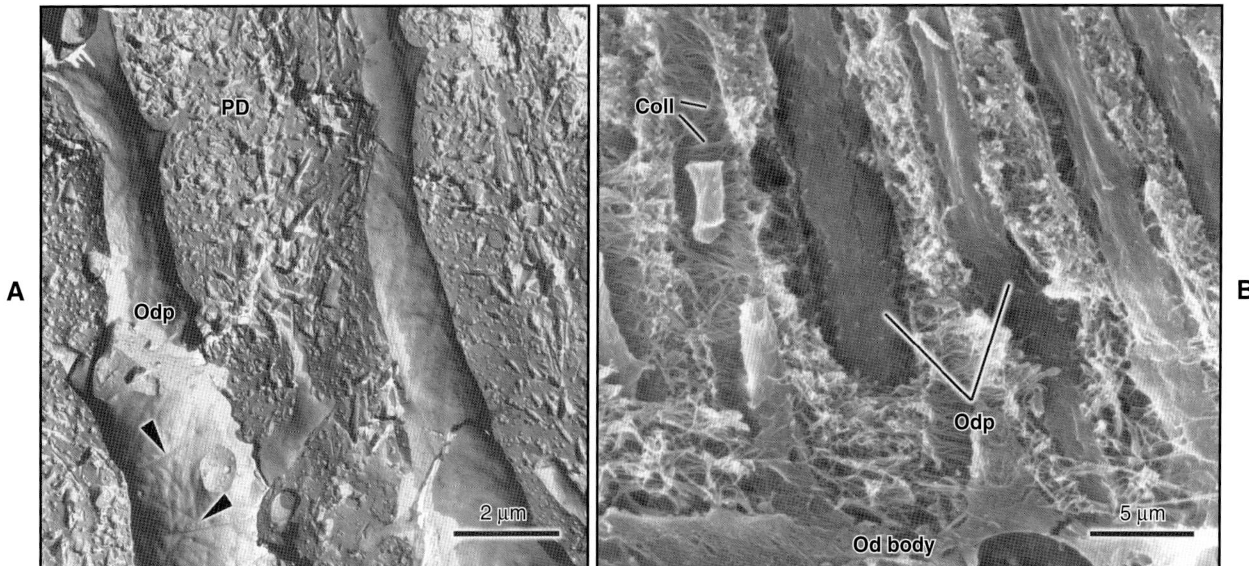

Fig. 8.48 Freeze-fracture (A) and scanning electron microscope (B) preparations illustrating the odontoblast process *(Odp)* near its point of emergence from the cell body. The process is surrounded by the collagen *(Coll)* fibrils of predentin *(PD)*. The fibrils are associated intimately with the process, and in certain areas they imprint the membrane *(arrowheads)*. *Od*, Odontoblast.

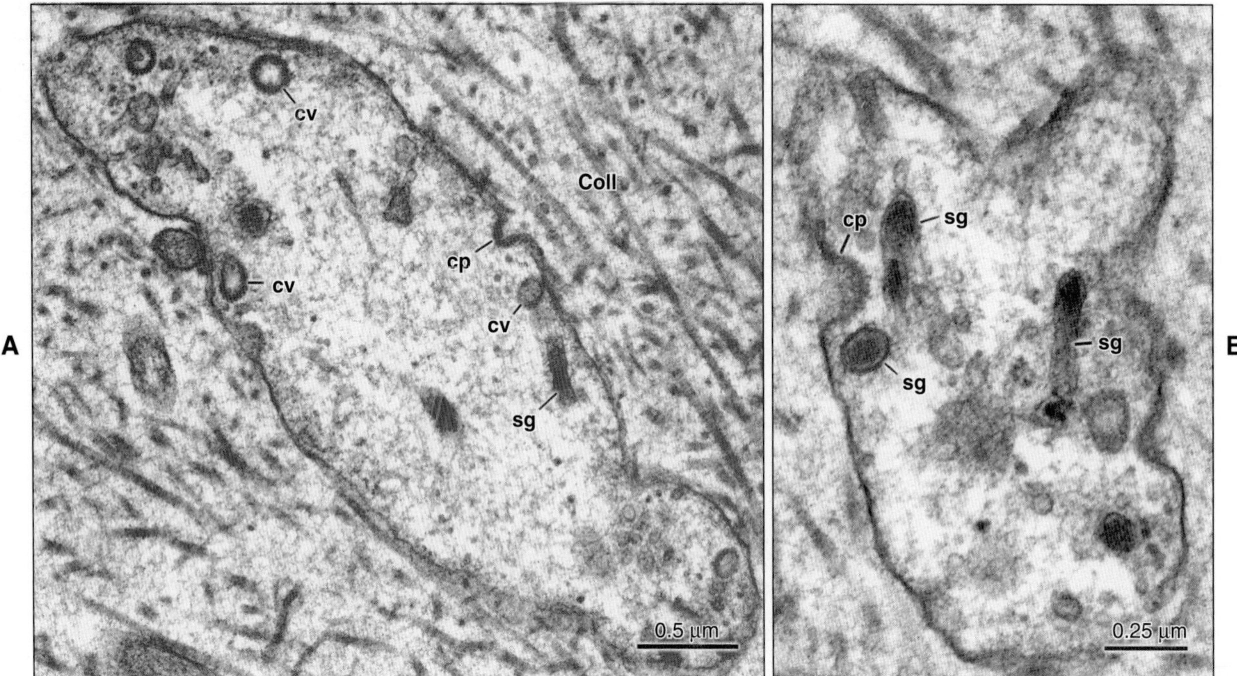

Fig. 8.49 (A, B) Two views of cross-cut odontoblast processes at the level of predentin, close to the cell body. The processes are surrounded by collagen *(Coll)* fibrils and contain elongated and round secretory granules *(sg)*, coated pits *(cp)*, and vesicles *(cv)* suggestive of intense pinocytotic activity along the cell membrane. (B) Same image as in (A) except at a higher magnification.

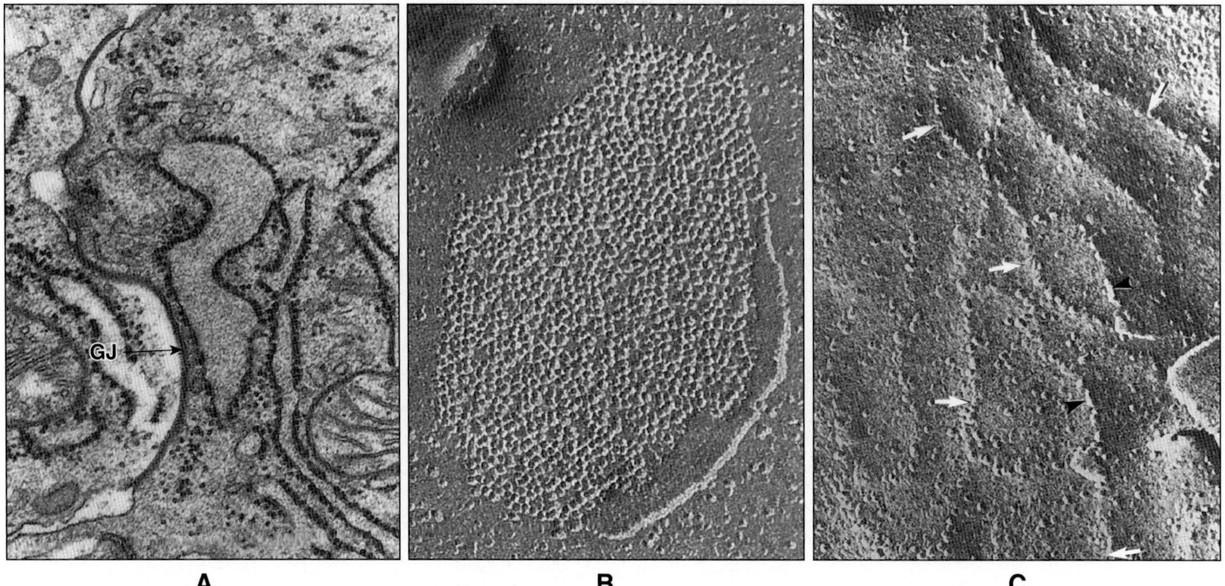

Fig. 8.50 Junctions between odontoblasts. (A) Electron micrograph showing a gap junction *(GJ)*. (B) Freeze fracture of a GJ. (C) Freeze fracture of a tight junction consisting of extensive and branched rows of zipperlike particles *(arrows)*. (A, C, Courtesy M. Weinstock; B, from Arana-Chavez VE, Katchburian E: Development of tight junctions between odontoblasts in early dentinogenesis as revealed by freeze-fracture, *Anat Rec* 248:332–338, 1997.)

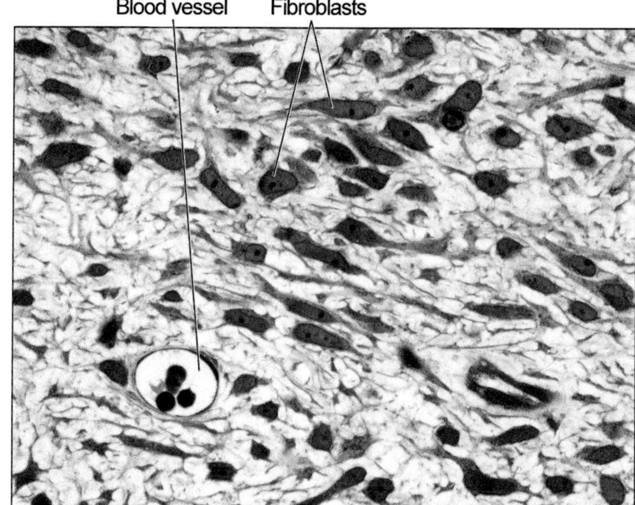

Fig. 8.51 Light microscopic appearance of fibroblasts in the dental pulp.

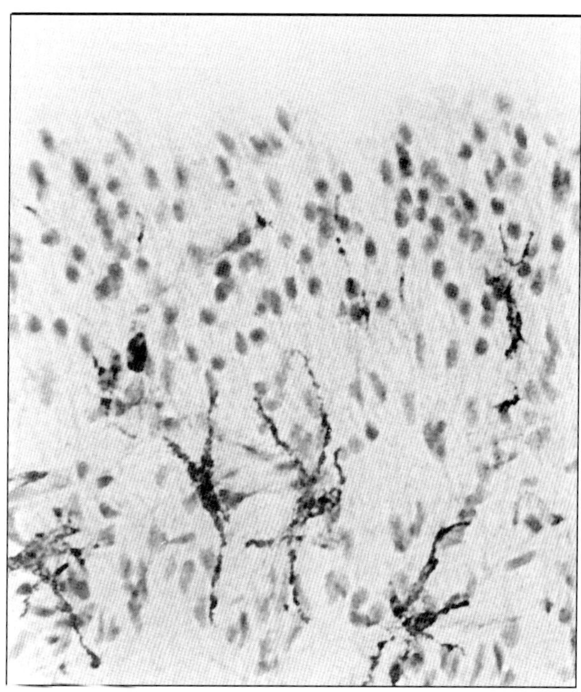

Fig. 8.53 Dendritic cells in the odontoblast layer. (Courtesy G. Bergen-[illegible])

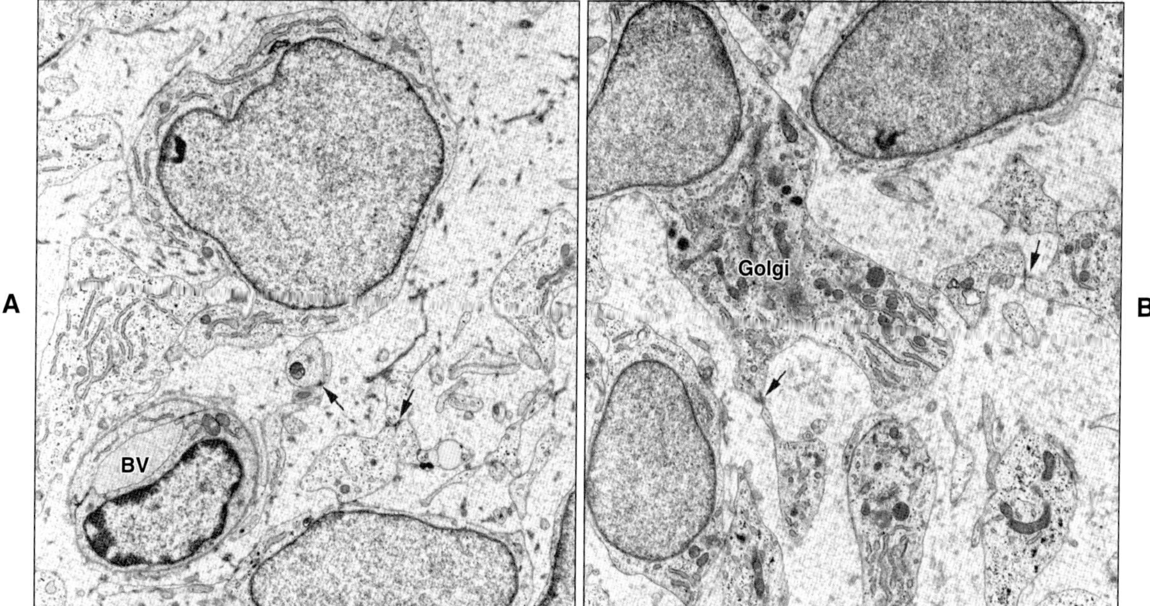

Fig. 8.52 (A, B) Transmission electron microscope images of young pulp from a rat incisor. Fibroblasts show a well-developed Golgi complex *(Golgi)* and extensive cell processes that establish desmosomal contacts *(arrows)* with processes of adjacent cells. At this early stage, few collagen fibrils occur, and the extracellular matrix consists mainly of ground substance. *BV,* Blood vessel.

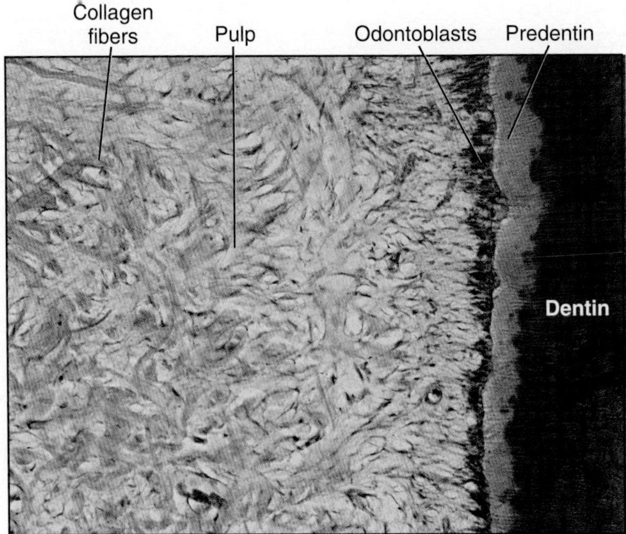

Fig. 8.54 Histologic preparation specially stained to reveal collagen. With age the collagen becomes more abundant and aggregates to form larger fiber bundles.

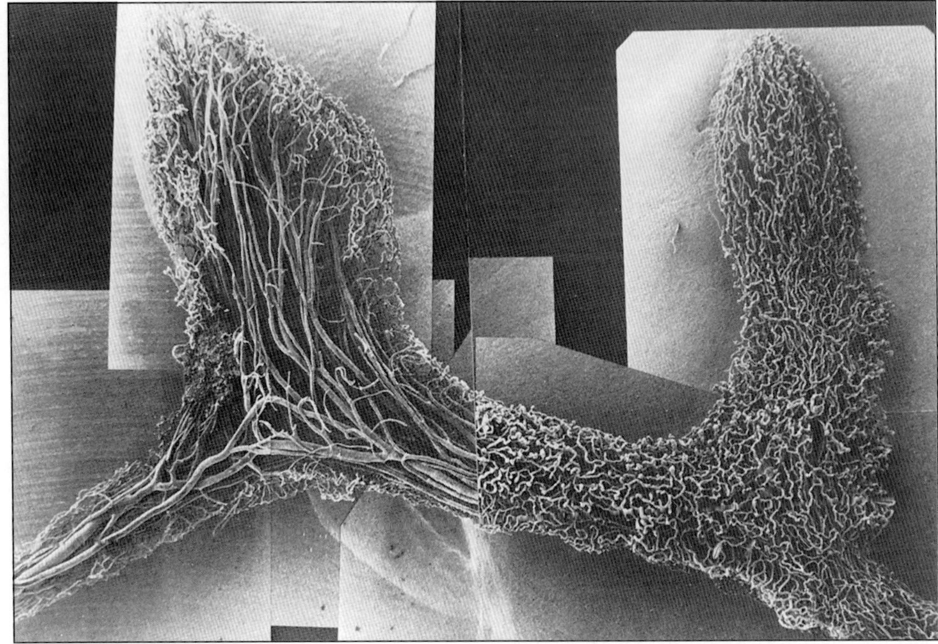

Fig. 8.55 Resin cast of the vasculature of a canine molar. On the right the peripheral vasculature can be seen. On the left this vasculature has been removed to show the central pulp vessels and their peripheral ramifications. (Courtesy K. Takahashi.)

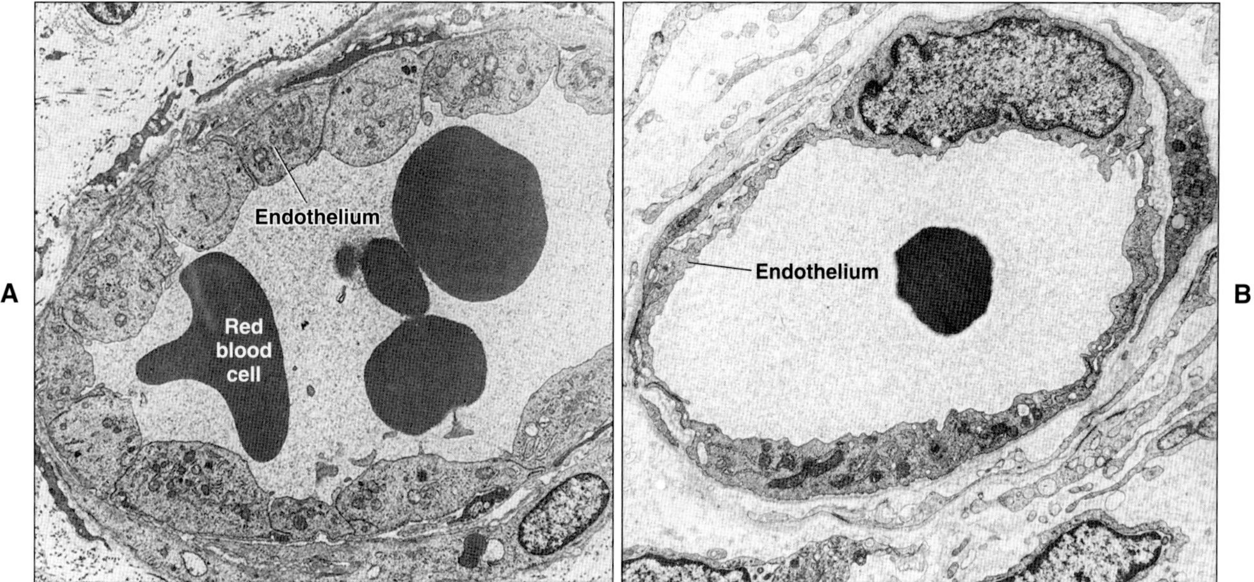

Fig. 8.56 Electron micrographs of an arteriovenous shunt in dental pulp. Such a shunt is characterized by bulging endothelial cells (A) that contrast with the flattened endothelial lining cells of venules (B).

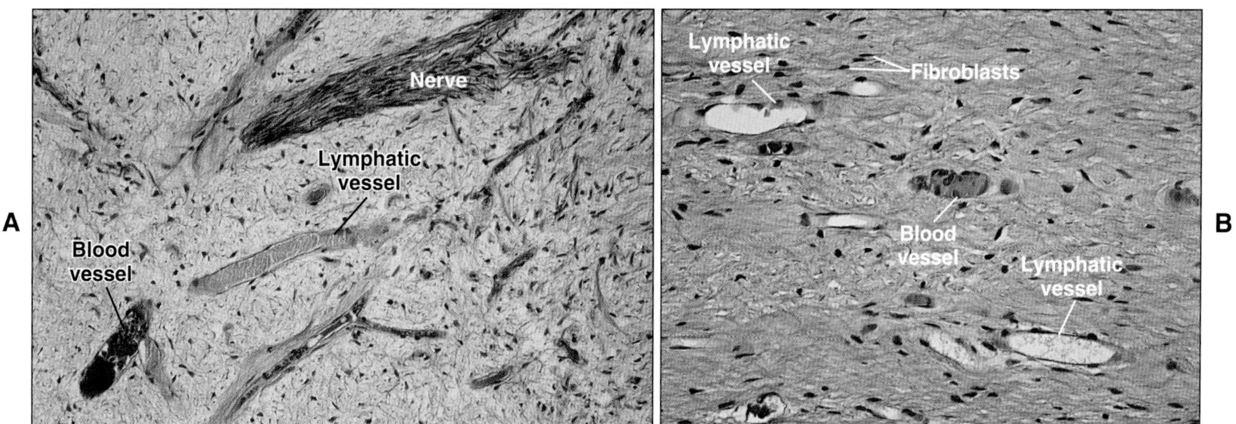

Fig. 8.57 Lymphatic vessels in the dental pulp (A, B). These have a thin wall and, distinct from blood vessels, they contain no blood cells.

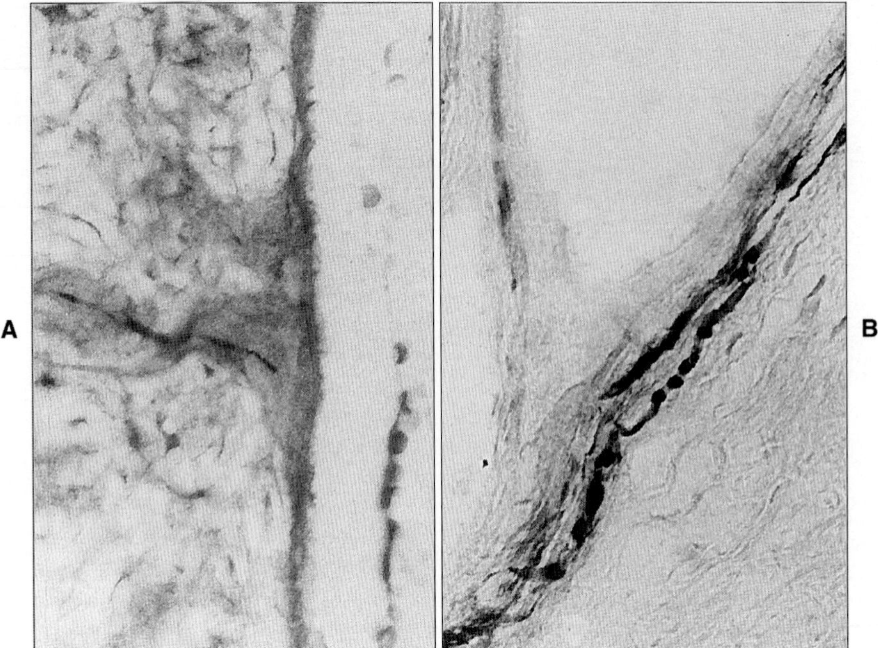

Fig. 8.58 (A) Free nerve endings terminating in the vascular wall of a capillary. (B) Varicose nerve endings terminating on an arteriole. (From Okamura K, et al.: An immunohistochemical and ultrastructural study of vasomotor nerves in the microvasculature of human dental pulp, *Arch Oral Biol* 40:47–53, 1995.)

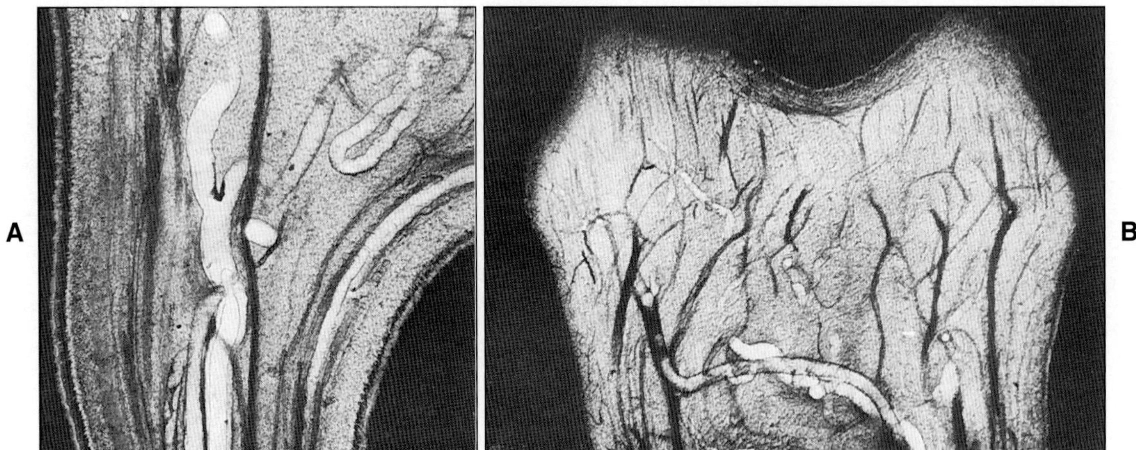

Fig. 8.59 Photomicrographs of a tooth showing the general pattern of distribution of nerves and vessels in the root canal (A) and in the pulp chamber (B). (From Bernick S: Vascular and nerves changes associated with the healing of the human pulp, *Oral Surg Oral Med Oral Pathol* 33:983–1000, 1972.)

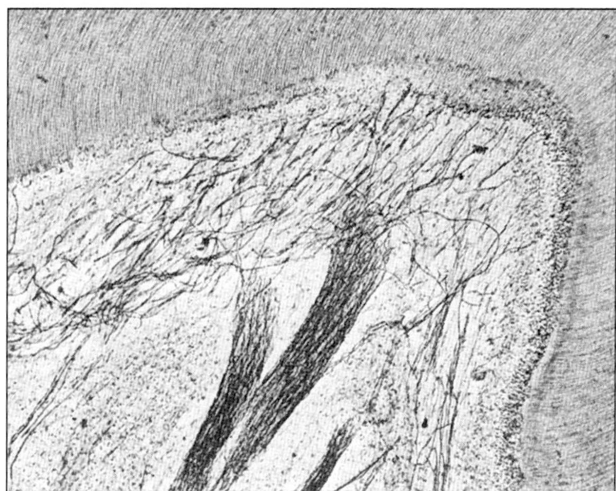

Fig. 8.60 Plexus of Raschkow in a silver-stained demineralized section. The ascending nerve trunks branch to form this plexus, which is situated beneath the odontoblast layer. (From Bernick S: Innervation of teeth. In Finn SB, editor: *Biology of the dental pulp organ,* Tuscaloosa, 1968, University of Alabama Press.)

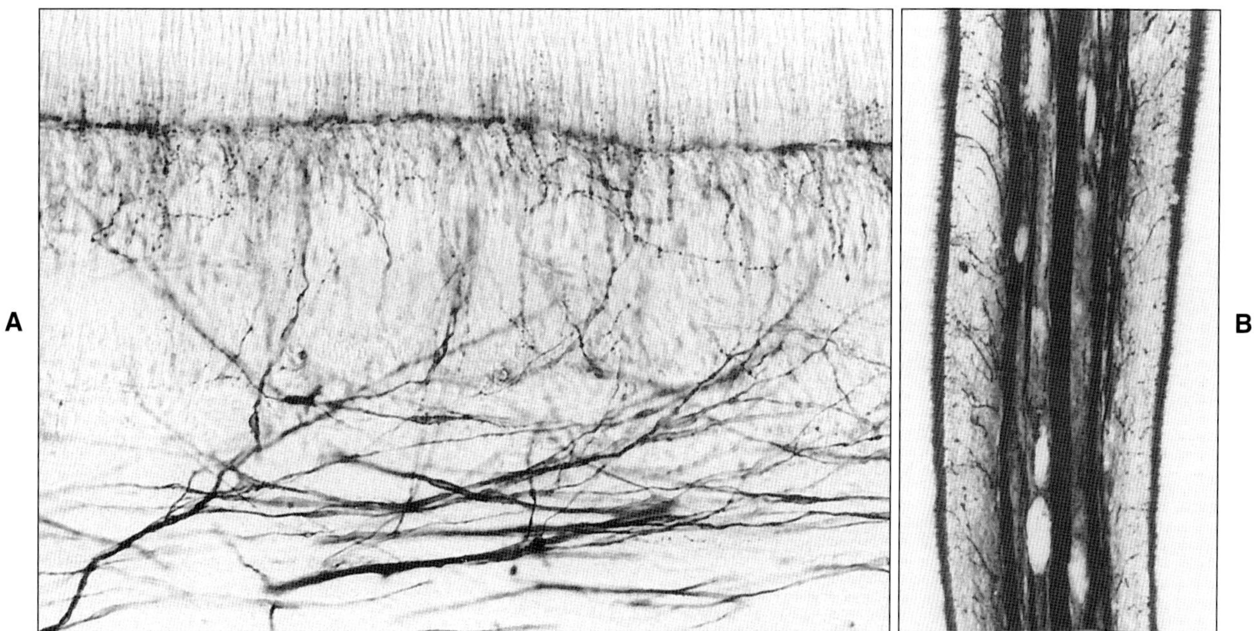

Fig. 8.61 (A) Dentin innervation demonstrated by immunocytochemical staining of nerve growth factor receptor (NGFR). NGFR is present in some of the dentinal tubules, suggesting that nerves extend into them. (B) Nerves in radicular pulp. Side branches are directed to the dentin, and a plexus of Raschkow is absent. (A, From Maeda T, et al.: Immunocytochemical localization of nerve growth factor receptor (NGFR) in human teeth, *Proc Finn Dent Soc* 88(1):S557–S562, 1992; B, from Maeda T, et al.: Dense innervation of human radicular dental pulp as revealed by immunocytochemistry for protein gene-product 9.5, *Arch Oral Biol* 39:563–568, 1994.)

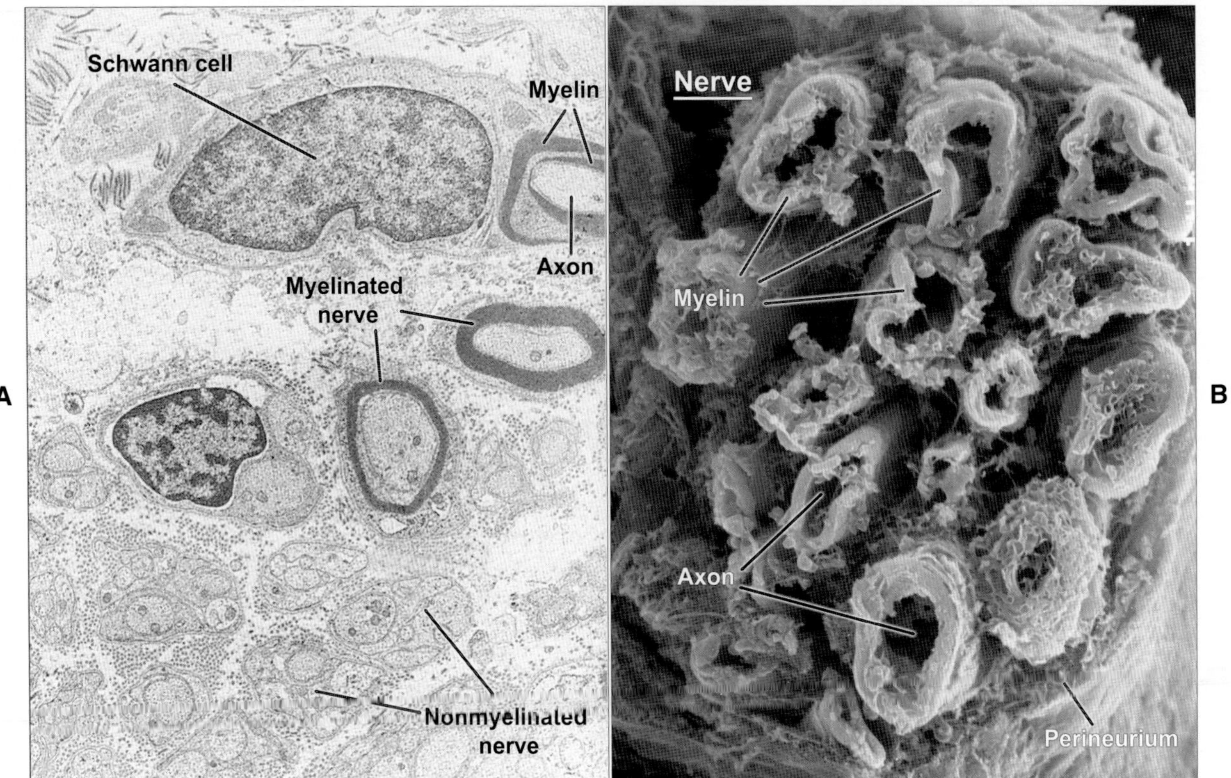

Fig. 8.62 (A) Transmission electron micrograph showing a mixture of myelinated and nonmyelinated nerves in pulp. (B) Scanning electron micrograph of a nerve with myelinated axons. Myelin forms an insulating sheath around axons.

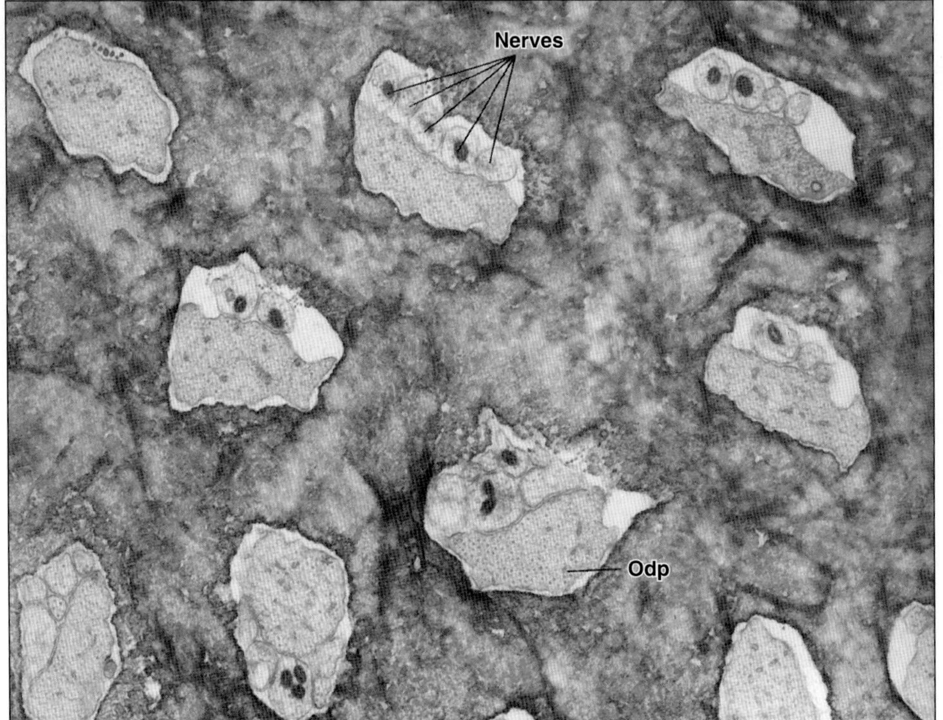

Fig. 8.63 Electron micrograph of pulpal horn dentin seen in cross section. Some of the tubules contain an odontoblast process *(Odp)* and neural elements. (Courtesy R. Holland.)

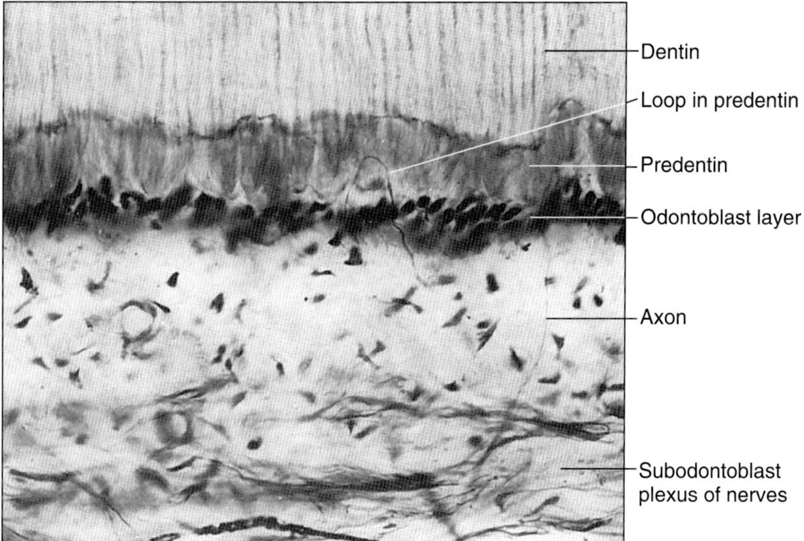

Fig. 8.64 A nerve fibril arising from the plexus of Raschkow is shown passing between the odontoblasts and looping within the predentin. (From Bernick S: Innervation of teeth. In Finn SB, editor: *Biology of the dental pulp organ*, Tuscaloosa, 1968, University of Alabama Press.)

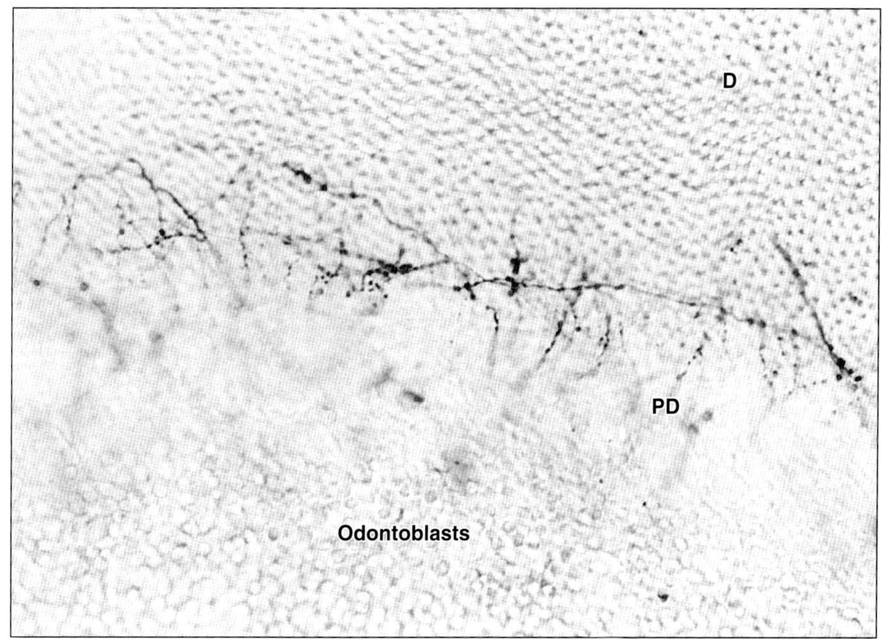

Fig. 8.65 Nerve at the predentin-dentin *(PD, D)* junction demonstrated by staining for nerve growth factor receptor in a tangential section. Its extensive ramification is notable. (From Maeda T, et al.: Immunocytochemical localization of nerve growth factor receptor (NGFR) in human teeth, *Proc Finn Dent Soc* 88(Suppl 1): S557–S562, 1992.)

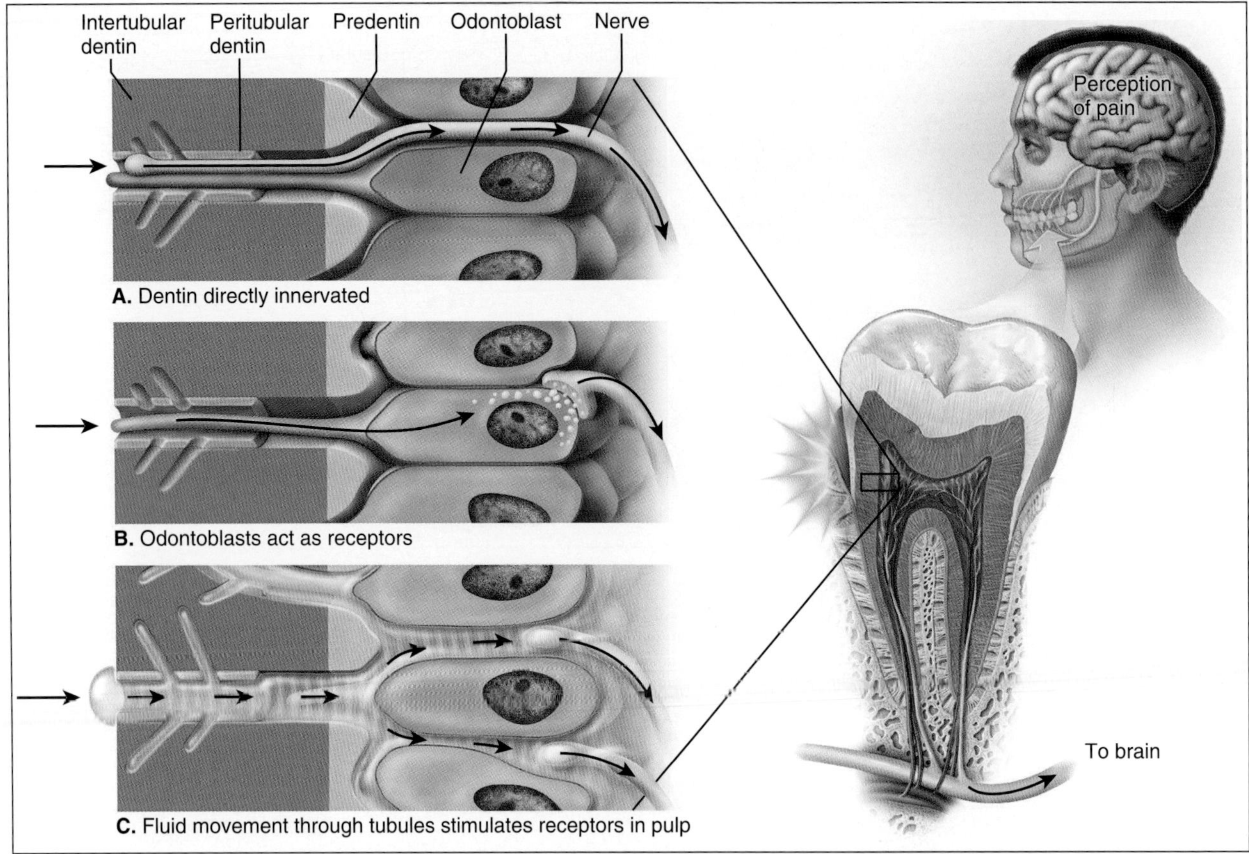

Fig. 8.66 Three theories of dentin sensitivity. *A* suggests that the dentin is innervated directly. *B* suggests that the odontoblast acts as a receptor. *C* suggests that the receptors at the base of odontoblasts are stimulated directly or indirectly by fluid movement through the tubules.

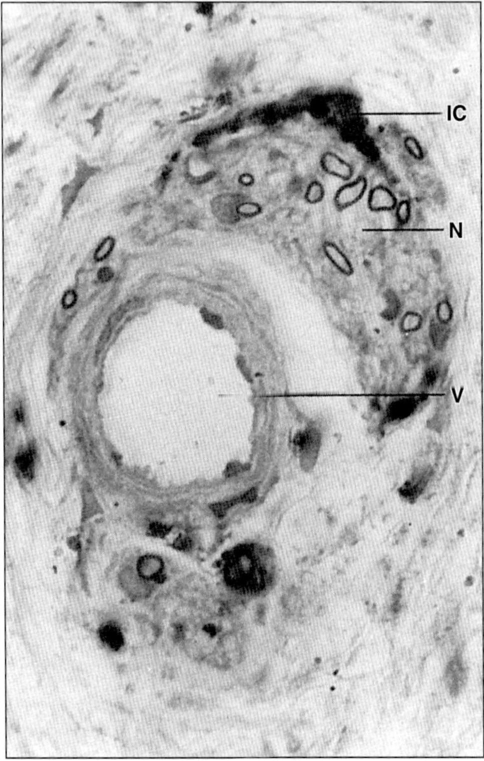

Fig. 8.67 Association between immunocompetent cell *(IC)*, vascular *(V)*, and neural elements *(N)*. (From Yoshiba N, et al.: Immunohistochemical localization of HLA-DR-positive cells in unerupted and erupted normal and carious human teeth, *J Dent Res* 75:1585–1589, 1996.)

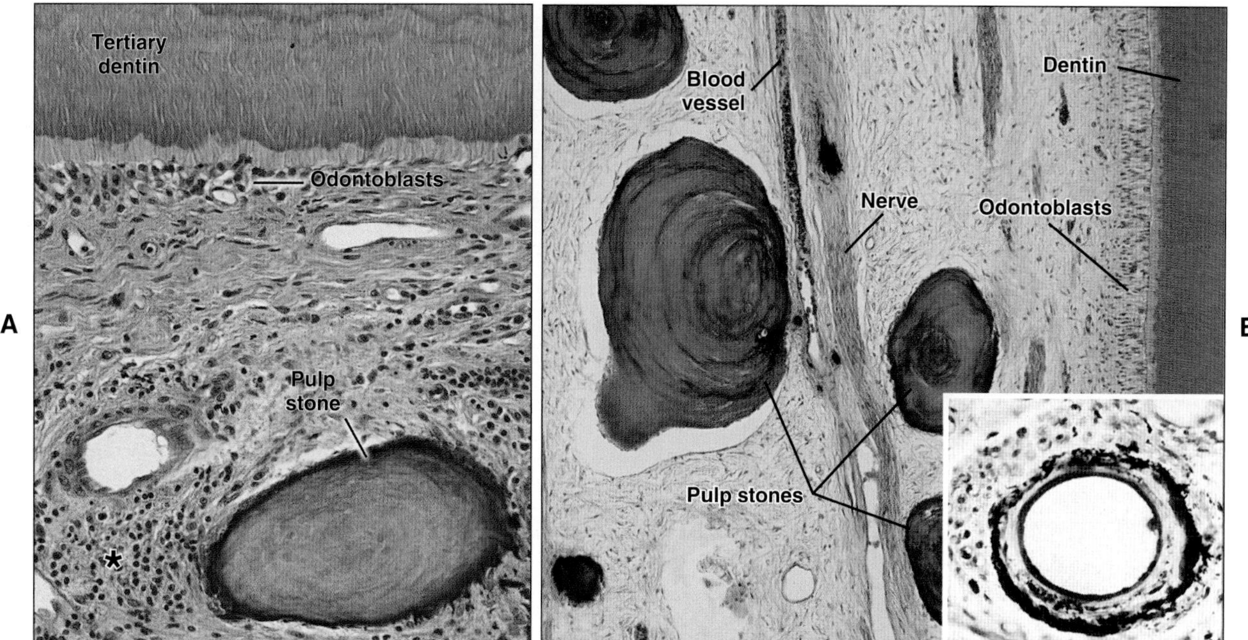

Fig. 8.68 Free (false) pulp stones. (A) The presence of tertiary dentin and a strong mononuclear inflammatory cell infiltrate *(*)* are indicative of a carious lesion. (B) Multiple stones in an aged pulp. Dystrophic calcification is beginning in a vessel wall *(inset)*. (A, Courtesy P. Tambasco de Oliveira; inset, from Bernick S: Age changes in the blood supply to human teeth, *J Dent Res* 46:544–550, 1967.)

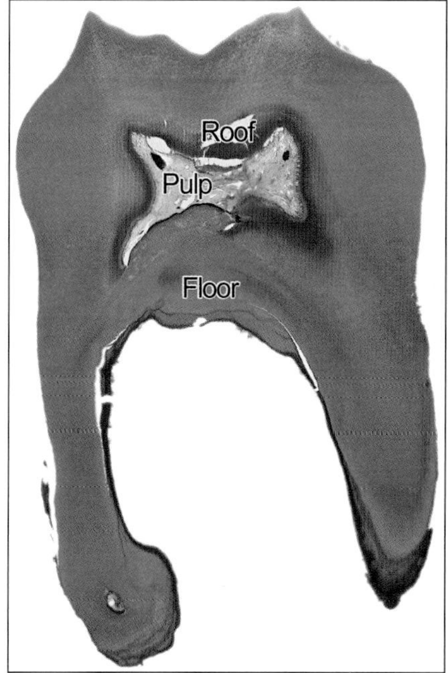

Fig. 8.69 Decreased pulp volume with age. The pulp has been reduced considerably by the continued deposition of dentin on the pulp chamber floor and tertiary dentin formation on the roof.

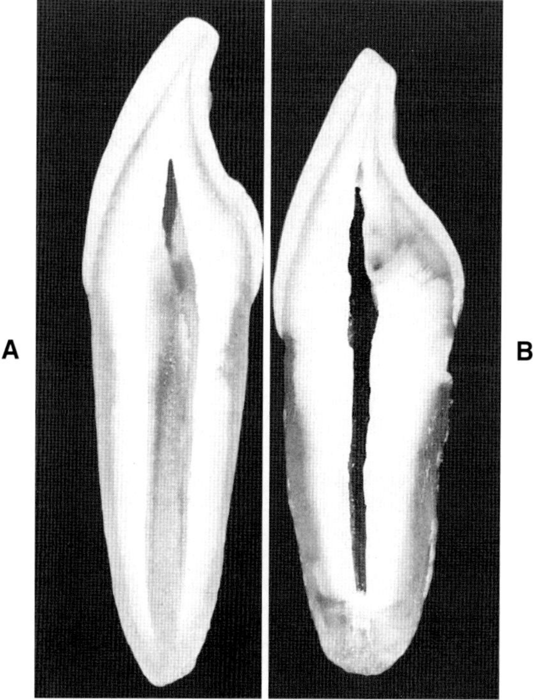

Fig. 8.70 Difference in pulp volume between a young tooth (A) and an older tooth (B).

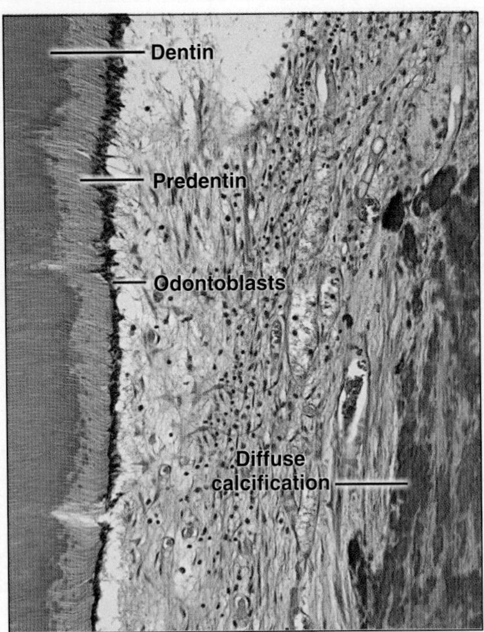

Fig. 8.71 Diffuse calcification associated with collagen bundles in the center of the pulp chamber. (Courtesy P. Tambasco de Oliveira.)

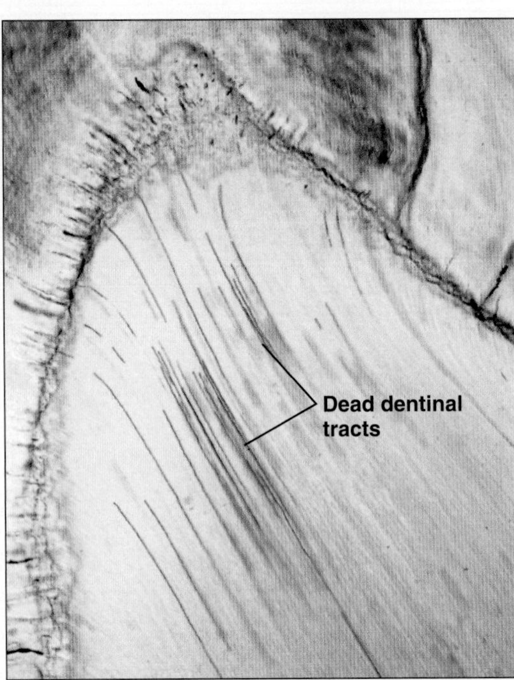

Fig. 8.72 Dead tracts in a ground section. Under transmitted illumination the tracts appear dark because trapped air in them refracts the light

RECOMMENDED READING

Brännström M, Aström A: The hydrodynamics of the dentine: its possible relationship to dentinal pain, *Int Dent J* 22:219, 1972.

Butler WT: Dentin matrix proteins, *Eur J Oral Sci* 106:204, 1998.

Goldberg M, et al.: Dentin: structure, composition and mineralization, *Front Biosci (Elite Ed)* 3:711–735, 2011.

Huang GT: Dental pulp and dentin tissue engineering and regeneration: advancement and challenge, *Front Biosci (Elite Ed)* 3:788–800, 2011.

Linde A: Structure and calcification of dentin. In Bonucci E, editor: *Calcification in biological systems*, Boca Raton, FL, 1992, CRC Press.

Linde A, Lundgren T: From serum to the mineral phase: the role of the odontoblast in calcium transport and mineral formation, *Int J Dev Biol* 39:213, 1995.

MacDougall M, et al.: Molecular basis of human dentin diseases, *Am J Med Genet A* 140:2536, 2006.

Miura M, et al.: SHED: stem cells from human exfoliated deciduous teeth, *Proc Natl Acad Sci USA* 100:5807–5812, 2003.

Qin C, et al.: Post-translational modifications of sibling proteins and their roles in osteogenesis and dentinogenesis, *Crit Rev Oral Biol Med* 15:126, 2004.

Ruch JV, et al.: Odontoblast differentiation, *Int J Dev Biol* 39:51, 1995.

Shimono M, et al.: *Dentin/pulp complex*, Tokyo, Japan, 1996, Quintessence.

Volponi AA, et al.: Stem cell-based biological tooth repair and regeneration, *Trends Cell Biol* 20:715–722, 2010.

Yamakoshi Y, et al.: Dentin glycoprotein: the protein in the middle of the dentin sialophosphoprotein chimera, *J Biol Chem* 280:17472, 2005.

9

Periodontium

Antonio Nanci

OUTLINE

The periodontium is defined as those tissues supporting and investing the tooth and consists of cementum, periodontal ligament (PDL), bone lining the alveolus (socket), and that part of the gingiva facing the tooth. Proper functioning of the periodontium is achieved only through structural integrity and interaction between these various tissues. Together these tissues form a specialized fibrous joint (gomphosis), the components of which are of ectomesenchymal origin (except the gingiva). The widespread occurrence of periodontal diseases and the realization that periodontal tissues lost to disease can be repaired have resulted in considerable effort to understand the factors and cells regulating the formation, maintenance, and regeneration of the periodontium. This chapter describes the histologic events leading to the formation of supporting tissues (Fig. 9.1), except for the dentogingival junction, which is covered under oral mucosa (see Chapter 12).

CEMENTUM

Cementum is a hard, avascular connective tissue that covers the roots of teeth (Fig. 9.2). It is classified according to the presence or absence of cells within its matrix and the origin of the collagen fibers of the matrix. The development of cementum has been subdivided into a prefunctional stage, which occurs throughout root formation, and a functional stage, which begins when the tooth is in occlusion and continues throughout life. Several varieties of cementum exist. The beginning student, however, needs only to think of the two main forms of cementum that have different structural and functional characteristics: (a) acellular cementum, which provides attachment for the tooth, and (b) cellular cementum, which has an adaptive role in response to tooth wear and movement and is associated with repair of periodontal tissues.

Biochemical Composition

Four mineralized tissues are found in the oral cavity, and three of these—enamel, dentin, and cementum—are components of the tooth. Their characteristics and biochemical composition are summarized in Table 1.1. The composition of cementum is similar to that of bone. Cementum is approximately 45% to 50% hydroxyapatite by weight, and the remaining portion is collagen and noncollagenous matrix proteins. Type I collagen is the predominant collagen of cementum; in cellular intrinsic fiber cementum (intrinsic referring to the endogenous origin of the fibers), it constitutes up to 90% of the organic components, and, just as in bone, it accommodates a substantial part of mineral deposition. Type I collagen is also the major collagen within the PDL region, and its main function is to structure the fiber bundles that anchor the tooth to the bone and distribute masticatory forces. Other collagens associated with cementum include type III, a less cross-linked collagen found in high concentrations during development and during repair and regeneration of mineralized tissues but is reduced with maturation of this tissue, and type XII collagen, a fibril-associated collagen with interrupted triple helices that bind to type I collagen and to noncollagenous proteins. Type XII collagen is found in high concentrations in ligamentous tissues, including the PDL, with lower levels noted in cementum. This nonfibrillar collagen interacts with type I collagen and may assist in maintaining a functional and mature PDL that can withstand the forces of occlusion. Trace amounts of other collagens, including types V, VI, and XIV, also are found in extracts of mature cementum; however, these may be contaminants from the PDL region produced by PDL fibroblasts associated with collagen fibers inserted into cementum. Noncollagenous proteins identified in cementum also are associated with bone and include the following: alkaline phosphatase, bone sialoprotein, dentin matrix protein 1, dentin sialoprotein, fibronectin, osteocalcin, osteonectin,

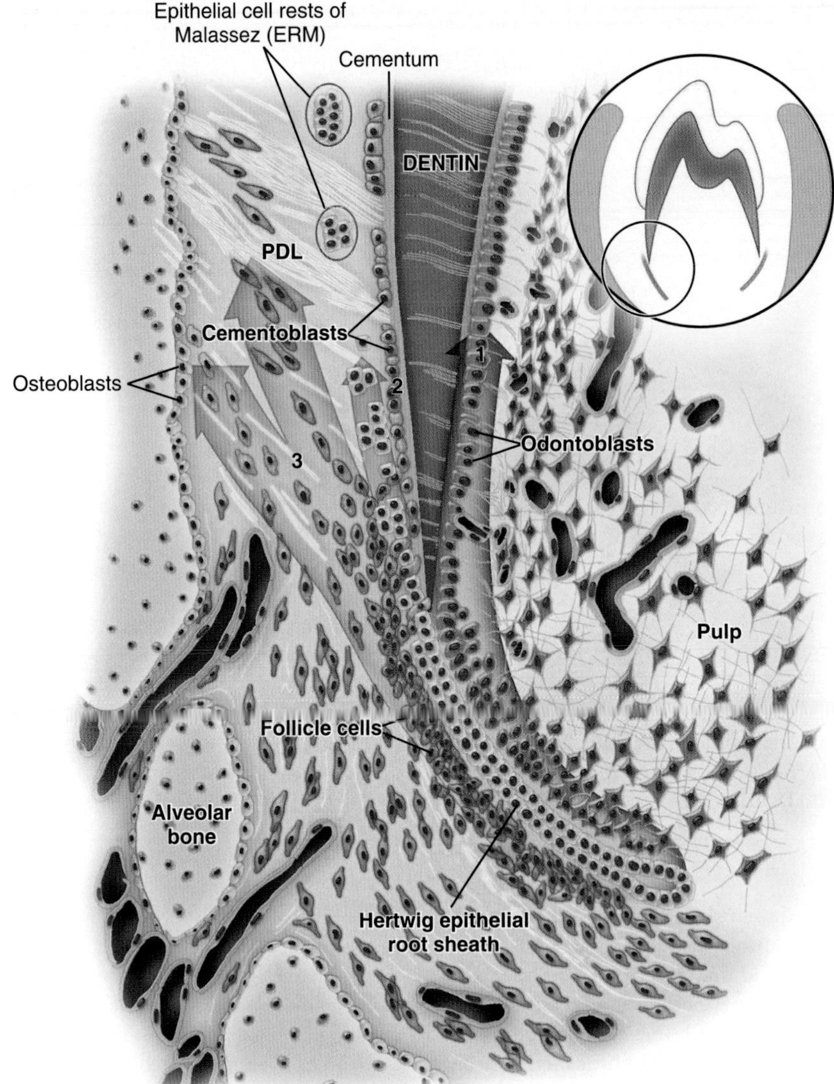

Fig. 9.1 Summary of *(1)* the differentiation of odontoblasts from ectomesenchymal cells in the radicular pulp, *(2)* the fragmentation of Hertwig epithelial root sheath with residual portions forming the epithelial rests of Malassez, and *(3)* the ensuing differentiation of cementoblasts from Hertwig epithelial root sheath cells or follicle cells, and the follicle contribution to the formation of the fiber bundles of the periodontal ligament *(PDL)* and, possibly, osteoblasts.

osteopontin, proteoglycans, proteolipids, tenascin, and several growth factors. Two apparently unique cementum molecules, an adhesion molecule (cementum attachment protein) and an insulin-like growth factor (IGF), have been identified. In addition to producing the listed common matrix proteins, the expression of the osteoblast-specific bone-restricted interferon-inducible transmembrane (IFITM)–like (BRIL) membrane protein, a member of the IFITM protein family (see Chapter 6), adds additional support for similarity between these two cell types.

Initiation of Cementum Formation

Although cementum formation takes place along the entire root, its initiation is limited to the advancing root edge (Fig. 9.3). At this site, Hertwig epithelial root sheath (HERS), which derives from the coronoapical extension of the inner and outer enamel epithelium (see Chapter 5), is believed to send an inductive message possibly by secreting some enamel proteins or other epithelial product to the facing ectomesenchymal pulp cells. These cells differentiate into odontoblasts and produce a layer of predentin (Fig. 9.4; see also Fig. 9.3). The next series of events results in formation of cementum on the root surface; however, the specific trigger factors responsible for promoting its formation still are unresolved. Current theories include the following: (1) Soon after deposition of dentin, HERS becomes interrupted, and ectomesenchymal cells from the inner portion of the dental follicle then can come in contact with the predentin; (2) infiltrating dental follicle cells receive a reciprocal inductive signal from the dentin and/or the surrounding HERS cells and differentiate into cementoblasts; or (3) HERS cells transform into cementoblasts (a process discussed subsequently). During these processes, some cells from the fragmented root sheath form discrete masses surrounded by a basal lamina known as *epithelial cell rests of Malassez* (ERMs), which persist in the mature PDL (Figs. 9.5 and 9.6). Evidence is increasing that these rests are not simply residual cells but, instead, may participate in maintenance and regeneration of periodontal tissues. If some HERS cells remain attached to the forming root surface, they can produce focal deposits of enamel-like material called *enamel pearls* (Fig. 9.7), which are most commonly found in the area of root furcation.

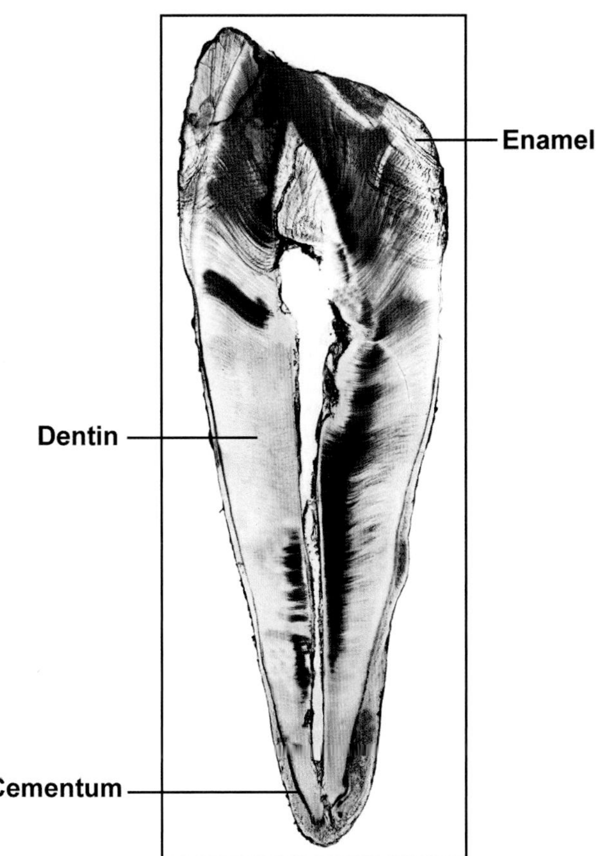

Fig. 9.2 Ground section of a premolar showing the distribution of cementum around the root. Increasing amounts of cementum occur around the apex.

Origin of Periodontal Cells and Differentiation of Cementoblasts

Several factors need to be fully determined to better understand the periodontium, including the following:

1. What are the precursors of cementoblasts and PDL fibroblasts?
2. Do cementoblasts express unique gene products, or are they simply positional osteoblasts?
3. Are acellular and cellular cementum phenotypically distinct tissues?
4. What factors promote cementoblast differentiation?
5. What regulates formation of the PDL vs. cementogenesis, thus providing a balance between cementum, PDL, and alveolar bone?

Answers to these questions are important not only to understand normal formation processes, but also to envisage novel, targeted therapeutic approaches for periodontal diseases.

The long-standing view is that precursor cells for cementoblasts and PDL fibroblasts reside in the dental follicle and that factors within the local environment regulate their ability to function as cementoblasts that form root cementum or as fibroblasts of the PDL. Cells involved in regenerating periodontal tissues include stem cells migrating from the vascular region and local progenitor cells. In addition, there is now increasing evidence that epithelial cells from HERS may undergo epithelial-mesenchymal transformation into cementoblasts during development. Such transformation is a fundamental process in developmental biology, as seen in Chapter 2 during neural crest cell migration, and in Chapter 3 during medial edge fusion of the palatal shelves. Structural and immunocytochemical data support the possibility that at least in part cementoblasts are transformed from epithelial cells of HERS. In rodents, initial formation of acellular cementum takes place in the presence of epithelial cells, and some studies have shown that

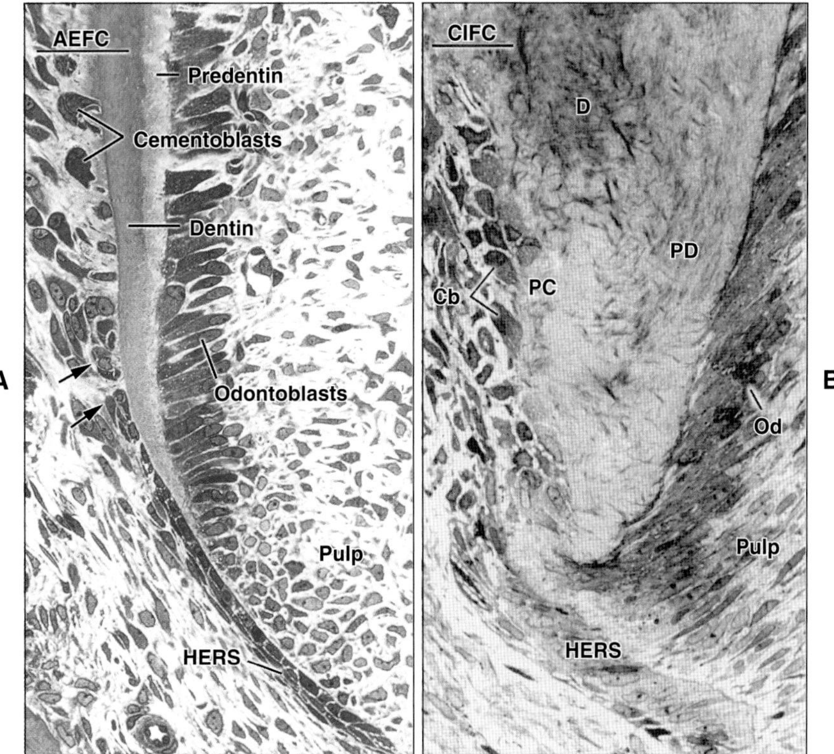

Fig. 9.3 Histologic sections of the advancing root edge in (A) a rat during acellular extrinsic fiber cementum *(AEFC)* formation and (B) a human during cellular intrinsic fiber cementum *(CIFC)* formation. In the rat, Hertwig epithelial root sheath *(HERS)* is still present when radicular dentin *(D)* calcifies; in fact, deposition of acellular cementum starts on mineralized dentin, often in the presence of cells with epithelial characteristics *(arrows)*. In human teeth, acellular and cellular cementum are deposited before the surface layer of dentin mineralizes. *Cb*, Cementoblast; *Od*, odontoblast; *PC*, precementum; *PD*, predentin.

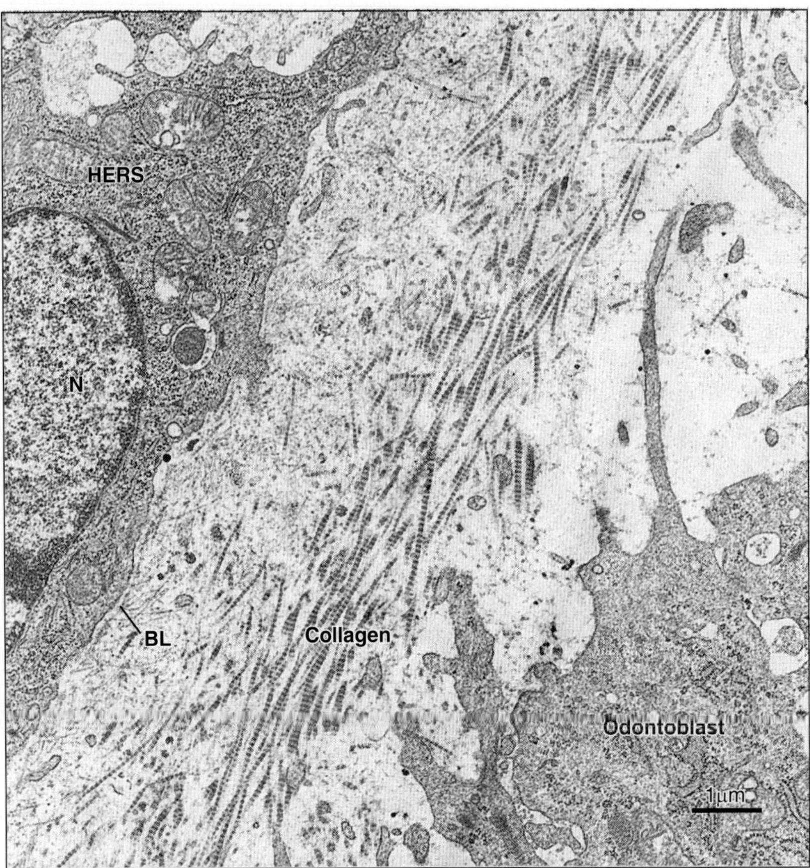

Fig. 9.4 Electron micrograph of early root dentinogenesis. The large collagen fibril bundles are first deposited parallel and at a distance from the basal lamina *(BL)* that supports Hertwig epithelial root sheath *(HERS)*. *N*, Nucleus.

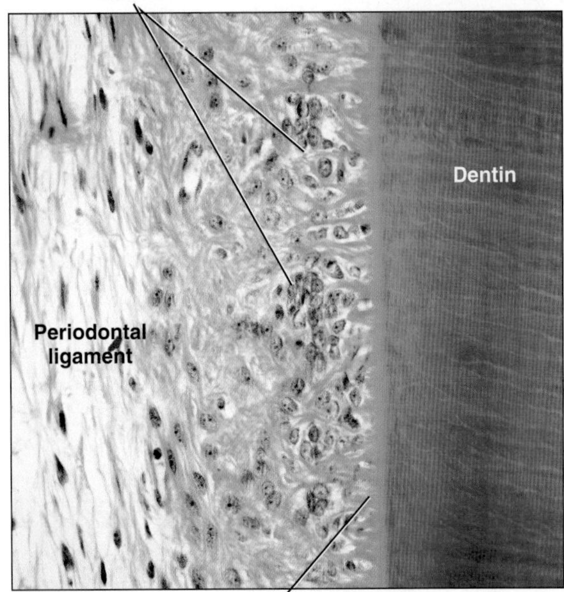

Fig. 9.5 Initial cementum formation. The first increment of cementum forms against the root dentin surface. Epithelial cell rests of Malassez (remnants of the root sheath) can be seen within the follicular tissue.

enamel organ–derived cells are capable of producing mesenchymal products, such as type I collagen, bone sialoprotein, and osteopontin.

Uncertainty still exists as to whether acellular (primary) and cellular (secondary) cementum are produced by distinct populations of cells expressing spatiotemporal behaviors that result in the characteristic histologic differences between these tissues. This potential cellular and formative distinctiveness is highlighted in mice null for the tissue-nonspecific alkaline phosphatase gene or rats treated with bisphosphonates. In these animals, acellular cementum formation is affected significantly, whereas cellular cementum appears to develop normally. In hypophosphatemic mice, formation of acellular cementum can be rescued by enzyme replacement therapy for tissue-nonspecific alkaline phosphatase. This suggests differences in cell types or factors controlling development of these two varieties of cementum. In the human counterpart, hypophosphatasia, characterized by low levels of alkaline phosphatase, cementum formation appears to be limited or nonexistent, not exclusive to acellular versus cellular. In contrast, in mice with mutations in genes that maintain extracellular pyrophosphate levels, such as *ank* and *PC-1*, resulting in limited levels of pyrophosphate, formation of cellular cementum occurs even at early stages of root development. These findings suggest an important role for phosphate in controlling the rate of cementum formation.

Molecular Factors Regulating Cementogenesis

To understand the specific role of phosphate and other molecules, additional studies that focus on defining the cells and factors controlling development, maintenance, and regeneration of

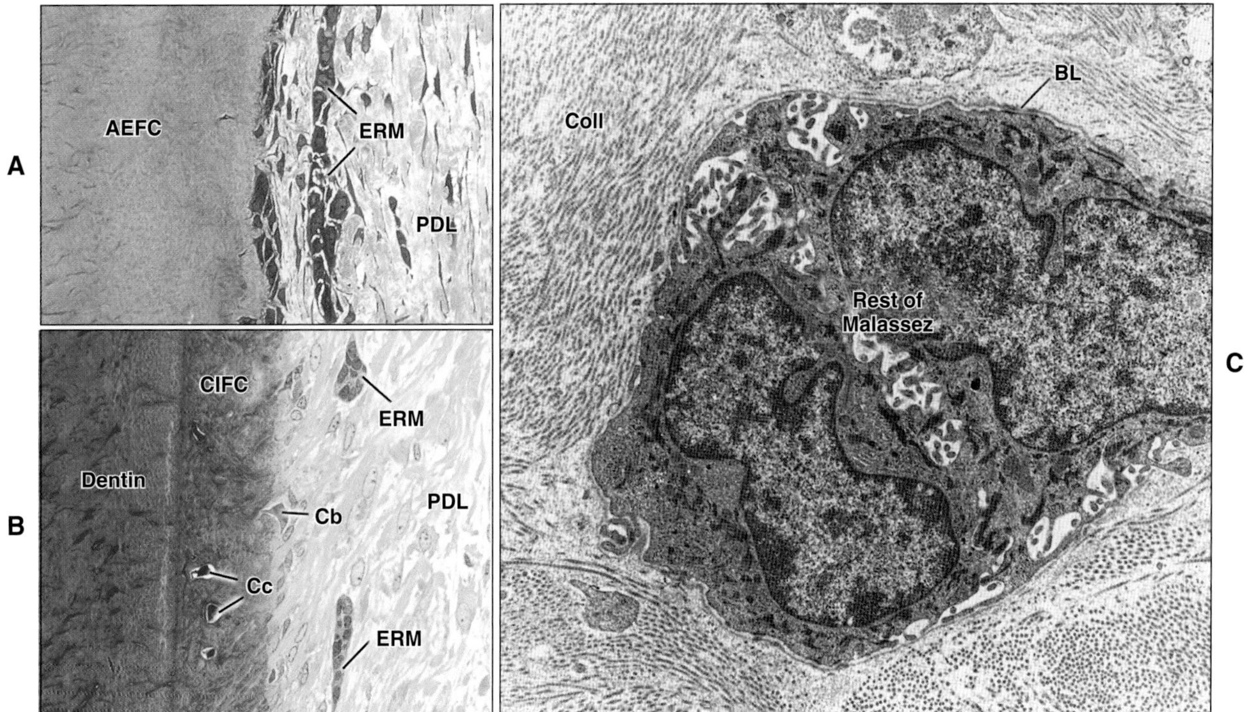

Fig. 9.6 Light micrographs taken along the forming root in (A) a human tooth and (B) a porcine one. Epithelial cell rests of Malassez *(ERMs)* are seen close to the tooth surface. These can appear as long strands or more discrete elongated or spherical groups of cells. The size of the cells and their staining density may vary. (C) Electron micrograph of an epithelial rest. The scarcity of cytoplasmic organelles and basal lamina *(BL)* surrounding it are notable. *AEFC,* Acellular extrinsic fiber cementum; *Cb,* cementoblast; *Cc,* cementocyte; *CIFC,* cellular intrinsic fiber cementum; *Coll,* collagen fibrils; *PDL,* periodontal ligament.

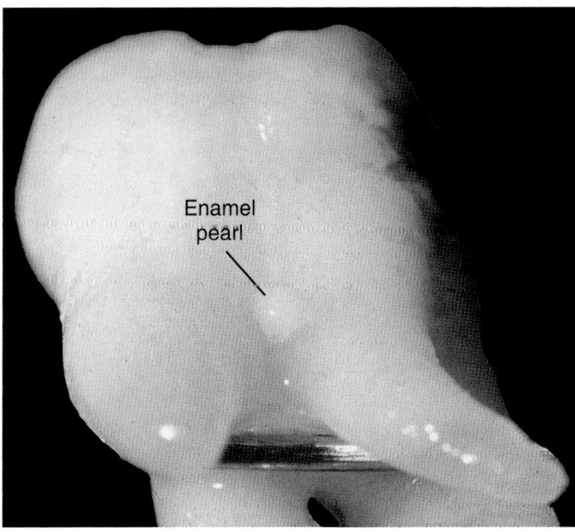

Fig. 9.7 Enamel pearls appear as spheric masses and develop ectopically in the area of root furcations.

periodontal tissues are required. Some of the factors known to be involved in controlling these events are discussed next and are summarized in Table 9.1.

Bone Morphogenetic Proteins

Bone morphogenetic proteins (BMPs) are members of the transforming growth factor β (TGF-β) superfamily that act through transmembrane serine and threonine protein kinase receptors. These signaling molecules have a variety of functions during morphogenesis and cell differentiation, and in teeth they are considered to be part of the network of epithelial-mesenchymal signaling molecules regulating initiation of crown formation. The roles for BMPs in root development, including whether they are implicated in epithelial-mesenchymal signaling, and the signal pathways and transcription factors involved in modulating their behavior remain to be defined. However, several of the BMPs, including BMP2, BMP4, and BMP7, are known to promote differentiation of preosteoblasts and putative cementoblast precursor cells. In addition, BMPs have been used successfully to induce periodontal regeneration in a number of experimental models and in certain clinical situations.

Epithelial Factors

Epithelial-mesenchymal interactions are required for formation of the tooth crown, and epithelial factors are implicated. The same two populations of cells involved in crown morphogenesis (i.e., epithelial and ectomesenchymal cells) also take part in root formation. The possibility that such interactions also are required for development of periodontal tissues and that some of the same signaling molecules are involved is thus a logical assumption. Prospective candidates include enamel proteins, parathyroid hormone–related protein, and basal lamina constituents. In the case of enamel proteins, the debate centers around the fact that enamel proteins have not been detected consistently along forming roots. However, this does not rule out a transient expression at early stages of root formation where they could influence odontoblast and/or cementoblast differentiation. Along this line, an enamel matrix derivative, consisting predominantly of amelogenin molecules, is used clinically to stimulate repair and regeneration, and although much has been discovered over the past 20 years, its mechanism of action remains to be determined.

TABLE 9.1 Some Key Molecules in the Periodontium

	Suggested Function Related to Cementogenesis
Growth Factors	
Transforming growth factor β superfamily (including bone morphogenetic proteins)	These factors are reported to promote cell differentiation and subsequently cementogenesis during development and regeneration.
Platelet-derived growth factor (PDGF) and insulin-like growth factor (IGF)	Existing data suggest that PDGF alone or in combination with IGF promotes cementum formation by altering cell cycle activities.
Fibroblast growth factors	Suggested roles for these factors are promoting cell proliferation and migration and vasculogenesis—all key events for formation and regeneration of periodontal tissues.
Adhesion Molecules	
Bone sialoprotein Osteopontin	These molecules may promote adhesion of selected cells to the newly forming root. Bone sialoprotein may be involved in promoting mineralization, whereas osteopontin may regulate the extent of crystal growth.
Epithelial/enamel proteins	Epithelial-mesenchymal interactions may be involved in promoting follicle cells along a cementoblast pathway. Some epithelial molecules may promote periodontal repair directly or indirectly.
Collagens	Collagens, especially types I and III, play key roles in regulating periodontal tissues during development and regeneration. In addition, type XII may assist in maintaining the periodontal ligament space vs. continuous formation of cementum.
Gla Proteins	
Matrix Gla protein/bone Gla protein (osteocalcin)	These proteins contain γ-carboxyglutamic acid, hence the name *Gla* proteins. Osteocalcin is a marker for cells associated with mineralization (i.e., osteoblasts, cementoblasts, odontoblasts) and is considered to be a regulator of crystal growth. It has also been proposed to act as a hormone regulating energy metabolism through several synergistic functions favoring pancreatic β cell proliferation, increasing insulin secretion (in the pancreas) and sensitivity in peripheral tissues, and promoting energy expenditure (in brown adipose tissue) and testosterone production by Leydig cells in testes. Matrix Gla protein appears to play a significant role in preventing abnormal ectopic calcification.
Transcription Factors	
Runt-related transcription factor 2 Osterix	As for osteoblasts, these may be involved in cementoblast differentiation.
Signaling Molecules	
Osteoprotegerin Receptor-activated nuclear factor κB ligand Receptor-activated nuclear factor κB	These molecules mediate bone and root resorption by osteoclasts.
Sclerostin	Antagonist of Wnt and promotes cementum formation
Wingless-related integration site (Wnt)	Regulates stem cell populations and differentiation of cementoblasts
Cementum-Specific Proteins	
Cementum protein 1 (cementum-derived protein 23)	May play a role as a local regulator of cell differentiation and extracellular matrix mineralization.

Major Matrix Proteins With Cell Adhesion Motifs

Bone sialoprotein and osteopontin are multifunctional molecules associated with cementum formation during development and in repair and regeneration of periodontal tissues. They contain the cell adhesion motif arginine-glycine-aspartic acid and thereby are believed to promote adhesion of selected cells onto the newly forming root. Present data further suggest that both proteins may be implicated in regulating mineral formation on the root surface. The balance between the activities of these two molecules may contribute to establishing and maintaining an unmineralized PDL between cementum and alveolar bone. No major developmental root anomalies have been reported in the osteopontin knockout mouse model. On the other hand, bone sialoprotein expression affects acellular cementum formation (see Box 9.1) and periodontal attachment possibly by promoting mineralization at the root surface to anchor PDL fibers.

Gla Proteins

Proteins enriched in γ-carboxyglutamic acid (Gla), a calcium-binding amino acid, are known as *Gla proteins.* Bone Gla protein (osteocalcin) is a marker for maturation of osteoblasts, odontoblasts, and cementoblasts and is considered to regulate the extent of mineralization. Also, this osteoblast-derived hormone may regulate insulin secretion, insulin sensitivity, and energy expenditure. Matrix Gla protein (MGP) has been identified in periodontal tissues and, based on its suggested role as an inhibitor of mineralization, may act to preserve the PDL width. Mice null for MGP exhibit substantial ectopic calcification. However, periodontal development and tooth formation appear to be normal in MGP-null mice; thus additional studies are required to define the role of MGP within periodontal tissues.

Transcription Factors

As shown in Chapter 6, runt-related transcription factor 2 (Runx2), also known as *core binding factor alpha 1 (Cbfa1),* and osterix, downstream from Runx2, have been identified as master switches for differentiation of osteoblasts. Runx2 now has been found to be expressed in dental follicle cells, PDL cells, and cementoblasts. Based on similarities between cementoblasts (at least in cellular cementum) and osteoblasts, it is likely that both factors may be involved in cementoblast differentiation. The exact factors triggering expression or activation of these key transcription factors currently are being investigated; BMPs already have been identified as factors promoting expression of Runx2.

BOX 9.1 Bone sialoprotein is important for periodontal mineralization and function

The periodontium is a complex structure that provides tooth attachment and protection of underlying connective tissues. Acellular cementum is critical for attachment of the tooth root to the surrounding alveolar bone. Cementum anchors Sharpey's fibers, which are the embedded extremities of unmineralized periodontal ligament (PDL) fibers. The mechanisms underlying the carefully controlled regulation of the hard-soft tissue interfaces of the cementum-PDL-alveolar bone have remained a persistent mystery of periodontal biology. Evidence has been accumulating that selective expression of certain enzymes and extracellular matrix (ECM) proteins helps to precisely guide mineralization of cementum and bone, while sparing the PDL to remain as an unmineralized connective tissue. One such protein is proposed to be bone sialoprotein (BSP).

BSP has long been used as a marker for both cementum and bone. Cementoblasts (cells that make cementum) and osteoblasts (cells that make bone) strongly express the *BSP* gene and protein during development, but expression is absent in cells of the PDL. BSP is a secreted, acidic phosphoprotein associated with mineralized tissues. It was first identified several decades ago as a major, non-collagenous component of the bone. Based on its close association with the mineralized bone ECM, it was hypothesized that BSP might regulate mineralization of bones and teeth. The amino acid sequence of BSP provided information about its potential roles. BSP has several evolutionarily conserved amino acid domains that contribute to its functions, as shown by cell-free and in vitro cell experiments.[1] BSP harbors a collagen-binding domain that may direct its localization and interactions with the surrounding collagenous ECM of cementum and bone. There are also two or more (depending on species) polyglutamic acid domains that carry a high negative charge and are thought to promote initiation and growth of hydroxyapatite mineral. An arginine glycine aspartic acid (RGD) integrin-binding domain initiates cell signaling that may lead to changes in cell migration, attachment, and/or differentiation.

The in vivo importance of BSP was not clear until creation of a mouse model where *BSP* was genetically deleted.[2] Knockout animals allow inference of a gene's function by investigation of the consequences of the target gene's removal. Loss of BSP resulted in periodontal defects (Box 9.1, Fig. 1) that included acellular cementum hypoplasia or aplasia and cellular cementum and alveolar bone hypomineralization in mice.[3] With the reduced ability of acellular cementum to anchor Sharpey's fibers, PDL became detached and disorganized, and the tooth-bone connection was effectively reduced or severed. Periodontal detachment led to a long junctional epithelium and an influx of odontoclasts that extensively resorbed the cervical root surface. Increased numbers of osteoclasts progressively destroyed alveolar bone levels in mice lacking BSP. Periodontal breakdown led to tooth mobility, malocclusion, and tooth loss. While this collection of manifestations in some ways resembles the periodontal destruction that accompanies cases of severe periodontitis, the primary defect in the absence of BSP is structural rather than infection and inflammation-mediated.

The importance of BSP in alveolar bone mineralization was also revealed in the BSP knockout mouse model. With removal of *BSP*, large regions of hypomineralized alveolar bone accumulated during development and alveolar bone was marked by a persistently low mineral density.[4] These mineralization defects were possibly more profound than effects of BSP knockout on bones of the appendicular skeleton, such as femurs and tibias. This finding suggests that BSP is more critical for intramembranous ossification of alveolar bone than endochondral ossification of the long bones. The role of BSP in alveolar bone was further tested using a challenge model where first maxillary molars were extracted to study alveolar bone healing in the remaining socket. Compared to healthy controls, mice lacking BSP showed severe and persistent defects in alveolar bone healing.[5] Both the quantity and quality of new bone was dramatically reduced in the absence of BSP confirming its requirement for proper alveolar bone healing.

These results indicate BSP is an essential and non-redundant factor for cementum and alveolar bone mineralization. Enamel (which does not contain BSP) and dentin are spared any developmental effects of BSP knockout, confirming distinct regulatory mechanisms for mineralization among the four unique dentoalveolar hard tissues. These studies of BSP also serve to communicate the profound importance of acellular cementum for periodontal stability and function. BSP emerges as one of the (probably many) factors that selectively directs cementum and bone mineralization within the periodontium. Future studies are needed to identify mechanisms of action of BSP, and how it relates to other regulators of mineralization that work within the periodontal region. Ultimately, studies of periodontal development like this one aim to identify factors and mechanisms that may be repurposed to promote periodontal repair and regeneration.

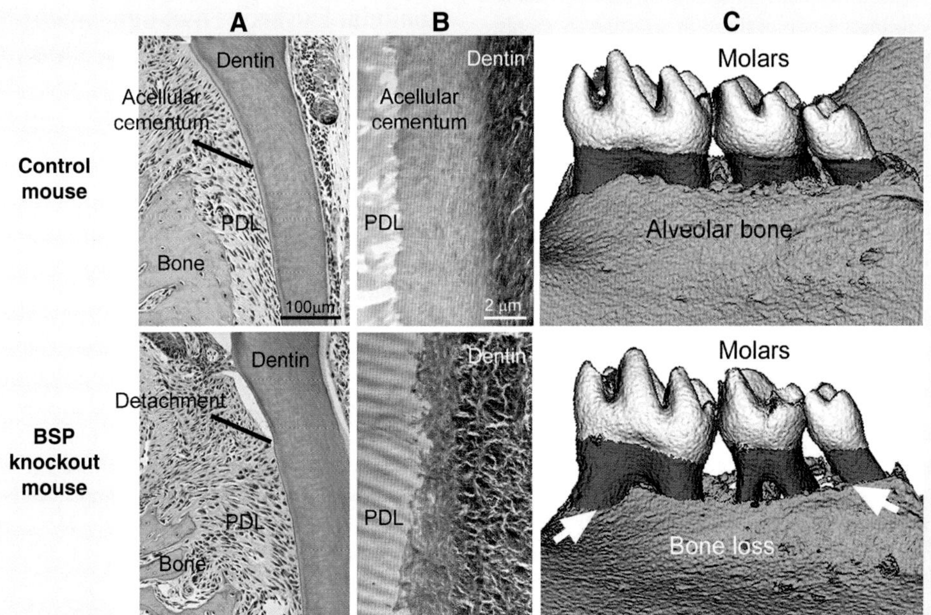

Box 9.1 Fig. 1 Periodontal defects arising from genetic knockout of bone sialoprotein (BSP) in mice. (A) Decalcified histology (H&E stain) of molar teeth shows detachment of periodontal ligament (PDL) in BSP knockout mice due to reduced strength of attachment to the root surface. (B) Transmission electron microscopy of molar teeth shows reduced layer of acellular cementum in BSP knockout mice. (C) Micro-computed tomography images reveal substantial alveolar bone loss in BSP knockout mice as a result of periodontal defects. (A and B, Adapted from Foster BL, et al.: Mineralization defects in cementum and craniofacial bone from loss of bone sialoprotein, *Bone* 78:150–164, 2015; C, Adapted from Ao M, et al.: Overlapping functions of bone sialoprotein and pyrophosphate regulators in directing cementogenesis, *Bone* 105:134–147, 2017.)

Continued

BOX 9.1 Bone sialoprotein is important for periodontal mineralization and function—cont'd

Recommended Reading

1. Goldberg HA, Hunter GK: Functional domains of bone sialoprotein. In Goldberg M, editor: *Phosphorylated extracellular matrix proteins of bone and dentin*, Bentham Science Publishers, 2012, pp 266–282.
2. Malaval L, et al.: Bone sialoprotein plays a functional role in bone formation and osteoclastogenesis, *J Exp Med* 205(5):1145–1153, 2008, Epub 2008/05/07. PubMed PMID: 18458111; PMCID: PMC2373846.
3. Foster BL, et al.: Deficiency in acellular cementum and periodontal attachment in bsp null mice, *J Dent Res* 92(2):166–172, 2013, Epub 2012/11/28. PubMed PMID: 23183644; PMCID: PMC3545692 authorship and/or publication of this article.
4. Foster BL, et al.: Mineralization defects in cementum and craniofacial bone from loss of bone sialoprotein, *Bone* 78:150–164, 2015, Epub 2015/05/13. PubMed PMID: 25963390; PMCID: PMC4466207.
5. Chavez MB, et al.: Bone sialoprotein is critical for alveolar bone healing in mice, *J Dent Res* 102(2):187–196, 2023, PubMed PMID: WOS:000885695700001.

Brian L. Foster, *PhD*
Division of Biosciences,
College of Dentistry,
The Ohio State University

TABLE 9.2 Type, Distribution, and Function of Cementum

Type	Origin of Fibers	Location	Function
Acellular (primary)	Extrinsic (some intrinsic fibers initially)	From cervical margin to the apical third	Anchorage
Cellular (secondary)	Intrinsic	Middle to apical third and furcations	Adaptation and repair
Mixed (alternating layers of acellular and cellular)	Intrinsic and extrinsic	Apical portion and furcations	Adaptation
Acellular afibrillar	—	Spurs and patches over enamel and dentin	No known function along the cementoenamel junction

Wnt Signaling

Wingless-related integration site (Wnt) molecules are small, secreted glycoproteins that act extracellularly to regulate many different processes such as development, growth, patterning, stemness, and cancer. The Wnt signaling pathway is evolutionarily conserved and extraordinarily complex (see Chapter 6. Wnt reporter and lineage-tracing strains of mice have allowed researchers to create molecular maps of Wnt responsiveness in the craniofacial tissues, and these patterns of Wnt signaling colocalize with various stem or progenitor populations in alveolar bone, the PDL, and the cementum. Osterix is believed to control cementoblast proliferation by maintaining a low level of Wnt. Inactivation of the Wnt signaling antagonist sclerostin leads to an increase in cementum formation. Phosphate/pyrophosphate levels have also been shown in vitro to influence Wnt signaling. Thus Wnt proteins offer a tremendous potential for promoting periodontal tissue formation and regeneration (see Yin in Recommended Reading).

Other Factors

Other molecules that are found within the developing and mature periodontal tissues include alkaline phosphatase, several growth factors (e.g., IGF, TGF-β, and platelet-derived growth factor), metalloproteinases, and proteoglycans. The significance of alkaline phosphatase to cementum formation has long been appreciated and is discussed in a previous section. Proteoglycans accumulate at the dentin-cementum junction, and it has been proposed that, together with noncollagenous matrix proteins such as bone sialoprotein and osteopontin, they may mediate initial mineralization and fiber attachment.

Mineralized tissues such as bone are turning over continually and require a delicate balance between formative and resorptive cells. Two key factors that have emerged as critical to this balance are osteoprotegerin and receptor-activated nuclear factor κB ligand (RANKL). Both are produced by osteoblasts and PDL fibroblasts. As discussed in more detail in Chapter 6, RANKL activates osteoclasts by binding to specific cell-surface receptors (RANK), whereas osteoprotegerin acts as a decoy interfering with the binding of RANKL to RANK. Growth factors and cytokines in the local region of the periodontium have been shown to modulate expression of osteoprotegerin and RANKL and thus may be important for controlling osteoclastic-mediated bone and root resorption; thus they may be attractive factors in designing therapeutic agents to regulate the behavior of this cell.

Equally important to the process of cell maturation and function are the timed expression of specific cell-surface receptors and the ability of certain factors to regulate their expression and, subsequently, the signaling pathways mediated by ligand-receptor interactions.

CEMENTUM VARIETIES

Table 9.2 lists the various types of cementum along with the origin, location, and function of each.

Acellular Extrinsic Fiber Cementum (Primary Cementum)

Cementoblasts that produce acellular extrinsic fiber cementum differentiate in proximity to the advancing root edge. During root development in human teeth, the first cementoblasts align along the newly formed but not yet mineralized mantle dentin (predentin) surface after disintegration of HERS (Fig. 9.8A and B). These first cementoblasts exhibit fibroblastic characteristics, extend cell processes into the unmineralized dentin, and initially deposit collagen fibrils within it so the dentin and cementum fibrils intermingle. Mineralization of the mantle dentin starts internally and does not reach the surface until mingling has occurred. Mineralization then spreads across into cementum under the regulatory influence of noncollagenous matrix proteins, thereby establishing the cementodentinal junction. In rodents, initial cementum deposition occurs onto the already mineralized dentin surface, preventing the intermingling of fibers (see Fig. 9.3A).

Initial acellular extrinsic fiber cementum consists of a mineralized layer with a short fringe of collagen fibers implanted perpendicular to the root surface (see Fig. 9.8D). The cells on the root surface then migrate away from the surface but continue to deposit collagen so that the fine fiber bundles lengthen and thicken. These cells also secrete noncollagenous matrix proteins that fill in the spaces between the collagen fibers (Fig. 9.9). This activity continues until about 15 to 20 μm of cementum has been formed, at which time the forming PDL fiber bundles become stitched to the fibrous fringe. Thereafter, the surface cells, now clearly defined as cementoblasts, will synthesize and secrete only noncollagenous matrix proteins, and the collagen fibrils that embed in the cementum layer will be formed by PDL fibroblasts. Although this cementum variety is called *acellular extrinsic fiber cementum,* whether its initial part should be classified instead as having intrinsic fibers is debatable. As described previously, the

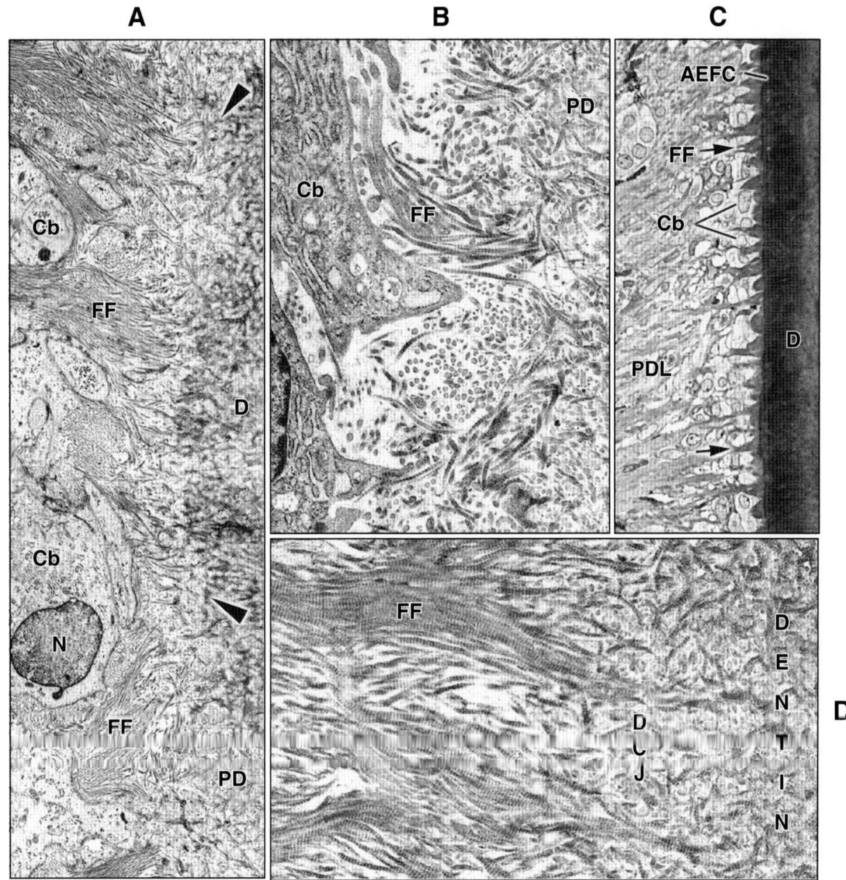

Fig. 9.8 Early human acellular extrinsic fiber cementogenesis *(AEFC)*. (A) Intermingling of collagen fiber bundles with those at the unmineralized dentin (predentin *[PD]*) surface. Arrowheads indicate the external dentin mineralization front. (B) Details of the intermingling. (C) The final connection between collagen fiber bundles of acellular (primary) cementum and dentin *(D)* surface is shown. (D) The fibrous fringe *(FF)* extending from cementum. *Cb,* Cementoblast; *DCJ,* dentinocemental junction; *N,* nucleus; *PDL,* periodontal ligament. (Courtesy D.D. Bosshardt.)

collagenous matrix of the first-formed cementum results from cementum-associated cells and is elaborated before the PDL forms; therefore the collagen is of local or intrinsic origin. This cementum variety develops slowly as the tooth is erupting and is considered to be acellular because the cells that form it remain on its surface (see Fig. 9.8C).

With the light microscope, acellular extrinsic fiber cementum seems relatively structureless (Fig. 9.10A); however, two sets of striations can be seen with special stains or polarized light. The striations running parallel to the root surface indicate incremental deposition, whereas the short striations at right angles to the root surface indicate the inserted mineralized PDL collagen fiber bundles (Fig. 9.11). With the electron microscope, these collagen bundles can be seen clearly to enter cementum, where they become fully mineralized. No well-defined layer of cementoid, akin to osteoid or predentin, can be distinguished on the surface of this cementum. However, the principal PDL fibers, or at least their cementum-related portion, may be regarded as equivalent to the cementoid. The overall degree of mineralization of this cementum is about 45% to 60%, but soft x-ray examination reveals that the innermost layer is less mineralized and that the outer layers are characterized by alternating bands of more and less mineral content that run parallel to the root surface.

Cellular Intrinsic Fiber Cementum (Secondary Cementum)

In some teeth (see the following discussion), after at least half the root is formed, a more rapidly formed and less mineralized variety of cementum (cellular intrinsic fiber cementum) is deposited on the unmineralized dentin surface near the advancing root edge (see Fig. 9.3B) as for acellular cementum. Differentiating cementoblasts deposit the collagen fibrils into the unmineralized dentin so that fibrils from both layers intermingle. These cells also manufacture various noncollagenous matrix proteins that fill in the spaces between collagen fibrils, regulate mineral deposition, and together with the mineral impart cohesion to the cementum layer (Fig. 9.12). A layer of unmineralized matrix (cementoid), which calcifies gradually, is present at the surface of the mineralized cementum matrix, with a mineralization front between the two layers (Figs. 9.13 and 9.14; see also Fig. 9.12). In contrast to osteoid or predentin, cementoid is not as regular and readily discernible. As cementum deposition progresses, cementoblasts become entrapped in the extracellular matrix they secrete (Fig. 9.15; see also Fig. 9.12). These entrapped cells with reduced secretory activity are called *cementocytes,* and similar to osteocytes they reside in a lacuna. Histologic studies suggest that incorporation of cementoblasts within cementum is more haphazard than that of osteoblasts within bone. Cementocytes have processes that lodge in canaliculi that communicate but do not form a syncytium that extends all the way to the surface, as is the case within bone (see Fig. 9.12A). Nourishment of the cells is believed to occur essentially by diffusion, and cementocytes in deeper layers may not be vital. With the electron microscope, cementocytes present a variable picture, depending on the distance of their location from the cement surface and their nutritional supply from the PDL. Loss of intracellular organelles and cell death is progressive in the deeper layers of cellular cementum. Although such features are consistent with loss of cell function, they also may reflect poor tissue preservation in the deeper layers. After a rapid initial phase

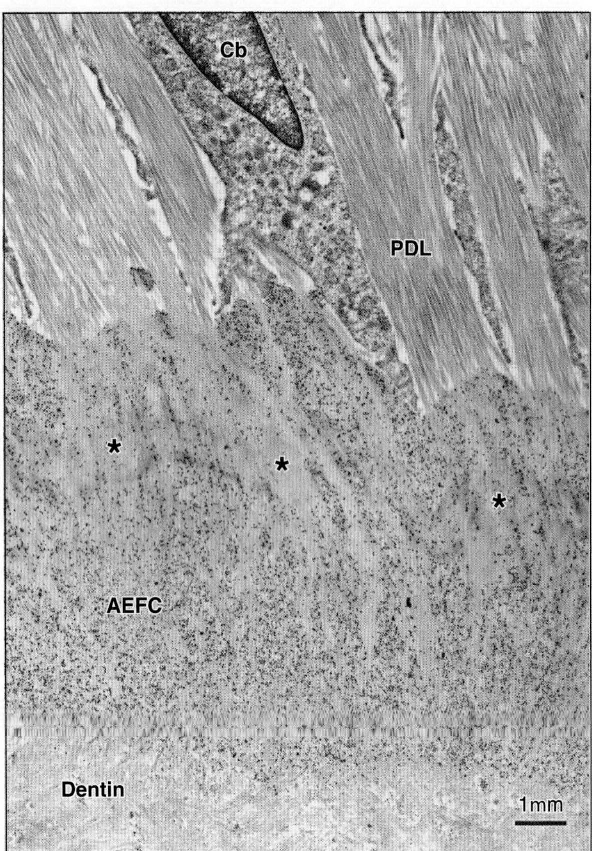

Fig. 9.9 Colloidal gold immunocytochemical preparation illustrating the presence and distribution of osteopontin *(black dots)*, a major noncollagenous matrix protein, in rat acellular extrinsic fiber cementum *(AEFC)*. This protein accumulates between the inserted portions of the extrinsic collagen fibers *(*)* and is more concentrated near dentin, where collagen fibers are sparse and more loosely arranged. *Cb*, Cementoblast; *PDL*, periodontal ligament.

of matrix formation, the deposition rate slows and secretion occurs in a more directional manner. This may sometimes lead to the formation of a layer of acellular intrinsic fiber cementum because the cells are not engulfed in their matrix but remain on its surface. In some species, disaggregating HERS cells get trapped near the cementodentinal junction, and cellular cementum forms around and above them.

Collagen fibrils are deposited haphazardly during the rapid phase; however, subsequently, the bulk of fibrils organize as bundles oriented parallel to the root surface (see Fig. 9.14). When the PDL becomes organized, cellular cementum continues to be deposited around the ligament fiber bundles, which become incorporated into the cementum and partially mineralized, thereby creating cellular mixed fiber cementum. This constitutes the bulk of secondary cementum, and with the light microscope, this tissue is identified easily because of (1) inclusion of cementocytes within lacunae with processes in canaliculi directed toward the tooth surface (see Fig. 9.12A and 9.15), (2) its laminated structure, and (3) the presence of cementoid on its surface. The intrinsic fibers are mineralized uniformly, whereas the extrinsic fiber bundles are mineralized variably, with many having a central, unmineralized core.

Cellular (secondary) cementum differs from acellular (primary) cementum in a number of ways. Not only are structural differences obvious in that the cells are incorporated into the matrix, but also the phenotype of the cells producing them may differ. Furthermore, secondary cementum is involved in tooth attachment in a minor and secondary way (this variety of cementum is usually absent from incisor and canine teeth) and is confined to the apical and interradicular regions of the tooth.

Acellular Afibrillar Cementum

The acellular afibrillar cementum variety consists of an acellular and afibrillar mineralized matrix with a texture similar to the one constituting the bulk of acellular extrinsic fiber cementum or the one found among the collagen fibrils of fibrillar cementum varieties and of bone. This cementum lacks collagen and hence plays no role in tooth attachment. It is deposited over enamel and dentin in proximity to the cementoenamel junction (Fig. 9.16A).

The cells responsible for the production of acellular afibrillar cementum still have not been identified with precision. For a long time, this cementum variety was believed to represent a developmental anomaly formed as the result of local disruptions in the reduced enamel epithelium that permit follicular cells to come into contact with the enamel surface and differentiate into cementoblasts. This concept has come under questioning because the enamel organ itself has been demonstrated to be able to produce mesenchymal proteins found in bone and cementum. Hence the reduced enamel epithelium need not obligatorily retract from the enamel surface to result in deposition of afibrillar cementum.

Researchers also have reported that HERS may produce epithelial products that accumulate on the forming root surface to form a layer, referred to as *intermediate cementum*. To date, however, no study has demonstrated the consistent presence of a distinct matrix layer between dentin and cementum proper. These may actually correspond to the situation where acellular afibrillar cementum forms on top of enamel (see later). The apparent presence of a layer along the radicular dentin surface in some histologic preparations (see Fig. 9.11C and D) does not consist of enamel proteins and may result from the way dentin and cementum collagen interface and the packing density of noncollagenous matrix proteins among the collagen fibrils.

Distribution of Cementum Varieties Along the Root

In humans, acellular afibrillar cementum is limited to the cervical enamel surface and occurs as spurs extending from acellular extrinsic fiber cementum or as isolated patches on the enamel surface close to the cementoenamel junction. Acellular extrinsic fiber cementum, which becomes the principal tissue of attachment, extends from the cervical margin of the tooth and covers two-thirds of the root and often more. Indeed, in incisors and canines, this form of cementum is often the only one found, and it extends to the apical foramen. At the cervical margin, the cementum is approximately 50 μm thick and increases in thickness as it progresses apically to approximately 200 μm. Cellular cementum is confined to the apical third and interradicular regions of premolar and molar teeth. Cellular cementum is often absent from single-rooted teeth, which indicates that its presence is not essential for tooth support. Both fibrillar cementum varieties can overlap. As mentioned before, the type of cementum formed during periodontal wound healing appears to be cellular in origin.

CEMENTOENAMEL JUNCTION

Classically, in approximately 30% of human teeth the cementum and enamel meet as a butt joint, forming a distinct cementoenamel junction at the cervical margin; 10% have a gap between the cementum and enamel, exposing root dentin; and in about 60% the cementum overlaps the enamel. This information was obtained from the study of ground sections (see Fig. 9.16), but studies with a scanning electron microscope indicate that the cementoenamel junction may exhibit all

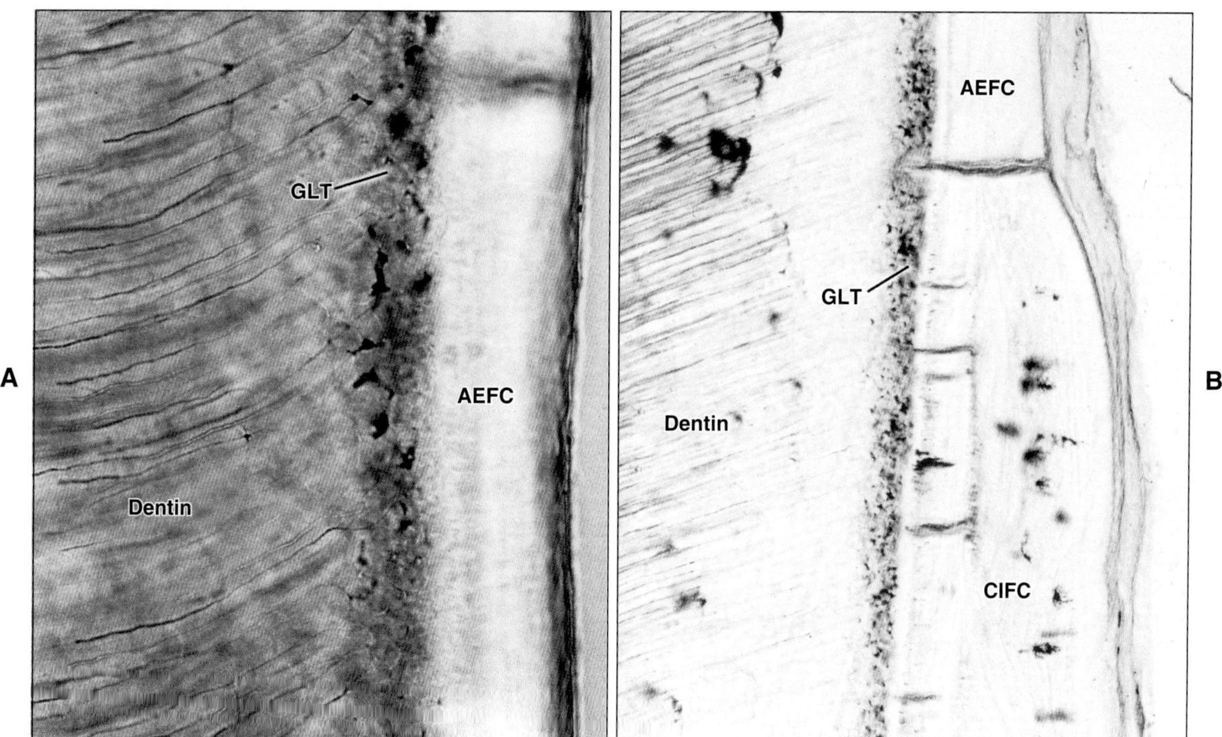

Fig. 9.10 Ground sections of human teeth examined by transmitted light illustrating (A) acellular extrinsic fiber cementum *(AEFC)* and (B) the transition between the former and cellular intrinsic fiber cementum *(CIFC)*. Both appear as a translucent, structureless layer. Cementocytes *(dark, rounded structures)* are present in the cellular intrinsic fiber cementum. *GLT,* Granular layer of Tomes (see Chapter 8).

of these forms and shows considerable variation when traced circumferentially. The exposure of root dentin at the cervical margin can lead to sensitivity at this site. It has also been suggested that such morphology may result in increased risk for idiopathic osteoclast-mediated root resorption and root surface caries.

ATTACHMENT OF CEMENTUM ONTO DENTIN

The attachment mechanism of cementum to dentin is of biologic interest and of clinical relevance because pathologic alterations and clinical interventions may influence the nature of the exposed root surface and hence the quality of the new attachment that forms when repair cementum is deposited. The mechanism by which these hard tissues bind together is essentially the same for acellular extrinsic fiber cementum and cellular intrinsic fiber cementum. Mineralization of the mantle dentin starts internally and does not reach the surface until the collagen fibrils of dentin and cementum have had the time to blend together. Mineralization then spreads through the surface layer of dentin, across the dentin-cementum junction, and into cementum, essentially resulting in an amalgamated mass of mineral. Although initiation of dentin mineralization occurs in relation to matrix vesicles in the radicular predentin, the subsequent spread of mineral deposition is under the regulatory influence of the various noncollagenous matrix proteins. From a biomechanical perspective, this arrangement appears optimal for a strong union between dentin and cementum. In acellular extrinsic fiber cementum of rodent teeth, cementum is deposited onto mineralized dentin, making amalgamation of dentin and cementum impossible and establishing a weakened interface. Indeed, histologic sections of rodent teeth often show a separation between dentin and cementum in the cervical third of the root. Interestingly, repair cementum adheres well to the root surface if a resorptive phase precedes new matrix deposition, implying that odontoclasts not only remove mineral and matrix but most likely also precondition the root surface. One possibility is that odontoclasts generate an organic matrix fringe with which the matrix of reparative cementum then can blend, thereby recapitulating the developmental sequence.

ALVEOLAR PROCESS

The alveolar process is the bone of the jaws that contains the sockets (alveoli) for the teeth (Fig. 9.17). The alveolar process consists of an outer (buccal and lingual) cortical plate, a central spongiosa, and bone lining the alveolus (alveolar bone). The cortical plate and alveolar bone meet at the alveolar crest (usually 1.5–2 mm below the level of the cementoenamel junction on the tooth it surrounds). Alveolar bone comprises inner and outer components. It is perforated by many foramina, which transmit nerves and vessels, and is sometimes referred to as the *cribriform plate.* Radiographically, alveolar bone also is referred to as the *lamina dura* because of an increased radiopacity (Fig. 9.18). This increased radiopacity is a result of the presence of thick bone without trabeculations that x-rays must penetrate and not of increased mineral content.

The bone directly lining the socket (inner aspect of alveolar bone) is referred to as *bundle bone.* Embedded within this bone are the extrinsic collagen fiber bundles of the PDL (Fig. 9.19), which, as in cellular cementum, are mineralized only at their periphery. Bundle bone thus provides attachment for the PDL fiber bundles that insert into it. Histologically, bundle bone generally is described as containing less intrinsic collagen fibrils than lamellar bone and exhibiting a coarse-fibered texture. Bundle bone is apposed to an outer layer of lamellar bone, but in some cases the alveolar bone can be made up almost completely of bundle bone. This is a simplistic description, however,

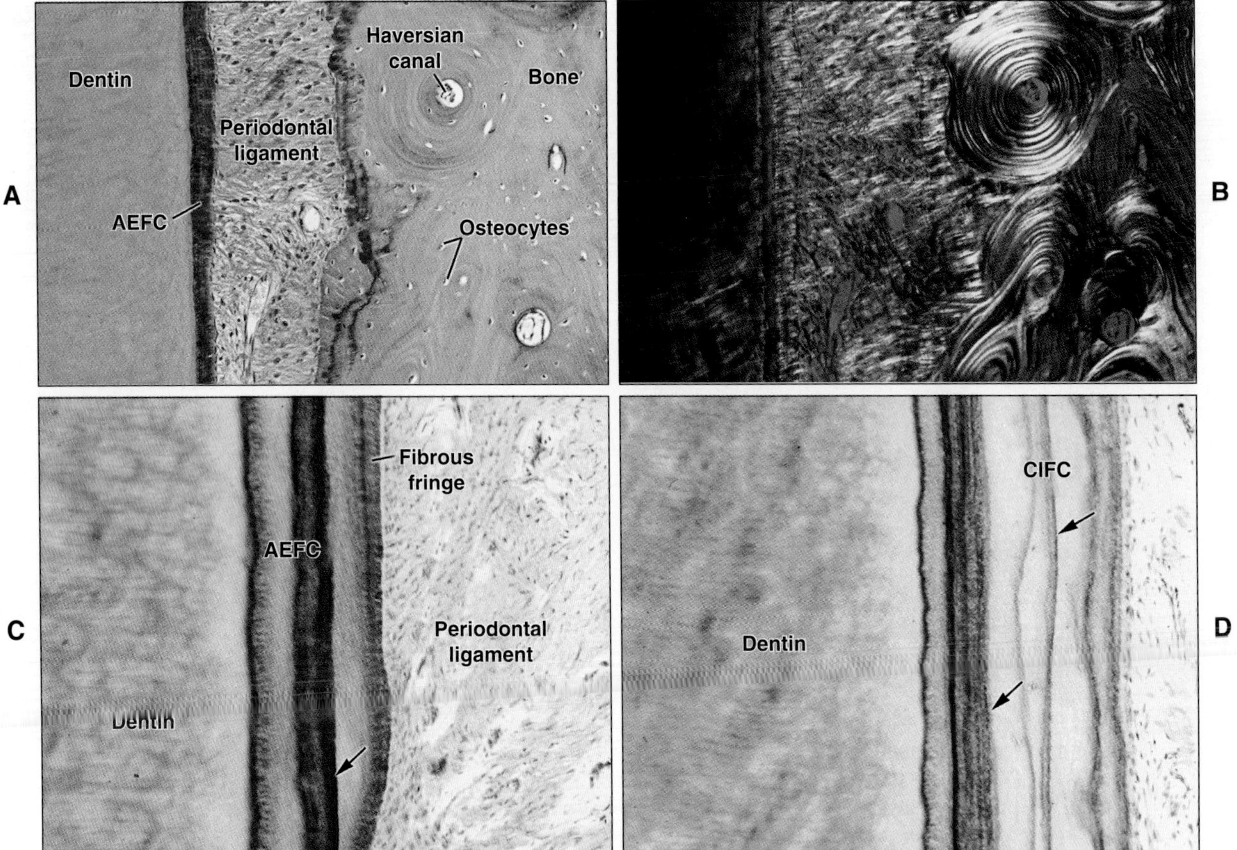

Fig. 9.11 Histologic section examined by (A) transmitted and (B) polarized light. Polarized microscopy reveals perpendicular striations in the cementum layer and in the surface of alveolar bone. These correspond to the sites of insertion of collagen fiber bundles. (C, D) Longitudinal *(arrows)* and perpendicular lines are also visible with some histologic stains. The longitudinal layering can appear as thin or thicker lines, essentially denoting the interface between successive layers of cementum. *AEFC,* Acellular extrinsic fiber cementum; *CIFC,* cellular intrinsic fiber cementum. (A, B, Courtesy P. Tambasco de Oliveira.)

because the tooth constantly is making minor movements, and therefore the bone of the socket wall constantly must adapt to many forms of stress. Thus practically all histologic forms of bone can be observed lining the alveolus, even in the same field in the same section (Fig. 9.20). This considerable variation reflects the functional plasticity of alveolar bone.

The cortical plate consists of surface layers of lamellar bone supported by compact Haversian system bone of variable thickness. The cortical plate is generally thinner in the maxilla and thickest on the buccal aspect of mandibular premolars and molars. The trabecular (spongy) bone occupying the central part of the alveolar process also consists of lamellae with Haversian systems occurring in the larger trabeculae. Yellow marrow, rich in adipose cells, generally fills the intertrabecular spaces, although sometimes there can be red or hematopoietic marrow. Trabecular bone is absent in the region of the anterior teeth, and, in this case, the cortical plate and alveolar bone are fused together. The important part of this complex in terms of tooth support is the bundle bone.

PERIODONTAL LIGAMENT

Understanding the cell populations and their function in healthy, mature periodontal tissues is required for developing predictable regenerative therapies. Investigations to date suggest that the PDL region in health contains a heterogeneous population of mesenchymal cells and that some cells within this population, when triggered appropriately, can differentiate toward an osteoblast or cementoblast phenotype (i.e., promote formation of bone and cementum). In addition, perivascular and endosteal fibroblasts, again when appropriately induced, have the capacity to form PDL, cementum, and bone. Compelling evidence exists indicating that populations of cells within the PDL, during development and during regeneration, secrete factors that can regulate the extent of mineralization. Thus factors secreted by PDL fibroblasts may inhibit mineralization and prevent the fusion of tooth root with surrounding bone, a situation referred to as *ankylosis.* Although much research is still to be done, current knowledge has enabled development of improved strategies for attracting and maintaining cells at a regeneration site.

The PDL is soft, specialized connective tissue situated between the cementum covering the root of the tooth and the bone forming the socket wall. The PDL ranges in width from 0.15 to 0.38 mm, with its thinnest portion around the middle third of the root (Figs. 9.21 and 9.22). The average width is 0.21 mm at 11 to 16 years of age, 0.18 mm at 32 to 52 years of age, and 0.15 mm at 51 to 67 years of age, showing a progressive decrease with age. The PDL is a connective tissue particularly well adapted to its principal function, supporting the teeth in their sockets while permitting them to withstand the considerable forces of mastication. The PDL also has the important function, in addition to attaching teeth to bone, of acting as a sensory receptor, which is necessary for the proper positioning of the jaws during normal function.

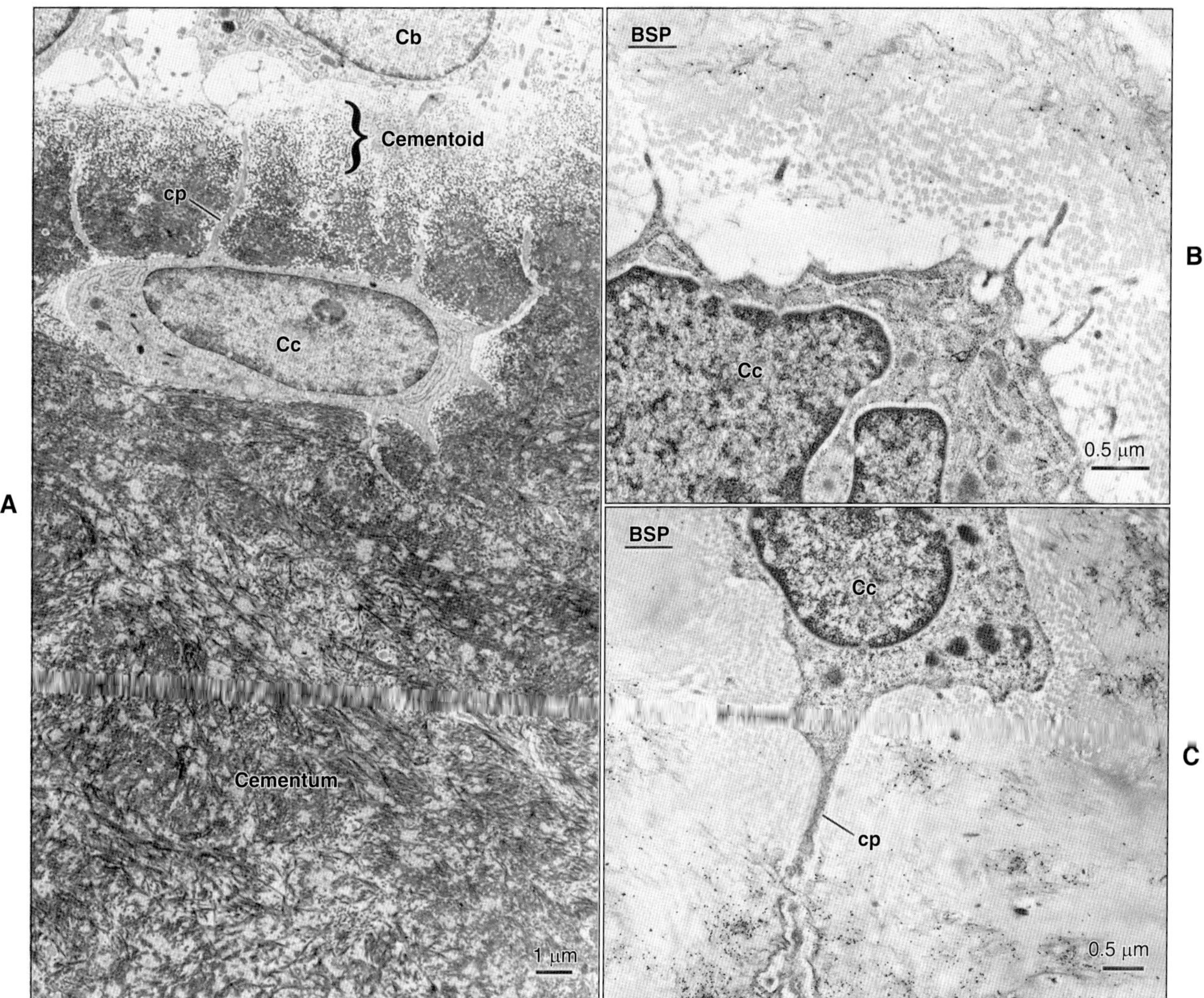

Fig. 9.12 Cellular intrinsic fiber cementum from (A, C) rat and (B) human being. (A) Cementoblasts *(Cbs)* line the cementum surface and are apposed against a layer of unmineralized matrix (cementoid). (A–C) Cementocytes *(Ccs)* reside within lacunae in cementum and can adopt various shapes. (A) The cell processes *(cps)* of cementocytes generally are directed toward the surface. (B, C) Immunocytochemical preparations for bone sialoprotein *(BSP)*. This noncollagenous matrix protein (indicated by the presence of *black dots*) accumulates among the mineralized collagen in regions that are generally more electron dense.

Apart from recognition that the PDL is formed within the developing dental follicle region, the exact timing of events associated with the development of an organized PDL varies among species, with individual tooth families, and between deciduous and permanent teeth. What follows is a generalized account from several studies undertaken largely on primates. At the commencement of formation, the ligament space consists of unorganized connective tissue with short fiber bundles extending into it from the bone and cemental surfaces (Fig. 9.23). Next, ligament mesenchymal cells begin to secrete collagen (mostly type I), which assembles as collagen bundles extending from the bone and cementum surfaces to establish continuity across the ligament space and thereby secure an attachment of the tooth to bone. In addition to collagen, several noncollagenous proteins are secreted that appear to play a role in the maintenance of the PDL space, but this still remains an unresolved question. Eruptive tooth movement and the establishment of occlusion then modify this initial attachment. For example, before the tooth erupts, the crest of the alveolar bone is above the cementoenamel junction, and the developing fiber bundles of the PDL are directed obliquely. Because the tooth moves during eruption, the level of the alveolar crest comes to coincide with the cementoenamel junction, and the oblique fiber bundles just below the free gingival fibers become horizontally aligned. During the process of tooth eruption, osteoclast precursors are activated by a variety of factors secreted by cells within the local environment, including RANKL/osteoprotegerin ligand and macrophage colony–stimulating factor. Functional osteoclasts are critical for the formation of marrow spaces within bone and for tooth eruption. When the tooth finally comes into function, the alveolar crest is positioned nearer the apex. The horizontal fibers (alveolar crest fibers) have become oblique once more, with the difference that now the cemental attachment has reversed its relation to the alveolar attachment and is positioned in a coronal direction, as opposed to its previous apical direction (Fig. 9.24). Only after the teeth come into function do the fiber bundles of the PDL thicken appreciably.

When the periodontium is exposed to increased function, the width of the PDL can increase by as much as 50%, and the principal fiber bundles also increase greatly in thickness. The bony trabeculae supporting the alveoli also increase in number and in thickness, and the alveolar bone itself becomes thicker. Conversely, a reduction in function leads to changes that are the opposite of those described for

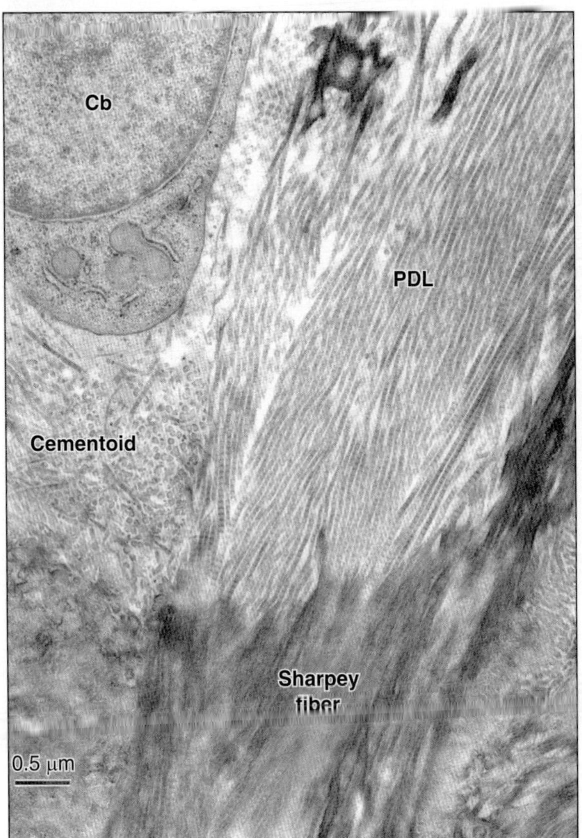

Fig. 9.13 Electron micrograph illustrating the insertion of periodontal ligament *(PDL)* fiber bundles into cellular intrinsic fiber cementum. Cementoid is seen at the surface of mineralized cementum. *Cb,* Cementoblast.

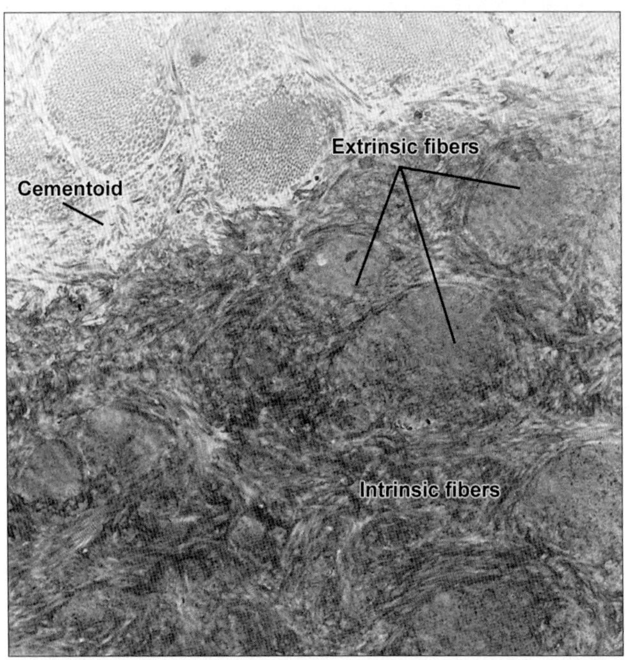

Fig. 9.14 Electron micrograph of an oblique section through the periodontal ligament–cementum interface. The distinction between extrinsic and intrinsic fibers within cementum is readily apparent, the intrinsic fibers essentially surrounding the embedded portions of the extrinsic fibers, which constitute Sharpey's fibers. (Courtesy M.A. Listgarten.)

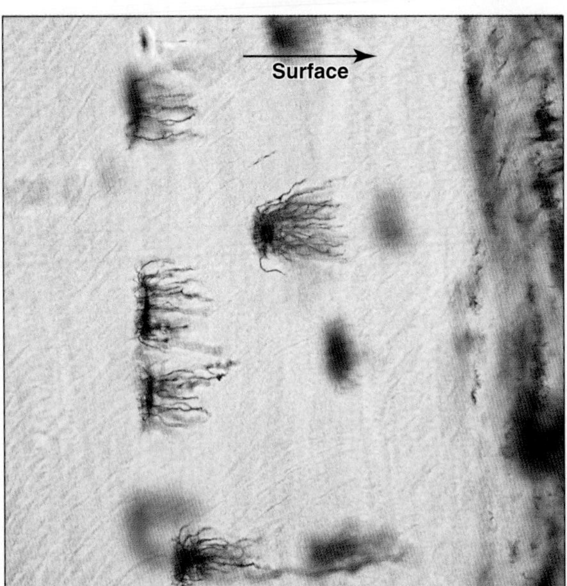

Fig. 9.15 Cementocyte lacunae in ground section. Most of the canaliculi point toward the tooth surface *(arrow)*. The indistinct dark patches are other cementocyte lacunae deeper within the ground section (and consequently out of focus).

excess function. The ligament narrows, the fiber bundles decrease in number and thickness, and the trabeculae become fewer. This reduction in width of the PDL is caused mostly by the deposition of additional cementum (Fig. 9.25).

Similar to all other connective tissues, the PDL consists of cells and an extracellular compartment of collagenous fibers and a noncollagenous extracellular matrix. The cells include osteoblasts and osteoclasts (technically within the ligament but functionally associated with bone), fibroblasts, ERMs, macrophages, undifferentiated mesenchymal cells, stem cells, and cementoblasts (also technically within the ligament but functionally associated with cementum). The extracellular compartment consists of well-defined collagen fiber bundles (Fig. 9.26) embedded in an amorphous background material (ground substance) consisting of, among others, glycosaminoglycans, glycoproteins, and glycolipids.

Fibroblasts

The principal cells of the PDL are fibroblasts. Although fibroblasts look alike microscopically, heterogeneous cell populations exist between different connective tissues and within the same connective tissue. In the case of the PDL, its fibroblasts are characterized by an ability to achieve an exceptionally high rate of turnover of proteins within the extracellular compartment—in particular, collagen. PDL fibroblasts are large cells with an extensive cytoplasm containing an abundance of organelles associated with protein synthesis and secretion (i.e., rough endoplasmic reticulum, Golgi complex, and many secretory granules). Ligament fibroblasts also have a well-developed cytoskeleton (see Chapter 4) with a particularly prominent actin network, the presence of which is believed to indicate the functional demands placed on the cells, requiring change in shape and migration. Ligament fibroblasts also show frequent cell-to-cell contacts of the adherens and the gap junction types. Fibroblasts are aligned along the general direction of the fiber bundles and have extensive processes that wrap around the bundles. The collagen fibrils of the fiber bundles are being remodeled continuously. The fibroblast achieves remodeling of collagen; it is capable of simultaneously synthesizing and degrading collagen (see Chapter 4). Because of the exceptionally high rate of turnover of collagen in

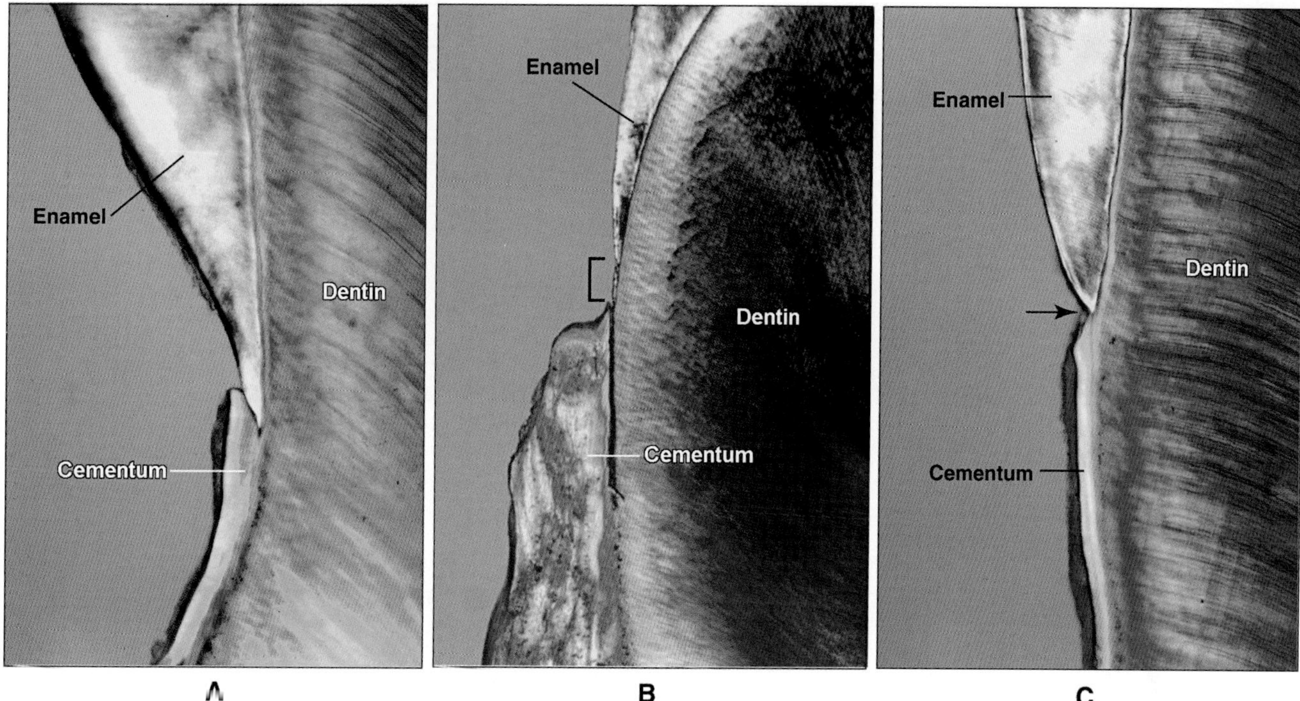

Fig. 9.16 Three configurations of the cementoenamel junction in ground sections. (A) Cementum overlaps the enamel. (B) A deficiency of cementum (*bracket*) leaves root dentin exposed. (C) A butt joint is visible (*arrow*). (B, C, Courtesy P. Tambasco de Oliveira.)

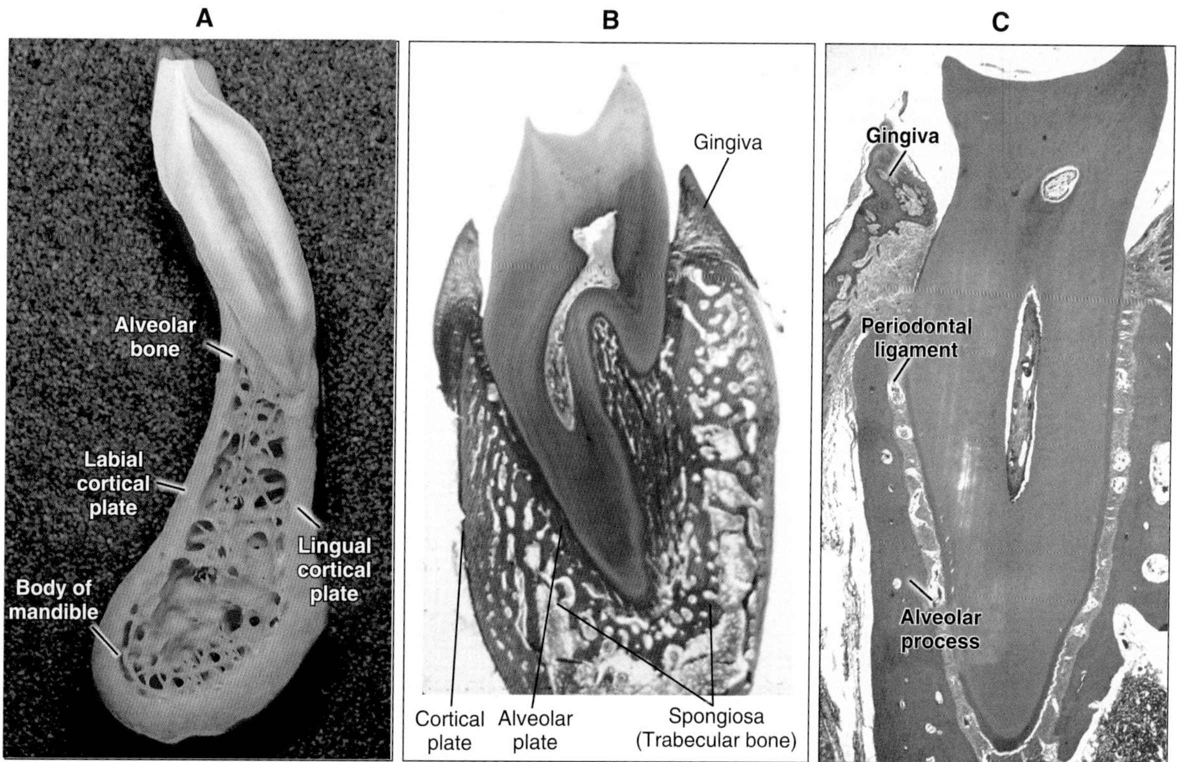

Fig. 9.17 (A) Trabecular bone is found between the lingual cortical plate and alveolar bone in the region of the apical third of the root and in the body of the mandible. (B, C) Histologic sections illustrating (B) a thick alveolar process with an abundant spongiosa (trabecular bone) between the cortical plates and alveolar bone and (C) a thin alveolar process lacking distinct trabecular bone. (A, Courtesy P. Tambasco de Oliveira.)

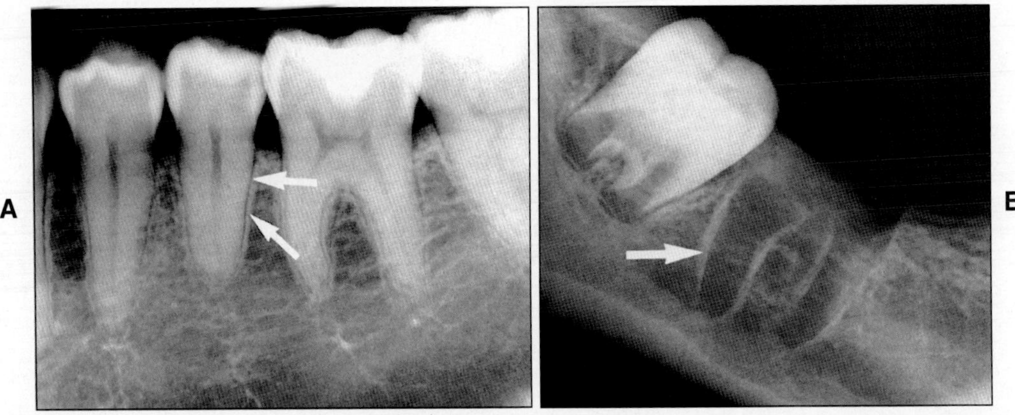

Fig. 9.18 The lamina dura *(arrows)* appears as a thin opaque layer around teeth (A) and around a recent extraction socket (B). (From White SC, Pharoah MJ: *Oral radiology: principles and interpretation*, ed 6, St. Louis, MO, 2009, Mosby.)

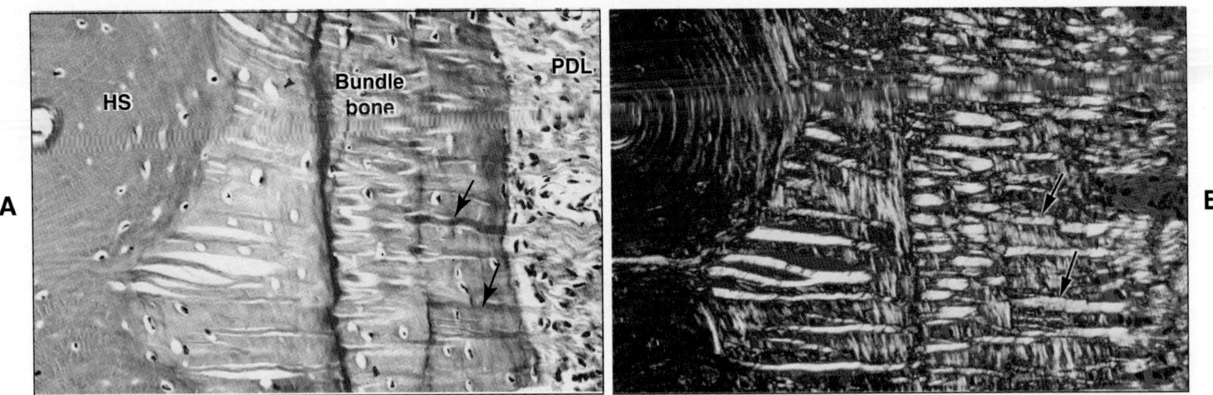

Fig. 9.19 Histologic preparations of alveolar bone examined by (A) transmitted and (B) polarized light microscopy. Periodontal ligament *(PDL)* fiber bundles *(arrows)* insert into the bone lining the alveolar socket, giving it the name bundle bone. The inserted fibers are referred to as *Sharpey's fibers* and appear refringent under polarized light. Bundle bone is apposed to trabecular bone with Haversian systems *(HS)*. (Courtesy P. Tambasco de Oliveira.)

the ligament, any interference with fibroblast function by disease rapidly produces a loss of the supporting tissue of a tooth. Importantly, in inflammatory situations, such as those associated with periodontal diseases, an increased expression of matrix metalloproteinases occurs that aggressively destroys collagen. Thus attractive therapies for controlling tissue destruction may include host modulators that have the capacity to inhibit matrix metalloproteinases.

Fibroblast contractility probably is of greatest significance during posteruptive tooth movements. These include functional movements during mastication, accommodation for growth of the jaws, and compensation for occlusal and interproximal wear. Fibroblasts are associated intimately with the fibrous components of their matrix and respond to changes in tension and compression in the matrix. Integrins, which bind to extracellular matrix components, serve as mechanotransducers to transmit the stimulus to the cell. In addition to contraction, the response of the cell may encompass the pulling of collagen fibrils back toward the cell, the movement of cell processes or individual receptors on the processes, or a combination of all these events. The fibroblasts and the collagen align parallel to the direction of the principal strain in the matrix, which probably accounts for the highly ordered arrangement of PDL fiber bundles.

Mechanical stress also is a significant stimulus for extracellular matrix production by fibroblasts; the repetitive stress to which the PDL is subjected presumably contributes to the high rates of collagen turnover in this tissue. This rapid turnover of matrix components allows the PDL to adapt to the demands of functional tooth movements. Localized changes in tensile and compressive forces during growth, and the mesial drift resulting from interproximal wear, stimulate bone and cementum formation or resorption. In contrast, the absence of these forces, such as when a tooth has no opponent, results in decreased matrix production, increased collagenase (matrix metalloproteinase 1) secretion, and a thinning of the PDL.

Epithelial Cells

The epithelial cells in the PDL are remnants of HERS (the ERMs). They occur close to the cementum as clusters or strands of cells and are easily recognized in histologic sections because their nuclei generally stain deeply (see Fig. 9.6) and immunohistochemically by their expression of cytokeratin 14 and 19 (Fig. 9.27). Some believe they form a network around roots that possibly interconnect with the junctional epithelium (see Fig. 9.27). ERMs have been proposed to play a role in periodontal maintenance and to represent a stem cell compartment capable of

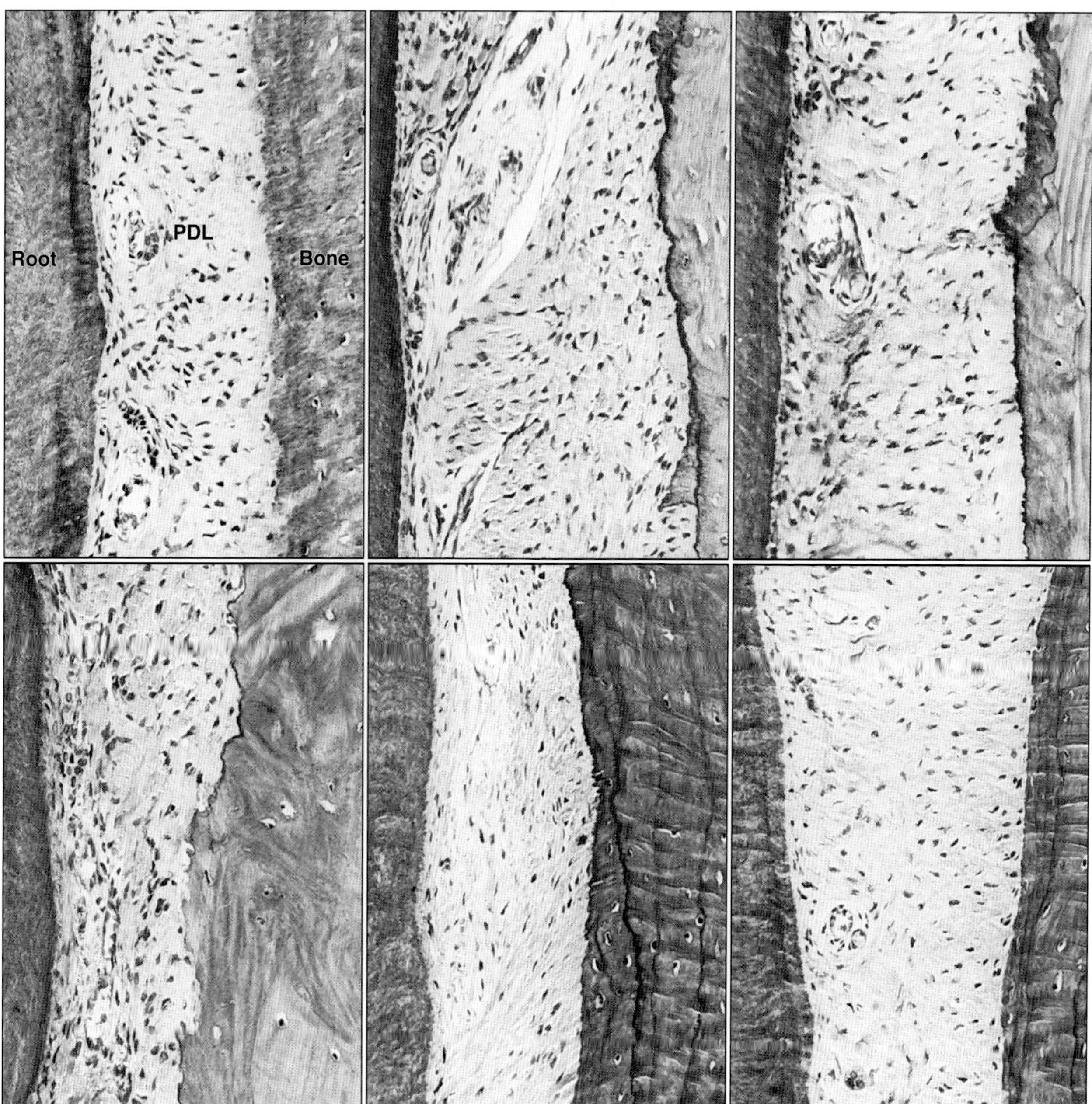

Fig. 9.20 Photomicrographs of the periodontal ligament *(PDL)* region from a single tooth. The considerable variation in morphology of the bone lining this alveolus is produced by the resorption and deposition of bone as it responds to functional demands placed on it. The root surface is always on the left and bone on the right.

giving rise to many if not all cell types found in the periodontium. It has been shown that under certain circumstances they can be activated and produce epithelial and mesenchymal matrix proteins that are implicated in the mineralization of tooth and bone matrices. When periodontal integrity is compromised (see Nishio et al., in Recommended Reading), ERMs are activated very early on and dramatically upregulate the expression of the matricellular-like protein odontogenic ameloblast–associated protein (see Chapters 7 and 12 for discussion on this protein).

Undifferentiated Mesenchymal Cells

An important cellular constituent of the PDL is the undifferentiated mesenchymal cell or progenitor cell; these cells have a perivascular location. Although they have been demonstrated to be a source of new cells for the PDL, whether a single progenitor cell gives rise to daughter cells that differentiate into fibroblasts, osteoblasts, and cementoblasts or whether separate progenitors exist for each cell line is not known. The fact that new cells are being produced for the PDL while cells of the ligament are in a steady state means that this production of new cells must be balanced by migration of cells out of the ligament or cell death. Selective deletion of ligament cells occurs by apoptosis (see Chapter 7 for description of this process), and this process provides cell turnover, which, in the rat PDL, involves approximately 2% of the population at any time.

Stem Cells

Pluripotent stem cells are present in the PDL, which represents an easily accessible source of stem cells compared with those found in pulp. These postnatal mesenchymal stem cells have the capacity of self-renewal and

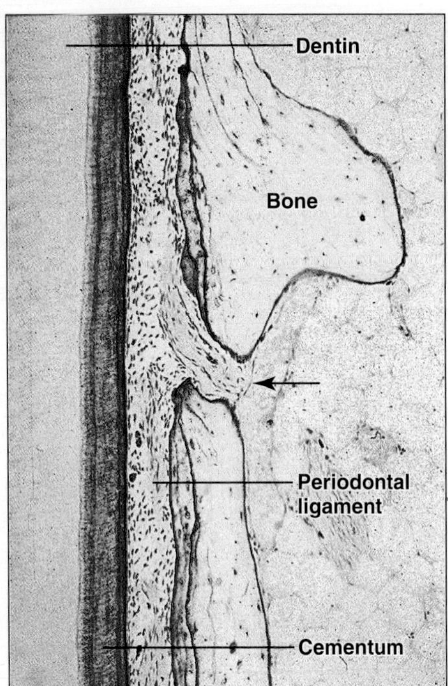

Fig. 9.21 Longitudinal section along the tooth root. Note the perforation *(arrow)* in the alveolar bone that transmits neurovascular bundles.

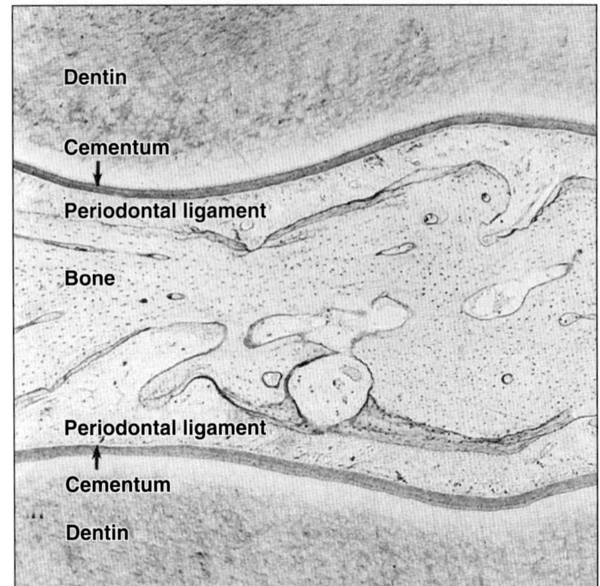

Fig. 9.22 Periodontal ligament in a cross section between two teeth.

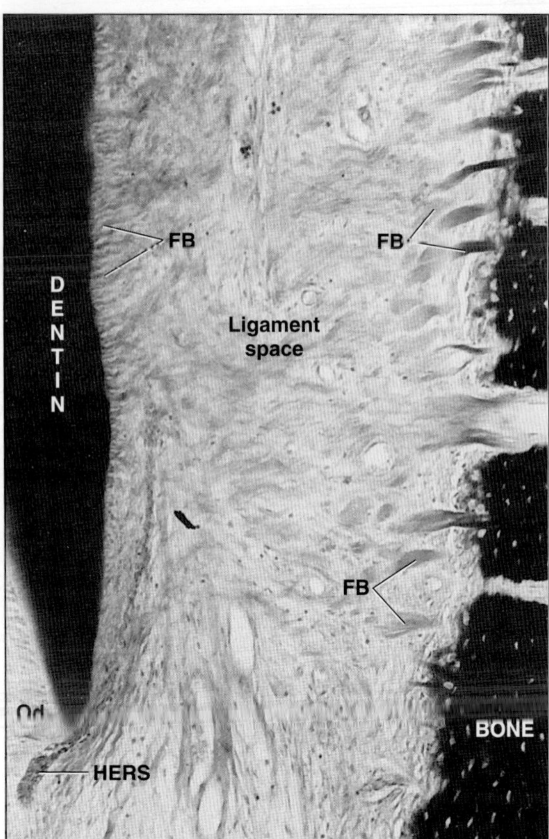

Fig. 9.23 The developing periodontal ligament. Fiber bundles *(FB)* extend into the unorganized ligament space from the cement and alveolar bone surfaces. *HERS,* Hertwig epithelial root sheath; *Od,* odontoblasts.

have the potential to differentiate into adipogenic, cementogenic, osteogenic, and chondrogenic cells. Some believe that PDL stem cells express distinctive mesenchymal and embryonic markers.

Bone and Cementum Cells

Although technically situated within the PDL, bone and cementum cells are associated properly with the hard tissues they form and are discussed with these tissues.

Fibers

The predominant collagens of the PDL are types I, III, and XII, with individual fibrils having a smaller average diameter than tendon collagen fibrils. This difference is believed to reflect the short half-life of ligament collagen, meaning that they have less time for fibrillar assembly.

Most collagen fibrils in the PDL are arranged in definite and distinct fiber bundles. Each bundle resembles a spliced rope; individual strands can be remodeled continually, whereas the overall fiber maintains its architecture and function. In this way the fiber bundles are able to adapt to the continual stresses placed on them. These bundles are arranged in groups that can be seen easily in an appropriately stained light microscope section (Figs. 9.28 and 9.29). Those bundles running between the tooth and bone represent the principal fiber bundles of the PDL. These bundles are as follows:

1. The alveolar crest group, attached to the cementum just below the cementoenamel junction and running downward and outward to insert into the rim of the alveolus
2. The horizontal group, just apical to the alveolar crest group and running at right angles to the long axis of the tooth from cementum to bone, just below the alveolar crest
3. The oblique group, by far the most numerous in the PDL and running from the cementum in an oblique direction to insert into bone coronally
4. The apical group, radiating from the cementum around the apex of the root to the bone, forming the base of the socket
5. The interradicular group, found only between the roots of multirooted teeth and running from the cementum into the bone, forming the crest of the interradicular septum (see Fig. 9.28)

At each end, all the principal collagen fiber bundles of the PDL are embedded in cementum or bone (see Figs. 9.5, 9.8, 9.11, 9.13, 9.19, and 9.23). The embedded portion is referred to as *Sharpey's fibers.* Sharpey's

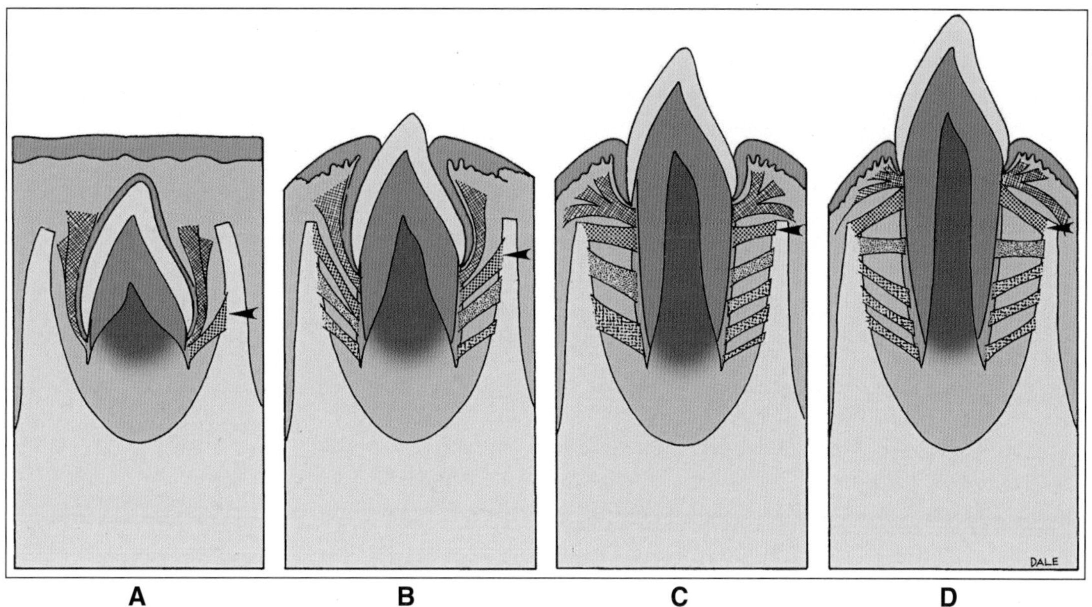

Fig. 9.24 The development of principal fiber groupings in the periodontal ligament. The group of alveolar crest fibers *(arrowheads),* first forming in (A), are initially oblique (B), then horizontal (C), and then oblique again (D).

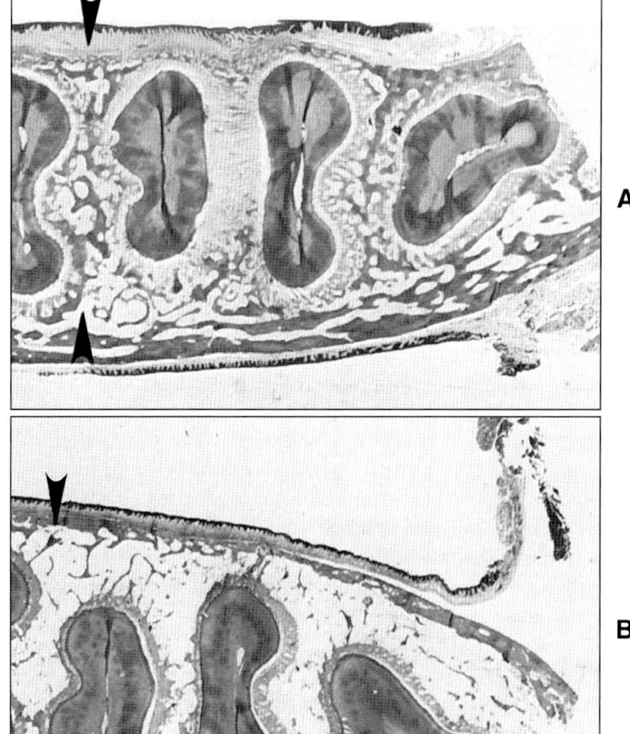

Fig. 9.25 Photomicrographs of the effect of nonfunction on the supporting apparatus of the tooth. (A) Normal appearance of tissues supporting the teeth. (B) Effect of nonfunction for 6 months. The loss of bone in the area *(arrowheads)* is notable. A narrowing of the ligament also can be distinguished. (Courtesy D.C. Picton.)

fibers, in primary acellular cementum, are mineralized fully; those in cellular cementum and bone generally are mineralized only partially at their periphery. Occasionally, Sharpey's fibers pass uninterruptedly through the bone of the alveolar process to continue as principal fibers of an adjacent PDL, or they may mingle buccally and lingually with the fibers of the periosteum that cover the outer cortical plates of the alveolar process. Sharpey's fibers pass through the alveolar process only when the process consists entirely of compact bone and contains no Haversian systems, which is not common.

Although not strictly part of the PDL, other groups of collagen fibers are associated with maintaining the functional integrity of the periodontium. These groups are found in the lamina propria of the gingiva and collectively form the gingival ligament (see Figs. 9.28 and 9.29). Five groups of fiber bundles compose this ligament:

1. Dentogingival group. These are the most numerous fibers, extending from the cervical cementum to the lamina propria of the free and attached gingivae.
2. Alveologingival group. These fibers radiate from the bone of the alveolar crest and extend into the lamina propria of the free and attached gingivae.
3. Circular group. This small group of fibers forms a band around the neck of the tooth, interlacing with other groups of fibers in the free gingiva and helping to bind the free gingiva to the tooth (see Fig. 9.28).
4. Dentoperiosteal group. Running apically from the cementum over the periosteum of the outer cortical plates of the alveolar process, these fibers insert into the alveolar process or the vestibular muscle and floor of the mouth.
5. Transseptal fiber system. These fibers run interdentally from the cementum just apical to the base of the junctional epithelium of one tooth over the alveolar crest and insert into a comparable region of the cementum of the adjacent tooth. Together these fibers constitute the transseptal fiber system, collectively forming an interdental ligament connecting all the teeth of the

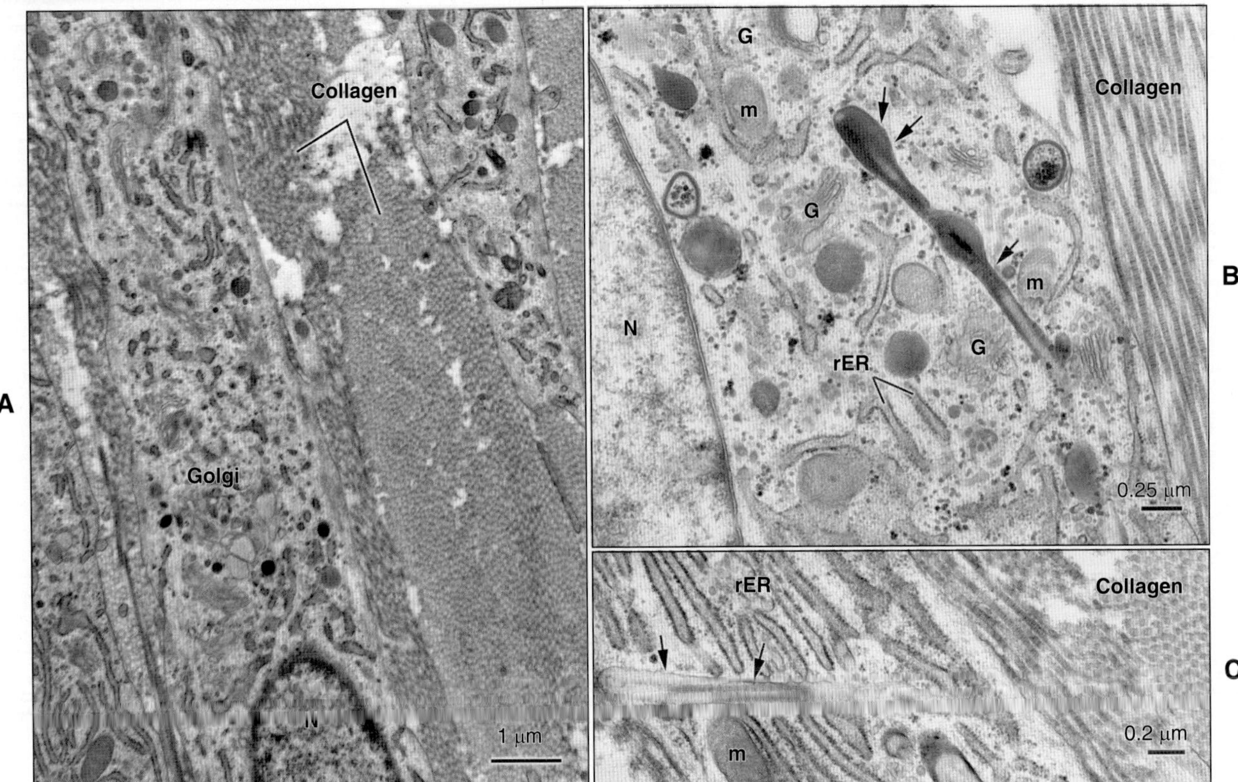

Fig. 9.26 Electron micrographs of the periodontal ligament in a pig. (A) Elongated fibroblasts can be seen alternating with distinctive collagen fiber bundles. The clear areas are occupied by ground substance. (B, C) The periodontal ligament undergoes turnover and remodeling, during which matrix synthesis and breakdown take place. Some collagen degradation takes place intracellularly following its internalization *(arrows)*. *G,* Golgi complex; *m,* mitochondria; *N,* nucleus; *rER,* rough endoplasmic reticulum.

arch (Fig. 9.30). The supracrestal fibers, particularly the transseptal fiber system, have been implicated as a major cause of postretention relapse of orthodontically positioned teeth. The inability of the transseptal fiber system to undergo physiologic rearrangement has led to this conclusion. Although the rate of turnover is not as rapid as in the PDL, studies have shown that the transseptal fiber system is capable of turnover and remodeling under normal physiologic conditions, as well as during therapeutic tooth movement. A sufficiently prolonged retention period after orthodontic tooth movement then would seem reasonable to allow reorganization of the transseptal fiber system to ensure the clinical stability of tooth position.

Elastic Fibers

The three types of elastic fibers are elastin, oxytalan, and elaunin (see Chapter 4). Only oxytalan fibers are present within the PDL; however, elaunin fibers may be found within fibers of the gingival ligament.

Oxytalan fibers (Fig. 9.31) are bundles of microfibrils that are distributed extensively in the PDL. The fibers run more or less vertically from the cementum surface of the root apically, forming a three-dimensional branching meshwork that surrounds the root and terminates in the apical complex of arteries, veins, and lymphatic vessels. The fibers also are associated with neural and vascular elements. Oxytalan fibers are numerous and dense in the cervical region of the ligament, where they run parallel to the gingival group of collagen fibers. Although their function has not been determined fully, they are believed to regulate vascular flow in relation to tooth function. Because they are elastic, they can expand in response to tensional variations, with such variations then registered on the walls of the vascular structures.

Ground Substance

Ground substance is an amorphous background material that binds tissue and fluids, the latter serving for the diffusion of gases and metabolic substances. Ground substance is a major constituent of the PDL, but few studies have been undertaken to determine its exact composition. What information exists indicates similarity to most other connective tissues in terms of its components, with some variation in ratios, so that in the ligament, dermatan sulfate is the principal glycosaminoglycan. The PDL ground substance has been estimated to be 70% water and is believed to have a significant effect on the ability of the tooth to withstand stress loads. An increase in tissue fluids occurs within the amorphous matrix of the ground substance in areas of injury and inflammation.

Blood Supply

For a connective tissue, the PDL is exceptionally well vascularized, which reflects the high rate of turnover of its cellular and extracellular constituents. The main blood supply of connective tissue is from the superior and inferior alveolar arteries. These arteries pursue an intraosteal course and give off alveolar branches that ascend within the bone as interalveolar arteries. Numerous branches arise from the interalveolar vessels to run horizontally, penetrate the alveolar bone, and enter the PDL space. Because they enter the ligament, they are called *perforating arteries,* and they are more abundant in the PDL of posterior teeth than in that of anterior teeth and are in greater numbers

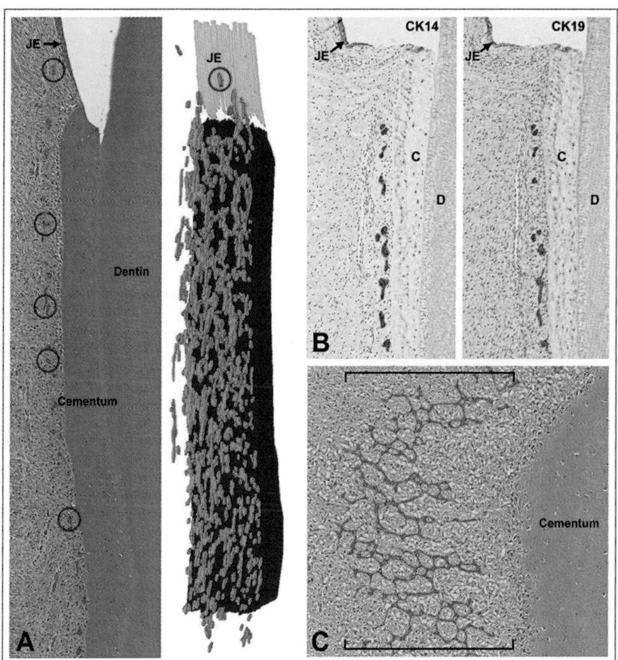

Fig. 9.27 (A) Epithelial cell rests of Malassez generally appear as isolated islands *(circles)* along the root surface. Three-dimensional reconstruction from serial sections, however, clearly demonstrates that these islands are part of an intricate network that surrounds the tooth roots and that extends into the junctional epithelium *(JE)*. (B) Immunohistochemical preparations showing that these cell clusters *(brown areas)* are rich in cytokeratin 14 and 19 (*CK14* and *CK19*). (C) This network can also be seen in fortuitous tangential sections to the tooth surface. (C, courtesy C. Rivest.)

in mandibular than in maxillary teeth. In single-rooted teeth, these arteries are found most frequently in the gingival third of the ligament, followed by the apical third.

This pattern of distribution has clinical importance. In the healing of extraction wounds, new tissue invades from the perforations, and the formation of a blood clot occupying the socket is more rapid in its gingival and apical areas. Within the ligament, these arteries occupy areas (or layers) of loose connective tissue called *interstitial areas* between the principal fiber bundles. Vessels course in an apical-occlusal direction with numerous transverse connections (Fig. 9.32). Fenestrated capillaries occur.

Many arteriovenous anastomoses occur within the PDL, and venous drainage is achieved by axially directed vessels that drain into a system of retia (or networks) in the apical portion of the ligament consisting of large-diameter venules (see Fig. 9.32). Lymphatic vessels tend to follow the venous drainage.

Nerve Supply

The use of radioautographic and immunocytochemical labeling of neural proteins has greatly improved knowledge about the innervation of the PDL over what previously was based on the results of somewhat unpredictable silver staining techniques. Although species differences have been reported, a general pattern of ligament innervation seems to exist (Fig. 9.33). First, the general anatomic configuration is applicable to all teeth, with nerve fibers running from the apical region toward the gingival margin and being joined by fibers entering laterally through the foramina of the socket wall (see Fig. 9.21). These latter fibers divide into two branches, one extending apically and the other gingivally. Second, regional variation occurs in the termination of neural elements, with the apical region of the ligament containing more nerve endings than elsewhere (except for the upper incisors, where not only is the innervation generally denser than in molars but also further dense distributions of neural elements exist in the coronal half of the labial PDL as well as apically, suggesting that the spatial arrangement of receptors is a factor in determining the response characteristics of the ligament). Third, the manner in which these nerve fibers terminate is being clarified. Four types of neural terminations now have been described (Fig. 9.34). The first (and most common) are free nerve endings that ramify in a treelike configuration. These nerve endings are located at regular intervals along the length of the root, suggesting that each termination controls its own territory, and extend to the cementoblast layer. These nerve endings originate largely from unmyelinated fibers but carry with them a Schwann cell envelope with processes that project into the surrounding connective tissue (Fig. 9.35). Such endings are believed to be nociceptors and mechanoreceptors. The second type of nerve terminal is found around the root apex and resembles Ruffini corpuscles. These nerves appear to be dendritic and end in terminal expansions among the PDL fiber bundles. By electron microscopy, such receptors can be seen to have subdivided further into simple and compound forms, the former consisting of a single neurite and the latter of several terminations after branching. Both receptors have ensheathing Schwann cells that are especially close to collagen fiber bundles (Fig. 9.36), which provide morphologic evidence of their known physiologic function as mechanoreceptors. An incomplete fibrous capsule sometimes is found associated with the compound receptors. The third type of nerve terminal is a coiled form found in the midregion of the PDL, the function and ultrastructure of which have not yet been determined. The fourth type (the least common) is found associated with the root apex and consists of spindlelike endings surrounded by a fibrous capsule.

The autonomic supply of the PDL has not yet been fully determined, and the few descriptions available concern sympathetic supply. No evidence indicates the existence of a parasympathetic supply. The many free nerve terminals observed in close association with blood vessels are believed to be sympathetic and to affect regional blood flow.

Adaptation to Functional Demand

The structural components of the periodontium have been presented. (The gingiva facing teeth are described in Chapter 12.) Together these components form a functional system that provides an attachment for the tooth to the bone of the jaw while permitting the teeth to withstand the considerable forces of mastication.

A remarkable capacity of the PDL is that it maintains its width more or less over time. The balance between formation and maintenance of mineralized tissues, bone, and cementum versus soft connective tissues of the PDL requires finely regulated control over cells in the local area. Several situations in which this balance is disrupted result in a variety of abnormal pathologic conditions (e.g., lack of tooth eruption because of ankylosis of teeth with surrounding bone, often associated with an osteoclast defect, and lack of cementum formation resulting in exfoliation of teeth, as observed in hypophosphatasia).

Compelling evidence exists indicating that populations of cells within the PDL, during development and during regeneration, secrete molecules that can regulate the extent of mineralization and prevent the fusion of the tooth root with surrounding bone. At the cell level, it has been reported that Msx2 (Msh homeobox 2) prevents the osteogenic differentiation of PDL fibroblasts by repressing

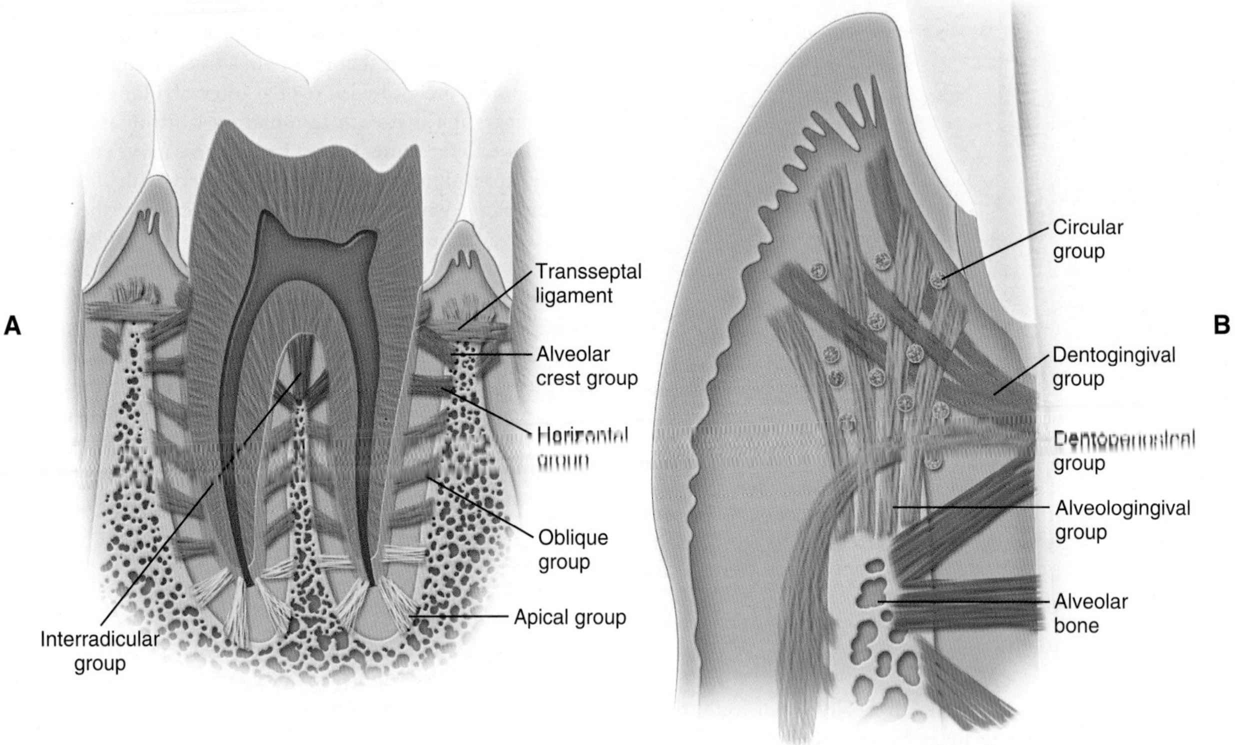

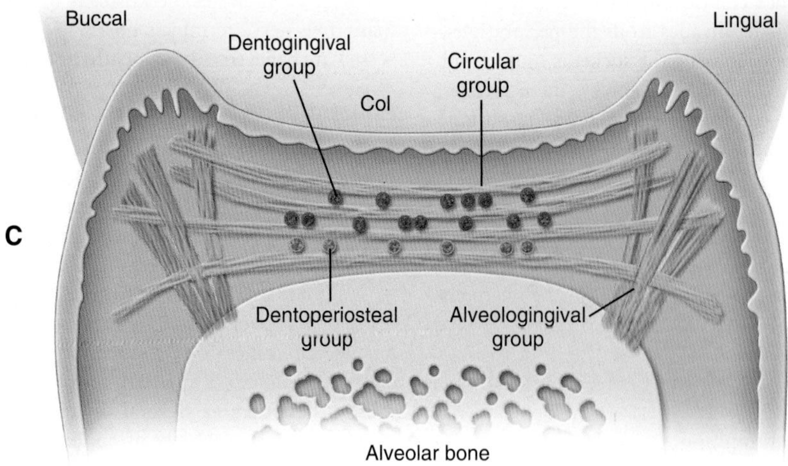

Fig. 9.28 The arrangement of the principal fiber groups within the periodontium. (A) Principal fiber groups. (B) Fiber groups of the gingival ligament. (C) Gingival ligament fibers as seen interproximally related to the gingival col.

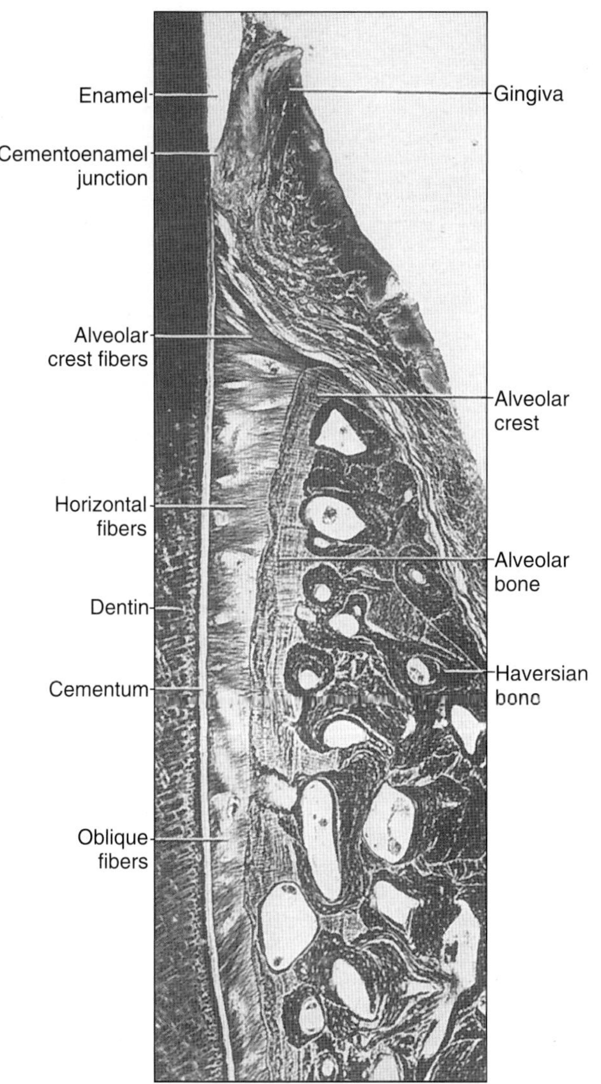

Fig. 9.29 Silver-stained section of some fiber groups of the gingival and periodontal ligaments.

Runx2 transcriptional activity. Indeed, Msx2 may play a central role in preventing ligaments and tendons, in general, from mineralizing. At this point, the issue of how the PDL stays uncalcified while it is trapped between two calcified tissues remains unresolved and will require more attention.

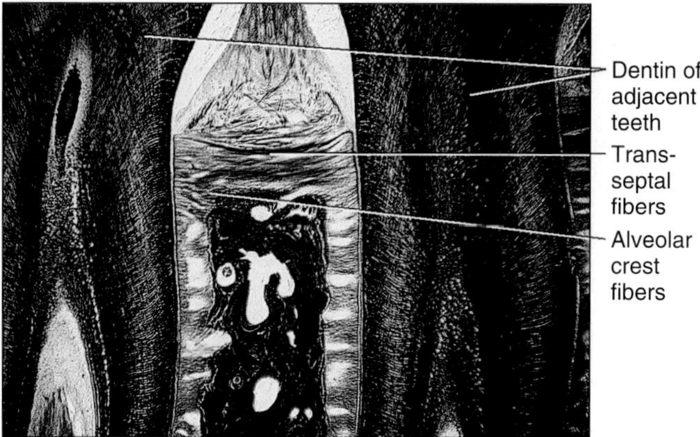

Fig. 9.30 Histology of alveolar crest fibers extending from the cementum of the cervical region to the alveolar bone. Periodontal fibers penetrate alveolar bone, and transseptal fibers extend from the tooth on the left to the right. (From Avery JA, Chiego Jr DJ: *Essentials of oral histology and embryology,* ed 3, St. Louis, MO, 2006, Mosby.)

The PDL also has the capacity to adapt to functional changes. When the functional demand increases, the width of the PDL can increase by as much as 50%, and the fiber bundles also increase greatly in thickness. Conversely, a reduction in function leads to narrowing of the ligament and a decrease in number and thickness of the fiber bundles. These functional modifications of the PDL also implicate corresponding adaptive changes in the bordering cementum and alveolar bone.

Another major function of the periodontium is sensory, although the nature of this function of the PDL still is being debated. When teeth move in their sockets, undoubtedly they distort receptors in the PDL and trigger a response. Thus the PDL contributes to the sensations of touch and pressure on the teeth; in addition, the spatial distribution of receptors is significant. What is equally certain, however, is that the ligament receptors are not the only organs from which sensations arise. For example, when teeth are tapped, vibrations are passed through the bone and detected in the middle ear. Debate also exists about the exact physiologic function of these receptors. Stimulation of the teeth causes a reflex jaw opening, and likewise, stimulation of periodontal mechanoreceptors initiates this response. Whether such a reflex is required for the normal masticatory process or is a protective mechanism to prevent forces applied to the teeth from reaching potentially damaging levels is not known.

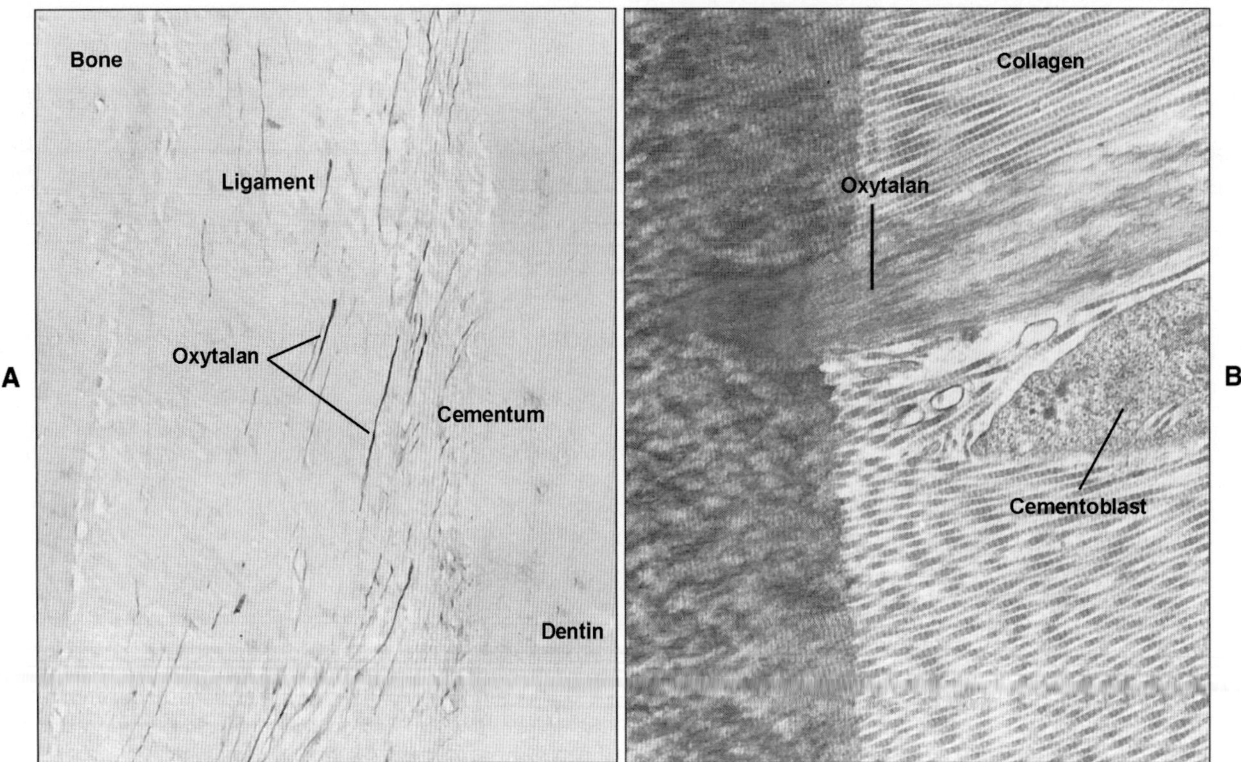

Fig. 9.31 Oxytalan fibers seen through (A) the light microscope and (B) the electron microscope. These fibers run in an oblique direction, often from the cementum to blood vessels.

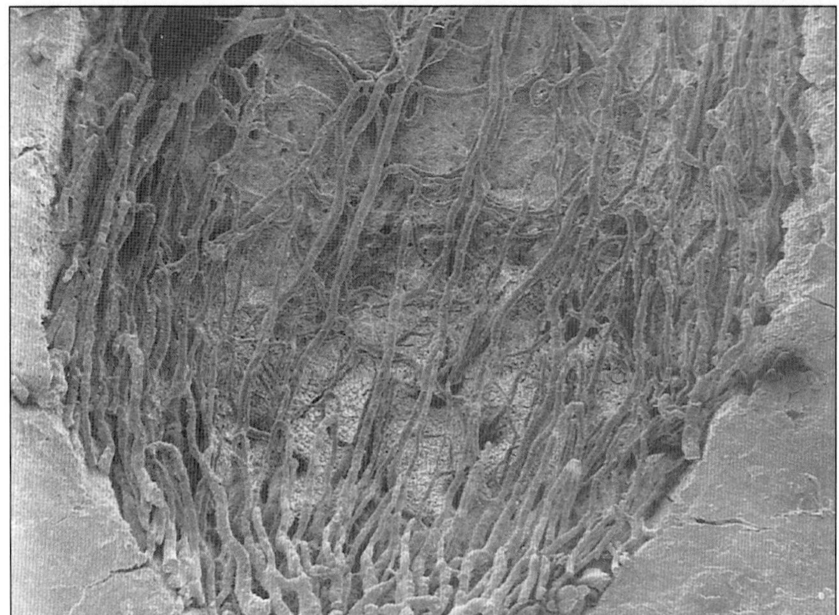

Fig. 9.32 Corrosion cast demonstrating the extensive vasculature of the periodontal ligament. Many transverse connections and the thickened venous network at the apex are visible. (From Selliseth NJ, Selvig KA: The vasculature of the periodontal ligament: a scanning electron microscopic study using corrosion casts in the rat, *J Periodontol* 65:1079–1087, 1994.)

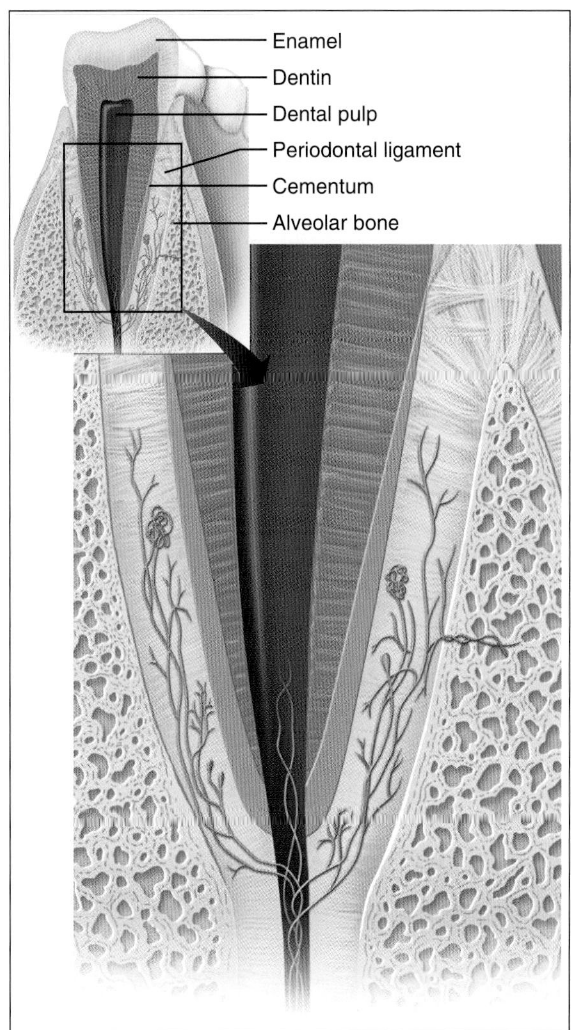

Fig. 9.33 General pattern of periodontal ligament innervation.

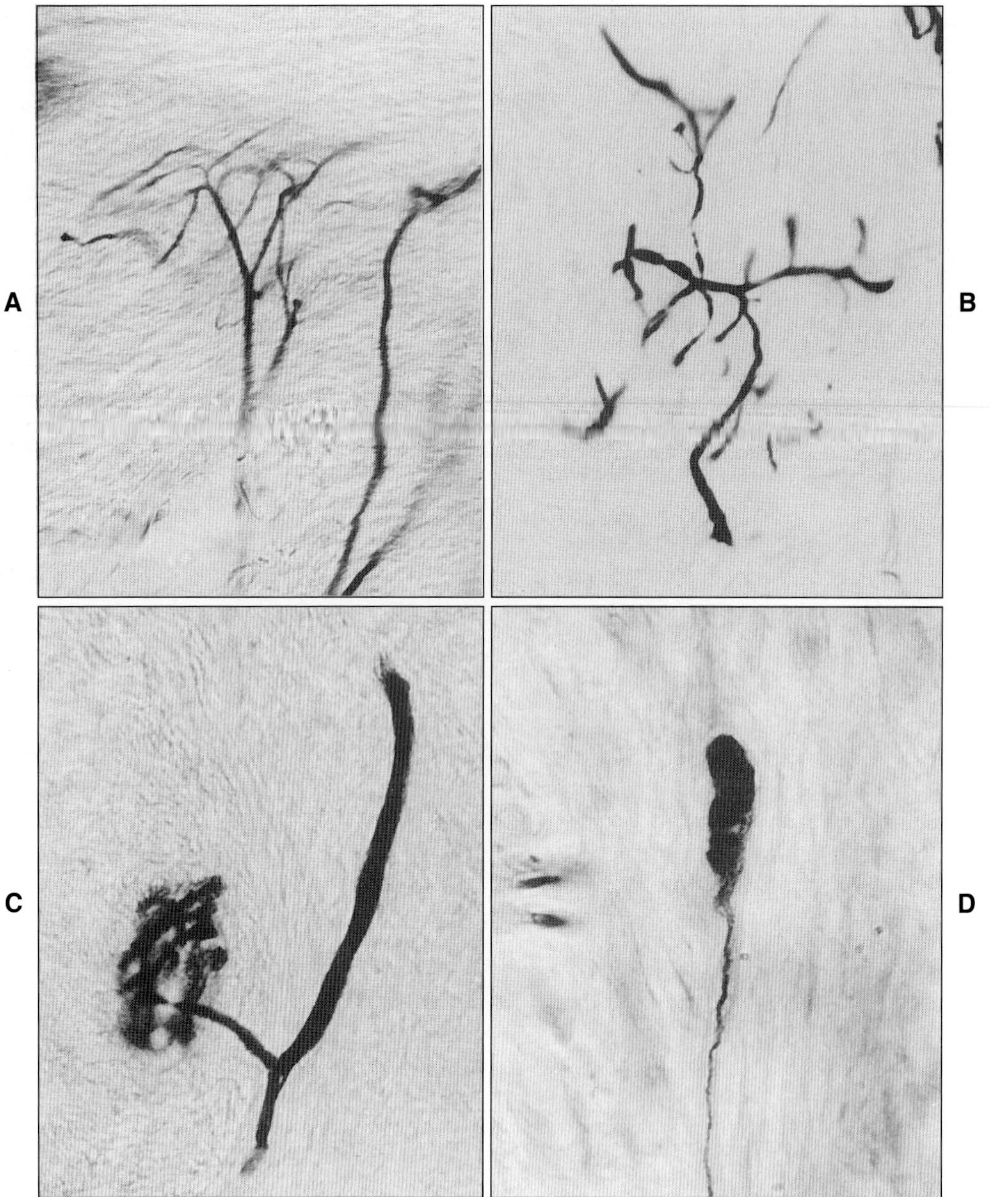

Fig. 9.34 The four types of nerve endings found in a human periodontal ligament. (A) Free endings with tree-like ramifications. (B) Ruffini ending. (C) Coiled ending. (D) Encapsulated spindle-type ending. (From Maeda T, et al.: Nerve terminals in human periodontal ligament as demonstrated by immunohistochemistry for neurofilament protein (NFP) and S-100 protein, *Arch Histol Cytol* 53:259–265, 1990.)

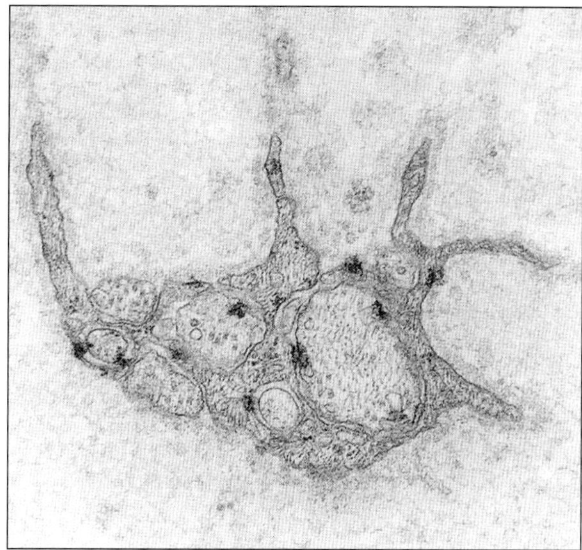

Fig. 9.35 Electron micrograph of a free nerve ending in a human periodontal ligament with an associated Schwann cell sending fingerlike projections into the connective tissue. (From Lambrichts I, et al.: Morphology of neural endings in the human periodontal ligament: an electron microscopic study, *J Periodontal Res* 27:191–196, 1992.)

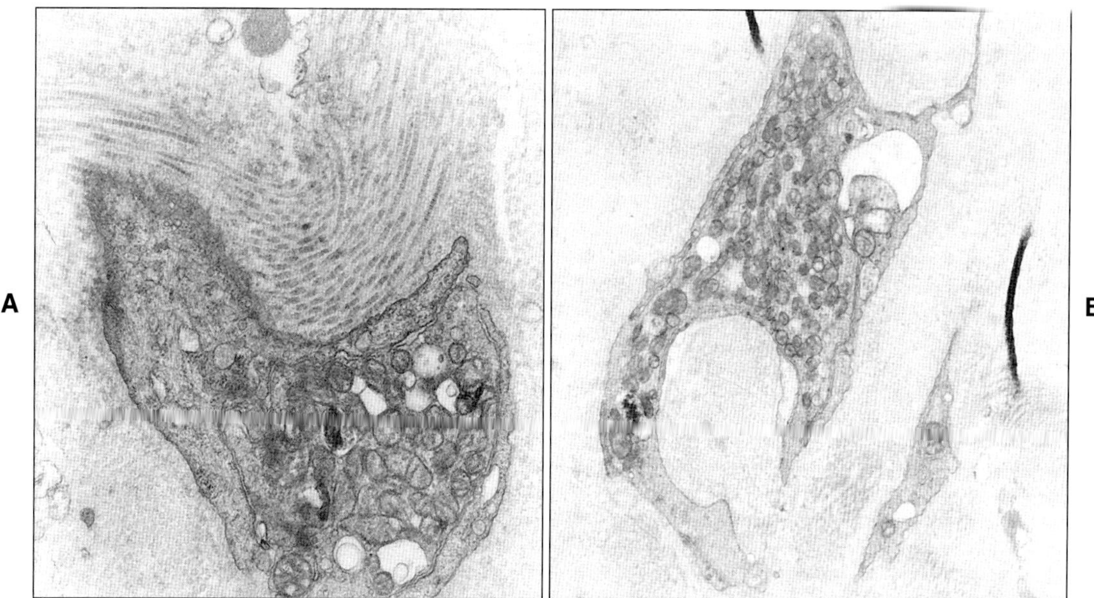

Fig. 9.36 Electron micrographs illustrating the close relationship of Ruffini-like endings with collagen fiber bundles. (A) Insertion of collagen fibrils into the basal lamina of a Schwann cell. (B) Neurite embracing a bundle of collagen fibrils. (From Lambrichts I, et al.: Morphology of neural endings in the human periodontal ligament: an electron microscopic study, *J Periodontal Res* 27:191–196, 1992.)

RECOMMENDED READING

Bartold PM, Narayanan AS: Molecular and cell biology of healthy and diseased periodontal tissues, *Periodontol 2000* 40:29–49, 2006.

Beertsen W, et al.: The periodontal ligament: a unique, multifunctional connective tissue, *Periodontol 2000* 13:20–40, 1997.

Bosshardt DD: Are cementoblasts a subpopulation of osteoblasts or a unique phenotype? *J Dent Res* 84:390–406, 2005.

Diekwisch TG: The developmental biology of cementum, *Int J Dev Biol* 45(5–6):695–706, 2001.

Lekic PC, et al.: Is fibroblast heterogeneity relevant to the health, diseases, and treatments of periodontal tissues? *Crit Rev Oral Biol Med* 8:253–268, 1997.

Nanci A, Bosshardt DD: Structure of periodontal tissues in health and disease, *Periodontol 2000* 40:11–28, 2006.

Nishio C, et al.: Disruption of periodontal integrity induces expression of apin by epithelial cell rests of Malassez, *Periodontal Res* 45(6):709–713, 2010.

Polimeni G, et al.: Biology and principles of periodontal wound healing/regeneration, *Periodontol 2000* 41:30–47, 2006.

Saffar JL, et al.: Alveolar bone and the alveolar process: the socket that is never stable, *Periodontol 2000* 13:76–90, 1997.

Ten Cate AR: The development of the periodontium: a largely ectomesenchymally derived unit, *Periodontol 2000* 13:9–19, 1997.

Wesselink PR, Beertsen W: The prevalence and distribution of rests of Malassez in the mouse molar and their possible role in repair and maintenance of the periodontal ligament, *Arch Oral Biol* 38:399–403, 1993.

Yin X, et al.: Wnt signaling and its contribution to craniofacial tissue homeostasis, *J Dent Res* 94:1487–1494, 2015.

10

Physiologic Tooth Movement: Eruption and Shedding

Antonio Nanci

OUTLINE

The jaws of an infant can accommodate only a few small teeth. Because teeth, when formed, cannot increase in size, the larger jaws of the adult require not only more but also bigger teeth. This accommodation is accomplished with two dentitions. The first is the deciduous or primary dentition, and the second is the permanent or secondary dentition (Figs. 10.1 and 10.2).

The early development of teeth has been described already, and the point has been made that the teeth develop within the tissues of the jaw (Fig. 10.3). For teeth to become functional, considerable movement is required to bring them into the occlusal plane. The movements teeth make are complex and may be described in general terms as follows:

Preeruptive tooth movement. Made by the deciduous and permanent tooth germs within tissues of the jaw before they begin to erupt.

Eruptive tooth movement. Made by a tooth to move from its position within the bone of the jaw to its functional position in occlusion. This phase sometimes is subdivided into intraosseous and extraosseous components.

Posteruptive tooth movement. Maintaining the position of the erupted tooth in occlusion while the jaws continue to grow and compensate for occlusal and proximal tooth wear.

Superimposed on these movements is a progression from primary to permanent dentition involving the shedding (exfoliation) of the deciduous dentition. Although this categorization of tooth movement is convenient for descriptive purposes, what is being described is a complex series of events occurring in a continuous process to move the tooth in a three-dimensional space.

PREERUPTIVE TOOTH MOVEMENT

When the deciduous tooth germs first differentiate, they are extremely small, and a good deal of space is available for them in the developing jaw. Because they grow rapidly, however, they become crowded. A lengthening of the jaws, which permits the deciduous second molar tooth germs to move backward and the anterior germs to move forward gradually, alleviates this crowding. At the same time, the tooth germs are moving bodily outward and upward (or downward, as the case may be) with the increasing length, width, and height of the jaws.

The origin of the successional permanent teeth was described in Chapter 5. Those tooth germs develop on the lingual aspect of their deciduous predecessors in the same bony crypt. From this position they shift considerably as the jaws develop. For example, the incisors and canines eventually occupy a position in their own bony crypts on the lingual side of the roots of their deciduous predecessors, and the premolar tooth germs, also in their own crypts, finally are positioned between the divergent roots of the deciduous molars (Figs. 10.4 and 10.5).

The permanent molar tooth germs, which have no predecessors, develop from the backward extension of the dental lamina. At first, little room is available in the jaws to accommodate these tooth germs. In the upper jaw the molar tooth germs develop first, with their occlusal surfaces facing distally, and then swing into position only when the maxilla has grown sufficiently to provide room for such movement (Fig. 10.6). In the mandible the permanent molars develop with their axes showing a mesial inclination, which becomes vertical only when sufficient jaw growth has occurred.

These preeruptive movements of deciduous and permanent tooth germs place the teeth in a position within the jaw for eruptive movement. These preeruptive movements of teeth are a combination of two factors: (1) total bodily movement of the tooth germ and (2) growth in which one part of the tooth germ remains fixed while the rest continues to grow, leading to a change in the center of the tooth germ. This growth explains, for example, how the deciduous incisors maintain their position relative to the oral mucosa as the jaws increase in height.

Preeruptive movements occur in an intraosseous location and are reflected in the patterns of bony remodeling within the crypt wall. For example, during bodily movement in a mesial direction, bone resorption occurs on the mesial surface of the crypt wall, and bone deposition occurs on the distal wall as a filling-in process. During eccentric growth, only bony resorption occurs, thus altering the shape of the crypt to accommodate the altering shape of the tooth germ. Little is known about the mechanisms that determine preeruptive tooth movements, including whether remodeling of bone to position the bony crypt is important as a mechanism or merely represents an adaptive response.

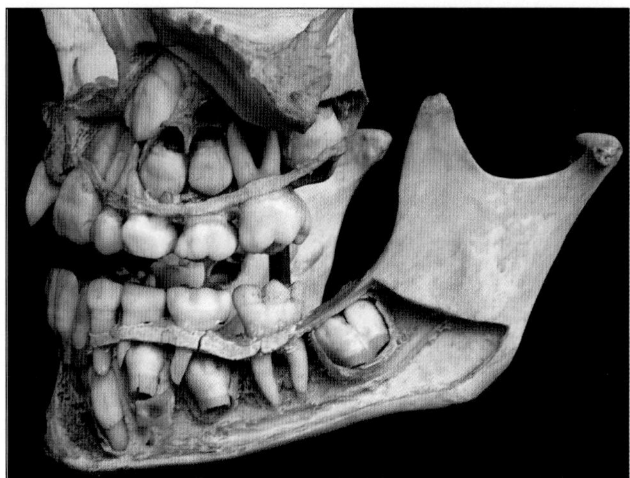

Fig. 10.1 Dried skull of an 8-year-old child. The outer cortical plate has been cut away to show the mixed dentition. (Courtesy M. Schmittbuhl.)

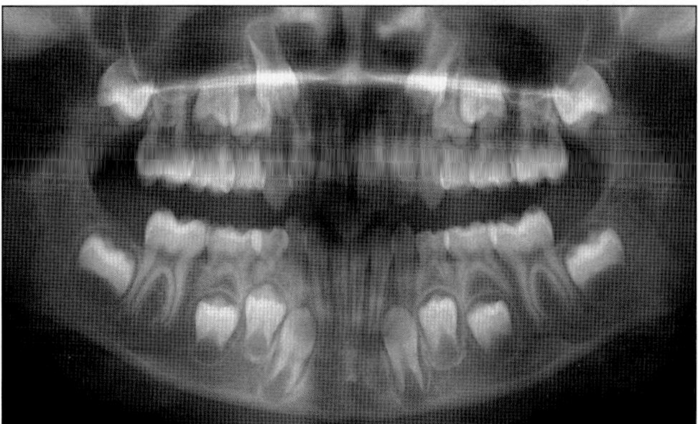

Fig. 10.2 Panoramic radiograph of the mixed dentition of a 7-year-old child. (Courtesy M. Schmittbuhl.)

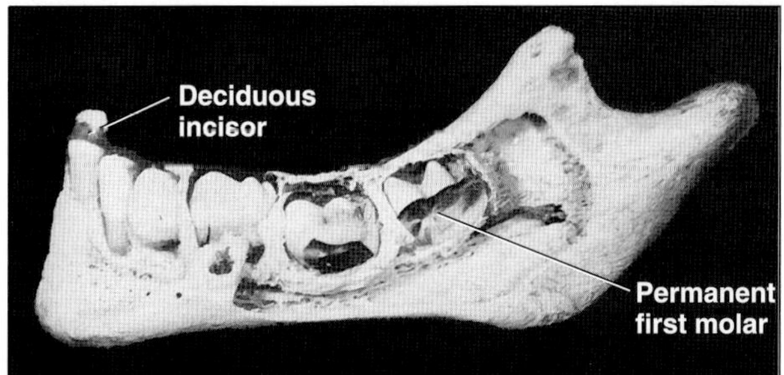

Fig. 10.3 Dried mandible of a 6-month-old child. The teeth occupy most of the body of the mandible. The first deciduous incisor has erupted. The amount of crown formation in the permanent first molar is notable.

ERUPTIVE TOOTH MOVEMENT

The mechanisms of eruption for deciduous and permanent teeth are similar, resulting in the axial or occlusal movement of the tooth from its developmental position within the jaw to its final functional position in the occlusal plane. The actual eruption of the tooth when it breaks through the gum is only one phase of eruption.

Histologic Features

Histologically, many changes occur in association with and for the accommodation of tooth eruption. The periodontal ligament (PDL)

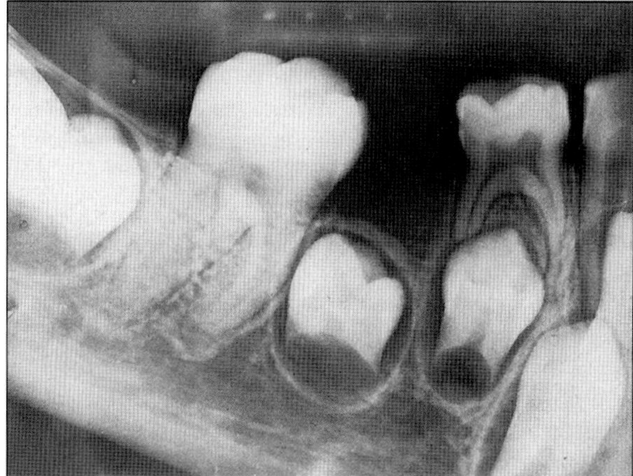

Fig. 10.4 Radiograph of a 7-year-old child's jaw. The permanent first premolar is erupting between the divergent roots of the deciduous first molar. The deciduous second molar has been lost early, which could lead to a tipping of the permanent first molar and prevent eruption of the permanent second premolar. (Courtesy M. Schmittbuhl.)

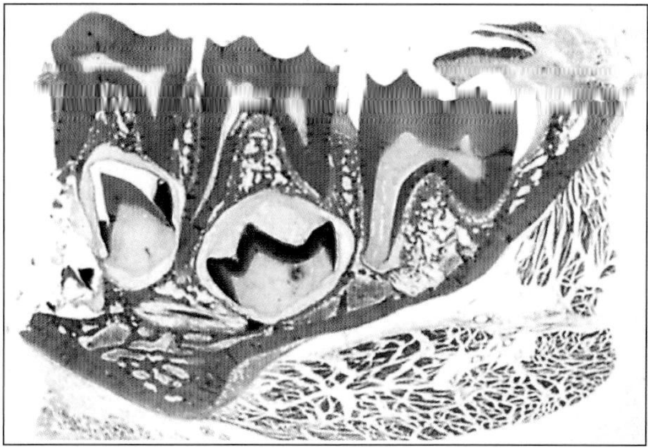

Fig. 10.5 Histologic section showing teeth from the permanent dentition developing between the roots of the corresponding deciduous teeth. The roots of the molar on the lefthand side are being resorbed.

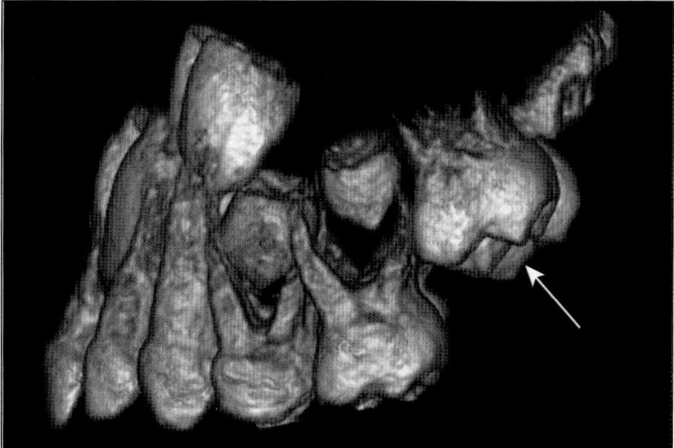

Fig. 10.6 Computed tomography reconstruction of maxillary teeth showing the developing third molar with its occlusal surface facing backward *(arrow)*. (Courtesy M. Schmittbuhl.)

develops only after root formation has been initiated; when established, the PDL must be remodeled to accommodate continued eruptive tooth movement. The remodeling of PDL fiber bundles is achieved by the fibroblasts, which simultaneously synthesize and degrade the collagen fibrils as required across the entire extent of the ligament. Recall also that the fibroblast has a cytoskeleton, which enables it to contract. This contractility is a property of all fibroblasts but is especially well developed in PDL fibroblasts, which have been demonstrated to exert stronger contractile forces than, for example, gingival or skin fibroblasts. Ligament fibroblasts exhibit numerous contacts with one another of the adherens type and exhibit a close relationship to PDL collagen fiber bundles.

The architecture of the tissues in advance of erupting successional teeth differs from that found in advance of deciduous teeth. The fibrocellular follicle surrounding a successional tooth retains its connection with the lamina propria of the oral mucous membrane by means of a strand of fibrous tissue containing remnants of the dental lamina (gubernacular cord). In a dried skull, holes can be identified in the jaws on the lingual aspects of deciduous teeth. These holes, which once contained the gubernacular cords, are termed *gubernacular canals* (Figs. 10.7 and 10.8). As the successional tooth erupts, its gubernacular canal is widened rapidly by local osteoclastic activity, delineating the eruptive pathway for the tooth. The rate of eruption depends on the phase of movement. During the intraosseous phase, the rate can attain 10 mm/day; it increases to about 75 mm/day once the tooth escapes from its bony crypt. This rate persists until the tooth reaches the occlusal plane, indicating that soft connective tissue provides little resistance to tooth movement.

When the erupting tooth appears in the oral cavity, it is subjected to environmental factors that help determine its final position in the dental arch. Muscle forces from the tongue, cheeks, and lips play on the tooth, as do the forces of contact of the erupting tooth with other erupted teeth. The childhood habit of thumb sucking is an obvious example of environmental influence of tooth position.

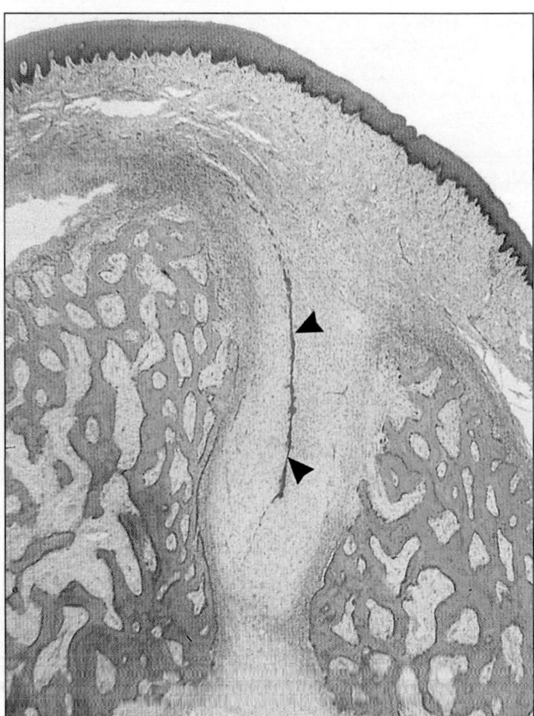

Fig. 10.7 Gubernacular canal and its contents in histologic section. The canal is filled with connective tissue that connects the dental follicle to the oral epithelium. Strands of epithelial cells *(arrowheads)*, remnants of the dental lamina, are often present.

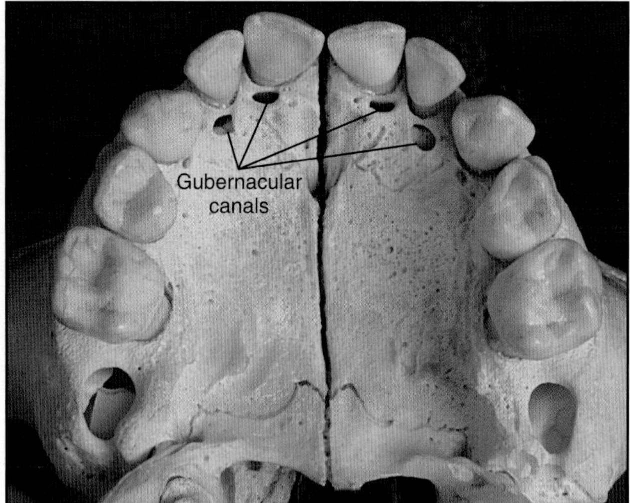

Fig. 10.8 Dried skull of a 5-year-old child. The gubernacular canals are located behind the upper deciduous incisors. (Courtesy M. Schmittbuhl.)

Mechanisms of Eruptive Tooth Movement

Eruptive mechanisms are not yet understood fully, but it is generally believed that eruption is a multifactorial process in which cause and effect are difficult to separate. Numerous theories for tooth eruption have been proposed; among these, root elongation, alveolar bone remodeling, and, to some extent, formation of the PDL provide the most plausible explanation for tooth eruption in human beings. An excellent critical review on the factors involved in tooth eruption has been written by Marks and Schroeder (see Recommended Reading).

Root Formation

At first glance, root formation appears to be an obvious cause of tooth eruption because it undoubtedly causes an overall increase in the length of the tooth that must be accommodated by the growth of the root into the bone of the jaw, by an increase in jaw height, or by the occlusal movement of the crown. Although the last movement is what occurs, it does not follow that root growth is responsible. Indeed, clinical observation, experimental studies, and histologic analysis argue strongly against such a conclusion. For example, if a continuously erupting tooth (e.g., the guinea pig molar) is prevented from erupting by being pinned to bone, root growth continues and is accommodated by resorption of some bone at the base of the socket and by a buckling of the newly formed root. This experiment yields two conclusions: (1) that root growth produces a force and (2) that this force is sufficient to produce bone resorption. Thus although root growth can produce a force, it cannot be translated into eruptive tooth movement unless some structure exists at the base of the tooth capable of withstanding this force; because no such structure exists, some other mechanism must move the tooth to accommodate root growth. The situation is substantiated further by the facts that rootless teeth erupt, that some teeth erupt a greater distance than the total length of their roots, and that teeth still will erupt after the completion of root formation.

In conclusion, root formation per se is not required for tooth eruption, although root formation, under certain circumstances, may accelerate tooth eruption. Depending on the rate at which the root elongates, the basal bone will resorb or form to maintain a proper relationship between the root and bone.

Bone Remodeling

Bone remodeling of the jaws has been linked to tooth eruption in that, as in the preeruptive phase, the inherent growth pattern of the mandible or maxilla supposedly moves teeth by the selective deposition and resorption of bone in the immediate neighborhood of the tooth. The strongest evidence in support of bone remodeling as a cause of tooth movement comes from a series of experiments in dogs. When the developing premolar is removed without disturbing the dental follicle, or if eruption is prevented by wiring the tooth germ down to the lower border of the mandible, an eruptive pathway still forms within the bone overlying the enucleated tooth as osteoclasts widen the gubernacular canal. If the dental follicle is removed, however, no eruptive pathway forms. Furthermore, if a metal or silicone replica replaces the tooth germ, and as long as the dental follicle is retained, the replica will erupt, with the formation of an eruptive pathway. These observations should be analyzed carefully. First, they clearly demonstrate that an eruptive pathway can form in bone without a developing and growing tooth. Second, they show that the dental follicle is involved. The conclusion cannot be drawn that the demonstration of an eruptive pathway forming within bone means that bony remodeling is responsible for tooth movement unless coincident bone deposition also can be demonstrated at the base of the crypt, and prevention of such bone deposition can be shown to interfere with tooth eruption. Careful studies using tetracyclines as markers of bone deposition have shown that the predominant activity in the fundus of an alveolus in a number of species (including human beings) is bone resorption. In humans, for instance, the base of the crypt of the permanent first and third molars continually resorbs as these teeth erupt, although in the second premolar and molar, some bone deposition on the crypt floor occurs. In the case of the demonstrated eruption of an inert replica, one might think that only bony remodeling could bring this about, but as discussed next, evidence indicates that follicular tissue is responsible for this movement. In addition, some recent studies are showing that alveolar bone growth at the base of the crypt is required for molar tooth eruption in rats. Clearly, the intraosseous tooth eruption needs further attention. Irrespective of whether bone growth is a primary moving force, it is generally agreed that the dental follicle is needed for eruption to occur and that, as discussed next, it modulates bone remodeling.

Dental Follicle

Investigations indicate a pattern of cellular activity involving the reduced dental epithelium and the follicle associated with tooth eruption, which facilitates connective tissue degradation and bone resorption as the tooth erupts. In osteopetrotic animals, which lack colony-stimulating factor 1 (CSF1; a factor that stimulates differentiation of osteoclasts), eruption is prevented because no mechanism for bone removal exists. Local administration of this factor permits the differentiation of osteoclasts, and eruption occurs. The reduced enamel epithelium also secretes proteases, which assist in the breakdown of connective tissue to produce a path of least resistance. Expression of bone morphogenetic protein 6 in the dental follicle may also be essential for promoting alveolar bone growth at the base of the crypt.

It is believed that there is signaling between the reduced enamel epithelium and dental follicle. This signaling could explain the remarkable consistency of eruption times because the enamel epithelium likely is programmed as part of its functional life cycle. Signaling also helps explain why radicular follicle, which is not associated with reduced enamel epithelium, does not undergo degeneration but instead participates in the formation of the PDL.

Periodontal Ligament

Formation and renewal of the PDL have been considered factors in tooth eruption because of the traction power that fibroblasts have and because of experimental results using the continuously erupting rat incisor. The situation is different in teeth with a limited growth period in which the presence of a PDL does not always correlate with resorption. Cases occur in which a PDL is present and the tooth does not erupt, and cases occur in which rootless teeth erupt.

Molecular Determinants of Tooth Eruption

As mentioned, tooth eruption is a tightly regulated process involving the tooth organ (dental follicle, enamel organ) and surrounding alveolar tissues. Tooth movement results from a balance between tissue destruction (bone, connective tissue, and epithelium) and tissue formation (bone, PDL, and root). During bone remodeling, osteoclasts are recruited; these derive from circulating monocytes that are attracted chemically at the site where bone resorption takes place. The follicle produces CSF1, a growth factor that promotes the differentiation of monocytes into macrophages and osteoclasts. Furthermore, interleukin-1α, a promoter of bone resorption, is synthesized by the enamel organ in response to epidermal growth factor and induces follicular cells to produce CSF1. Monocyte chemotactic protein 1 (Mcp1) also may be involved in attracting monocytes along the path of tooth eruption.

As discussed in Chapter 6, osteoclastogenesis is regulated through signaling via the receptor-activated nuclear factor κB (RANK)/RANK ligand (RANKL)/osteoprotegerin pathway. Osteoprotegerin inhibits osteoclast formation, and its expression is downregulated in the apical portion of the dental follicle. Finally, differentiation of osteoblasts at the base of the alveolar crypt is accentuated. The runt-related transcription factor 2 (Runx2) is involved in osteoblast differentiation and function, and, as expected, it is expressed at a high level in the basal portion of the dental follicle. Transforming growth factor β (TGF-β) downregulates expression of Runx2 in the apical portion of the dental follicle, favoring bone removal along the surface where the tooth erupts. Epidermal growth factor, which increases the level of expression of TGF-β, has been shown to accelerate incisor eruption in rodents.

Table 10.1 lists the various molecules that have been proposed to take part in the paracrine signaling cascade of eruption. Understanding their role may one day offer the possibility to correct eruption effects and achieve molecular orthodontic movements. Along this line, it has been shown using local gene transfer that RANKL accelerates and osteoprotegerin diminishes orthodontic tooth movement in rats.

TABLE 10.1 Putative Molecules Implicated in the Tooth Eruption Signaling Cascade

Molecule	Abbreviation
Bone morphogenetic protein 2	BMP2
Epidermal growth factor	EGF
Epidermal growth factor receptor	EGFR
Colony-stimulating factor-1	CSF1
Colony-stimulating factor-1 receptor	CSF1R
Interleukin-1α	IL1α
Interleukin-1 receptor	IL1R
c-Fos	
Nuclear factor κB	NF-κB
Monocyte chemotactic protein 1	MCP1
Transforming growth factor-α	TGF-α
Transforming growth factor-β1	TGF-β1
Parathyroid hormone–related protein	PTHrP
Osteoprotegerin	OPG
Receptor activator of nuclear factor κB ligand	RANKL
Runt-related transcription factor 2	Runx2

From Wise GE, et al.: Cellular, molecular, and genetic determinants of tooth eruption, *Crit Rev Oral Biol Med* 13:323–334, 2002.

POSTERUPTIVE TOOTH MOVEMENT

Posteruptive movements are those made by the tooth after it has reached its functional position in the occlusal plane. They may be divided into three categories: (1) movements to accommodate the growing jaws, (2) those to compensate for continued occlusal wear, and (3) those to accommodate interproximal wear.

Accommodation for Growth

Posteruptive movements that accommodate the growth of the jaws are completed toward the end of the second decade, when jaw growth ceases. They are seen histologically as a readjustment of the position of the tooth socket, achieved by the formation of new bone at the alveolar crest and on the socket floor to keep pace with the increasing height of the jaws. Studies have shown that this readjustment occurs between 14 and 18 years of age, when active movement of the tooth takes place. The apices of the teeth move 2 to 3 mm away from the inferior dental canal (regarded as a fixed reference point). This movement occurs earlier in females than in males and is related to the burst of condylar growth that separates the jaws and teeth, permitting further eruptive movement.

Although such movement is seen as remodeling of the socket, one must not assume it brings about tooth movement. The same arguments that apply to bony remodeling for preeruptive and eruptive tooth movement apply in this case.

Compensation for Occlusal Wear

The axial movement that a tooth makes to compensate for occlusal wear most likely is achieved by the same mechanism as eruptive tooth movement. Notably, these axial posteruptive movements are made when the apices of the permanent lower molars are formed fully and the apices of the second premolar and molar are almost complete, which indicates again that root growth is not the factor responsible for axial eruptive tooth movement and further emphasizes the role of the PDL. Compensation for occlusal wear often is stated to be achieved by continued cementum deposition around the apex of the tooth; however, the deposition of cementum in this location occurs only after the tooth has moved.

Accommodation for Interproximal Wear

Wear also occurs at the contact points between teeth on their proximal surfaces; its extent can be considerable (>7 mm in the mandible). This interproximal wear is compensated for by the process of mesial or approximal drift. Mesial drift and an understanding of its probable causes are important to the practice of orthodontics because the maintenance of tooth position after treatment depends on the extent of such drift. The forces causing mesial drift are multifactorial and include an anterior component of occlusal force, contraction of the transseptal ligament between teeth, and soft tissue pressure.

Anterior Component of Occlusal Force

When teeth are brought into contact (e.g., in clenching the jaws), an anteriorly directed force is generated. This force can be demonstrated easily by placing a steel strip between the teeth and showing that more force is required to remove it when the jaws are clenched. This anterior force is the result of the mesial inclination of most teeth and the summation of intercuspal planes (producing a forward-directed force). In the case of incisors, which are inclined labially, any anterior component of force would be expected to move them in the same direction. The incisors move mesially, but this can be explained by the billiard ball analogy (Fig. 10.9). When cusps are selectively ground, the direction of occlusal force can be enhanced or reversed. Paradoxically, one experiment designed to demonstrate this anterior component of force also showed that other factors are involved. When opposing teeth were removed, thereby eliminating the biting force, the mesial migration of teeth was slowed but not halted, indicating the presence of some other force. The transseptal fibers of the PDL have been implicated.

Contraction of the Transseptal Ligament

The PDL plays an important role in maintaining tooth position. The suggestion has been made that its transseptal fibers (running

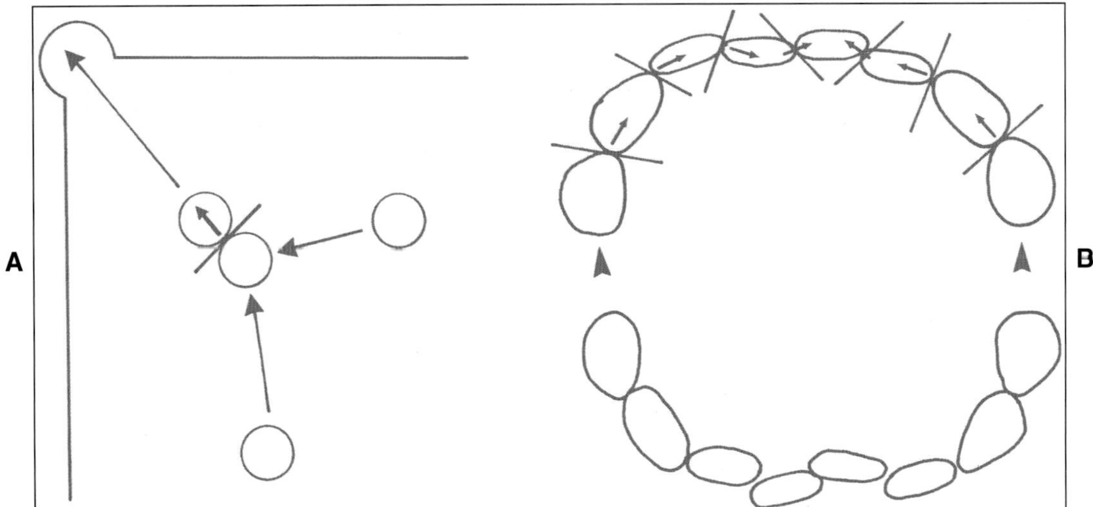

Fig. 10.9 Billiard ball analogy. (A) If the two touching balls are in line with the pocket, no matter how the first ball is struck, the second will enter the pocket because it travels at right angles to the common tangent between the two balls. (B) In a young dentition the arrowheads indicate the anterior component of force, which drives the first premolars against the canines. Following the example of the billiard balls, the canines and incisors all move in directions at right angles to the common tangents drawn through the contact points *(arrows)*. (From Osborn J. In Poole DFG, Stack MV, editors: *The eruption and occlusion of teeth,* Proceedings of the 27th Symposium of the Colston Research Society, London, 1976, Butterworth Heinemann.)

between adjacent teeth across the alveolar process) draw neighboring teeth together and maintain them in contact, and some supporting evidence exists. For example, relapse of orthodontically moved teeth can be reduced if a fiberotomy removing the transseptal ligament is cut. Also, in experimental demonstration, in bisected teeth the two halves separate from each other, but if the transseptal ligaments are cut previously, this separation does not occur. Furthermore, remodeling by collagen phagocytosis has been demonstrated in the transseptal ligament, with the rate of turnover increasing during orthodontic tooth movement; however, this only shows that the transseptal ligament is capable of adaptation. A simple and elegant experiment indicates that the cause of mesial drift is multifactorial: Grinding away proximal contacts provides room for a tooth to move, after which teeth move to reestablish contact. If teeth also are ground out of occlusion and their proximal surfaces are disked, the rate of drift is slowed.

Soft Tissue Pressures

The pressures generated by the cheeks and tongue may push teeth mesially. When such pressures are eliminated, however, by constructing an acrylic dome over the teeth, mesial drift still occurs, which suggests that soft tissue pressure does not play a major role (if any) in creating mesial drift. Nevertheless, soft tissue pressure influences tooth position, even if it does not cause tooth movement.

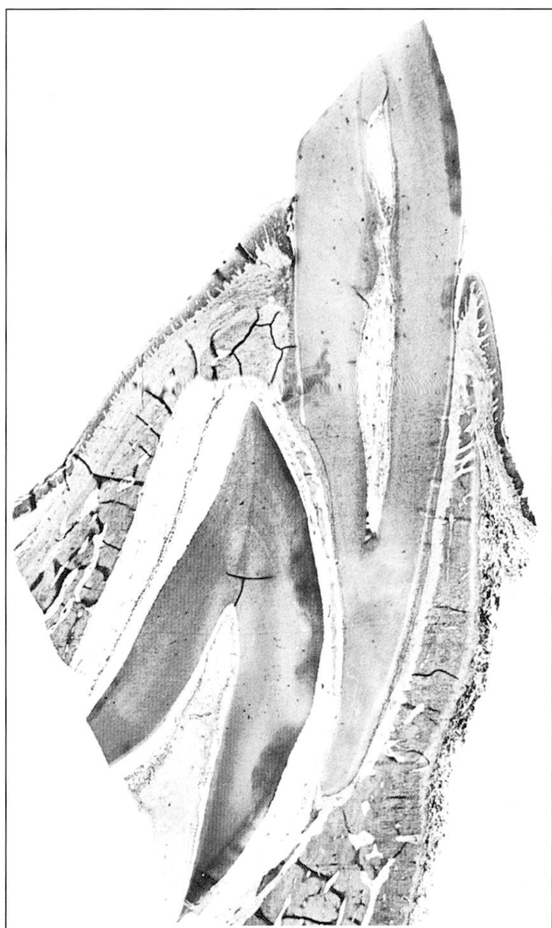

Fig. 10.10 Photomicrograph of the relative positions of deciduous and permanent canines. Resorption occurs on the lingual aspect of the deciduous canine, and the tooth often is shed with much of its lingual root intact.

SHEDDING OF TEETH

As the permanent incisors, canines, and premolars develop, increase in size, and begin to erupt, they influence the pattern of resorption of the deciduous teeth and their exfoliation (shedding). For instance, the permanent incisors and canines develop lingually to the deciduous teeth and erupt in an occlusal and vestibular direction. Resorption of deciduous tooth roots occurs on the lingual surface, and these teeth are shed with much of their pulp chamber intact (Figs. 10.10 and 10.11). Permanent premolars develop between the divergent roots of deciduous molars and erupt in an occlusal direction. Hence the resorption of interradicular dentin takes place with some resorption of the pulp chamber, coronal dentin, and sometimes enamel (Figs. 10.12 and 10.13).

Odontoclast

The resorption of dental hard tissue is achieved by cells with a histologic nature similar to that of osteoclasts, but because of their involvement in the removal of dental tissue they are called *odontoclasts* (Figs. 10.14 and 10.15). Odontoclasts derive from the monocyte and migrate from blood vessels to the resorption site where they fuse to form the characteristic multinucleated odontoclast with a clear attachment zone and ruffled border.

Less is known about the resorption of the soft tissues of the tooth (i.e., the pulp and PDL) as it sheds. Although active root resorption is taking place, coronal pulp appears normal, and odontoblasts still line the surface of the predentin. When root resorption is almost complete, these odontoblasts degenerate, and mononuclear cells emerge from the pulpal vessels and migrate to the predentin surface where they fuse with other mononuclear cells to form odontoclasts actively engaged in the removal of dentin (Fig. 10.16). Just before exfoliation, resorption ceases as the odontoclasts migrate away from the dentin surface, and

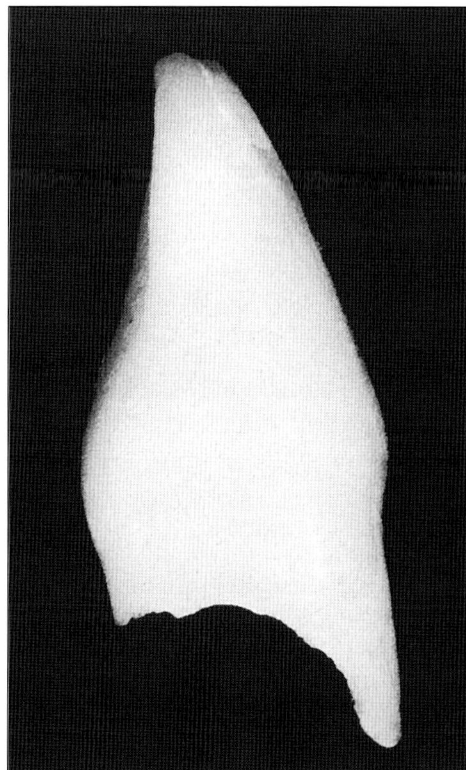

Fig. 10.11 Exfoliated deciduous canine. This tooth is shed with a considerable portion of its root remaining on the buccal aspect.

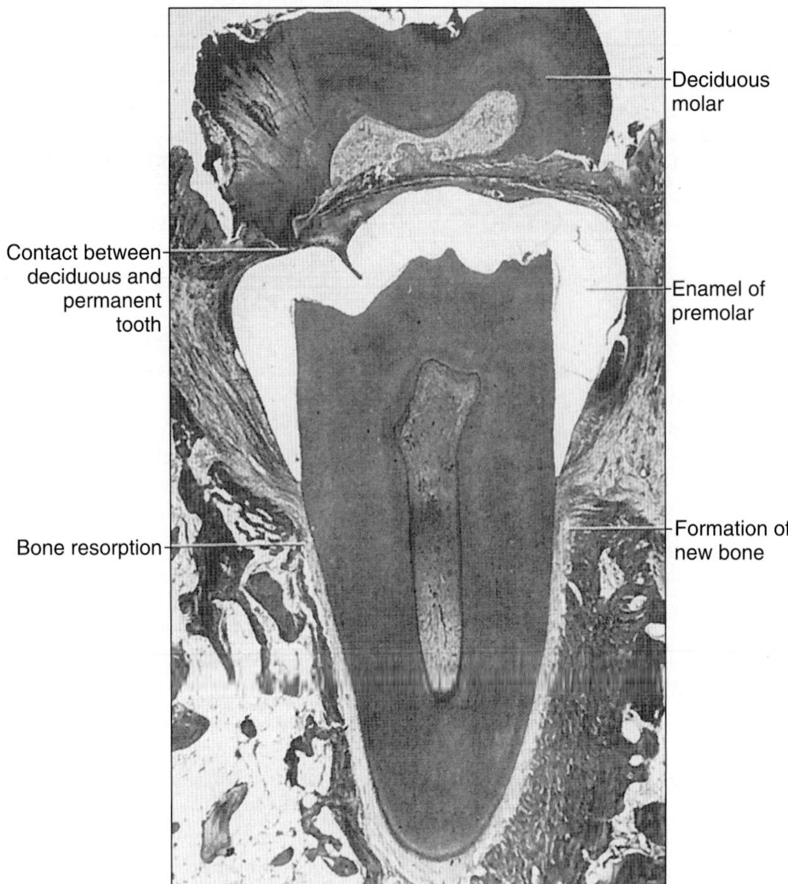

Fig. 10.12 Roots of a primary molar completely resorbed. Dentin is in contact with the premolar enamel. (Courtesy E.A. Grimmer.)

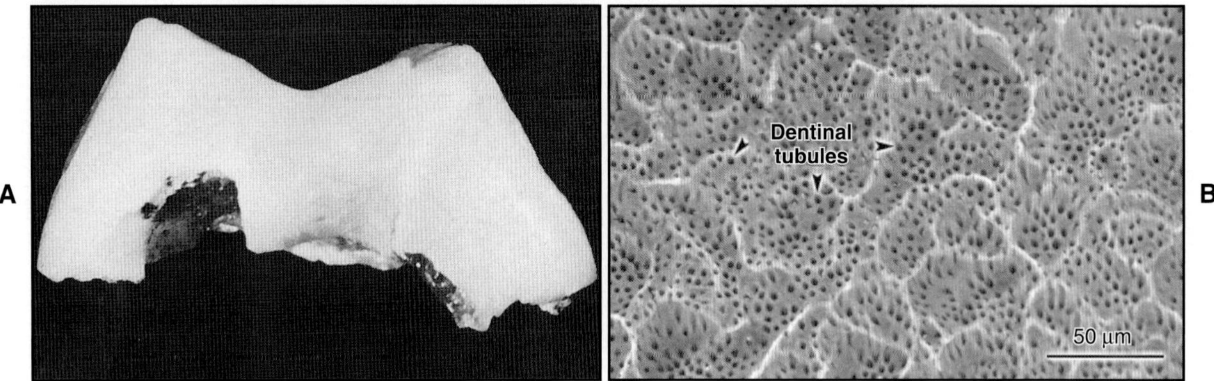

Fig. 10.13 (A) Exfoliated deciduous molar. The roots have been lost completely, and the enamel and coronal dentin have eroded. (B) Scanning electron microscope view of the eroded dentin surface showing the numerous resorption lacunae created by odontoclasts.

the remaining pulp cells now deposit a cementlike tissue on it (Fig. 10.17). The tooth then sheds, with some pulpal tissue intact.

Simple observation of histologic sections shows that the loss of PDL fibers is abrupt. Electron microscopic investigation confirms this finding and shows that cell death in this region occurs without inflammation. Cell death assumes at least two forms. In one instance, fibroblasts exhibit signs of interference with normal cellular processes such as secretion (Fig. 10.18), as well as other cytotoxic alterations that eventually lead to necrosis and cell death. This process is induced in response to local cell insult. In the other, ligament fibroblasts exhibit morphologic features characteristic of apoptotic cell death (Fig. 10.19). Apoptosis (see Chapter 7) has been well described and involves condensation of the cell with its ultimate phagocytosis by neighboring macrophages or undamaged fibroblasts. The finding of apoptotic cell death in the resorbing PDL suggests that shedding teeth also is a programmed event. Support for this conclusion is obtained from the study of tooth eruption in monozygotic twins, which indicates that shedding is determined mostly (80%) by genetic factors (with the remaining determinants being local).

Pressure

Obviously pressure from the erupting successional tooth plays a role in shedding the deciduous dentition. For instance, if a successional

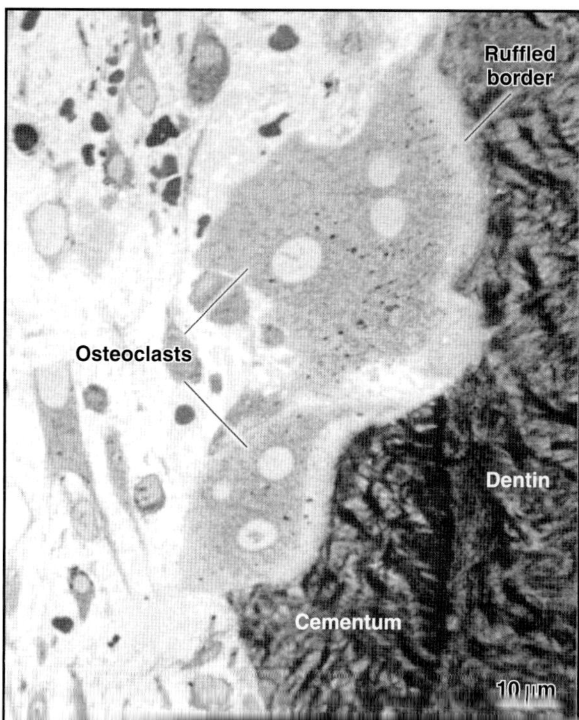

Fig. 10.14 Root resorption induced by orthodontic forces in a human premolar. Cementum and dentin have been resorbed by odontoclasts that line the root surface. These large, multinucleated cells with a ruffled border resemble osteoclasts.

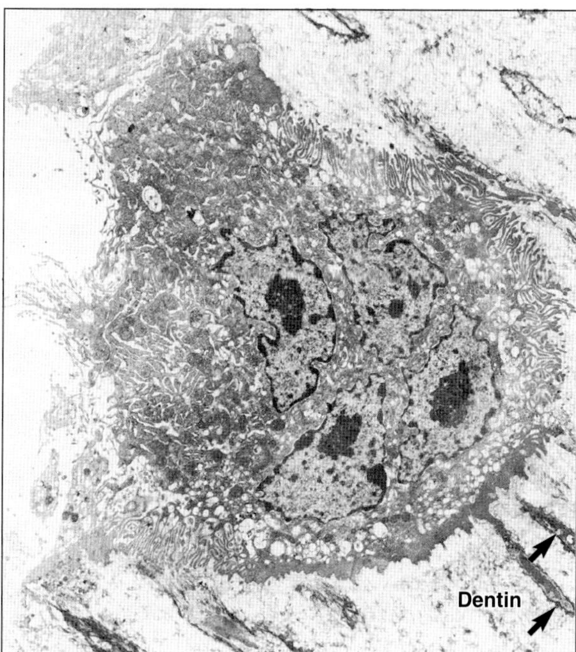

Fig. 10.15 Fine structure of the odontoclast. This cell is resorbing dentin and sends extensions *(arrows)* into the dentinal tubules. The ruffled or brush border can be seen, as can the multinucleated character of the cell. (From Freilich LS: Ultrastructure and acid phosphatase cytochemistry of odontoclasts: effects of parathyroid extract, *J Dent Res* 50:1047–1055, 1971.)

tooth germ is missing congenitally or occupies an aberrant position in the jaw, shedding of the deciduous tooth is delayed. Yet the tooth usually is shed. The suggestion also has been made that increased force applied to a deciduous tooth can initiate its resorption. Growth of the face and jaws and the corresponding enlargement in size and strength of the muscles of mastication probably increase the forces applied to the deciduous teeth so that the supporting apparatus of the tooth, in particular the PDL, is damaged and tooth resorption is initiated (Fig. 10.20).

The superimposition of local pressure and masticatory forces on physiologic tooth resorption is likely to determine the pattern and rate of deciduous tooth shedding. Pressure from an erupting permanent tooth results in some root loss, which, in turn, means loss of supporting tissue. As the support of the tooth diminishes, the tooth is less able to withstand the increasing masticatory forces, and thus the process of exfoliation is accelerated.

Pattern of Shedding

In general, the pattern of exfoliation is symmetric for the right and left sides of the mouth. Except for second molars, the mandibular primary teeth are shed before their maxillary counterparts. The exfoliation of all four secondary primary molars is practically simultaneous. Exfoliation occurs in females before it does in males. The greatest discrepancy between the sexes is observed for the mandibular canines and the least for the maxillary central incisors. The sequence of shedding in the mandible follows the anterior-to-posterior order of the teeth in that jaw. In the maxilla, the first molar exfoliating before the canine disrupts this sequence.

In summary (Fig. 10.21), physiologic tooth movement is a complex and multifactorial process. Several related events take place involving bone remodeling and soft tissue removal. Failure of such events to proceed properly delays or prevents eruption. Active tooth eruption begins in a dynamic intraosseous environment that undergoes bone formation and resorption, events that are regulated by the dental follicle and enamel organ. Although the force for eruptive tooth movement might be considered to have been identified, the controlling mechanisms remain to be defined fully. The consistency of eruption dates for the human dentition is remarkable (the so-called 6-year molars as a descriptor for the permanent first molars testifying to this) and surely indicates the involvement of programmed development. The ability of orthodontists to manage clinically and intervene during tooth resorption is limited and includes extraction of primary teeth, surgical removal of bone, and incising of ligaments. A better understanding of the molecular mediators of eruption, and, in particular, of the role of products produced by the reduced enamel organ certainly will increase clinical options. Because the eruption pathway created by osteoclasts determines, at least initially, the direction of tooth eruption and hence its three-dimensional positioning in the forming jaw, one even may question whether using some of these mediators to manage the final position and interrelation of teeth could be possible.

ABNORMAL TOOTH MOVEMENT

The steps leading to the development of the final permanent dentition are complex, requiring a balance among tooth formation, jaw growth, and the maintenance of function. Not surprisingly, disturbances in this process often indicate some local or systemic abnormality, and thus the patterns of tooth formation and eruption are of considerable diagnostic significance. The normal pattern is so remarkably consistent that permanent first molars (as just mentioned) often are referred to as 6-year molars because of their predictable time of eruption.

Earlier-than-normal tooth eruption is unusual. Sometimes babies are born with a central incisor that is erupted already, but this represents abnormal dental development, and the tooth is extracted

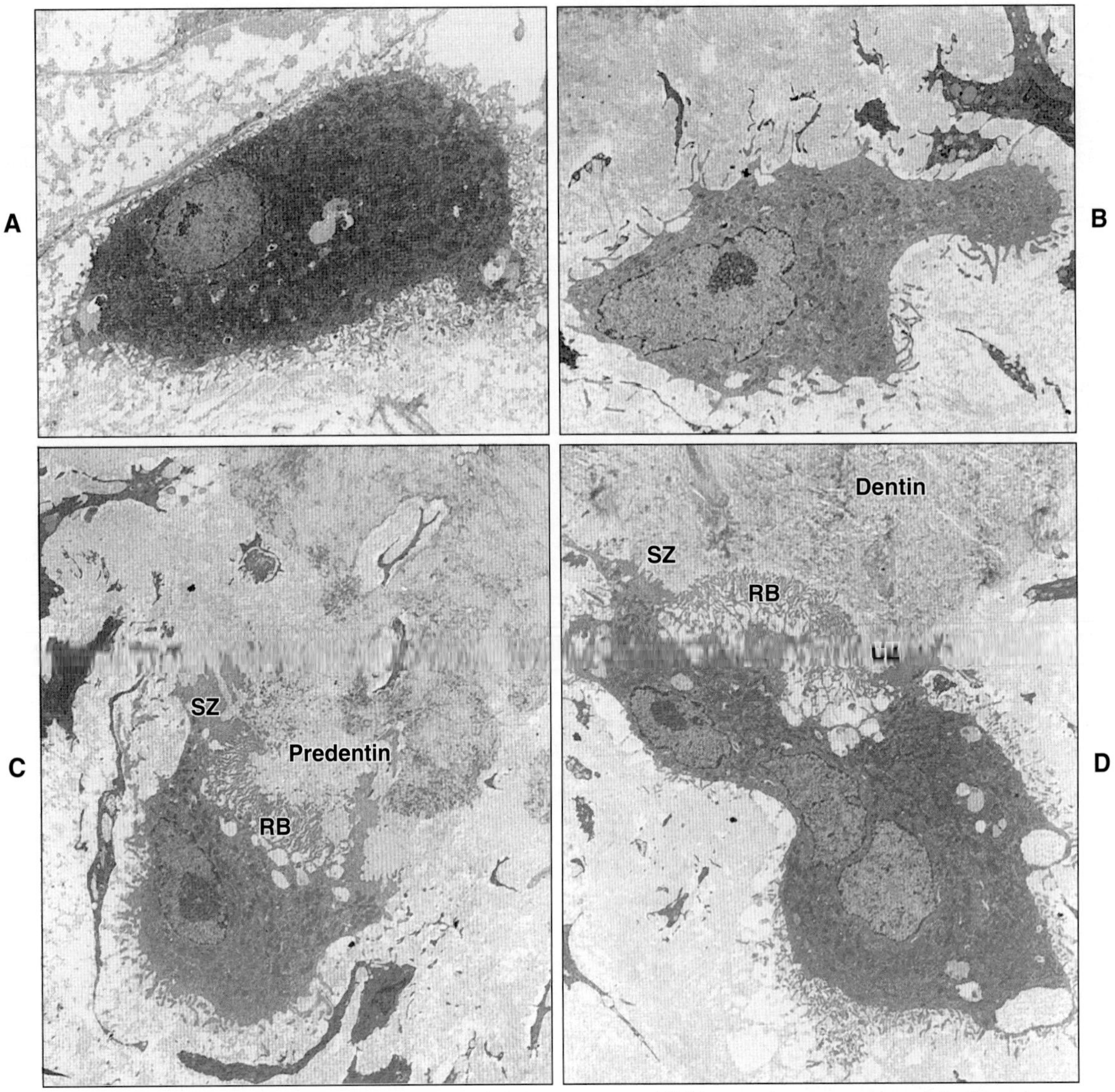

Fig. 10.16 Ultrastructure of odontoclasts and their precursors. (A) Mononuclear precursor cell in the pulp chamber. (B) Mononuclear precursor cell attached to the predentin surface. (C) Multinucleate odontoclast resorbing predentin. (D) Multinucleate odontoclast resorbing dentin. The sealing zones *(SZ)* and the ruffled border *(RB)* are notable in (C) and (D). (From Sahara N, et al.: Odontoclastic resorption at the pulpal surface of coronal dentin prior to shedding of human deciduous teeth, *Arch Histol Cytol* 55:273–285, 1992.)

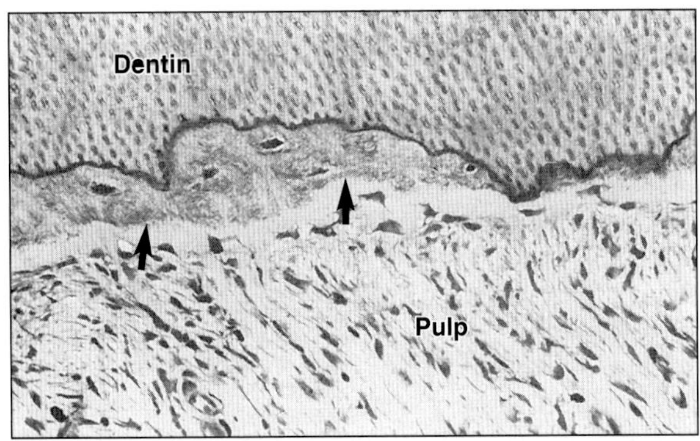

Fig. 10.17 Cementlike tissue *(arrows)* deposited on resorbed coronal dentin. (From Sahara N, et al.: Cementum-like tissue deposition on the resorbed pulp chamber wall of human deciduous teeth prior to shedding, *Acta Anat* 147:24–34, 1993.)

to permit suckling. The premature loss of a deciduous tooth occasionally leads to early eruption of its permanent successor. Delayed eruption of teeth is far more common and may be caused by congenital, systemic, or local factors (with local factors predominating). Congenital absence of teeth most commonly occurs with the permanent third molars. Systemic factors involving delays in tooth eruption may be caused by endocrine deficiencies, nutritional deficiencies, and some genetic factors. If teeth have not appeared in an infant during the first year, some underlying cause must be sought. Any systemic lesion delaying eruption of the permanent teeth usually has been identified before the sixth year, when the permanent first molars erupt.

Local factors preventing tooth eruption are many. Examples are early loss of a deciduous tooth with consequent drifting of the adjacent teeth to block the eruptive pathway (see Fig. 10.4) and eruption cysts (derived from the dental lamina). Crowding of teeth in small jaws often provides little room for eruption, with consequent impaction

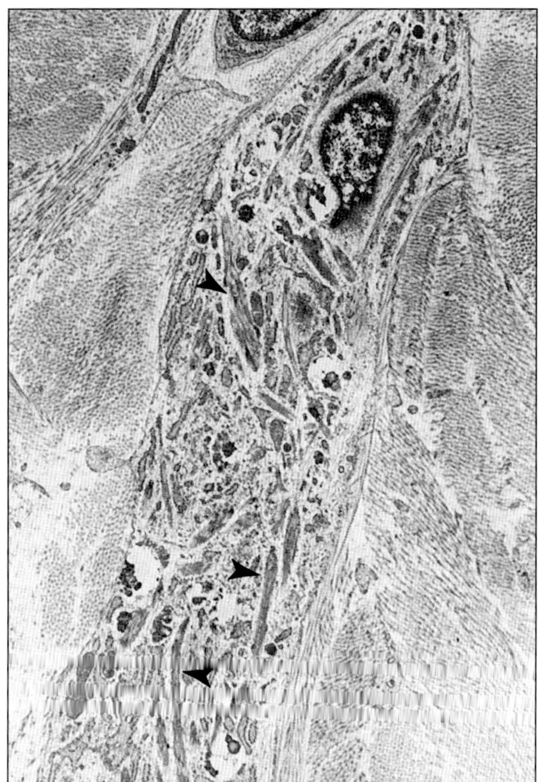

Fig. 10.18 Electron micrograph of a periodontal ligament fibroblast in an area preceding the root resorption front. The cytoplasm of the fibroblast is filled with collagen *(arrowheads)*, suggesting an interference with the protein synthetic and/or degradative cell physiology.

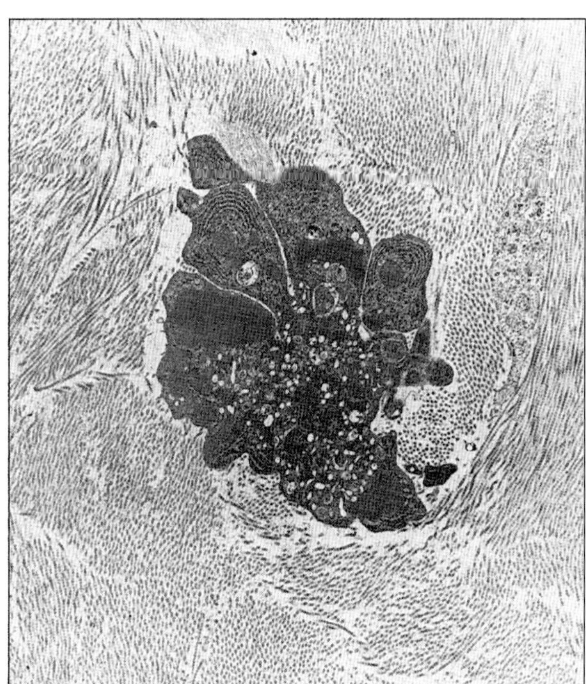

Fig. 10.19 A degenerated fibroblast in the periodontal ligament near the root resorption front. This appearance is characteristic of apoptotic (physiologic) cell death.

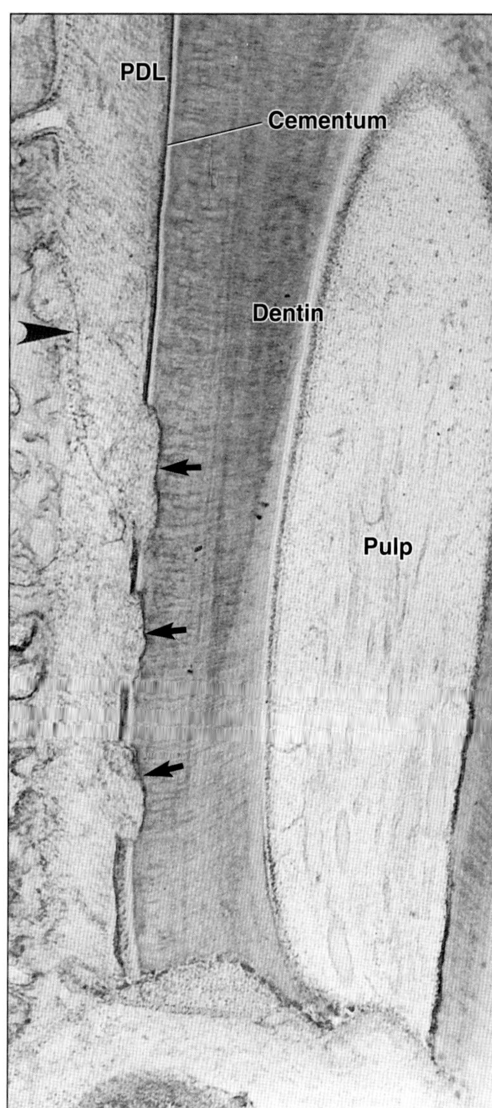

Fig. 10.20 Histology of root resorption. Tooth resorption is occurring at the apex of the root, and as a consequence, changes are seen in the periodontal ligament *(PDL)* as this structure becomes less able to cope with the forces applied to it. The downward and oblique orientation of the ligament fibers is progressively lost *(below arrowhead)*, and local pockets of cementum resorption occur *(arrows)*.

of the teeth (Fig. 10.22). The third molars are particularly prone to impaction because they erupt last, when the least room is available. The upper canine also commonly is impacted because of its late eruption (Fig. 10.23).

ORTHODONTIC TOOTH MOVEMENT

The supporting tissues of the tooth (i.e., the PDL and alveolar bone) have a remarkable plasticity that permits physiologic tooth movement and accommodates to the constant minor movements that the tooth makes during mastication. This plasticity of the supporting tissues of the tooth permits orthodontic tooth movement.

Theoretically, bringing about tooth movement without any tissue damage by using a light force, equivalent to the physiologic forces determining tooth position, to capitalize on the plasticity of the supporting tissues should be possible. The changes that happen under these circumstances are easy to describe: Differentiation of osteoclasts occurs, and they resorb bone of the socket wall on the pressure side. At the same time, remodeling of collagen fibers in the PDL occurs to accommodate the new tooth position. On the tension side, remodeling of collagen fiber bundles also takes place but in association with bone deposition on the socket wall. No changes occur in tooth structure (e.g., in the cementum). Whether current orthodontic techniques duplicate this ideal situation is doubtful; most involve some degree of tissue damage that varies because the forces applied to move the tooth are not distributed equally throughout the PDL.

Analyzing the tissue reactions in terms of a graph illustrating the typical pattern of orthodontic tooth movement is worthwhile (Fig. 10.24). An applied force results in immediate movement of the tooth, which, in turn, leads to areas of tension and compression within the PDL and to changes within the bone and ligament. Unlike physiologic tooth movement in which bone resorption of the alveolar wall occurs on its PDL aspect, orthodontic tooth movement also causes some internal or undermining resorption in which alveolar bone is remodeled from its endosteal face (Fig. 10.25).

This difference in resorption is caused by changes within the PDL resulting from compression. The ligament undergoes *hyalinization,* a term from light microscopy describing the loss of cells from an area of ligament because of trauma. Obviously if no cells are present, no bony remodeling can occur. Although hyalinization is present, tooth movement ceases. Only when new cells repopulate the hyalinized portion of the ligament and the bone is removed by osteoclasts does tooth movement begin again. This movement coincides with the active remodeling of ligament collagen by the newly arrived fibroblasts and the deposition of new bone. Obviously, heavier forces cause larger areas of hyalinization, a longer period of repair, and slower tooth movement.

Chapter 9 makes the point that orthodontic tooth movement is possible because of the greater resistance of cementum than bone to resorption. If both tissues were resorbed with equal facility, root loss would follow orthodontic movement; however, even when radiographs show no visible changes in the root surface, most teeth moved orthodontically undergo some degree of root resorption (Fig. 10.26), and resorption is followed by repair. This resorption is seen as small lacunae created by odontoclasts that are repaired rapidly by the formation of new cementum (Fig. 10.27). Because cementum is more resistant than bone to resorption, clinically demonstrable resorption usually occurs only after application of heavy force and the movement of teeth for more than 30 days.

In addition to changes within the periodontium, tooth movement demands remodeling of the adjacent gingival tissues (of which little is known) and some adaptation of pulpal tissue. The

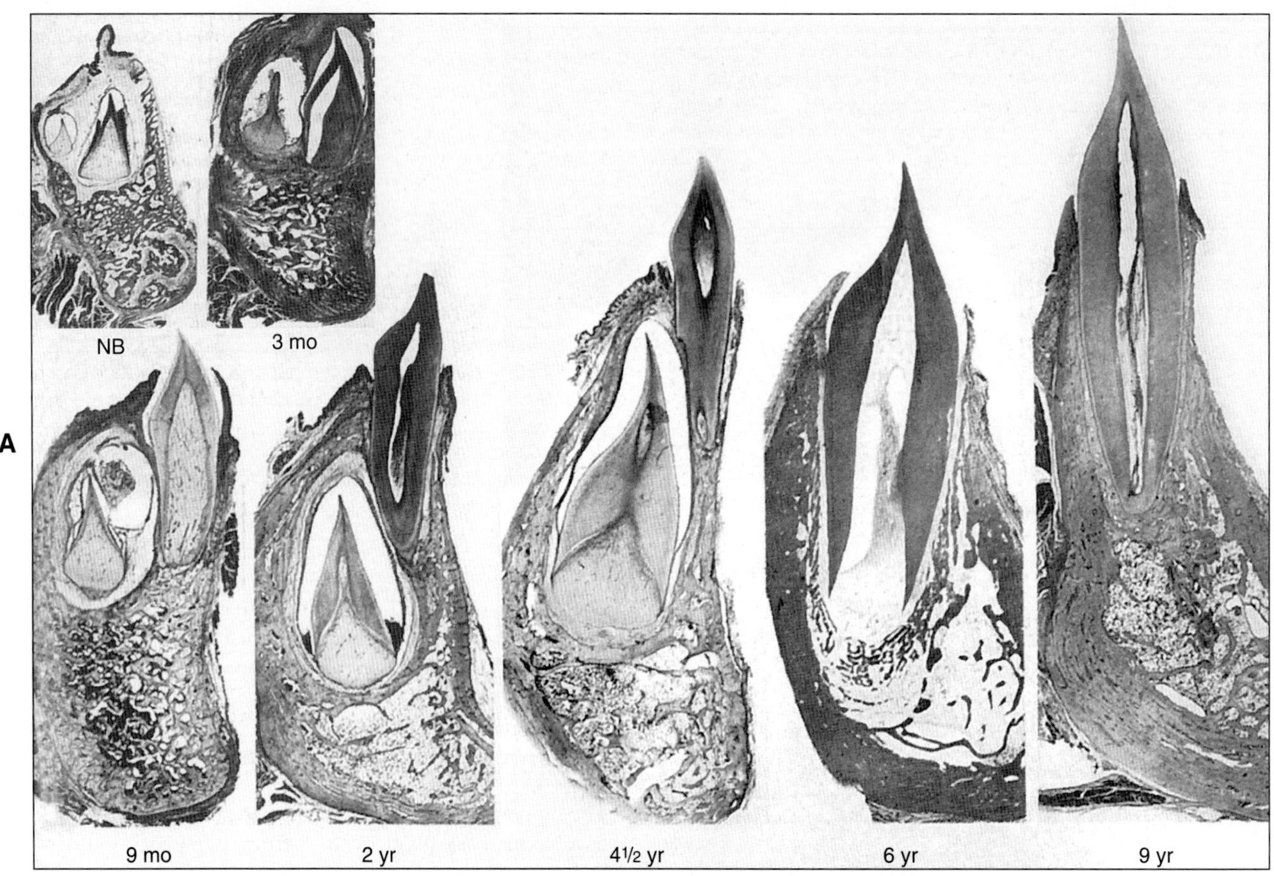

Fig. 10.21 Summary of preeruptive and eruptive tooth movement, including the pattern of tooth resorption. (A) Buccolingual sections through the central incisor region of the mandible at representative stages of development from birth *(NB)* to 9 years of age. At birth the deciduous and permanent tooth germs occupy the same bony crypt. Note how, by eccentric growth and eruption of the deciduous tooth, the permanent tooth germ comes to occupy its own bony crypt apical to the erupted incisor. At 4.5 years of age, resorption of the deciduous incisor has begun. At 6 years of age, the deciduous incisor has been shed, and its successor is erupting. The active deposition of new bone at the base of the socket is notable.

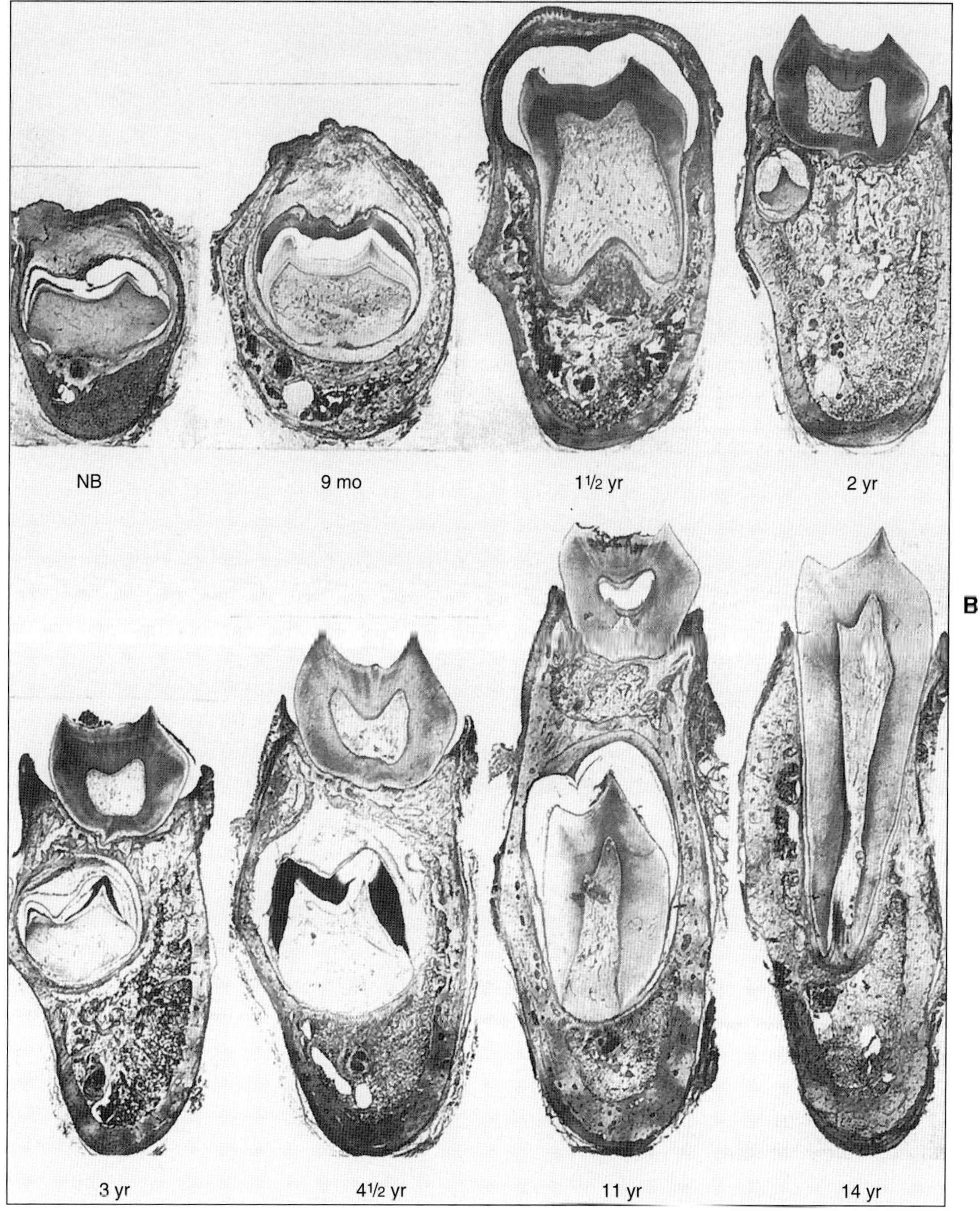

Fig. 10.21, cont'd (B) Buccolingual sections through the deciduous first molar and permanent first premolar of the mandible at representative stages of development from birth to 14 years of age. Note how the permanent tooth germ shifts its position. In the section of a 4.5-year-old mandible, the gubernacular canal is clearly visible. Lack of roots in the 2-, 3-, 4.5-, and 11-year-old sections results not from resorption but from the sections having been cut in the midline of a tooth with widely diverging roots. (From Bhaskar SN, editor: *Orban's oral histology and embryology*, ed 11, St. Louis, MO, 1991, Mosby.)

rapid a movement can lead to damage of the vessels supplying the pulp, resulting in eventual pulp necrosis, especially when the tooth is tilted too far. An interrupted force of some magnitude has little effect on the pulp, which is why removable appliances cause little or no pulp damage. With a fixed appliance providing a continuous force, some pulp damage usually occurs; because young pulp usually is involved and the forces are moderate, however, repair follows.

The development of a functional dentition from its inception through the deciduous to the permanent dentition has been described fully. Many of the key events in the process for both dentitions are summarized in Figs. 10.28 and 10.29.

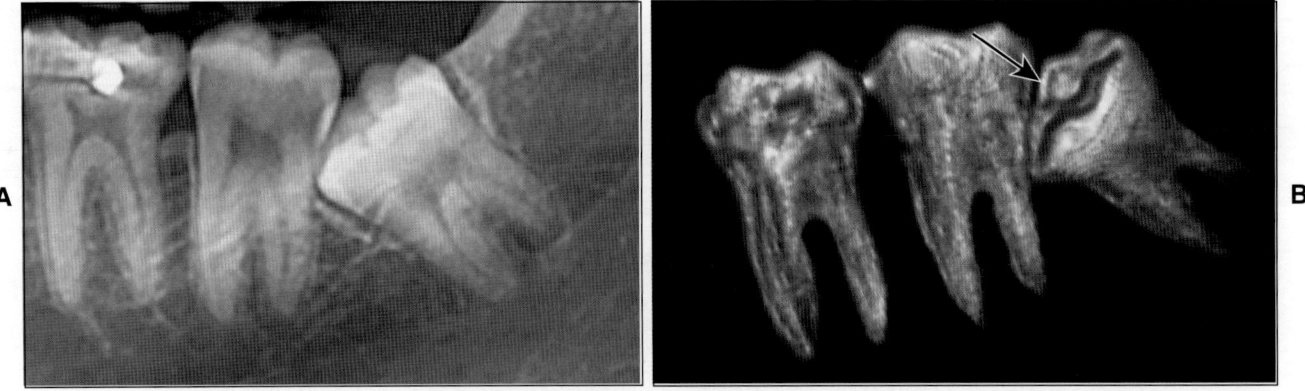

Fig. 10.22 Computed tomography scan slice (A) and three-dimensional reconstruction (B) of an impacted mandibular third molar *(arrow)*. (Courtesy M. Schmittbuhl.)

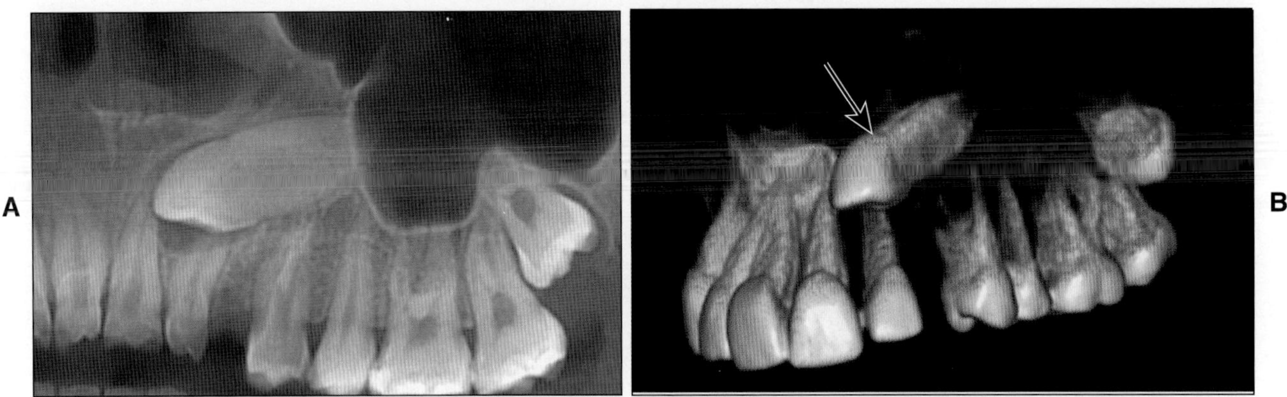

Fig. 10.23 Computed tomography scan slice (A) and three-dimensional reconstruction (B) of an impacted maxillary canine *(arrow)*. (Courtesy M. Schmittbuhl.)

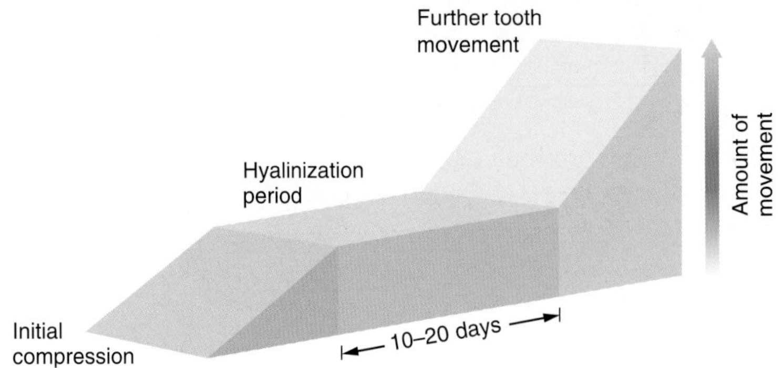

Fig. 10.24 Orthodontic tooth movement over time.

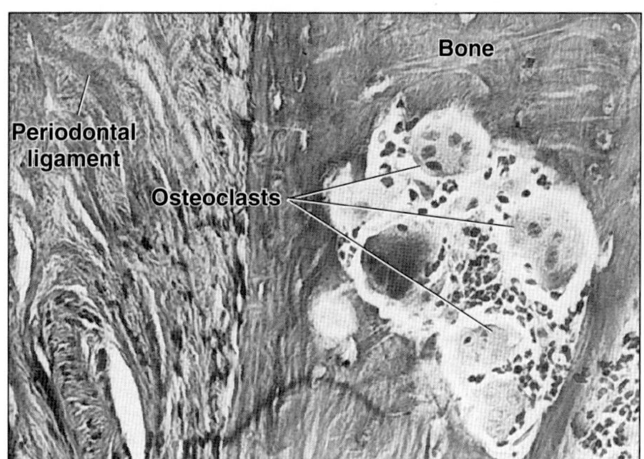

Fig. 10.25 Undermining resorption of alveolar bone 7 days after the beginning of tooth movement with a light tipping force. (From Buck DL, Church DH: A histologic study of human tooth movement, *Am J Orthod* 62:507–516, 1972.)

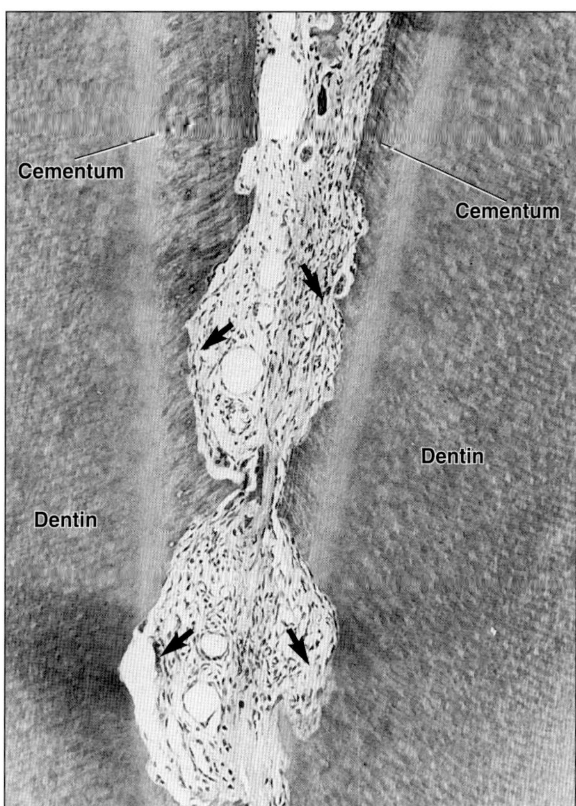

Fig. 10.26 Photomicrograph of the response of supporting tissues when the roots of teeth come into contact. The two teeth are tipping into contact as a consequence of malocclusion, but the same situation can be created by excessive orthodontic force. The interdental septum has been lost almost completely, and the root surfaces now are resorbing. Repair of these resorption bays *(arrows)* is possible if the drifting ceases.

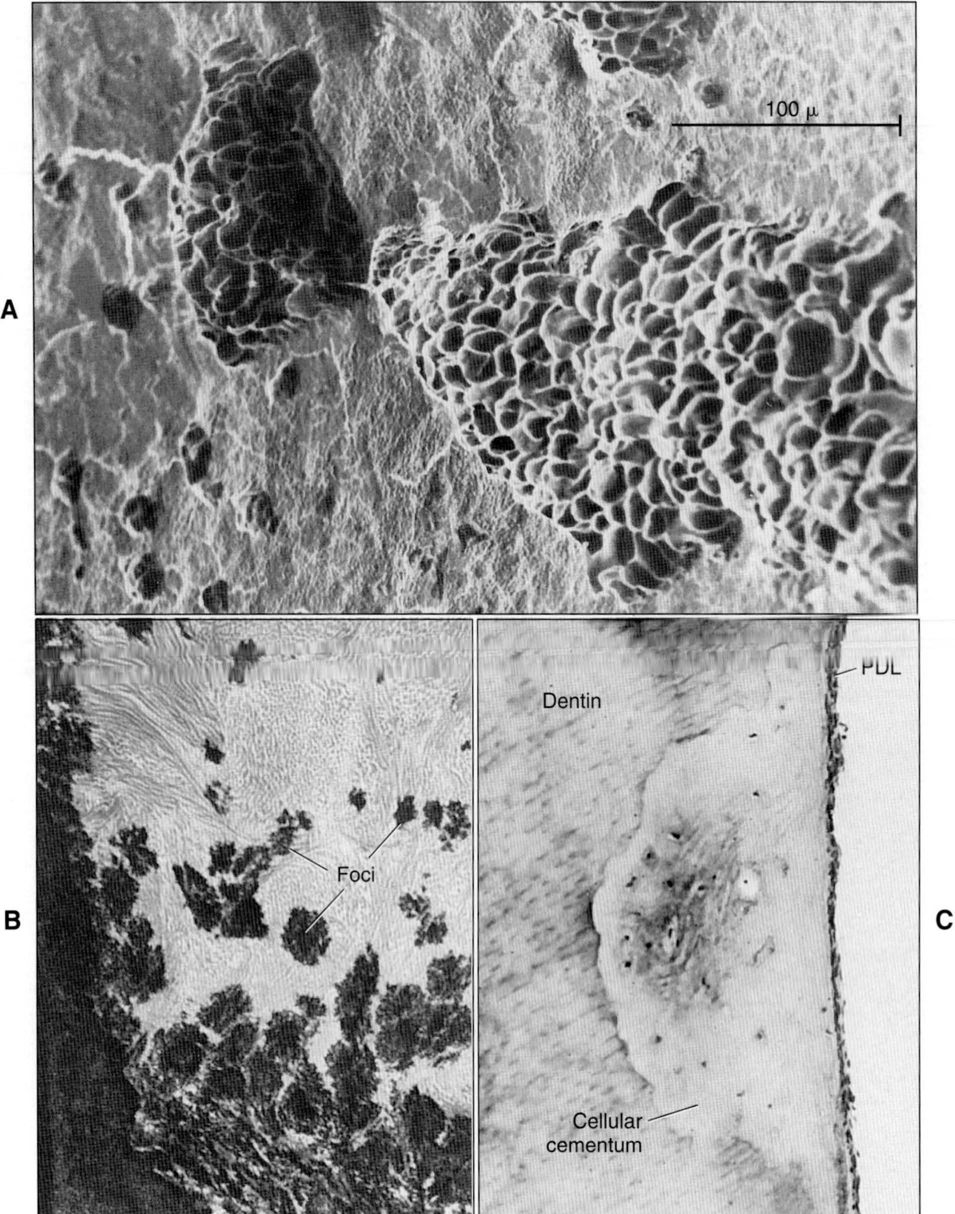

Fig. 10.27 Resorption and repair of the root surface. (A) Scanning electron micrograph of the root surface of a tooth used as an anchor for rapid maxillary expansion showing resorption lacunae on the root surface. (B) Transmission electron micrograph of a region of cementum repair illustrating the presence of mineralization foci in the collagenous tissue. (C) A light microscope picture of completed root surface repair. *PDL*, Periodontal ligament. (A, From Barber AF, Sims MR: Rapid maxillary expansion and external root resorption in man: a scanning electron microscope study, *Am J Orthod* 79:630–652, 1981; B, from Furseth R: The resorption processes of human deciduous teeth studied by light microscopy, microradiography and electron microscopy, *Arch Oral Biol* 13:417–431, 1968; C, from Langford SR, Sims MR: Root surface resorption, repair, and periodontal attachment following rapid maxillary expansion in man, *Am J Orthod* 81:108–115, 1982.)

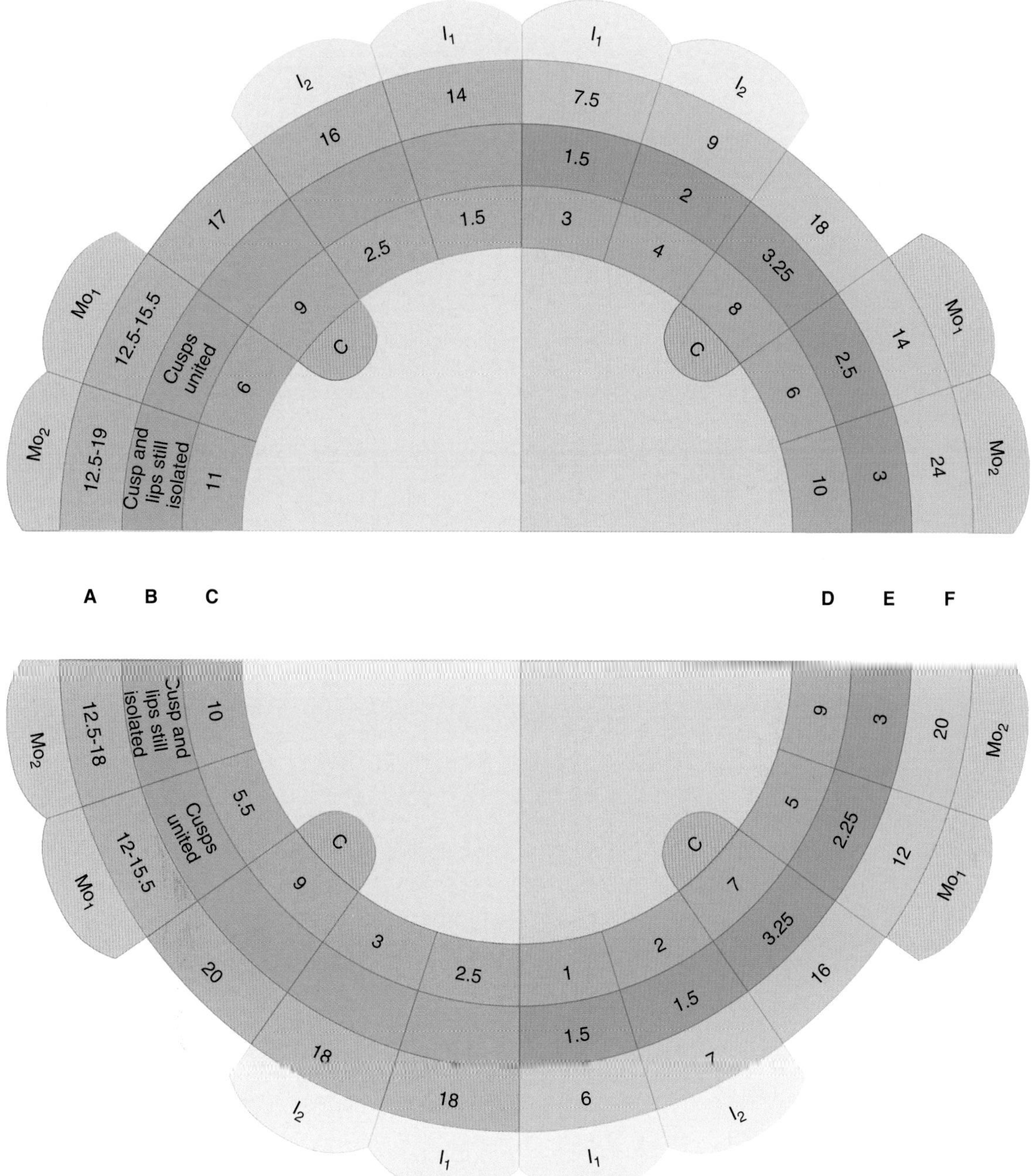

Fig. 10.28 Chronology of the human primary dentition. *(A)* Mineralization begins (weeks in utero). *(B)* Amount of enamel matrix found at birth. *(C)* Enamel complete (months). *(D)* Eruption sequence. *(E)* Root completed (years). *(F)* Emergence into the oral cavity (months). *C*, Canine; *I*, incisor; *Mo*, molar.

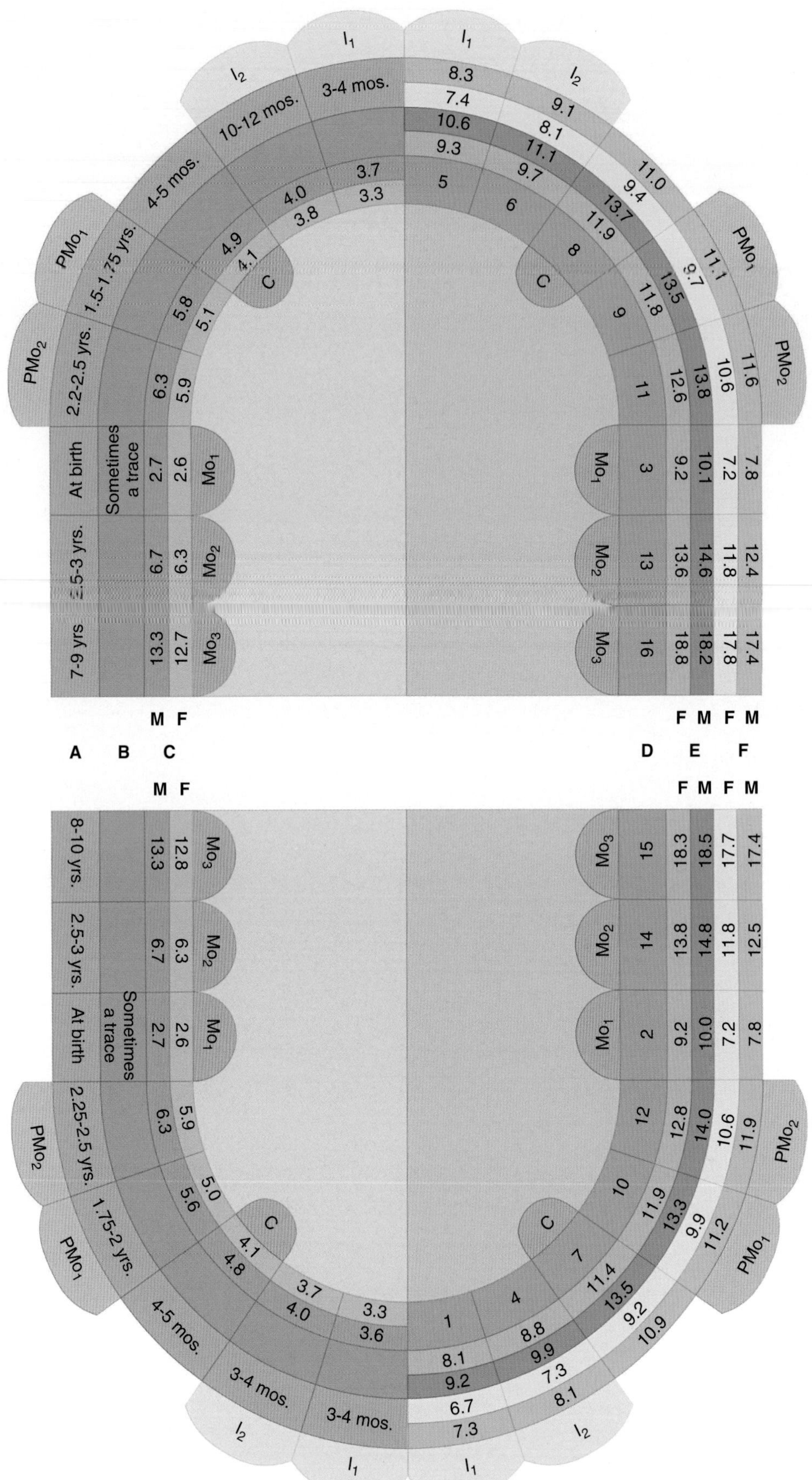

Fig. 10.29 Chronology of the human permanent dentition. *(A)* Mineralization begins. *(B)* Amount of enamel matrix at birth. *(C)* Enamel completed (years). *(D)* Eruption sequence. *(E)* Root completed (years). *(F)* Emergence into the oral cavity (years). *C*, Canine; *F*, female; *I*, incisor; *M*, male; *Mo*, molar; *PMo*, premolar.

RECOMMENDED READING

Cahill DR: Histological changes in the bony crypt and gubernacular canal of erupting permanent premolars during deciduous premolar exfoliation in beagles, *J Dent Res* 53:786–791, 1974.

Craddock HL, Youngson CC: Eruptive tooth movement—the current state of knowledge, *Br Dent J* 197:385–391, 2004.

Kardos TB: The mechanism of tooth eruption, *Br Dent J* 181:91–95, 1996.

Marks Jr SC, et al.: The mechanisms and mediators of tooth eruption: models for developmental biologists, *Int J Dev Biol* 39:223–230, 1995.

Marks Jr SC, Schroeder HE: Tooth eruption: theories and facts, *Anat Rec* 245:374–393, 1996.

Ten Cate AR, et al.: The role of fibroblasts in the remodeling of periodontal ligament during physiologic tooth movement, *Am J Orthod* 69:155–168, 1976.

Wise GE, King GJ: Mechanisms of tooth eruption and orthodontic tooth movement, *J Dent Res* 87:414–434, 2008.

Wise GE, et al.: Cellular, molecular and genetic determinants of tooth eruption, *Crit Rev Oral Biol Med* 13:323–334, 2002.

Wise GE, et al.: Requirement of alveolar bone formation for eruption of rat molars, *Eur J Oral Sci* 119:333–338, 2011.

11

Salivary Glands

Antonio Nanci, and Simon D. Tran

OUTLINE

The oral cavity is kept moist by a film of fluid called saliva that coats the teeth and the mucosa. Saliva is a complex fluid produced by the salivary glands. Individuals with a deficiency of salivary secretion experience difficulty eating, speaking, and swallowing and become prone to mucosal infections and rampant caries.

In human beings, three pairs of major salivary glands—the parotid, submandibular, and sublingual—are located outside the oral cavity, with extended duct systems through which the gland secretions reach the mouth. Numerous smaller minor salivary glands are located in various parts of the oral cavity (labial, lingual, palatal, buccal, glossopalatine, retromolar glands) typically located in the submucosal layer (Fig. 11.1), with short ducts opening directly onto the mucosal surface.

The composition of saliva is summarized in Table 11.1. The saliva produced by each major salivary gland, however, differs in amount and composition. The parotid glands secrete a watery saliva rich in enzymes such as amylase, proteins such as the proline-rich proteins, and glycoproteins. Submandibular saliva, in addition to the components already listed, contains highly glycosylated substances called *mucins.* The sublingual gland produces viscous saliva also rich in mucins. Oral fluid, which is referred to as *mixed (whole) saliva,* includes the secretions of the major glands, the minor glands, desquamated oral epithelial cells, microorganisms and their products, food debris, and serum components and inflammatory cells that gain access through the gingival crevice. Moreover, whole saliva is not the simple sum of all these components because many of the proteins are removed as they adhere to the surfaces of the teeth and oral mucosa, bind to microorganisms, or are degraded.

FUNCTIONS OF SALIVA

Saliva has many functions (Table 11.2), the most important being protection of the oral cavity.

Protection

Saliva protects the oral cavity in many ways. The fluid nature of saliva provides a washing action that flushes away nonadherent bacteria and other debris. In particular, the clearance of sugars from the mouth limits their availability to acidogenic plaque microorganisms. The mucins and other glycoproteins provide lubrication, preventing the oral tissues from adhering to one another and allowing them to slide easily over one another. The mucins also form a barrier against noxious stimuli, microbial toxins, and minor trauma.

Buffering

Bicarbonate and (to some extent) phosphate ions in saliva provide a buffering action that helps protect the teeth from demineralization caused by bacterial acids produced during sugar metabolism. Some basic salivary proteins also may contribute to the buffering action of saliva. Additionally, the metabolism of salivary proteins and peptides by bacteria produces urea and ammonia, which help to increase pH.

Pellicle Formation

Many of the salivary proteins bind to the surfaces of the teeth and oral mucosa, forming a thin film (salivary pellicle). Several proteins bind calcium and help to protect the tooth surface. Others have binding

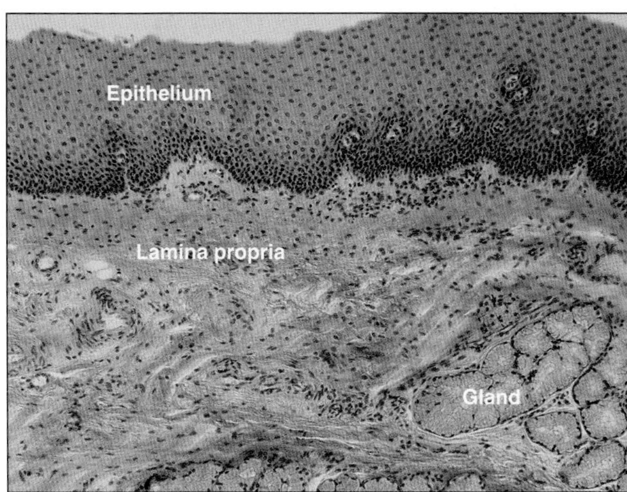

Fig. 11.1 Minor mucous salivary gland located in the submucosa below the epithelium of the oral cavity. The saliva secreted by minor salivary glands reaches the oral cavity through short ducts that connect the glands to the surface epithelium. (Courtesy B. Kablar.)

TABLE 11.1 Composition of Saliva

Parameter	Characteristics
Volume	600–1000 mL/day
Electrolytes	Na^+, K^+, Cl^-, HCO_3^-, Ca^{2+}, Mg^{2+}, HCO_3^{2-}, SCN^-, and F^-
Secretory proteins/ peptides	Amylase, proline-rich proteins, mucins, histatin, cystatin, peroxidase, lysozyme, lactoferrin, defensins, and cathelicidin-LL37
Immunoglobulins	Secretory immunoglobulin A (IgA); IgG, IgM
Small organic	Glucose, amino acids, urea, uric acid, and lipid molecules
Other components	Epidermal growth factor, insulin, cyclic adenosine monophosphate–binding proteins, and serum albumin

Flow Rate (mL/min)	Whole	Parotid	Submandibular
Resting	0.2–0.4	0.04	0.1
Stimulated	2–5	1–2	0.8
pH	6.7–7.4	6–7.8	

sites for oral bacteria, providing the initial attachment for organisms that form plaque.

Maintenance of Tooth Integrity

Saliva is supersaturated with calcium and phosphate ions. The solubility of these ions is maintained by several calcium-binding proteins, especially the acidic proline-rich proteins and statherin. At the tooth surface the high concentration of calcium and phosphate results in a posteruptive maturation of the enamel, increasing surface hardness and resistance to demineralization. Remineralization of initial caries lesions also can occur; this is enhanced by the presence of fluoride ions in saliva.

Antimicrobial Action

Saliva has a major ecologic influence on the microorganisms that colonize oral tissues. In addition to the barrier effect provided by mucins, saliva contains a spectrum of proteins with antimicrobial activity, such as the lysozyme, lactoferrin, peroxidase, and secretory leukocyte protease inhibitor. A number of small peptides that function by inserting into membranes and disrupting cellular or mitochondrial functions are present in saliva. These include α-defensins and β-defensins, cathelicidin-LL37, and the histatins. In addition to antibacterial and antifungal activities, several of these proteins and peptides exhibit antiviral activity. The major salivary immunoglobulin (secretory immunoglobulin A [IgA]) causes agglutination of specific microorganisms, preventing their adherence to oral tissues and forming clumps that are swallowed. Mucins and specific agglutinins also aggregate microorganisms.

TABLE 11.2 Functions of Saliva

Function	Effect	Active Constituents
Protection	Clearance	Water
	Lubrication	Mucins, glycoproteins
	Thermal/chemical insulation	Mucins
	Pellicle formation	Proteins, glycoproteins, mucins
	Tannin binding	Basic proline-rich proteins, histatins
Buffering	pH maintenance	Bicarbonate, phosphate, basic proteins, urea, ammonia
	Neutralization of acids	
Tooth integrity	Enamel maturation, repair	Calcium, phosphate, fluoride, statherin, acidic proline-rich proteins
Antimicrobial activity	Physical barrier	Mucins
	Immune defense	Secretory immunoglobulin A
	Nonimmune defense	Peroxidase, lysozyme, lactoferrin, histatin, mucins, agglutinins, secretory leukocyte protease inhibitor, defensins, and cathelicidin-LL37
Tissue repair	Wound healing, epithelial regeneration	Growth factors, trefoil proteins,
Digestion	Bolus formation	Water, mucins
	Starch, triglyceride digestion	Amylase, lipase
Taste	Solution of molecules	Water and lipocalins
	Maintenance of taste buds	Epidermal growth factor and carbonic anhydrase VI

Tissue Repair

A variety of growth factors and other biologically active peptides and proteins are present in small quantities in saliva. Under experimental conditions, many of these substances promote tissue growth and differentiation, wound healing, and other beneficial effects. However, the role of most of these substances in protection of the oral cavity is presently unknown.

Digestion

Saliva also contributes to the digestion of food. The solubilization of food substances and the actions of enzymes such as amylase and lipase begin the digestive process. The moistening and lubricative properties of saliva also allow the formation and swallowing of a food bolus.

Taste

Saliva functions in taste by solubilizing food substances so they can be sensed by taste receptors located in taste buds. Saliva produced by minor glands in the vicinity of the circumvallate papillae contains proteins that are believed to bind taste substances and present them to the taste receptors. Additionally, saliva contains proteins that have a trophic effect on taste receptors.

ANATOMY

The parotid gland is the largest salivary gland. The superficial portion of the parotid gland is located subcutaneously, in front of the external ear, and its deeper portion lies behind the ramus of the mandible. The parotid gland is associated intimately with peripheral branches of the facial nerve (cranial nerve VII) (Fig. 11.2A). The Stensen duct of the parotid gland runs forward across the masseter muscle, turns inward at the anterior border of the masseter, and opens into the oral cavity at a papilla opposite the maxillary second molar. A small amount of parotid tissue occasionally forms an accessory gland associated with Stensen duct, just anterior to the superficial portion. The parotid gland receives its blood supply from branches of the external carotid artery as they pass through the gland. The parasympathetic nerve supply to the parotid gland is mainly from the glossopharyngeal nerve (cranial nerve IX). The preganglionic fibers synapse in the otic ganglion; the postganglionic fibers reach the gland through the auriculotemporal nerve. The sympathetic innervation of all the salivary glands is provided by postganglionic fibers from the superior cervical ganglion, traveling with the blood supply.

The submandibular gland is situated in the posterior part of the floor of the mouth, adjacent to the medial aspect of the mandible and wrapping around the posterior border of the mylohyoid muscle (see Fig. 11.2B). The excretory (Wharton) duct of the submandibular gland runs forward above the mylohyoid muscle and opens into the mouth beneath the tongue at the sublingual caruncle, lateral to the lingual frenum. The submandibular gland receives its blood supply from the facial and lingual arteries. The parasympathetic nerve supply is derived mainly from the facial nerve (cranial nerve VII), reaching the gland through the lingual nerve and submandibular ganglion.

The sublingual gland is the smallest of the paired major salivary glands. The gland is located in the anterior part of the floor of the mouth between the mucosa and the mylohyoid muscle (see Fig. 11.2B). The secretions of the sublingual gland enter the oral cavity through a series of small ducts (ducts of Rivinus) opening along the sublingual fold and often through a larger duct (Bartholin duct) that opens with the submandibular duct at the sublingual caruncle. The sublingual gland receives its blood supply from the sublingual and submental arteries. The facial nerve (cranial nerve VII) provides the parasympathetic innervation of the sublingual gland also via the lingual nerve and submandibular ganglion.

The minor salivary glands, estimated to number between 600 and 1000, exist as small, discrete aggregates of secretory tissue present in the submucosa throughout most of the oral cavity. The only places they are not found are the gingiva and the anterior part of the hard palate. They are predominantly mucous glands, except for the lingual serous glands (Ebner glands) that are located in the tongue and open into the troughs surrounding the circumvallate papillae on the dorsum of the tongue and at the foliate papillae on the sides of the tongue.

Recently, bilateral mucous salivary glands (tubarial glands) were reported in the human nasopharynx using positron emission tomography/computed tomography with prostate-specific membrane antigen ligands. Their recognition as major salivary glands is still under discussion.

DEVELOPMENT

Similar to teeth, the individual salivary glands arise as a proliferation of oral epithelial cells, forming a focal thickening that grows into the underlying ectomesenchyme. Continued growth results in the formation of a small bud connected to the surface by a trailing cord of epithelial cells, with mesenchymal cells condensing around the bud (Fig. 11.3). Clefts develop in the bud, forming two or more new buds; continuation of this process, called branching morphogenesis, produces successive generations of buds and a hierarchic ramification of the gland.

Studies of analogous processes in experimental animals and studies of salivary gland development in vitro have revealed that the process of branching morphogenesis requires interactions between the epithelium and mesenchyme. Several factors that control the location of the branch points and the overall structure of the gland have been identified. Signaling molecules, including members of the fibroblast growth factor protein family, sonic hedgehog, transforming growth factor β, and their receptors, play a major role in the development of branches. The differential contraction of actin filaments at the basal and apical ends of the epithelial cells is believed to provide the physical mechanism underlying cleft formation, and the deposition of extracellular matrix components within the clefts apparently serves to stabilize them. The process of epithelial budding, which is the first step in branching morphogenesis, is due to a combination of strong cell-matrix adhesion (e.g., β1-integrin) and weak cell-cell adhesion by peripheral salivary epithelial cells. Finally, the specific mesenchyme associated with the salivary glands has been shown to provide the optimum environment for gland development.

The development of a lumen within the branched epithelium generally occurs in this order: (1) in the distal end of the main cord and in branch cords, (2) in the proximal end of the main cord, and (3) in the central portion of the main cord (Fig. 11.4). The lumina form within the ducts before they develop within the terminal buds. Some studies have suggested that lumen formation may involve apoptosis of centrally located cells in the cell cords, but further research is required to establish definitively a role for cell death in this process.

After development of the lumen in the terminal buds, the epithelium consists of two layers of cells. The cells of the inner layer eventually differentiate into the secretory cells of the mature gland, mucous or serous, depending on the specific gland. Some cells of the outer layer form the contractile myoepithelial cells that are present around the secretory end pieces and intercalated ducts. As the epithelial parenchymal components increase in size and number, the associated mesenchyme (connective tissue) is diminished, although a thin layer of connective tissue remains, surrounding each secretory end piece and duct of the adult gland. Thicker partitions of connective tissue (septa), continuous with the capsule and within which run the nerves and blood vessels supplying the gland, invest the excretory ducts and divide the gland into lobes and lobules (see Fig. 1.8).

The genes implicated in salivary gland development and their role have been investigated using knockout mouse models (Table 11.3).

The parotid glands begin to develop at 4 to 6 weeks of embryonic life, the submandibular glands at 6 weeks, and the sublingual and minor salivary glands at 8 to 12 weeks. The cells of the secretory end pieces and ducts attain maturity during the last 2 months of gestation. The glands continue to grow postnatally—with the volume proportion of acinar tissue increasing and the volume proportions of ducts, connective tissue, and vascular elements decreasing—up to 2 years of age.

STRUCTURE

As described in the previous section, a salivary gland consists of a series of branched ducts, terminating in spheric or tubular secretory end pieces or acini (see Fig. 1.7). An analogy can be made to a bunch of grapes, with the stems representing the ducts and the grapes

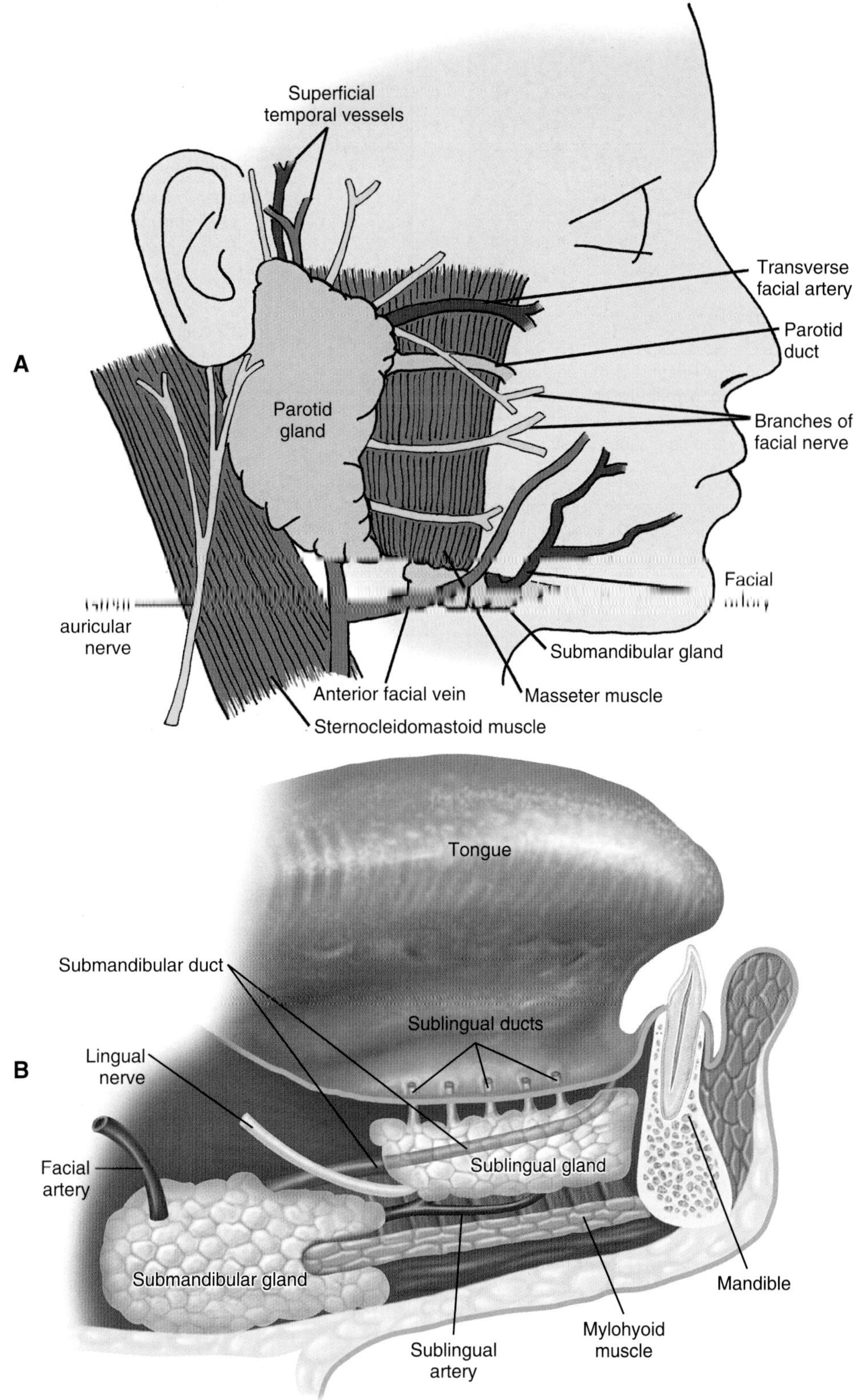

Fig. 11.2 Anatomy of the major salivary glands. (A) Parotid gland. (B) Submandibular and sublingual glands. The major glands are bilaterally paired and have long ducts that convey their saliva to the oral cavity. (From Hollinshead WH: The head and neck. In *Anatomy for surgeons,* vol 1, New York, NY, 1958, Hoeber.)

corresponding to the secretory end pieces. The main excretory duct, which empties into the oral cavity, divides into progressively smaller interlobar and intralobular excretory ducts that enter the lobes and lobules of the gland. The predominant intralobular ductal component is the striated duct, which plays a major role in modification of the primary saliva produced by the secretory end pieces. Connecting the striated ducts to the secretory end pieces are intercalated ducts, which branch once or twice before joining individual end pieces. The lumen

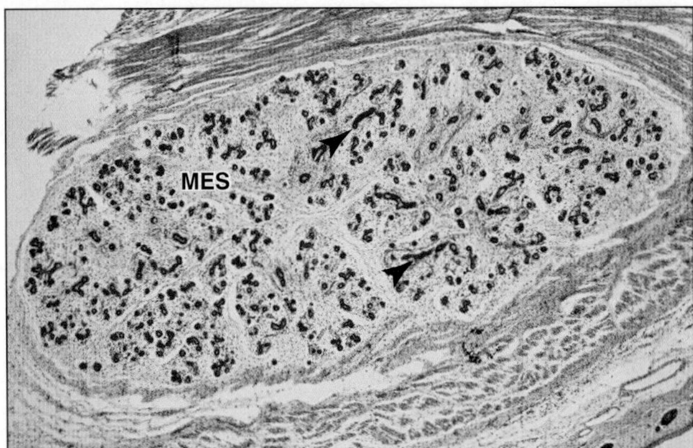

Fig. 11.3 Developing salivary gland. Proliferation of the epithelium into the underlying mesenchyme results in long epithelial cords *(arrowheads)* that undergo repeated dichotomous branching. The mesenchyme *(MES)* has condensed around the developing glandular epithelium.

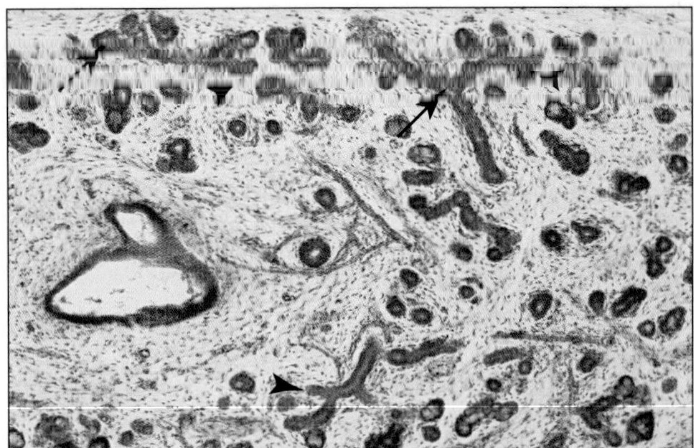

Fig. 11.4 Developing salivary gland. Lumen formation *(arrows)* has begun in the ducts. Branching of the distal ends of the epithelial cords is evident *(arrowheads)*.

TABLE 11.3 Mouse Gene Knockout Models and Salivary Gland Defects

Knockout Mouse Model	Defects in Salivary Glands
Adamts18	Reduced cleft formation and epithelial branching in embryonic submandibular gland
	Spontaneous submandibular gland scleroma (fibrosis, acinar atrophy), secretory dysfunction, and severe dental caries in adults
Ascl3	Smaller salivary glands but secrete saliva normally
	Lower level of cell proliferation
	Ascl3 cells are active proliferating progenitors but not the only precursors for salivary gland development
DLK1	Smaller salivary glands and weigh significantly less
	Reduced capacity to secrete saliva
Ehf	Distinct cellular phenotype with decreased granular convoluted tubules
	Increased accumulation of Sox9-positive intercalated ductal cell population
FGF10	Aplasia of salivary glands
FGFR2b	FGFR2b and FGF10 knockout mice are alike, suggesting that FGF10 is a ligand to FGFR2b during multiorgan development
Hs3st3b1	Reduced submandibular gland branching morphogenesis
	Reduced 3-O-sulfated heparan sulfate of myoepithelial cells
	Reduced secretory function
Lgr5	Disruption of salivary gland development
	Atypical number and localization of ducts
p63	Box development of several organs (e.g., tooth, salivary gland)
	Epithelial defects, including lack of skin, hair, mammary and prostate tissue, and salivary and lacrimal glands
	Involved in myoepithelial cell tumors
Sox9	Smaller initial buds of submandibular glands

of the end piece is continuous with that of the intercalated duct. In some glands, small extensions of the lumen (intercellular canaliculi) are found between adjacent secretory cells (Fig. 11.5). These intercellular canaliculi may extend almost to the base of the secretory cells and serve to increase the size of the secretory (luminal) surface of the cells.

Secretory Cells

The two main types of secretory cells present in salivary glands are serous cells and mucous cells. Serous and mucous cells differ in structure and in the types of macromolecular components that they produce and secrete. In general, serous cells produce proteins and glycoproteins (proteins modified by the addition of sugar residues [glycosylation]), many of which have well-defined enzymatic, antimicrobial, calcium-binding, or other activities. Typically, serous glycoproteins have N-linked (bound to the β-amide of asparagine) oligosaccharide side chains. The main products of mucous cells are mucins, which have a protein core (apomucin) that is organized into specific domains and is highly substituted with sugar residues. Mucins are therefore also glycoproteins, but they differ from most serous cell glycoproteins in the structure of the protein core, the nature (predominantly O-linked [i.e., to the hydroxyl groups of serine or threonine]) and extent of glycosylation, and their function. Mucins function mainly to lubricate and form a barrier on surfaces and to bind and aggregate microorganisms. Mucous cells secrete few, if any, other macromolecular components.

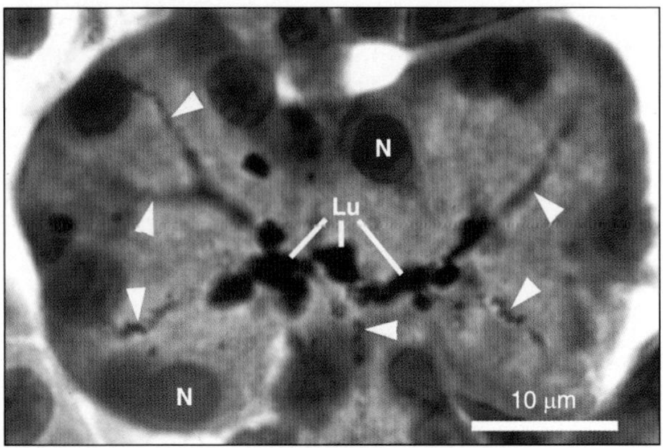

Fig. 11.5 Lumen and intercellular canaliculi in a serous end piece. The lumen *(Lu)* and intercellular canaliculi were filled with India ink. Arrowheads indicate intercellular canaliculi extending between adjacent cells. *N,* Nuclei of serous cells. (From Hand AR: Salivary glands. In Provenza DV, Seibel W, editors: *Oral histology: inheritance and development,* ed 2, Philadelphia, PA, 1986, Lea and Febiger.)

In recent years the distinction between serous cells and mucous cells has become somewhat blurred. Serous cells of some salivary glands are known to produce certain types of mucins, and some mucous cells are believed to produce certain nonglycosylated proteins. Additionally, advances in tissue preservation procedures have demonstrated that the structure of mucous and serous cells is similar and that the typical morphology of swollen, fused, and empty-appearing mucous granules is likely a result of artifactual changes occurring during chemical fixation.

Serous Cells

Secretory end pieces that are composed of serous cells are typically spherical and consist of 8 to 12 cells surrounding a central lumen (Fig. 11.6). The cells are pyramidal, with a broad base adjacent to the connective tissue stroma and a narrow apex forming part of the lumen of the end piece. The lumen usually has fingerlike extensions (intercellular canaliculi) located between adjacent cells that increase the size of the luminal surface of the cells. The spheric nuclei are located basally, and occasionally binucleated cells are seen. Numerous secretory granules in which the macromolecular components of saliva are stored are present in the apical cytoplasm (Figs. 11.7 and 11.8). The granules may have a variable appearance, ranging from homogeneously electron-dense to a combination of electron-dense and electron-lucent regions arranged in intricate patterns. The basal cytoplasm contains numerous cisternae of rough endoplasmic reticulum, which converge on a large Golgi complex located just apical or lateral to the nucleus (Fig. 11.9). Forming secretory granules of variable size and density are present at the *trans* face of the Golgi complex. These granules increase in size gradually as their content condenses, eventually forming the mature secretory granules. Serous cells also contain all the typical organelles found in other cells, including cytoskeletal components, mitochondria, lysosomes, and peroxisomes.

The plasma membranes of serous cells exhibit several specializations. The luminal surface, including the intercellular canaliculi, is studded with a few short microvilli. The lateral surfaces have occasional folds that interdigitate with similar processes from the adjacent cells. The basal surface is thrown into regular folds that extend laterally beyond the borders of the cell to interdigitate with folds of the adjacent cells. The folding of the cell membranes greatly increases the surface area of the cell. Serous cells, as well as mucous cells, also are joined to one another by a variety of intercellular junctions (see Chapter 4). A tight junction (zonula occludens), an adhering junction (zonula adherens), and a desmosome (macula adherens) form a junctional complex that separates the luminal surface from the basolateral surfaces of the cell. The tight junctions help maintain cell-surface domains and regulate the passage of material from the lumen to the intercellular spaces and vice versa. The tight junctions exhibit a selective permeability, allowing the passage of certain ions and water. Their permeability can be altered by specific neurotransmitters to allow the passage of larger molecules (up to several thousand Daltons in size). The adhering junctions, and desmosomes that also are found elsewhere along the lateral cell surfaces, serve to hold adjacent cells together. The secretory cells also are attached to the basal lamina and the underlying connective tissue by hemidesmosomes. Through interactions with cytoplasmic proteins and cytoskeletal elements, these cell-cell and cell-matrix junctions also function in signaling events that provide information to the cells about their immediate environment. Gap (communicating) junctions linking the cytoplasm of adjacent cells also are found along the lateral cell surfaces. These junctions allow the passage of small molecules between cells, such as ions, metabolites, and cyclic adenosine monophosphate (cAMP). They probably serve to coordinate the activity of all the cells within an end piece, creating a functional unit.

Mucous Cells

Secretory end pieces that are composed of mucous cells typically have a tubular configuration; when cut in cross section, these tubules appear as round profiles with mucous cells surrounding a central lumen of larger size than that of serous end pieces (Fig. 11.10). Mucous end pieces in the major salivary glands and some minor salivary glands have serous cells associated with them in the form of a demilune or crescent covering the mucous cells at the end of the tubule (Fig. 11.11). These serous demilune cells are in all respects similar to the serous end piece cells present in the same gland. Their secretions reach the lumen of the end piece through intercellular canaliculi extending between the mucous cells at the end of the tubule.

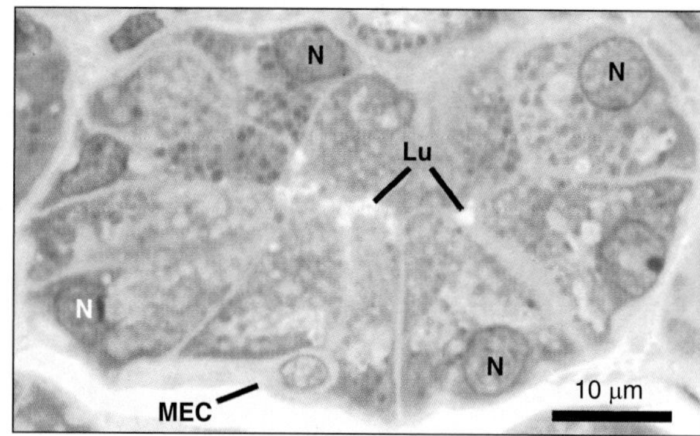

Fig. 11.6 Light micrograph of a serous end piece of the human submandibular gland stained with toluidine blue. The apical cytoplasm of the serous cells contains secretory granules of variable density. *Lu,* Lumen; *MEC,* myoepithelial cell; *N,* nucleus.

The most prominent feature of mucous cells is the accumulation in the apical cytoplasm of large amounts of secretory product (mucus), which compresses the nucleus and endoplasmic reticulum against the basal cell membrane. The secretory material appears unstained in routine histologic preparations, giving an empty appearance to the supranuclear cytoplasm. However, when special stains (e.g., periodic acid–Schiff stain, Alcian blue) that reveal sugar residues or acidic groups are used, the secretory material is strongly stained (see Fig. 11.11). In the electron microscope the mucous secretory granules appear swollen, their membranes are disrupted, and they often are fused with one another. Their content appears electron lucent but may include some finely filamentous or flocculent material (Fig. 11.12). As noted previously, the typical appearance of mucous granules probably is caused by artifacts induced during chemical fixation; when tissue samples are rapidly (a few milliseconds) frozen and subsequently prepared for electron microscopy, the mucous secretory granules are small, dense, have intact membranes, and do not fuse with one another.

Mucous cells have a large Golgi complex located mainly basal to the mass of secretory granules. Small granules form at the *trans* face of the Golgi complex, increase in size, and join the rest of the granules stored in the apical cytoplasm. The endoplasmic reticulum and most of the other organelles are limited mainly to the basal cytoplasm of the cell (Fig. 11.13; see also Fig. 11.12). Like serous cells, mucous cells are joined by a variety of intercellular junctions. Unlike serous cells, however, mucous cells lack intercellular canaliculi except for those covered by demilune cells.

Formation and Secretion of Saliva

The formation of saliva occurs in two stages. In the first stage, cells of the secretory end pieces and intercalated ducts produce primary saliva, which is an isotonic fluid containing most of the organic components and all of the water that is secreted by the salivary glands. In the second stage, the primary saliva is modified as it passes through the striated and excretory ducts, mainly by reabsorption and secretion of electrolytes. The final saliva that reaches the oral cavity is hypotonic.

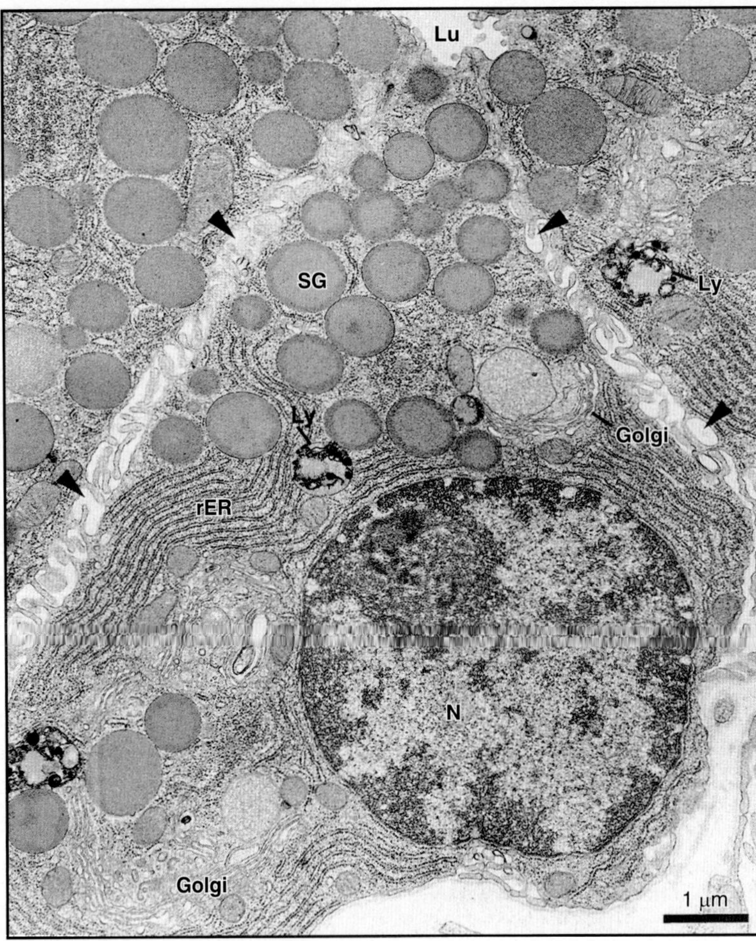

Fig. 11.7 Transmission electron micrograph of a serous cell of a rat parotid gland. The nuclei *(N)* and rough endoplasmic reticulum *(rER)* are located basally, and numerous electron-dense secretory granules *(SG)* are present in the apical cytoplasm. Portions of the Golgi complex *(Golgi)* are located apical and lateral to the nucleus. *Arrowheads* indicate intercellular spaces. *Lu,* Lumen; *Ly,* lysosomes. (From Hand AR: The effects of acute starvation on parotid acinar cells. Ultrastructural and cytochemical observations on ad libitum-fed and starved rats, *Am J Anat* 135:71–92, 1972.)

Macromolecular Components

Like other cells that are specialized for the synthesis and regulated secretion of proteins and glycoproteins, the cells of the secretory end pieces have abundant rough endoplasmic reticula and a large Golgi complex, and they store their products in membrane-bound granules in the apical cytoplasm. Secretory proteins are synthesized by ribosomes attached to the cisternae of the endoplasmic reticulum and translocated to the lumen of the endoplasmic reticulum. The proteins associate with other molecules (chaperones) that ensure proper folding of the protein, and posttranslational modifications such as disulfide bond formation and N- and O-linked glycosylation, are initiated. The proteins are transferred to the Golgi complex where they undergo further modification, followed by condensation and packaging into secretory granules (Fig. 11.14).

The secretory granules are stored in the apical cytoplasm until the cell receives an appropriate secretory stimulus. The granule membranes fuse with the cell membrane at the apical (luminal) surface, and the contents are released into the lumen by the process of exocytosis (Fig. 11.15). In salivary glands the sympathetic neurotransmitter norepinephrine usually is an effective stimulus of exocytosis. Norepinephrine binds to β-adrenergic receptors on the cell surface. Receptor activation, through guanosine triphosphate-binding proteins, stimulates adenylyl cyclase to produce cAMP. Increased cAMP levels activate protein kinase A, which phosphorylates other proteins in a cascade that eventually leads to granule exocytosis (Fig. 11.16). The fusion of the granule membrane with the cell membrane is mediated by the formation of a protein complex involving proteins of the granule membrane, proteins of the cell membrane, and proteins in the cytoplasm. After release of the granule content, the granule membrane is internalized by the cell as small vesicles, which may be recycled or degraded.

Fluid and Electrolytes

Release of water by the cells of the secretory end pieces is regulated principally by parasympathetic innervation. Binding of acetylcholine to muscarinic cholinergic receptors activates phospholipase C, resulting in the formation of inositol trisphosphate and the subsequent release of Ca^{2+} from intracellular stores. The increased Ca^{2+} concentration opens Cl^- channels in the apical cell membrane and K^+ channels in the basolateral membrane. The apical Cl^- efflux draws extracellular Na^+ into the lumen, probably through the tight junctions, to balance the electrochemical gradient. The osmotic gradient resulting from the increased luminal Na^+ and Cl^- concentration results in the movement of water into the lumen, probably through the cells via water channels (aquaporins) in the apical membrane and possibly through the tight junctions (see Fig. 11.16). A $Na^+/K^+/2Cl^-$ cotransporter and the

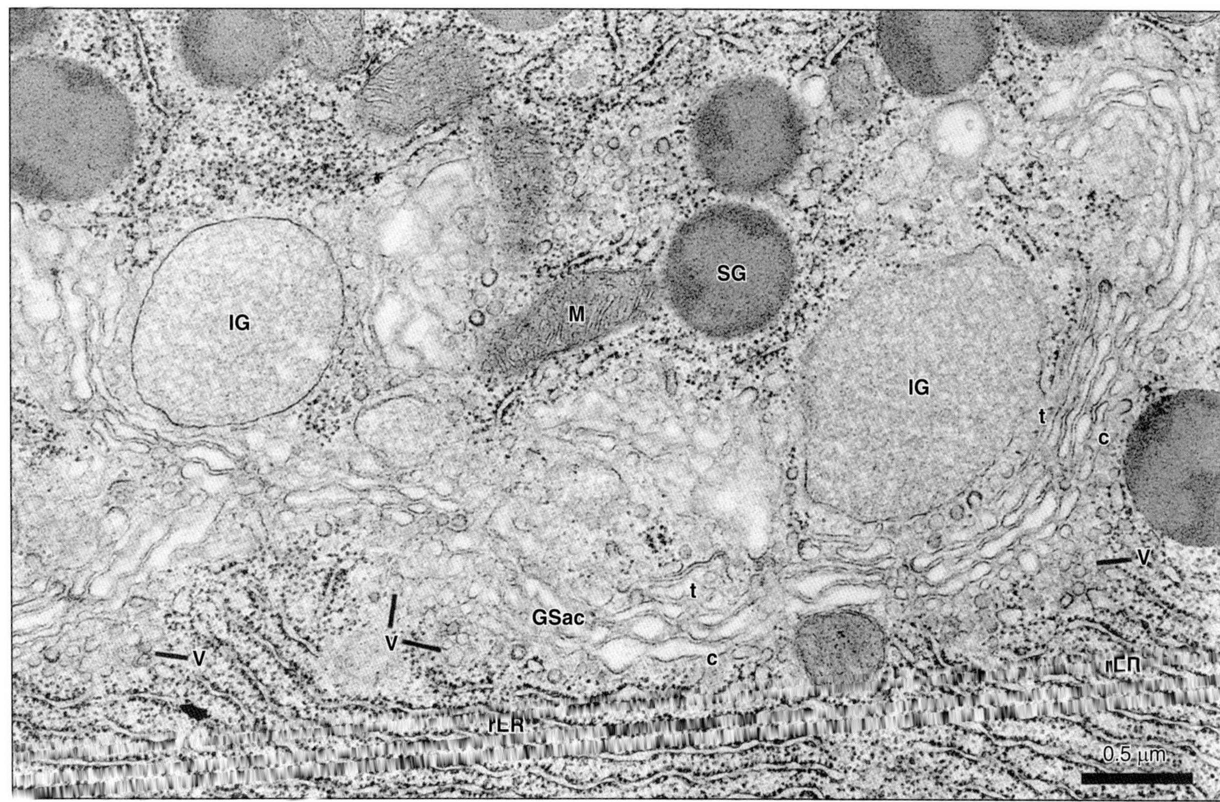

Fig. 11.8 Transmission electron micrograph of the Golgi complex of a serous cell of a rat parotid gland. The Golgi complex consists of several interconnected stacks of membranous saccules *(GSac)*. Small vesicles *(V)* are located between the rough endoplasmic reticulum *(rER)* and the cis face *(c)* of the Golgi complex, and immature granules *(IG)* of variable size and density are present at the *trans* face *(t)*. *M*, Mitochondrion; *SG*, mature secretory granules. (From Hand AR: Salivary glands. In Bhaskar SN, editor: *Orban's oral histology and embryology*, ed 11, St. Louis, MO, 1991, Mosby.)

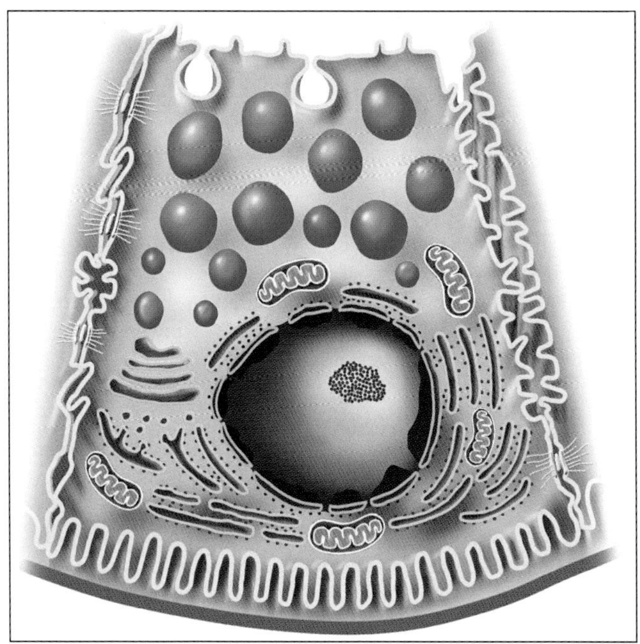

Fig. 11.9 Serous cell. Intercellular canaliculi are seen in longitudinal *(right)* and cross section *(left)*.

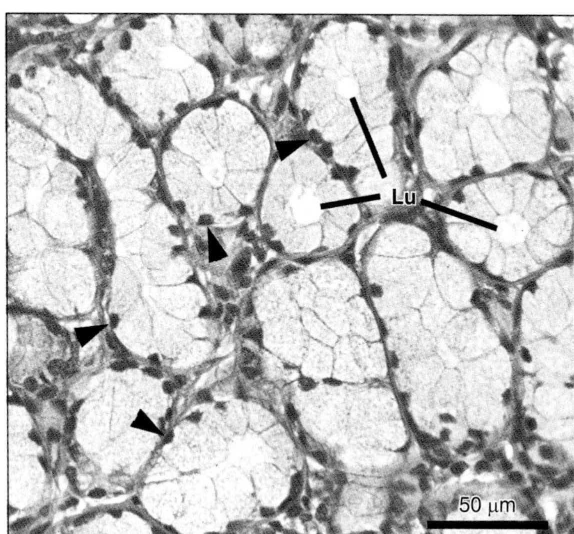

Fig. 11.10 Mucous cells in tubular secretory end pieces stained with hematoxylin and eosin. Poorly stained mucous secretory granules fill the cytoplasm, and the nuclei *(arrowheads)* are flattened and compressed against the basal surfaces of the cells. The lumina *(Lu)* are large compared with those of serous acini.

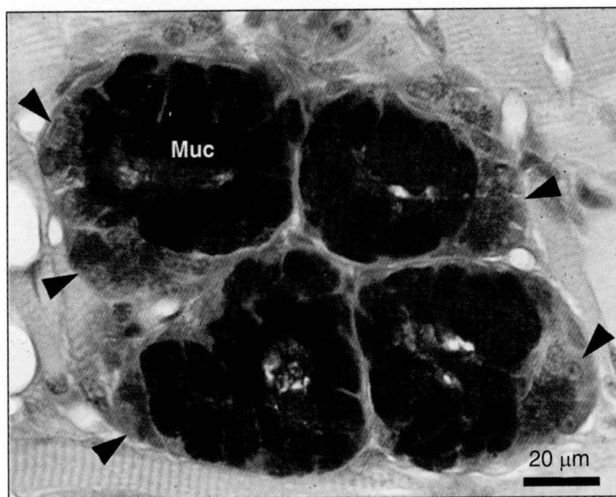

Fig. 11.11 Mucous end pieces with serous demilunes *(arrowheads)* in a minor salivary gland stained with periodic acid–Schiff, Alcian blue, and hematoxylin. The mucous secretory product *(Muc, dark purple)* stains strongly with periodic acid–Schiff and Alcian blue, whereas the glycoproteins of the serous demilune cells stain only with periodic acid–Schiff (magenta). (From Hand AR: Salivary glands. In Provenza DV, Seibel W, editors: *Oral histology, inheritance and development*, ed 2, Philadelphia, PA, 1986, Lea and Febiger.)

Na^+/K^+–adenosine triphosphatase in the basolateral membrane serve to maintain the intracellular ionic and osmotic balance during active secretion. Thus fluid secretion by the salivary glands is driven by the active transport of electrolytes.

Other receptors also are able to stimulate fluid secretion. Norepinephrine, acting via α-adrenergic receptors, and substance P activate the Ca^{2+}–phospholipid pathway just described. The cells also can secrete fluid using other electrolyte transport mechanisms. The apical Cl^- channel also is believed to transport HCO_3^- into the lumen. At high flow rates, salivary HCO_3^- concentrations increase significantly. A basolateral Na^+/H^+ exchanger serves to restore the intracellular pH after the acidification that occurs as a result of HCO_3^- secretion.

Other Mechanisms Modulating Saliva Secretion

The secretion of proteins and fluid and electrolytes by secretory end piece cells may be affected by other signaling molecules. Norepinephrine, acting via α-adrenergic receptors, and substance P, which binds to specific cell-surface receptors, activate the phospholipid-Ca^{2+} pathway described previously for muscarinic cholinergic stimulation, resulting in fluid and electrolyte secretion. Small amounts of protein are secreted in response to certain gastrointestinal hormones (e.g., gastrin and cholecystokinin) and other peptides released from autonomic nerve terminals, such as vasoactive intestinal polypeptide and neuropeptide Y. Substance P, vasoactive intestinal polypeptide, neuropeptide Y, and calcitonin gene–related peptide also exert effects on the glandular vasculature to regulate blood flow. Nitric oxide, produced by parasympathetic nerves, vascular endothelial cells, and glandular secretory cells, stimulates the production of cyclic guanosine monophosphate and the release of Ca^{2+} from intracellular storage sites in secretory cells. These mechanisms most likely act in concert with the β-adrenergic and muscarinic cholinergic signaling pathways to augment or modulate saliva secretion.

Extracellular adenosine triphosphate, which activates the P2X and P2Y purinergic receptors on secretory and duct cells, elevates intracellular Ca^{2+} levels. P2X receptors are nonselective cation channels that allow extracellular Ca^{2+} to enter the cell. P2Y receptors cause release of Ca^{2+} from intracellular storage sites via stimulation of phospholipase C and inositol trisphosphate formation. Purinergic receptors may serve to modulate saliva secretion induced by other signaling pathways; however, only in vitro studies of receptor function have been carried out, and the in vivo source of extracellular adenosine triphosphate is unknown. Thus the physiologic significance of purinergic receptor activation in salivary glands remains elusive.

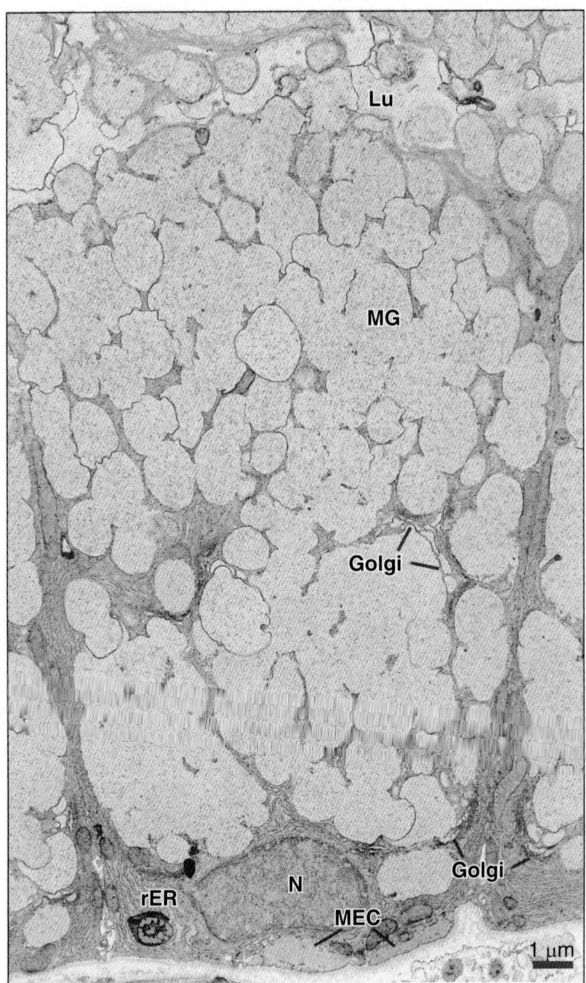

Fig. 11.12 Transmission electron micrograph of mucous cell of the mouse sublingual gland. The nucleus *(N)* and rough endoplasmic reticulum *(rER)* are located basally. The supranuclear cytoplasm is filled with pale mucous secretory granules *(MG)* that have a fine fibrillar content. Many granules have disrupted membranes and are fused with adjacent granules. The Golgi complex *(Golgi)* is large, and portions of it are located basally and centrally in the cell. Two myoepithelial cell processes *(MEC)* are present at the basal surface of the mucous cell. *Lu,* Lumen.

Myoepithelial Cells

Myoepithelial cells are contractile cells associated with the secretory end pieces and intercalated ducts of the salivary glands (Fig. 11.17). These cells are located between the basal lamina and the secretory or duct cells and are joined to the cells by desmosomes. Myoepithelial cells have many similarities to smooth muscle cells but are derived from epithelium. Myoepithelial cells present around the secretory end pieces have a stellate shape; numerous branching processes extend from the cell body to surround and embrace the end piece (Fig. 11.18). The processes are filled with filaments of actin and soluble myosin (Figs. 11.19 and 11.20). The cell membrane has numerous caveolae, which presumably function in initiating contraction. Most of the other cellular organelles are located in the perinuclear

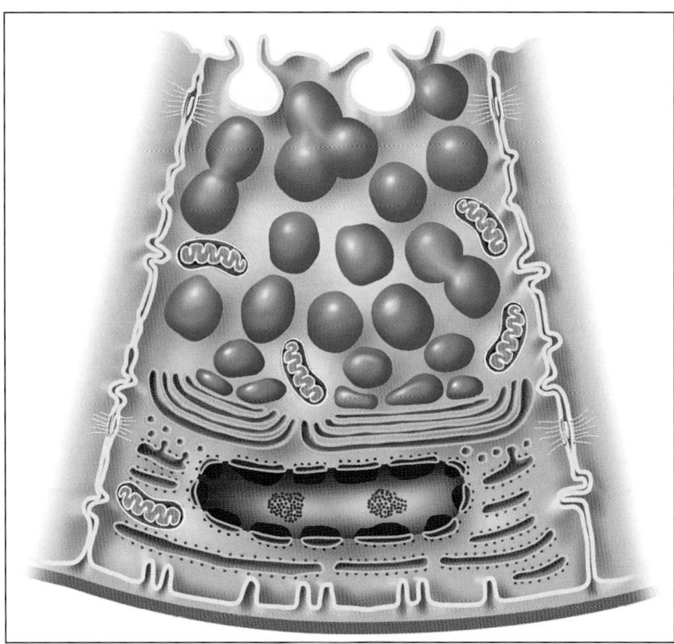

Fig. 11.13 Mucous cell

cytoplasm. Myoepithelial cells associated with the intercalated ducts have a more fusiform shape with fewer processes and tend to be oriented lengthwise along the duct.

Contraction of the myoepithelial cells is believed to provide support for the end pieces during active secretion of saliva. The cells also may help to expel the primary saliva from the end piece into the duct system. Contraction of the myoepithelial cells of the intercalated ducts may shorten and widen the ducts, helping to maintain their patency. Recent studies suggest that myoepithelial cells have additional functions that may be more important than their ability to contract. They provide signals to the acinar secretory cells that are necessary for maintaining cell polarity and the structural organization of the secretory end piece. The evidence also suggests that myoepithelial cells produce a number of proteins that have tumor suppressor activity, such as proteinase inhibitors (e.g., tissue inhibitor of metalloproteinases) and antiangiogenesis factors, and that these cells may provide a barrier against invasive epithelial neoplasms.

Ducts

The ductal system of salivary glands is a varied network of tubules that progressively increase in diameter, beginning at the secretory end pieces and extending to the oral cavity (see Fig. 11.7). The three classes of ducts are intercalated, striated, and excretory, each with differing structure and function. The ductal system is more than just a simple conduit for the passage of saliva; it actively participates in the production and modification of saliva.

Intercalated Ducts

The primary saliva produced by the secretory end pieces passes first through the intercalated ducts (Fig. 11.21). The first cells of the intercalated duct are directly adjacent to the secretory cells of the end piece, and the lumen of the end piece is continuous with the lumen of the intercalated duct. The intercalated ducts are lined by a simple cuboidal epithelium, and myoepithelial cell bodies and their processes typically are located along the basal surface of the duct. The overall diameter of the intercalated ducts is smaller than that of the end pieces, and their lumina are larger than those of the end pieces. Several ducts draining individual end pieces join to form larger intercalated ducts, and these may join again before emptying into the striated ducts. The length of the intercalated ducts in the different major and minor salivary glands varies.

The intercalated duct cells have centrally placed nuclei and a small amount of cytoplasm containing some rough endoplasmic reticulum and a small Golgi complex (Figs. 11.22 and 11.23). A few small secretory granules may be found in the apical cytoplasm, especially in cells located near the end pieces. The apical cell surface has a few short microvilli projecting into the lumen; the lateral surfaces are joined by apical junctional complexes and scattered desmosomes and gap junctions and have folded processes that interdigitate with similar processes of adjacent cells. Because of their small size and lack of distinctive features, intercalated ducts often are difficult to identify in routine histologic sections.

The intercalated ducts contribute macromolecular components, which are stored in their secretory granules, to the saliva. These components include lysozyme and lactoferrin; other currently unknown components probably also are secreted by these cells. A portion of the fluid component of the primary saliva likely is added in the intercalated duct region. Undifferentiated cells, thought to represent salivary gland stem cells, are believed to be present in the intercalated ducts. These cells may proliferate and undergo differentiation to replace damaged or dying cells in the end pieces and striated ducts.

Striated Ducts

The striated ducts, which receive the primary saliva from the intercalated ducts, constitute the largest portion of the duct system. These ducts are the main ductal component located within the lobules of the gland (i.e., intralobular) (Fig. 11.24). Striated duct cells are columnar, with a centrally placed nucleus and pale, acidophilic cytoplasm (Fig. 11.25). In well-preserved tissue, faint radially oriented lines or striations may be observed in the basal cytoplasm of the ducts. The overall diameter of the duct is greater than that of the secretory end pieces, and the lumen is larger than those of the secretory end pieces and intercalated ducts. A basal lamina encloses the striated duct, and a capillary plexus is present in the surrounding connective tissue.

The structure of the duct cells reflects an important function of these cells, which is the modification of the primary saliva by reabsorption

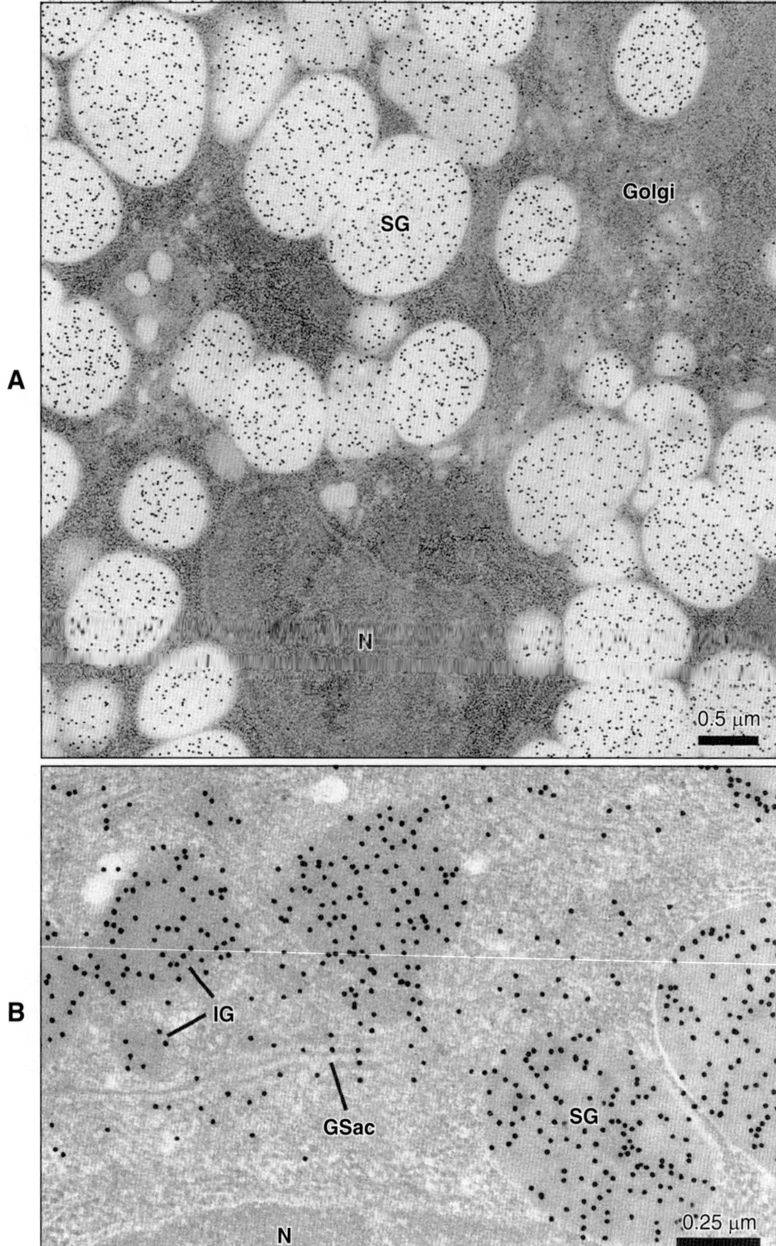

Fig. 11.14 Immunogold labeling of secretory proteins in salivary gland cells. (A) Parotid secretory protein in a serous cell of a rat parotid gland. The section was incubated with an antibody to parotid secretory protein and then with gold particles coupled to staphylococcal protein A to localize the bound antibody. Gold particles are present over the secretory granules *(SG)* and the Golgi complex *(Golgi)*, indicating the presence of parotid secretory protein in these organelles. (B) Submandibular gland secretory protein B (SMGB) in a serous demilune cell of a rat sublingual gland. The section was incubated with an antibody to the secretory protein, protein SMGB, and then was treated as in (A). Gold particles are present over the Golgi saccules *(GSac)* and immature *(IG)* and mature secretory granules *(SG)*. *N*, Nucleus.

and secretion of electrolytes. The basal striations of the duct cells, when observed by electron microscopy, result from the presence of numerous elongated mitochondria in narrow cytoplasmic partitions, separated by highly infolded and interdigitated basolateral cell membranes (Fig. 11.26). The apical cytoplasm may contain small secretory granules and electron-lucent vesicles. The granules contain kallikrein and perhaps other secretory proteins; the presence of vesicles suggests that the cells may participate in endocytosis of substances from the lumen. The duct cells also contain numerous lysosomes and peroxisomes, and deposits of glycogen commonly are present in the perinuclear cytoplasm. Adjacent cells are joined by well-developed tight junctions and junctional complexes but lack gap junctions. The structure of the striated duct cells is summarized in Fig. 11.27.

Excretory Ducts

The excretory ducts are located in the connective tissue septa between the lobules of the gland (i.e., in an extralobular or interlobular location). These ducts are larger in diameter than striated ducts and typically

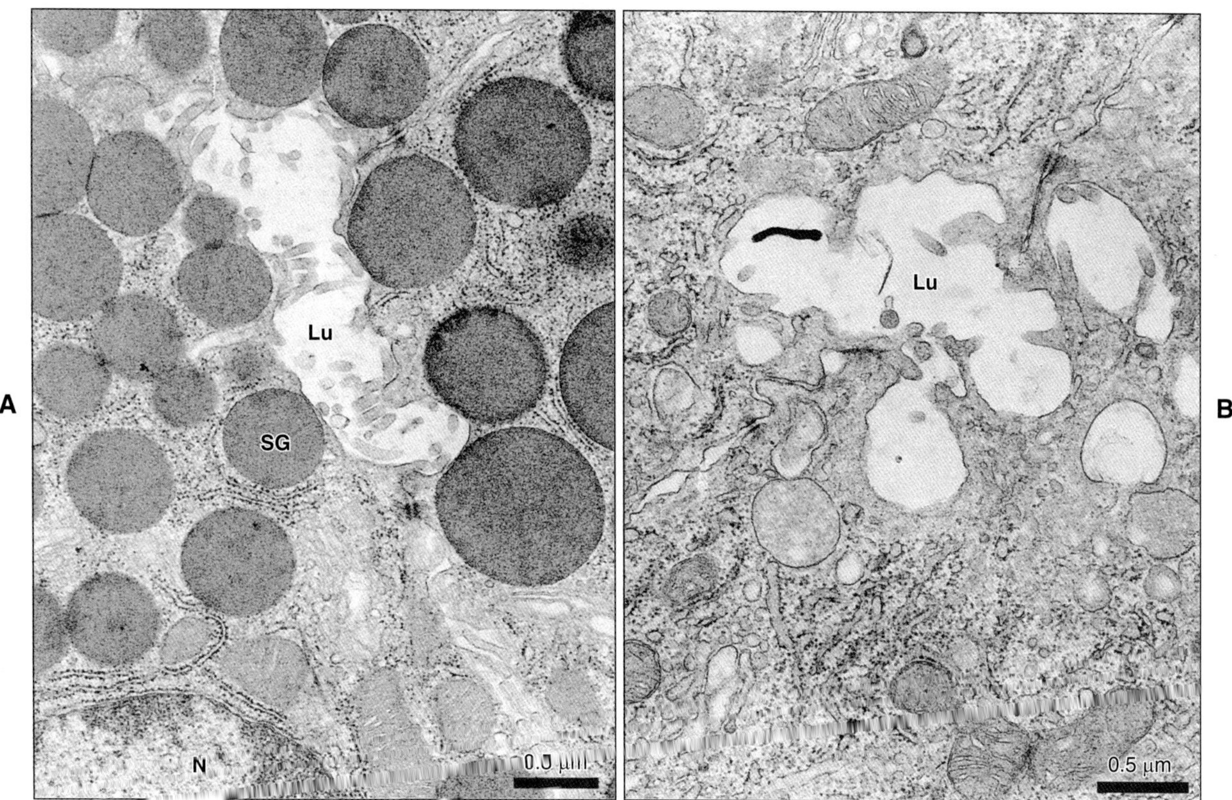

Fig. 11.15 Transmission electron micrographs of serous cells of the rat parotid gland demonstrating exocytosis of secretory granules *(SG)*. (A) The apical cytoplasm of resting (unstimulated) cells is filled with SG. (B) After administration of isoproterenol, a β-adrenergic drug, the cells are devoid of SG, and the lumen *(Lu)* is enlarged because of the fusion of granule membranes during exocytosis. *N,* Nucleus. (From Hand AR: Salivary glands. In Provenza DV, Seibel W, editors: *Oral histology: inheritance and development,* ed 2, Philadelphia, PA, 1986, Lea and Febiger.)

have a pseudostratified epithelium with columnar cells extending from the basal lamina to the ductal lumen and small basal cells that sit on the basal lamina but do not reach the lumen (Fig. 11.28A). As the smaller ducts join to form larger excretory ducts, the number of basal cells increases, and scattered mucous (goblet) cells may be present (see Fig. 11.28B). The epithelium of the main excretory duct may become stratified near the oral opening.

In the smaller excretory ducts the structure of the columnar cells is similar to that of the striated duct cells. As the ducts increase in size, the number of mitochondria and the extent of infolding of the basolateral membranes decrease. The basal cells have numerous bundles of intermediate filaments (tonofilaments) and are attached to the basal lamina by prominent hemidesmosomes. In some instances, basal cells may contain abundant actin filaments and have elongated processes similar to myoepithelial cells. Studies in experimental animals suggest that the columnar cells and the basal cells have a high rate of proliferation.

Small numbers of other types of cells are present in the excretory ducts and to some extent in the striated ducts. Tuft (caveolated or brush) cells, with long stiff microvilli and apical vesicles, are believed to be receptor cells of some type. Nerve endings occasionally are found adjacent to the basal portions of these cells. Other cells with pale cytoplasm and dense nuclear chromatin may be found toward the base of the duct epithelium. Some of these cells appear to be lymphocytes and macrophages. In other cases the cells have long branching processes that extend between the epithelial cells. These cells presumably are dendritic cells, or antigen-presenting cells, which are involved in immune surveillance and the processing and presentation of foreign antigens to T lymphocytes.

Ductal Modification of Saliva

In addition to conveying saliva from the secretory end pieces to the oral cavity, an important function of the striated and excretory ducts is the modification of the primary saliva produced by the end pieces and intercalated ducts occurring principally through reabsorption and secretion of electrolytes. The luminal and basolateral membranes have abundant transporters (Fig. 11.29) that function to produce a net reabsorption of Na^+ and Cl^-, resulting in the formation of hypotonic final saliva. The ducts also secrete K^+ and HCO_3^-, but little if any secretion or reabsorption of water occurs in the striated and excretory ducts. The final electrolyte composition of saliva varies, depending on the salivary flow rate. At high flow rates, saliva is in contact with the ductal epithelium for a shorter time, and Na^+ and Cl^- concentrations rise and K^+ concentration decreases. At low flow rates the electrolyte concentrations change in the opposite direction. The HCO_3^- concentration, however, increases with increasing flow rates, reflecting the increased secretion of HCO_3^- by the acinar cells to drive fluid secretion.

Electrolyte reabsorption and secretion by the striated and excretory ducts is regulated by the autonomic nervous system and by mineralocorticoids produced by the adrenal cortex. The sympathetic innervation has a more important role in regulating electrolyte transport in the ducts than in the acini because of a larger number of cAMP-regulated Cl^- channels (the cystic fibrosis transmembrane conductance regulator) in the luminal cell membrane.

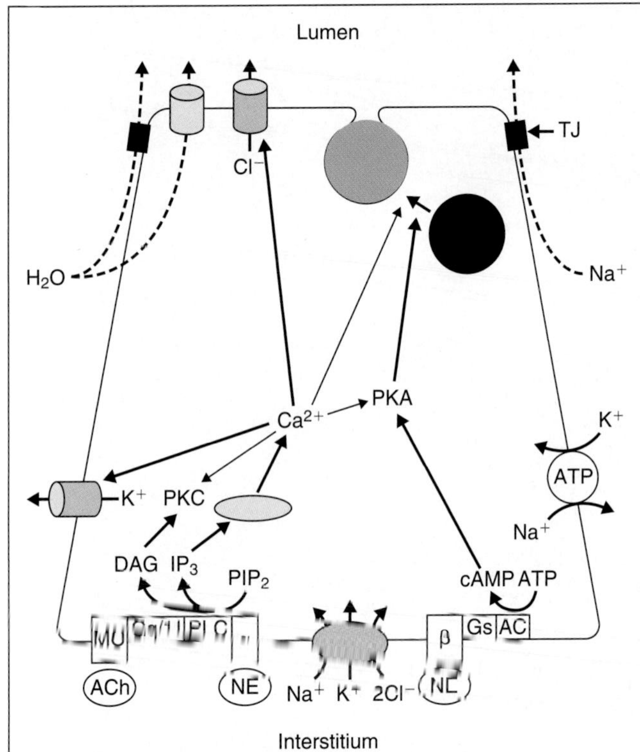

Fig. 11.16 Mechanisms of salivary secretion. Protein secretion occurs by exocytosis (i.e., the fusion of secretory granules with the luminal membrane to release their contents into the lumen). The binding of the sympathetic transmitter norepinephrine *(NE)* to β-adrenergic *(β)* receptors on the basolateral membrane activates a heterotrimeric G protein *(Gs)*, which, in turn, activates adenylyl cyclase *(AC)*, catalyzing the formation of cyclic adenosine monophosphate *(cAMP)* from adenosine triphosphate *(ATP)*. cAMP activates protein kinase A *(PKA)*, which phosphorylates other proteins in a cascade leading to exocytosis. Fluid and electrolyte secretion is stimulated mainly by the binding of the parasympathetic transmitter, acetylcholine *(ACh)* to muscarinic cholinergic *(MC)* receptors and by norepinephrine binding to α-adrenergic receptors *(α)*. These receptors activate a heterotrimeric G protein *(Gq/11)*, causing activation of phospholipase C *(PLC)*, which converts phosphatidylinositol bisphosphate *(PIP_2)* to inositol trisphosphate *(IP_3)* and diacylglycerol *(DAG)*. Inositol trisphosphate causes the release of Ca^{2+} from intracellular stores, probably the endoplasmic reticulum. The increased Ca^{2+} concentration opens Cl^- channels in the luminal membrane and K^+ channels in the basolateral membrane and activates the basolateral $Na^+/K^+/2Cl^-$ cotransporter. The increased luminal Cl^- is balanced by the movement of extracellular Na^{++} across the tight junctions *(TJ)*, and the resulting osmotic gradient pulls water into the lumen through the cell via the water channel aquaporin 5 and through the tight junction. The basolateral $Na^+/K^+/2Cl^-$ cotransporter and the Na^+/K^+–adenosine triphosphatase serve to maintain the intracellular electrolyte and osmotic balances. Calcium also stimulates exocytosis but to a lesser extent than cyclic adenosine monophosphate, and it modulates the activity of protein kinase A and protein kinase C *(PKC)*. Protein kinase C, in turn, modulates exocytosis and intracellular Ca^{2+} concentrations.

Connective Tissue

The connective tissue of the salivary glands includes a surrounding capsule, variably developed, that demarcates the gland from adjacent structures. Septa that extend inward from the capsule divide the gland into lobes and lobules and carry the blood vessels and nerves that supply the parenchymal components and the excretory ducts that convey saliva to the oral cavity (see Figs. 1.8 and 11.24). As in other locations, the cells of the connective tissue include fibroblasts, macrophages, dendritic cells, mast cells, plasma cells, adipose cells, and occasionally granulocytes and lymphocytes. Collagen and elastic fibers along with the glycoproteins and proteoglycans of the ground substance constitute the extracellular matrix of the connective tissue.

Within the lobules of the gland, finer partitions of connective tissue extend between adjacent secretory end pieces and ducts. These partitions carry the arterioles, capillaries, and venules of the microcirculation and the finer branches of the autonomic nerves that innervate the secretory and ductal cells. The same cellular and extracellular connective tissue components are present in these locations.

Plasma cells located adjacent to the secretory end pieces and intralobular ducts produce immunoglobulins that are translocated into the saliva by transcytosis. The main immunoglobulin present in saliva is secretory IgA, which is synthesized as a dimer complexed with an additional protein called J chain. The salivary gland epithelial cells have receptors for dimeric IgA on their basolateral membranes. The epithelial cells take up the receptor-bound IgA by endocytosis, and the vesicles containing the IgA move from the basolateral cytoplasm to the apical cytoplasm. The bound IgA, along with a portion of the receptor called secretory component, is released at the luminal surface of the cell. Small amounts of IgG and IgM also are secreted into the saliva.

Nerve Supply

The salivary glands are innervated by postganglionic nerve fibers of the sympathetic and parasympathetic divisions of the autonomic nervous system. Depending on the gland, preganglionic parasympathetic fibers originate in the superior or inferior salivatory nuclei in the brainstem and travel via the seventh (facial) and ninth (glossopharyngeal) cranial nerves to the submandibular and otic ganglia, where they synapse with postganglionic neurons that send their axons to the glands through the lingual and auriculotemporal nerves. Preganglionic sympathetic nerves originate in the thoracic spinal cord, synapse with postganglionic neurons in the superior cervical ganglion, and reach the glands traveling with the arterial blood supply. During development, the ability of sympathetic axons to reach their targets, and the survival of the postganglionic neurons, critically depend on neurotrophic factors synthesized by the cells of the developing glands.

Within the gland lobules, branches of the nerves follow the blood vessels, eventually forming a plexus of unmyelinated fibers adjacent to arterioles, ducts, and secretory end pieces (Fig. 11.30). The axons of each nerve bundle are invested by cytoplasmic processes of Schwann cells. Two different morphologic relationships between the nerves and the epithelial cells exist. In some cases, an axon leaves the nerve bundle, loses its Schwann cell investment, penetrates the epithelial basal lamina, and forms an expanded swelling (varicosity) in close contact (10–20 nm) with the basolateral membrane of the epithelial cell. In the most common relationship, the axon forms a varicosity but remains associated with the nerve bundle, and the Schwann cell covering is absent over the varicosity. In this type of innervation, the axonal varicosity is separated from the epithelial cells by 100 to 200 nm and the basal laminae surrounding the nerve bundle and the epithelial cell. The type of nerve–epithelial cell relationship (intraparenchymal and extraparenchymal, respectively) varies among the glands and among the different cells within a single gland. For example, intraparenchymal innervation occurs in the human submandibular gland and in the minor glands of the lip, whereas only extraparenchymal innervation occurs in the human parotid gland. Despite the different morphologic relationships, no functional differences between the two patterns of innervation are apparent.

Several varicosities may be present along the length of an axon, and a single nerve may innervate more than one epithelial cell. The

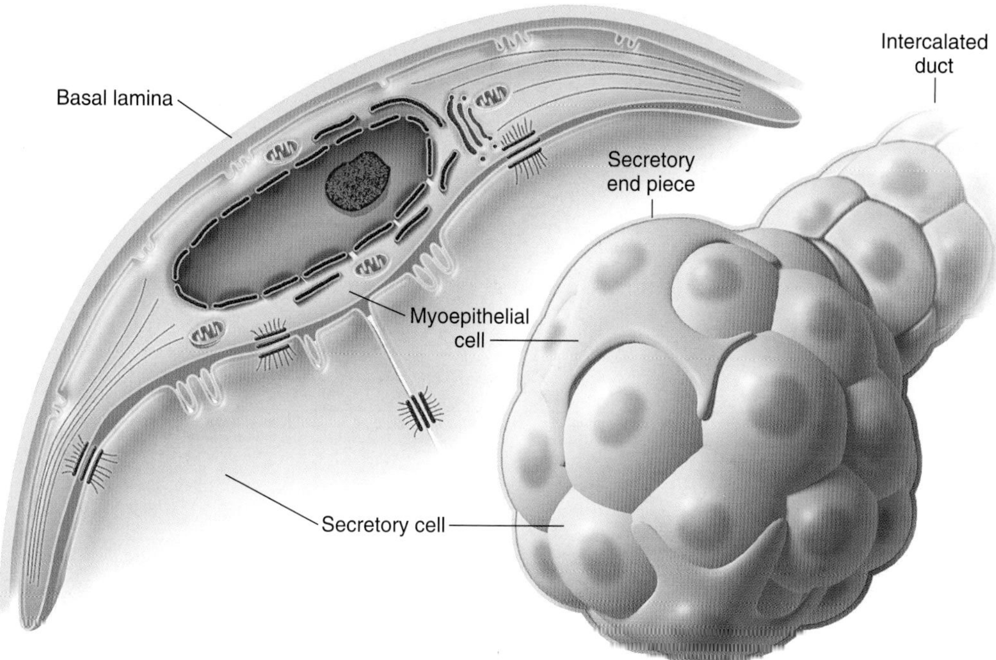

Fig. 11.17 Myoepithelial cells in section *(left)* and surface *(right)* views.

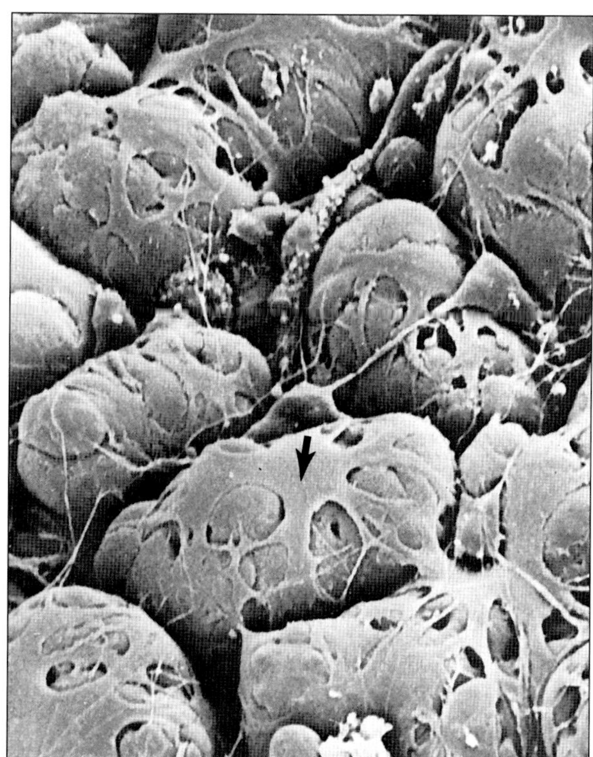

Fig. 11.18 Scanning electron micrograph of myoepithelial cells. The basal lamina has been digested away, revealing the basal surfaces of the acinar cells covered by myoepithelial cells *(arrow)* and their branching processes. (From Nagato T, et al.: A scanning electron microscope study of myoepithelial cells in exocrine glands, *Cell Tissue Res* 209:1–10, 1980.)

axonal varicosities contain small neurotransmitter vesicles; occasional larger, dense-cored vesicles; and mitochondria. These varicosities are believed to be the site of innervation of the gland cells and thus the site of neurotransmitter release. However, no specializations of the axonal or epithelial cell membranes occur at these sites as occur at synapses in the central nervous system. The main parasympathetic neurotransmitter is acetylcholine; the main sympathetic neurotransmitter is norepinephrine. Release of these transmitters and their interaction with cell-surface receptors initiate the response of the cells (i.e., fluid and electrolyte secretion, exocytosis, modulation of ductal transport processes, or contraction of myoepithelial cells or arteriolar smooth muscle cells).

Blood Supply

Rapid and sustained secretion of saliva, which is 99% water, necessitates an extensive blood supply to the salivary glands. One or more arteries enter the gland and give rise to smaller arteries and arterioles that tend to follow the path of the excretory ducts. The arterioles break up into capillaries that are distributed around the secretory end pieces and striated ducts. In some species the capillaries supplying the secretory end pieces and ducts arise from separate arterioles (i.e., a parallel arrangement), whereas in other species a venous portal system connects the capillary network around the end pieces with that around the ducts. An extensive capillary plexus, also arising from separate arterioles, exists around the excretory ducts. The endothelium of the capillaries and postcapillary venules is fenestrated.

The venous return, except as noted previously, generally follows the arterial supply. However, arteriovenous anastomoses occur in some glands. As blood flow increases during secretion (as much as fifteenfold during maximum secretion), more blood is diverted through these anastomoses, resulting in increased venous and capillary pressures. The resulting increase in fluid filtration across the capillary endothelium provides the fluid necessary to maintain secretion.

A

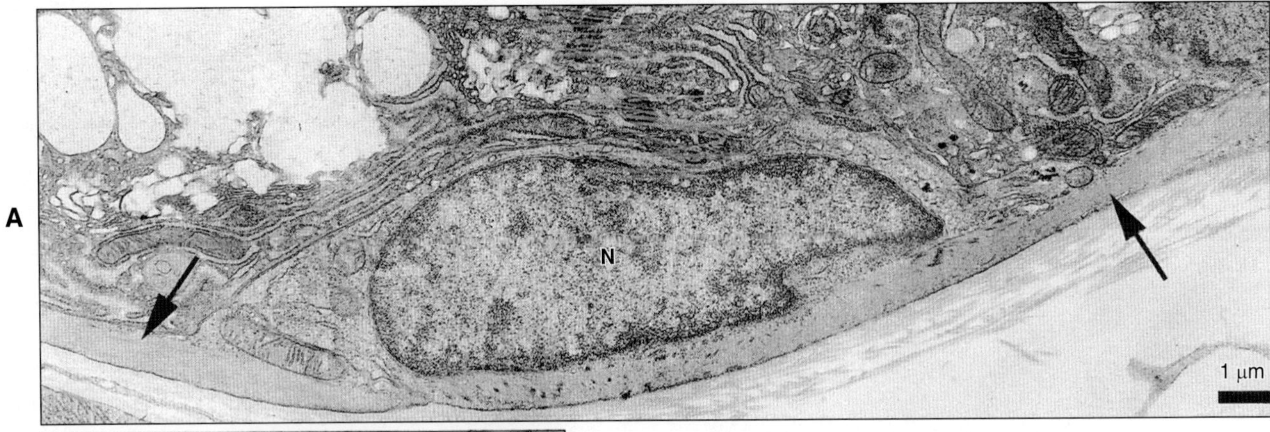

B

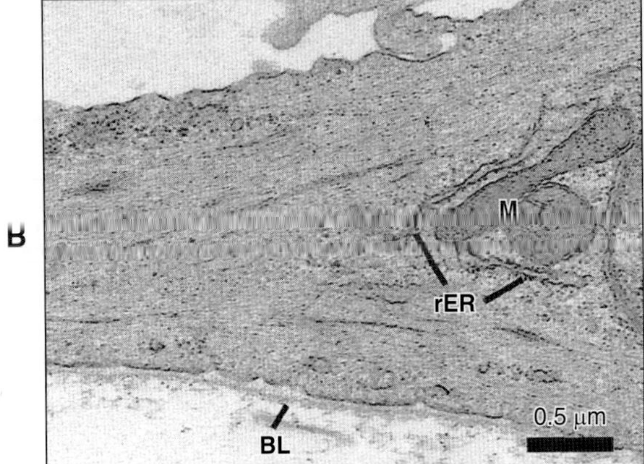

Fig. 11.19 (A) Transmission electron micrograph of a myoepithelial cell at the base of a mucous secretory cell of a rat sublingual gland. Processes of the cell *(arrows)* extend from both sides of the cell body. (B) The myoepithelial cell processes are filled with actin filaments. A few mitochondria *(M)* and short cisternae of rough endoplasmic reticulum *(rER)* are located in the perinuclear cytoplasm. The myoepithelial cell is located on the epithelial side of the basal lamina *(BL)*. *N,* Nucleus. (A, From Hand AR: Salivary glands. In Bhaskar SN, editor: *Orban's oral histology and embryology,* ed 11, St. Louis, MO, 1991, Mosby.)

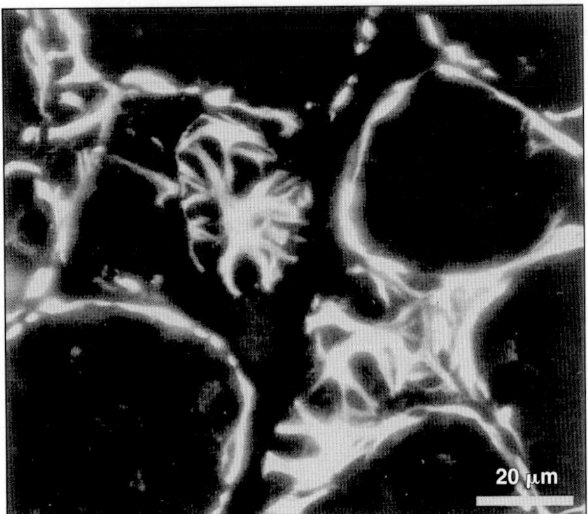

Fig. 11.20 Immunofluorescence of myosin in myoepithelial cells of the rat sublingual gland. The section was treated with an antibody to smooth muscle myosin, followed by a fluorescent-labeled secondary antibody. Tangential sections of acini reveal the branching nature of the myoepithelial cells. Myoepithelial cell processes cut in cross and longitudinal section surround adjacent acini. (Courtesy D. Drenckhahn, Würzburg, Germany. From Hand AR: Salivary glands. In Bhaskar SN, editor: *Orban's oral histology and embryology,* ed 11, St. Louis, MO, 1991, Mosby.)

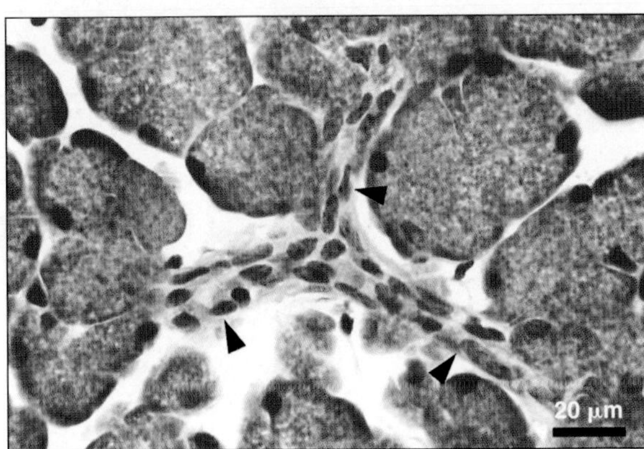

Fig. 11.21 Light micrograph of branching intercalated duct *(arrowheads)* joining several serous end pieces in the human submandibular gland. The duct cells are low cuboidal, and their cytoplasm stains lightly with eosin. The surrounding serous end piece cells stain with hematoxylin.

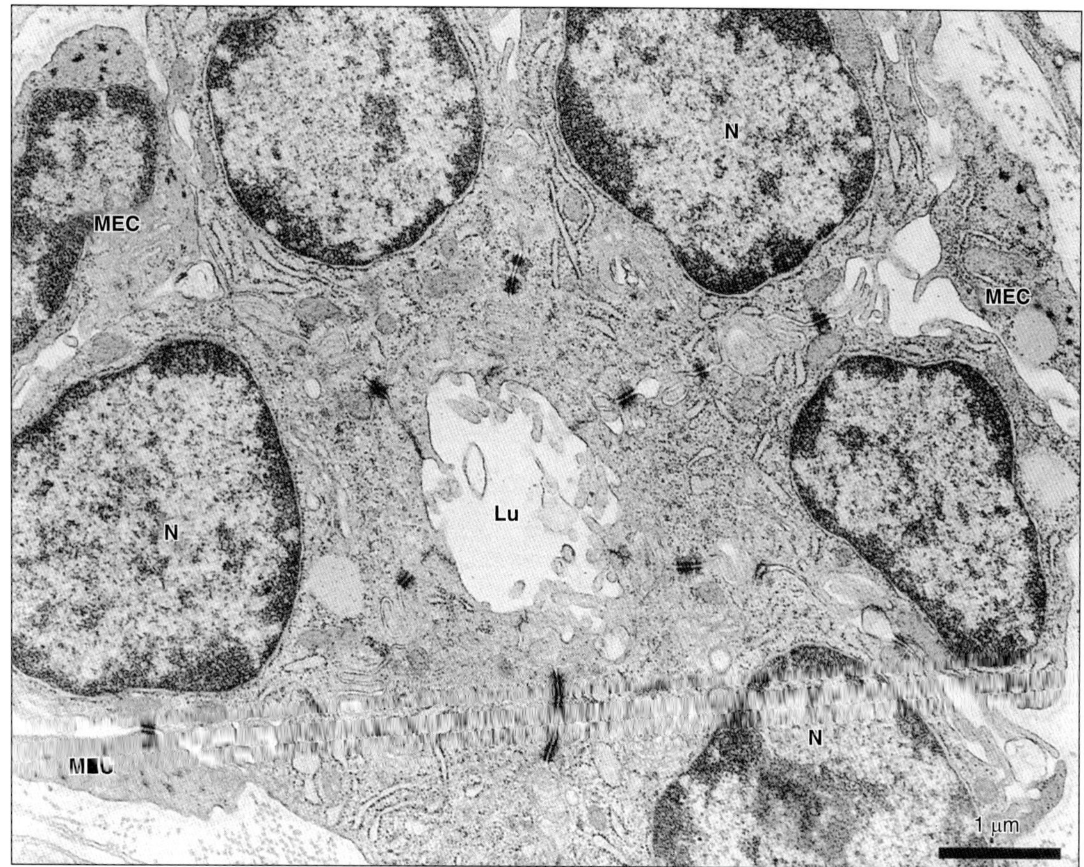

Fig. 11.22 Transmission electron micrograph of an intercalated duct of a rat parotid gland. The cuboidal cells have a few endoplasmic reticulum cisternae and a small Golgi complex and are joined by junctional complexes and numerous desmosomes. Myoepithelial cell processes *(MEC)* are present at the basal side of the duct cells. *Lu,* Lumen; *N,* nucleus. (From Hand AR: Salivary glands. In Bhaskar SN, editor: *Orban's oral histology and embryology,* ed 11, St. Louis, MO, 1991, Mosby.)

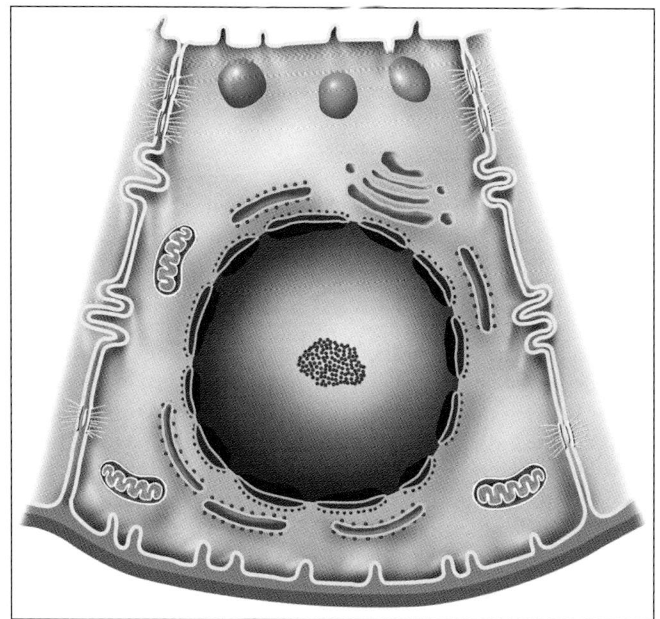

Fig. 11.23 Intercalated duct cell.

Summary of Salivary Gland Structure

Salivary glands consist of secretory end pieces that are composed of serous cells or mucous cells, or mucous end pieces capped by serous demilunes, and a system of ducts (intercalated, striated, and excretory) that modify the saliva produced by the end pieces and convey it to the oral cavity (Fig. 11.31). Contractile myoepithelial cells are distributed around the end pieces and intercalated ducts. The gland is supported by connective tissue, which carries the nerve, vascular, and lymphatic supplies to the parenchymal components and is the location of cells of the innate and adaptive immune systems.

HISTOLOGY OF THE MAJOR SALIVARY GLANDS

Parotid Gland

In the parotid gland the spheric secretory end pieces are all serous (Fig. 11.32). The pyramidally shaped acinar cells have a spheric, basally situated nucleus and surround a small, central lumen. The basal cytoplasm stains with basophilic dyes, and the secretory granules in the apical cytoplasm usually stain with acidophilic dyes. Fat cell spaces often are seen in sections of the parotid gland.

Intercalated ducts are numerous and long in the parotid gland. The ducts are lined with cuboidal epithelial cells and have lumina that are

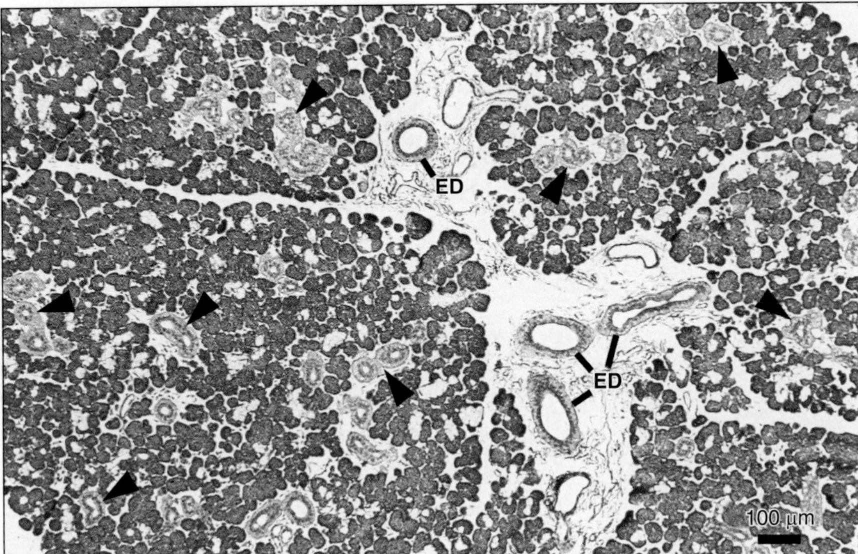

Fig. 11.24 Light micrograph of human submandibular gland stained with hematoxylin and eosin. Striated ducts *(arrowheads)* stain lightly with eosin and are readily identifiable at low power. The serous acini stain with hematoxylin. Larger excretory ducts *(ED)* are present in the interlobular connective tissue.

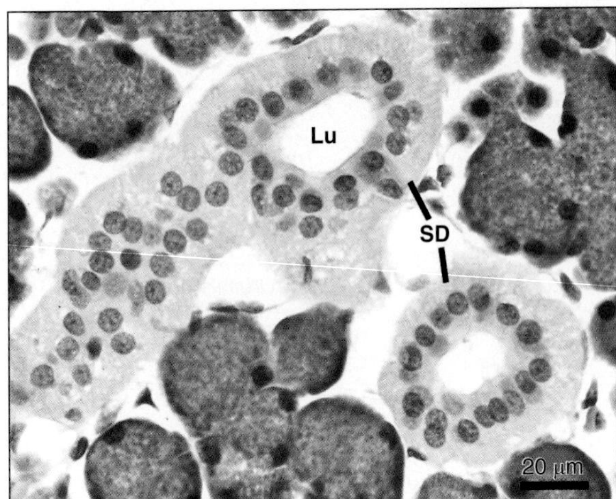

Fig. 11.25 Light micrograph of striated ducts *(SD)* in the human submandibular gland. The ducts have large lumina *(Lu)* and are lined by pale-staining, simple columnar epithelial cells with centrally placed nuclei and faint basal striations. The duct cell cytoplasm stains lightly with eosin.

larger than those of the acini. Nuclei of myoepithelial cells sometimes may be present at the basal surface of the ducts. The striated ducts are numerous and appear as slightly acidophilic, round, or elongated tubules of larger diameter than the end pieces. The ducts consist of a simple columnar epithelium, with round, centrally placed nuclei. Faint striations, representing the infolded basal cell membranes and mitochondria, may be visible below the nucleus. The lumina are large relative to the overall size of the ducts.

Submandibular Gland

The submandibular gland contains serous end pieces and mucous tubules capped with serous demilunes (Fig. 11.33); thus it is a mixed gland. Although the proportions of serous and mucous secretory end pieces may vary from lobule to lobule and among individual glands, serous cells significantly outnumber the mucous cells. The serous end pieces are similar in structure to those found in the parotid gland, with abundant secretory granules, a spherical nucleus, and basophilic cytoplasm. The mucous secretory cells are filled with pale-staining secretory material, and little cytoplasm is usually visible. The nucleus is compressed against the basal cell membrane and contains densely stained chromatin. The lumina of the mucous tubules are larger than those of serous end pieces. Serous demilune cells are similar in structure to the serous end piece cells, but they discharge their secretions into small intercellular canaliculi that extend between the mucous cells to reach the tubule lumen. The intercalated and striated ducts are less numerous than those in the parotid gland, but otherwise they are structurally similar.

Sublingual Gland

The sublingual gland also is a mixed gland, but mucous secretory cells predominate (Fig. 11.34). The mucous tubules and serous demilunes resemble those of the submandibular gland. Although serous end pieces may be present, they are rare, and most structures appearing as serous end pieces probably represent sections through demilunes that do not include the mucous tubule. The intercalated ducts are short and difficult to recognize. Intralobular ducts are fewer in number than in the parotid or submandibular glands, and some ducts may lack the infolded basolateral membranes characteristic of striated ducts.

HISTOLOGY OF THE MINOR SALIVARY GLANDS

Minor salivary glands consist of aggregates of secretory end pieces and ducts, organized into small lobulelike structures located in the submucosa or between muscle fibers of the tongue (Fig. 11.35; see also Fig. 11.1). The ducts draining individual glandular aggregates usually open directly onto the mucosal surface. The secretory end pieces of most minor glands are mucous or have a small serous component arranged as occasional demilunes. Intercalated ducts often are poorly developed, and the larger ducts may lack the typical infolded basolateral membranes of the striated ducts of the major glands. In contrast to the usual situation in the minor glands, the lingual serous glands (of Ebner) in the tongue below the circumvallate papillae are pure serous glands.

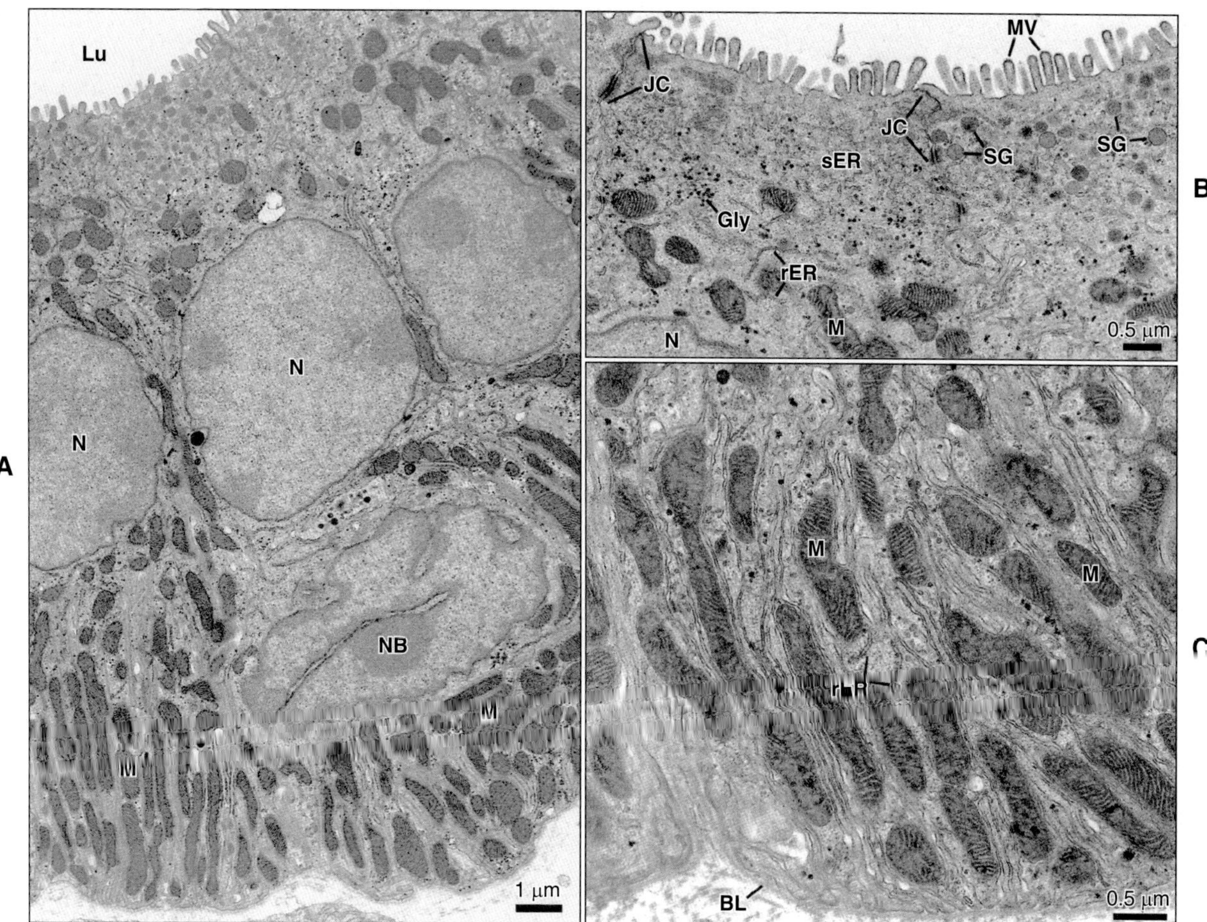

Fig. 11.26 Transmission electron micrographs of striated duct cells of the mouse parotid gland. (A) The columnar duct cells have centrally placed nuclei *(N)*, abundant mitochondria *(M)* between infolded basal membranes, and short microvilli on their apical surface. The basally located nucleus *(NB)* may belong to a dendritic (antigen-presenting) cell. (B) The apical cytoplasm contains irregular cisternae of smooth *(sER)* and rough *(rER)* endoplasmic reticulum, mitochondria near the nucleus, and scattered dense glycogen particles *(Gly)*. Some cells have an accumulation of small secretory granules *(SG)* near the apical membrane. Adjacent cells are held together by junctional complexes *(JC)*. (C) The basal region consists of partitions of cytoplasm containing mitochondria, a few endoplasmic reticulum cisternae, and glycogen particles separated from other cytoplasmic partitions by extensively infolded cell membranes. The narrow cytoplasmic processes extend laterally beyond the cell boundaries to interdigitate with similar processes from the adjacent cells. *BL,* Basal lamina; *Lu,* lumen; *MV,* microvilli. (A, From Park K, et al.: Defective fluid secretion and NaCl absorption in the parotid glands of Na+/H+ exchanger-deficient mice, *J Biol Chem* 276:27042–27050, 2001.)

Their secretions are released in regions with significant numbers of taste buds, specifically the troughs surrounding the vallate papillae and the clefts between the rudimentary foliate papillae on the sides of the tongue. They secrete digestive enzymes and proteins believed to play a role in the taste process. The fluid component of their secretions is presumed to cleanse the trough and prepare the taste receptors for a new stimulus.

Minor gland saliva typically is rich in mucins, various antibacterial proteins, and secretory immunoglobulins. The minor glands exhibit a continuous, slow secretory activity; thus they have an important role in protecting and moistening the oral mucosa, especially at night when the major salivary glands are mostly inactive.

CLINICAL CONSIDERATIONS

Age Changes

With age, a generalized loss of salivary gland parenchymal tissue occurs. A gradual reduction of up to 30% to 60% in the proportional acinar volume of the major salivary glands has been observed. The lost salivary cells often are replaced by adipose tissue. An increase in fibrous connective tissue and vascular elements also occurs. Changes of the duct system, including an increase in nonstriated intralobular ducts, dilatation of extralobular ducts, and degenerative and metaplastic changes, have been reported. Although decreased production of saliva often is observed in older persons, whether this is related directly to the reduction in parenchymal tissue is not clear. Some studies of healthy older individuals, in which the use of medications was controlled carefully, revealed little or no loss of salivary function, suggesting a large functional reserve capacity. Other studies suggest that although resting (unstimulated) salivary secretion is in the normal range, the volume of saliva produced during stimulated secretion is less than normal.

Diseases

Salivary glands may be influenced by a number of diseases, local and systemic. Several viruses (cytomegalovirus, Epstein-Barr virus, human herpesviruses 6 and 7) infect and replicate within salivary gland cells

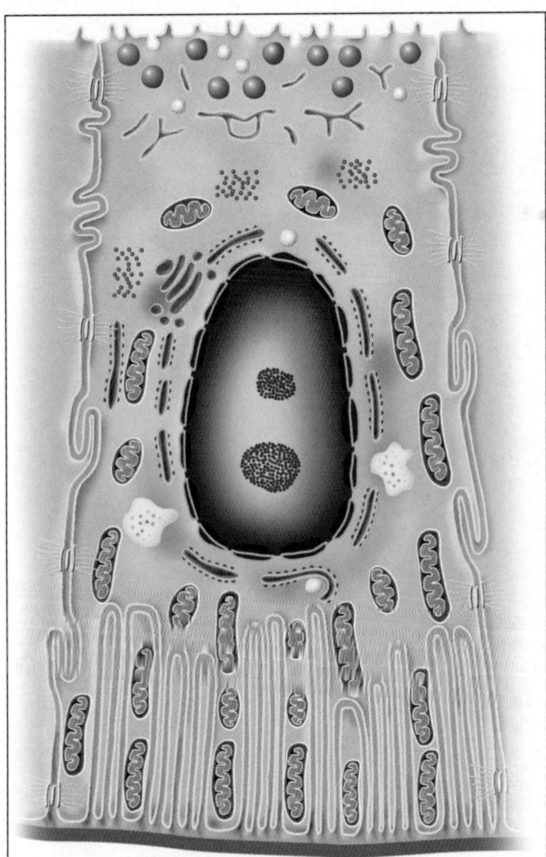

Fig. 11.27 Striated duct cell.

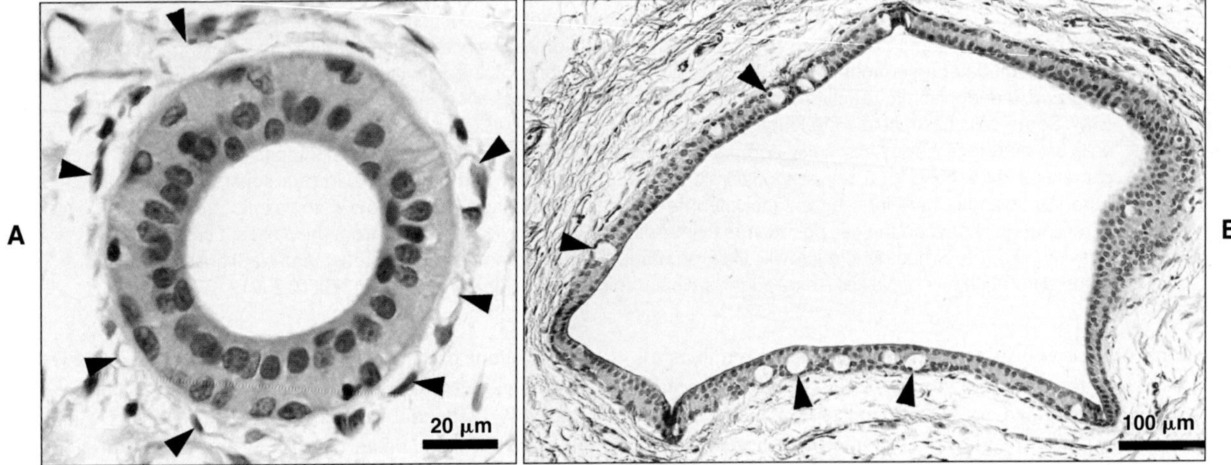

Fig. 11.28 Light micrographs of excretory ducts of the human submandibular gland stained with hematoxylin and eosin. (A) A small excretory duct in the interlobular connective tissue. The duct epithelium is pseudostratified with tall columnar cells and a few basal cells. Numerous capillaries and venules *(arrowheads)* are present around the duct. (B) A large excretory duct is surrounded by dense connective tissue. The pseudostratified epithelium contains several mucous goblet cells *(arrowheads)*.

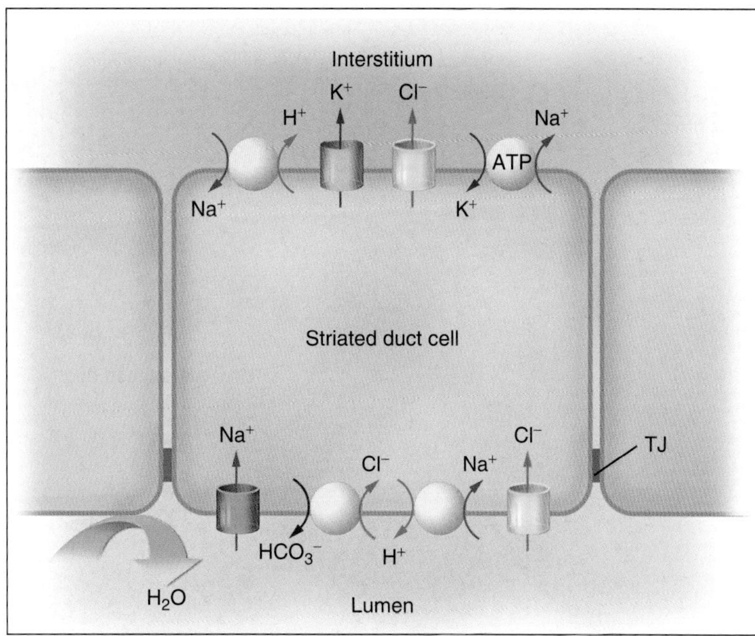

Fig. 11.29 Mechanisms of ductal modification of saliva. Striated duct cells reabsorb Na^+ and Cl^- mainly via channels in the luminal membrane. Na^+/H^+ and Cl^-/HCO_3^- exchangers provide additional mechanisms for uptake of these ions. Na^+ exits at the basolateral surface via the Na^+/K^+ adenosine triphosphatase *(ATP)*, and Cl^- exits via a channel. K^+ channels at the basolateral surface maintain electroneutrality, and the Na^+/H^+ exchanger compensates for intracellular acidification. The tight junctions *(TJ)* are relatively tight, and the duct cells are impermeable to water. (From Melvin JE: Chloride channels and salivary gland function, *Crit Rev Oral Biol Med* 10:199, 2009.)

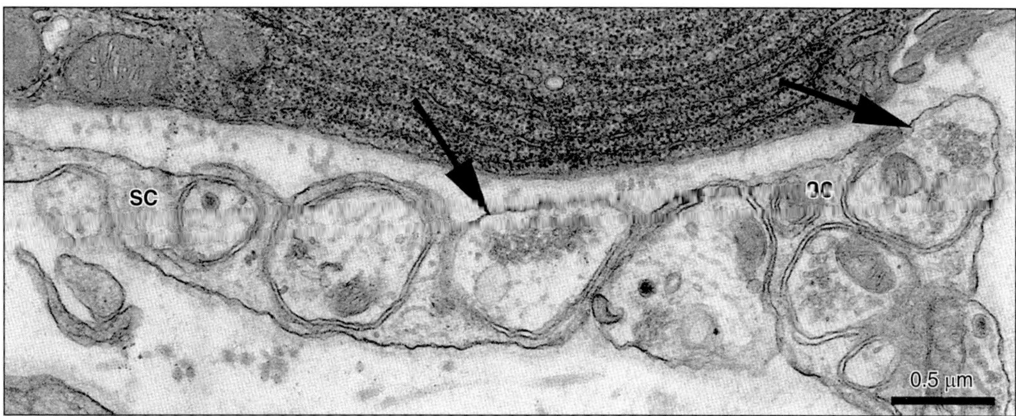

Fig. 11.30 Transmission electron micrograph of an autonomic nerve bundle in a rat submandibular gland. Unmyelinated axons are enclosed by Schwann cell *(SC)* cytoplasm. Innervation of the secretory cells occurs where axonal varicosities containing transmitter vesicles lack the SC covering *(arrows)*. (From Hand AR: Salivary glands. In Provenza DV, Seibel W, editors: *Oral histology: inheritance and development,* ed 2, Philadelphia, PA, 1986, Lea and Febiger.)

and are shed into saliva. Viral infections such as mumps and bacterial infections of individual glands may cause inflammation resulting in a painful swelling. Blockage of a duct may cause a transient swelling associated with eating as blood flow increases and saliva backs up in the gland. Ductal obstruction may result from the formation of sialoliths (stones), most common in the submandibular duct, or a mucous plug or the severing of the duct of a minor salivary gland by trauma. The salivary glands also may be affected by a variety of benign and malignant tumors.

The salivary glands may be affected in various endocrine, autoimmune, infectious, and genetic diseases. Diabetes may have significant effects on salivary glands and the secretion of saliva. Parotid gland swelling may occur, and salivary flow is reduced. Increased levels of glucose in saliva may influence plaque metabolism. Studies of experimental diabetes demonstrate changes in the expression of certain secretory proteins. Autoimmune diseases such as Sjögren syndrome, rheumatoid arthritis, or graft-versus-host disease occurring after tissue or organ transplantation may cause destruction

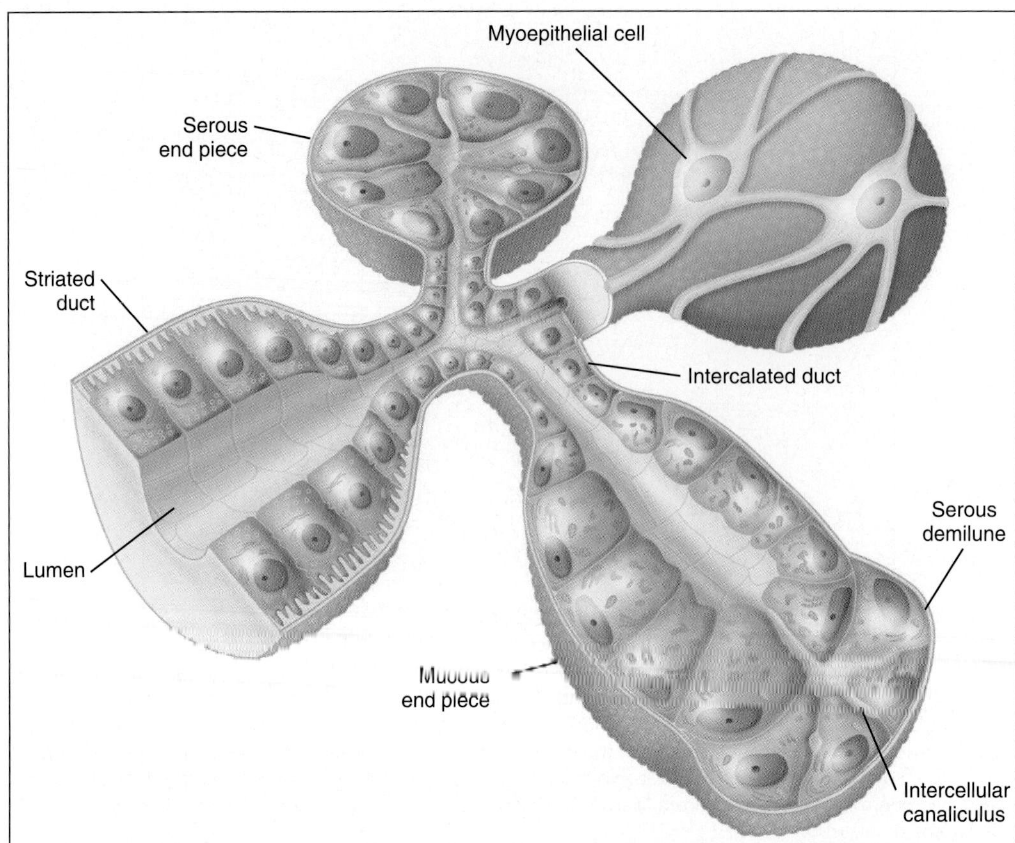

Fig. 11.31 Architecture of salivary gland ducts and secretory end pieces and the main features of the parenchymal cells. (From Hand AR: Salivary glands. In Bhaskar SN, editor: *Orban's oral histology and embryology,* ed 11, St. Louis, MO, 1991, Mosby.)

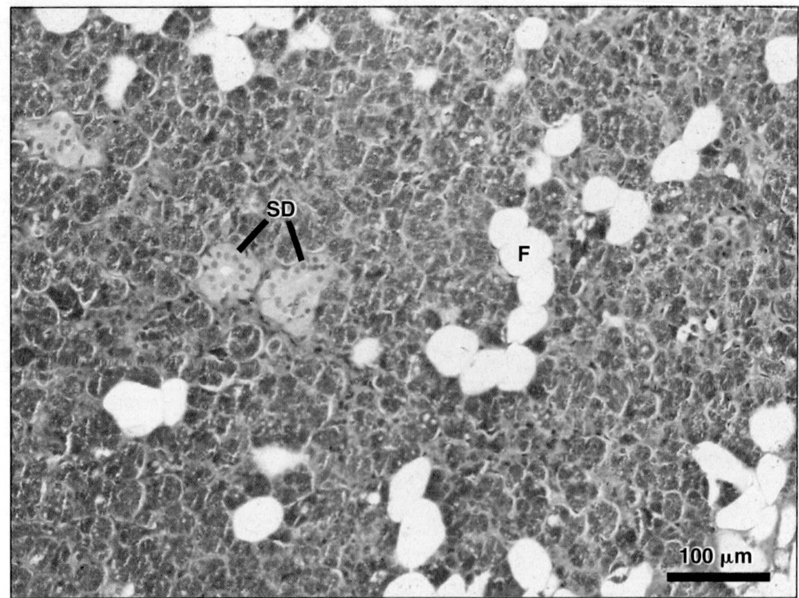

Fig. 11.32 Light micrograph of a human parotid gland, stained with hematoxylin and eosin. The secretory end pieces are all serous. *F,* Fat cells; *SD,* striated ducts.

of salivary tissue and reduced flow of saliva. Patients with adrenal diseases may have altered salivary electrolyte composition. Salivary function also is affected in individuals with acquired immune deficiency syndrome. Salivary flow rates are decreased, and lower levels of secretory immunoglobulins are present in saliva. Parotid gland enlargement may occur because of lymphadenopathy and lymphoepithelial cysts. Pathologic changes in salivary glands also are observed in individuals with cystic fibrosis. Salivary Na^+ and Cl^- concentrations are increased, and mucus-secreting glands may develop mucous plugs.

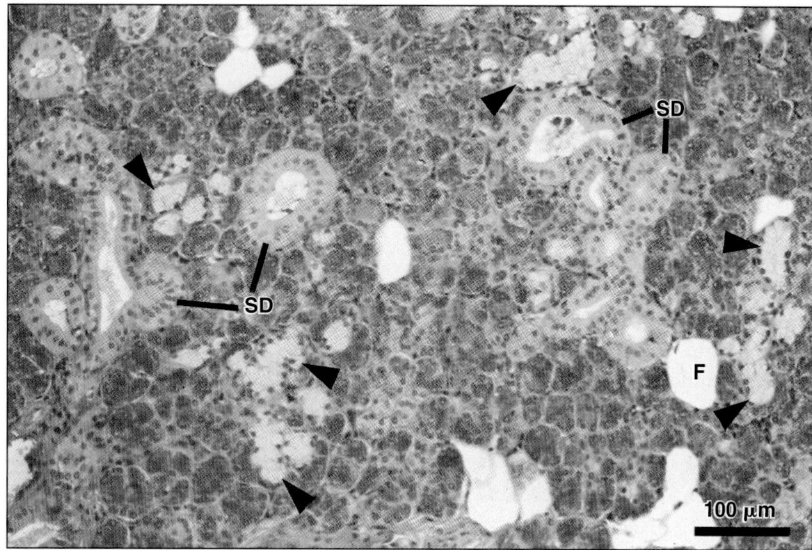

Fig. 11.33 Light micrograph of a human submandibular gland stained with hematoxylin and eosin. Serous secretory end pieces predominate, but a few mucous tubules *(arrowheads)* are present. Several lightly stained striated ducts *(SD)* are present. *F*, Fat cells.

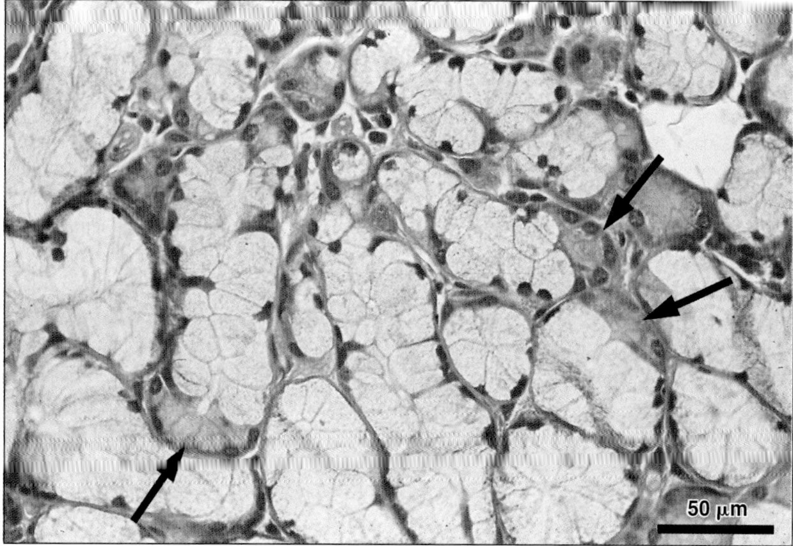

Fig. 11.34 Light micrograph of human sublingual gland stained with hematoxylin and eosin. Mucous tubules are abundant; many have serous demilunes *(arrows)*.

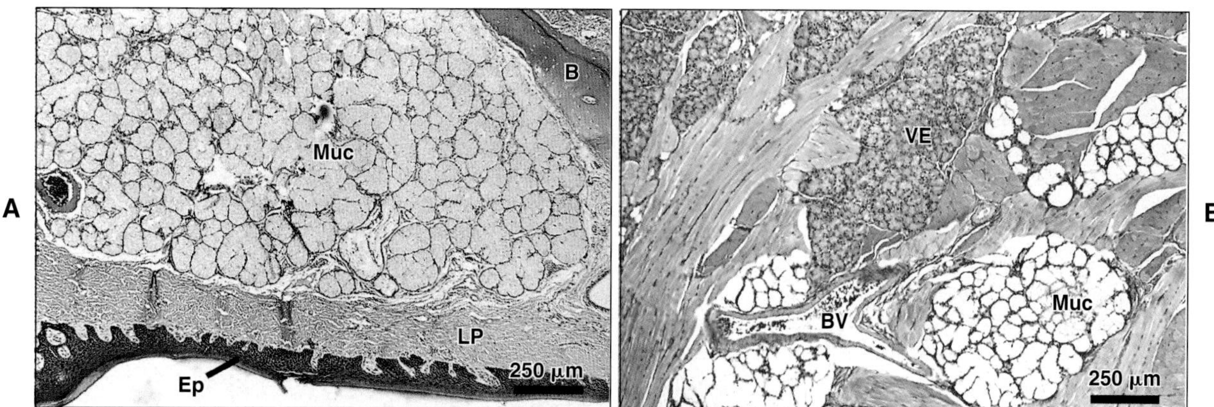

Fig. 11.35 Light micrographs of human minor salivary glands stained with hematoxylin and eosin. (A) Mucous gland *(Muc)* in the lateral portion of the hard palate. (B) Lingual serous (Ebner) glands *(VE)* and mucous glands located between muscle fibers in the posterior part of the tongue. *B*, Bone; *BV*, blood vessel; *Ep*, epithelium; *LP*, lamina propria.

Dry Mouth (Xerostomia)

Dry mouth (xerostomia) is a common clinical complaint. A loss of salivary function or a reduction in the volume of secreted saliva may lead to the sensation of oral dryness. Oral dryness occurs most commonly as a side effect of medications taken by the patient for other problems. Many drugs cause central or peripheral inhibition of salivary secretion. Destruction of salivary gland tissue is another common cause of xerostomia. Loss of gland function occurs after radiation therapy for head and neck cancer because the salivary glands often are included in the radiation field, and salivary gland cells are highly sensitive to the deleterious effects of radiation. Chemotherapy for cancer or associated with bone marrow transplantation also may cause reduced salivary function. Autoimmune diseases, in particular Sjögren syndrome, may cause progressive loss of salivary function from the invasion of lymphocytes into the gland and the destruction of epithelial cells.

The decreased volume of saliva in the mouth leads to drying of the oral tissues and loss of the protective effects of salivary buffers, proteins, and mucins. The oral tissues are more susceptible to infections, and speech, eating, and swallowing become difficult and painful. The teeth are highly susceptible to caries, especially near the gingival margin. Temporary relief is achieved by frequent sipping of water or artificial saliva. Patients who have some functional salivary tissue may benefit from pharmacologic therapy with oral parasympathomimetic drugs, such as pilocarpine, to increase salivary flow. In the future, satisfactory treatment of patients with xerostomia may include genetic modification of salivary gland cells to increase fluid and protein secretion and the use of stem cells to repair and regenerate the glands (see Box 11.1).

BOX 11.1 Stem Cells and Their Use to Regenerate Salivary Glands

Salivary epithelial cells are considered specialized and terminally differentiated cells with a slow turnover ranging between 50 and 125 days. During homeostasis there is an endogenous population of progenitor cells that can replace dying cells (Box 11.1 Fig. 1A). When salivary glands are injured, certain quiescent salivary cells regain their proliferative potential, while cells with mitotic activity can further transdifferentiate into additional cell types (see Box 11.1 Fig. 1B and C). In recent years, several populations of actively dividing salivary cells were identified through the use of injury-induced models. For example, by using a duct ligation model (to mimic a duct blocked by a salivary stone) or by using a radiation injury-induced model (to mimic ionizing radiation injury to healthy tissues experienced by head and neck cancer patients treated by radiotherapy), several cell populations that could partially regenerate the gland were identified. Such cells can be considered progenitor cells (with limited differentiation potential), while a small population of cells can also act as stem cells with the potential to generate most of the salivary cell phenotypes. In the acinar region, Mist1+ cells (a transcription factor used as a marker for salivary acinar cells) are responsible for acinar cell maintenance during homeostasis, ductal ligation, or radiation-injury response. A subset of these cells, expressing Sox2 and Sox9, can give rise to all the epithelial cells and are essential for acinar cell repair after radiation. In the ductal region, K5+/K14+ cells with Axin2 can respond readily to Wnt signals. These cells can transiently convert into stem cell–like c-KIT+ cells, which can give rise to both ductal and acinar cells. Myoepithelial cells (K14+/αSMA+) can also transdifferentiate to form acinar and intercalated duct cells (including c-KIT+ cells) in response to radiation injury but have a low proliferation potential.

When the injury is beyond the capacity of the salivary gland to regenerate itself, such as with patients experiencing severe dry mouth due to radiotherapy or Sjögren syndrome, experimental strategies using cell-based therapy, cell-free therapy, or three-dimensional (3D) organoids are being tested to repair and regenerate salivary glands.

Cell therapies using mesenchymal stem cells (MSCs) due to their immunomodulatory and antiinflammatory properties have become the most popular type of adult stem cells tested for regenerative therapies. The bone marrow and adipose tissues have been the two most preferred sources for MSCs, although other oral tissues such as the dental pulp and salivary glands possess MSCs as well. In clinical studies, MSCs derived from either the bone marrow or adipose tissue have been injected intravenously or intraglandularly into patients who had severe salivary hypofunction (dry mouth) due to radiotherapy or Sjögren syndrome. Results from the most promising clinical trials indicated a 30% to 50% increase in saliva secretion within 1 to 4 months after MSC treatment. Another type of cell therapy using peripheral blood-derived mononuclear cells (MNCs) is currently being tested in patients with radiation-induced xerostomia. MNCs are isolated from the patient's blood and cultured in vitro for 1 week with five specific factors to enhance their antiinflammatory and vasculogenic properties. These so-called effective MNCs are then injected back, intraglandularly, into the submandibular gland of the patient. Results from that clinical study will soon be published.

Numerous challenges remain with stem cell therapies, such as an insufficient number of cells isolated or expanded, factors that can affect the quality of the cells (e.g., donor age, health status), immune rejection if the cells are from another patient, or a possible unlimited proliferation of the transplanted stem cells. An alternative approach has been the use of cell-free therapies (i.e., use secretome of MSCs such as through the use of conditioned media, cell extracts, or exosomes). This approach is based on the premise that the paracrine factors released from stem cells are the active components responsible for their therapeutic action. Cell-free therapies, once successfully tested in clinical studies, would offer a product that can be stored for a longer term without losing its bioactive properties, would be easier to transport, and would have a reduced immune rejection.

In parallel to cell and cell-free experimental therapies that are currently being tested to restore salivary function, another category of treatment using stem cells that could soon be used to regenerate salivary glands is the use of 3D organoids for transplantation. Organoids are commonly derived from stem cells but can also be derived from partially digested tissues that contain some stem cells. Such culture conditions allow disease modeling as the extracellular environment can be mimicked to in vivo conditions. In the future, 3D salivary organoids may be used for transplantation. At the present time, this approach is limited to preclinical studies. There are three main components of a 3D culture: the scaffold, cells/tissues, and supplements (mainly growth factors). The scaffold provides an overall support to the cells for their optimal growth, interaction, and differentiation in a 3D plane. Ideal scaffold properties include optimal strength, porosity, biocompatibility, and low immunogenicity. The gold standard biomaterial for culturing salivary organoids is Matrigel, although hyaluronic acid, alginate, chitosan, silk, and synthetic materials such as polylactic acid, polylactic-coglycolic acid, polyglycolic acid, and polyethylene glycol have also been tested. More recently, bioengineered microchips with microbubble technology and magnetic bioassemblies exhibited favorable growth of salivary epithelial cells with the maintenance of their polarization (which is essential for salivary secretions). Using decellularized extracellular matrix (ECM), which is the ECM devoid of its original cells, can also provide a natural scaffold for salivary cells to grow into organoids. With all the recent advances in salivary cell culture and expansion, the path to developing new cell therapies to replace damaged salivary cells will soon become a clinical reality for patients.

Akshaya Upadhyay
McGill Craniofacial Tissue Engineering and Stem Cells Laboratory
Faculty of Dentistry
McGill University
Montreal, Quebec, Canada

Simon D. Tran
McGill Craniofacial Tissue Engineering and Stem Cells Laboratory
Faculty of Dentistry
McGill University
Montreal, Quebec, Canada

BOX 11.1 Stem Cells and Their Use to Regenerate Salivary Glands—cont'd

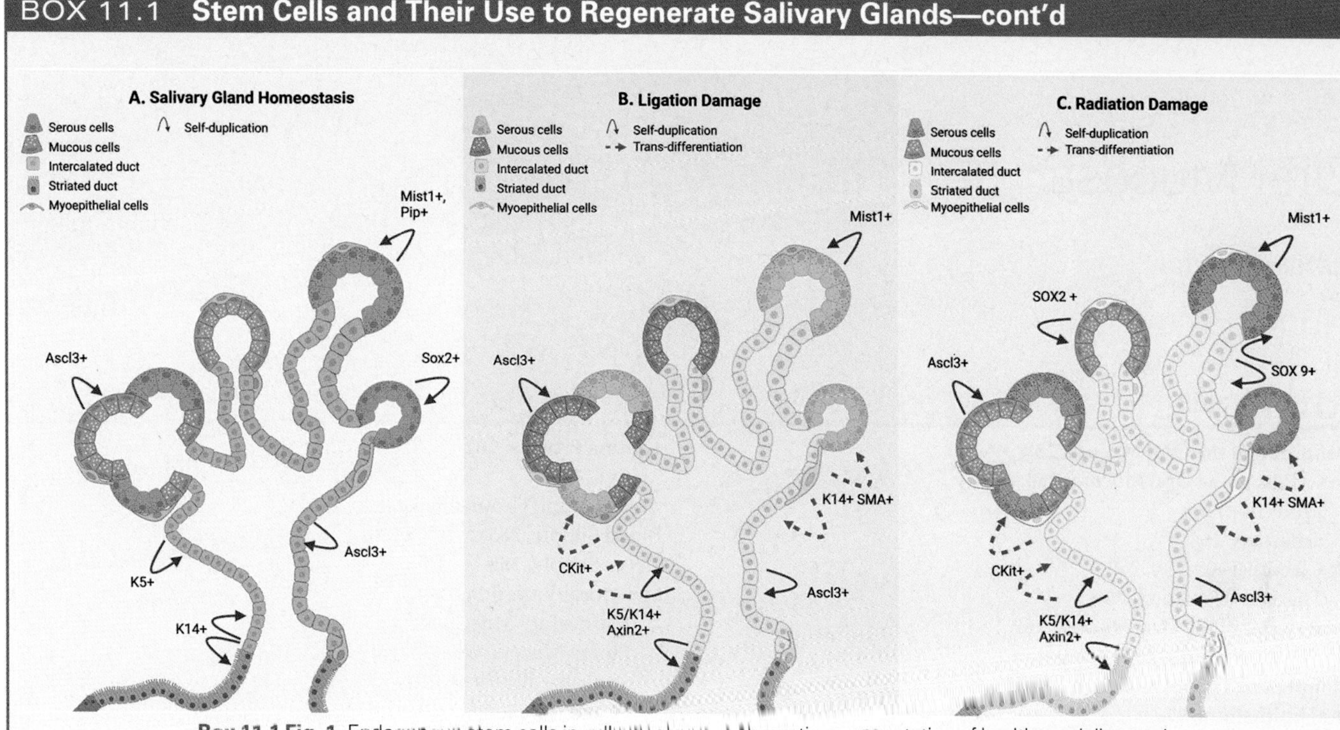

Box 11.1 Fig. 1 Endogenous stem cells in salivary glands. Schematic representation of healthy and diseased conditions in which stem and progenitor cells can repair and regenerate salivary glands. (A) Homeostasis involves maintenance and proliferation of salivary cells in a lineage restricted manner. Mist1 is positive for all acinar cells, and these cells proliferate to maintain the acinar cell population. A small proportion of Mist1 cells are also positive for Sox2 and possess the capacity to differentiate into both acinar and ductal cells. Ascl3-positive cells give rise to mucous acinar cells and ductal cells. K5/K14-positive cells are present in ductal and myoepithelial cells. (B) After ductal ligation injury, K5/14 cells expressing Axin2 (a ductal cell marker) and K14 expressing SMA (a myoepithelial cell marker) can transiently give rise to c-KIT cells, which are bipotent to form ductal or acinar cells. The remaining Mist1-positive cells can also repopulate acinar cells after ligation removal but in a reduced capacity. (C) After radiation injury, stem and progenitor cell populations described in (A) and (B) are injured and have a limited capacity to regenerate the salivary gland. An additional population of stem cells positive for Sox2 or Sox9 was identified to play a critical role in acinar cell repair. *Ascl3*, Achaete acute homolog-like 3 (also known as Sgn1, a basic helix-loop-helix transcription [bHLH] factor); *c-KIT*, also known as CD117, encodes the receptor tyrosine kinase (KIT); *K5/14*, keratin 5/14; Mist1, transcription factor belonging to the bHLH family of protein (also known as bhlha15); *Pip*, phosphatidylinositol phosphate; *SMA*, smooth muscle actin; *Sox2/9*, Sry-box transcription factor 2/9. (Created with BioRender.com.)

RECOMMENDED READING

Cutler LS: Functional differentiation of salivary glands. In Forte J, editor: *Handbook of physiology: salivary, pancreatic, gastric and hepatobiliary secretion*, vol 3, New York, NY, 1989, American Physiological Society.

Dobrosielski-Vergona K, editor: *Biology of the salivary glands*, Boca Raton, FL, 1993, CRC Press.

Dodds MW, et al.: Health benefits of saliva: a review, *J Dent* 33:223–233, 2005.

Hand AR: The secretory process of salivary glands and pancreas. In Riva A, Motta PM, editors: *Ultrastructure of the extraparietal glands of the digestive tract*, Boston, MA, 1990, Kluwer Academic.

Harunaga J, et al.: Dynamics of salivary gland morphogenesis, *J Dent Res* 90:1070–1077, 2011.

Marinkovic M, et al.: Autologous mesenchymal stem cells offer a new paradigm for salivary gland regeneration, *Int J Oral Sci* 15:18, 2023.

Melvin JE, et al.: Regulation of fluid and electrolyte secretion in salivary gland acinar cells, *Annu Rev Physiol* 67:445–469, 2005.

Proctor GB: The physiology of salivary secretion, *Periodontol 2000* 70:1, 2016.

Spielmann N, Wong DT: Saliva: diagnostics and therapeutic perspectives, *Oral Dis* 17:345–354, 2011.

Tandler B: Microstructure of the salivary glands, part I, *Microsc Res Tech* 26:1–19, 1993.

12

Oral Mucosa

Antonio Nanci

OUTLINE

DEFINITION OF THE ORAL MUCOSA

The term *mucous membrane* is used to describe the moist lining of the gastrointestinal tract, nasal passages, and other body cavities that communicate with the exterior. In the oral cavity, this lining is referred to as the *oral mucous membrane* or *oral mucosa*. At the lips, the oral mucosa is continuous with the skin; at the pharynx, the oral mucosa is continuous with the mucosa lining the rest of the gut. Thus the oral mucosa is located anatomically between skin and gastrointestinal mucosa and shows some properties of each.

The skin, oral mucosa, and intestinal lining consist of two separate tissue components: a covering epithelium and an underlying connective tissue.

FUNCTIONS OF THE ORAL MUCOSA

The structure of oral mucosa reflects a variety of adaptations that serve several functions. The major function is protection of the deeper tissues of the oral cavity; other functions include acting as a sensory organ, serving as the site of glandular activity, and secretion and thermal regulation.

Protection

As a surface lining, the oral mucosa separates and protects deeper tissues and organs in the oral region from the environment of the oral cavity. The normal activities of seizing food and biting and chewing expose the oral soft tissues to mechanical forces (compression, stretching, and shearing) and surface abrasions (from hard particles in the diet). The oral mucosa shows several adaptations of the epithelium and the connective tissue to withstand these insults. Furthermore, microorganisms that normally reside within the oral cavity would cause infection if they gained access to the tissues, and many of these produce substances that have a toxic effect on tissues. The epithelium of the oral mucosa acts as the major barrier to these threats.

Sensation

The sensory function of the oral mucosa provides considerable information about events within the oral cavity. In the mouth, receptors respond to temperature, touch, and pain; the tongue uniquely also has taste buds. Reflexes such as swallowing, gagging, retching, and salivating also are initiated by receptors in the oral mucosa.

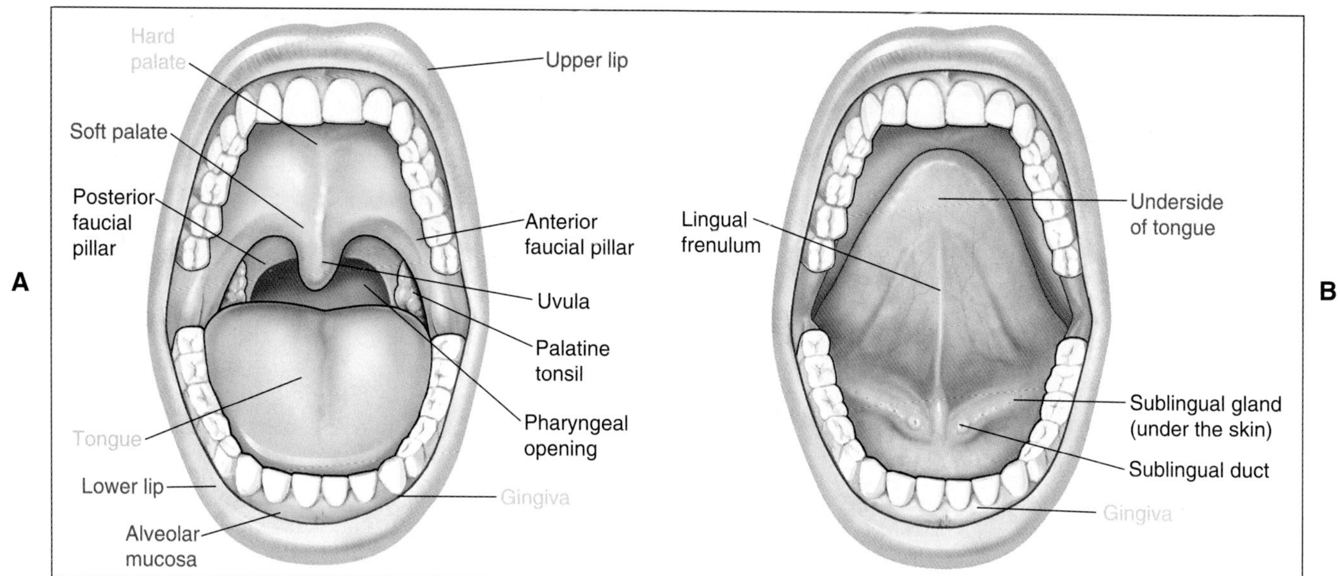

Fig. 12.1 Anatomic locations occupied by the three main types of mucosa in the oral cavity. (A) Supralingual view; (B) sublingual view. (From Thibodeau G, Patton K: *Anatomy and physiology*, ed 6, St. Louis, MO, 2007, Mosby.)

Glandular Activity

The salivary glands associated with the oral mucosa produce saliva, which contributes to the maintenance of a moist surface. The major salivary glands are situated distant from the mucosa, and their secretions pass through the mucosa via long ducts; however, many minor salivary glands are associated with the oral mucosa (the salivary glands are described fully in Chapter 11). Sebaceous glands are commonly present in the oral mucosa, but their secretions are probably insignificant.

Thermal Regulation

In some animals (such as the dog), considerable body heat is dissipated through the oral mucosa by panting; for these animals, the mucosa plays a major role in the regulation of body temperature. This is not the case for human oral mucosa, and no obvious specializations of the blood vessels exist for controlling heat transfer, such as arteriovenous shunts.

BOUNDARIES OF THE ORAL MUCOSA

The oral cavity consists of two parts: an outer vestibule bounded by the lips and cheeks and the oral cavity proper, which is separated from the vestibule by alveolar bone and gingiva. The hard and soft palates form the superior zone of the oral cavity proper, and the floor of the mouth and base of the tongue form the inferior border. Posteriorly the oral cavity is bounded by the pillars of the fauces and the tonsils. The oral mucosa shows considerable structural variation in different regions of the oral cavity, but three main types of mucosa can be identified according to their primary function: masticatory mucosa, lining mucosa, and specialized mucosa. Fig. 12.1 shows the anatomic location of each type, and the types are described fully later in the chapter. Quantitatively, the larger part of the oral mucosa is represented by lining mucosa, amounting to about 60% of the total area with masticatory mucosa and specialized mucosa occupying smaller areas (25% and 15%, respectively).

Clinical Features

Although the oral mucosa is continuous with the skin, it differs considerably in appearance. Generally, the oral mucosa is more deeply colored, most obviously at the lips (where the bright vermilion border contrasts with the skin tone). This coloration represents the combined effect of several factors: the concentration and state of dilation of small blood vessels in the underlying connective tissue, the thickness of the epithelium, the degree of keratinization, and the amount of melanin pigment in the epithelium. Color gives an indication as to the clinical condition of the mucosa; inflamed tissues are red because of dilation of the blood vessels, whereas normal healthy tissues are a paler pink.

Other features that distinguish the oral mucosa from skin are its moist surface and the absence of appendages. Skin contains numerous hair follicles, sebaceous glands, and sweat glands, whereas the oral mucosa essentially only has minor salivary glands. These glands are concentrated in various regions of the oral cavity, and the openings of their ducts at the mucosal surface are sometimes evident on clinical examination (Fig. 12.2B). Sebaceous glands are present in the upper lip and buccal mucosa in about three-quarters of adults and have been described occasionally in the alveolar mucosa and dorsum of the tongue (Fig. 12.3). Sebaceous glands appear as pale yellow spots (Fordyce spots).

The surface of the oral mucosa tends to be smoother and have fewer folds or wrinkles than the skin, but topographic features are readily apparent on clinical examination. The most obvious are the different papillae on the dorsum of the tongue and the transverse ridges (or rugae) of the hard palate. The healthy gingiva shows a pattern of fine surface stippling consisting of small indentations of the mucosal surface (see Fig. 12.2A). In many persons a slight whitish ridge occurs along the buccal mucosa in the occlusal plane of the teeth. This line (linea alba, "white line") is a keratinized region and may represent the effect of abrasion from rough tooth restorations or cheek biting.

The oral mucosa varies considerably in its firmness and texture. The lining mucosa of the lips and cheeks, for example, is soft and pliable, whereas the gingiva and hard palate are covered by a firm, immobile layer. These differences have important clinical implications for giving local injections of anesthetics or taking biopsies of oral mucosa. Fluid can be introduced easily into loose lining mucosa, but injection into the masticatory mucosa is difficult and painful. However, lining mucosa gapes when surgically incised and may require suturing, but

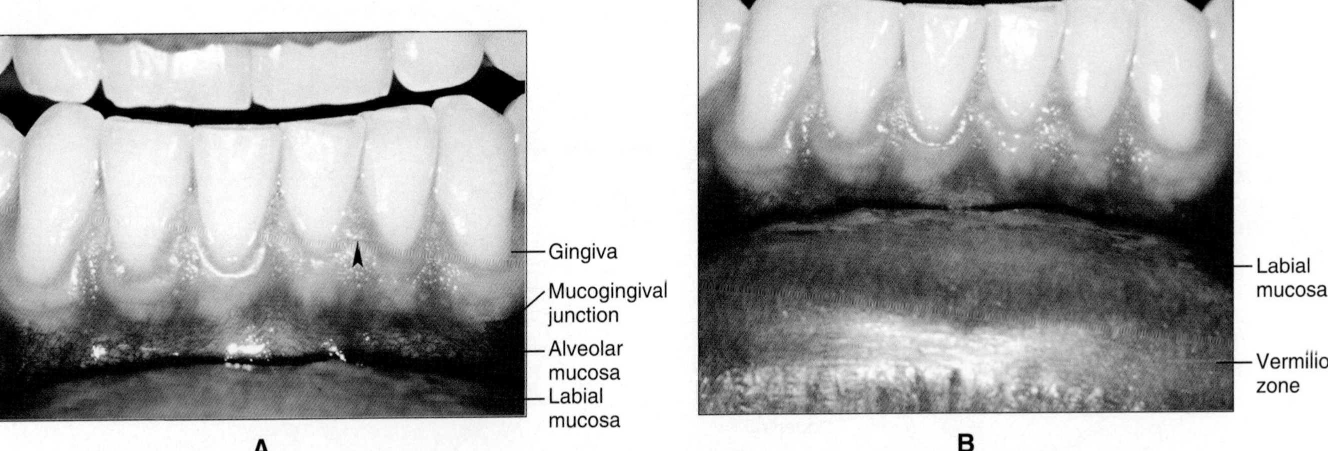

Fig. 12.2 Healthy oral mucosa. (A) Attached gingiva and the alveolar and labial mucosa. Gingival stippling is most evident in the interproximal regions *(arrowhead)*. The mucogingival junction between keratinized gingiva and nonkeratinized alveolar mucosa is clearly evident. (B) Vermilion zone adjoining the labial mucosa. Minor salivary gland ducts open to the surface in this region. (Courtesy A. Kauzman.)

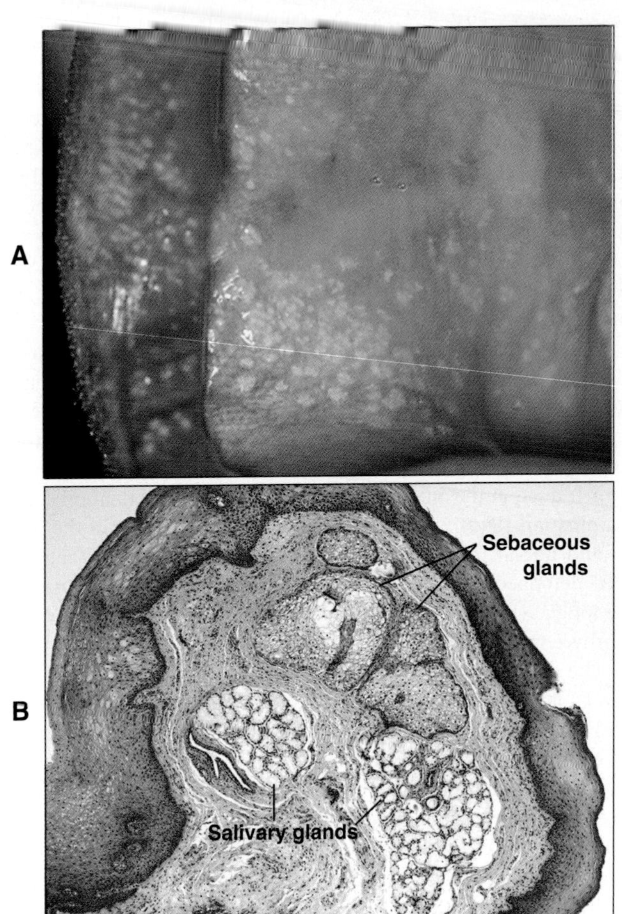

Fig. 12.3 Sebaceous glands in the mucosa of the cheek. (A) Clinically, these appear as clusters of yellowish spots called *Fordyce granules*. (B) Histologic section of a biopsy from this region. Note the presence of minor salivary glands in proximity to the sebaceous glands. (Courtesy A. Kauzman.)

masticatory mucosa does not. Similarly, the accumulation of fluid with inflammation is obvious and painful in masticatory mucosa, but in lining mucosa, the fluid disperses and inflammation may not be as evident or as painful.

COMPONENT TISSUES AND GLANDS

The two main tissue components of the oral mucosa are a stratified squamous epithelium (oral epithelium) and an underlying connective tissue layer (lamina propria) (Fig. 12.4). In the skin these two tissues are known as the *epidermis* and *dermis.* The interface between epithelium and connective tissue is usually irregular, and upward projections of connective tissue, called the connective tissue papillae, interdigitate with epithelial ridges or pegs (Fig. 12.5). There is a basal lamina at the interface between epithelium and connective tissue (see Fig. 12.5A).

Although the junction between oral epithelium and lamina propria is obvious, that between the oral mucosa and underlying tissue, or submucosa, is less easy to recognize compared with intestinal mucosa, which clearly is separated from underlying tissues by a layer of smooth muscle and elastic fibers (Fig. 12.6A). In many regions (e.g., cheeks, lips, and parts of the hard palate), a layer of loose fatty or glandular connective tissue containing the major blood vessels and nerves that supply the mucosa separates the oral mucosa from underlying bone or muscle. The layer represents the submucosa in the oral cavity (see Fig. 12.6B), and its composition determines the flexibility of the attachment of oral mucosa to the underlying structures. In regions such as the gingiva and parts of the hard palate, oral mucosa is attached directly to the periosteum of underlying bone, with no intervening submucosa (see Fig. 12.6C). This arrangement is called a *mucoperiosteum* and provides a firm, inelastic attachment.

The minor salivary glands are situated in the submucosa. Sebaceous glands are less abundant than salivary glands; they lie in the lamina propria and have the same structure as those present in the skin. The sebaceous glands produce a fatty secretion (sebum), the function of which in the oral cavity is unclear, although some claim that the sebum may lubricate the surface of the mucosa so that it slides easily against the teeth.

In several regions of the oral cavity there are nodules of lymphoid tissue that consist of crypts formed by invaginations of the epithelium into the lamina propria. These areas are infiltrated extensively by lymphocytes and plasma cells. Because of their ability to mount immunologic reactions, such cells play an important role in combating infections of the oral tissues. The largest accumulations of lymphoid tissue are found in the posterior part of the oral cavity where they form the lingual, palatine, and pharyngeal tonsils, often known collectively

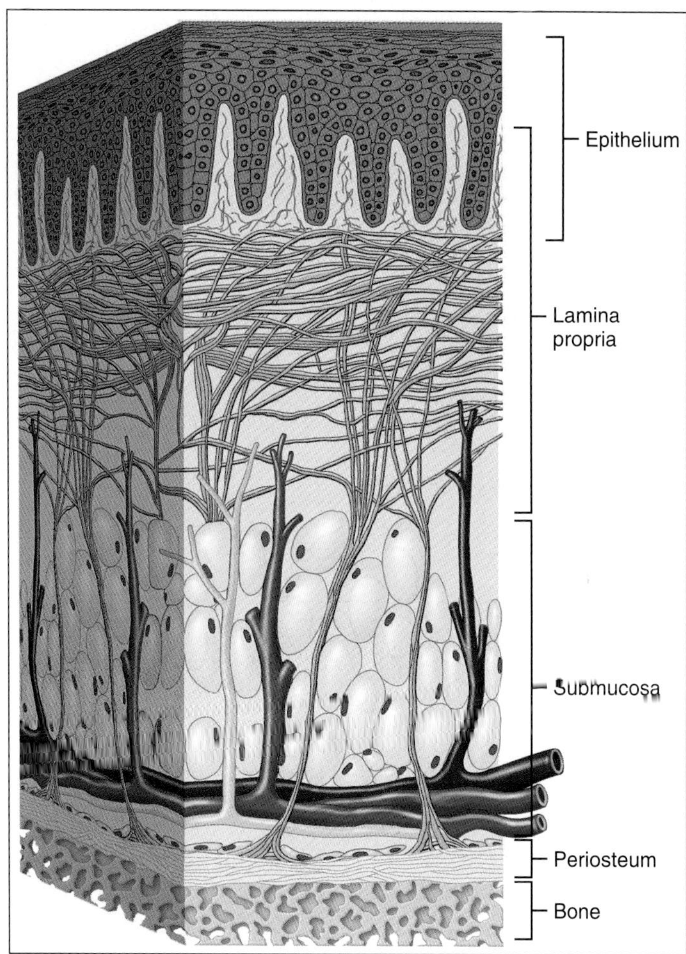

Fig. 12.4 Main tissue components of the oral mucosa.

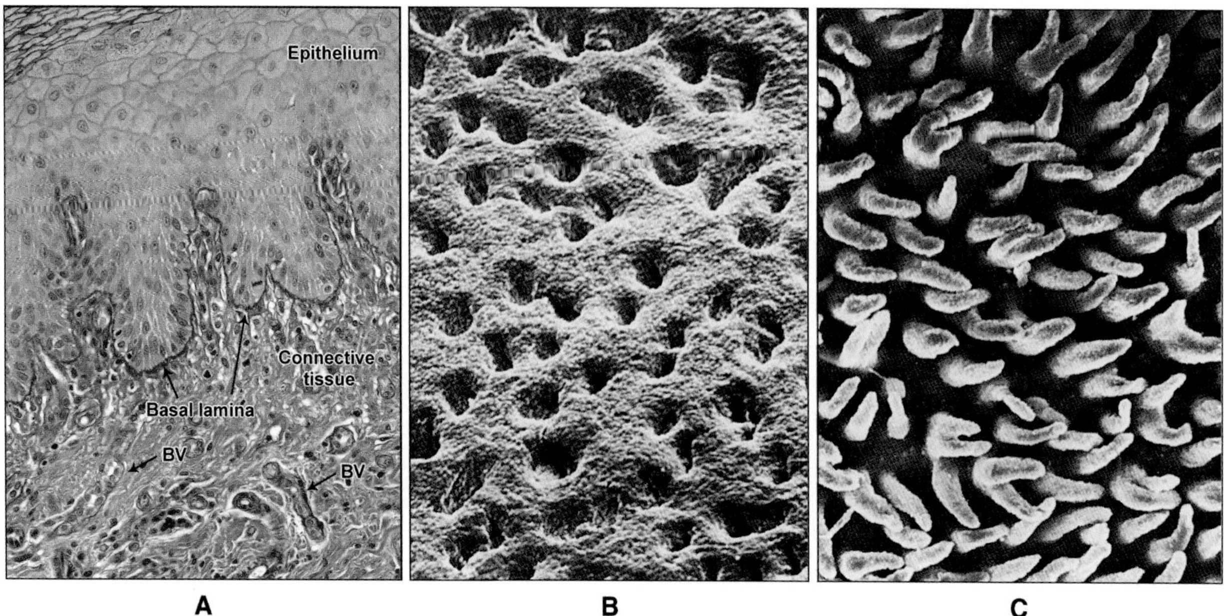

Fig. 12.5 Junction between epithelium and connective tissue. (A) Photomicrograph of section through cheek epithelium stained by the periodic acid–Schiff method, demonstrating the basal lamina at the interface between epithelium and connective tissue and their interdigitations. A similar basal lamina *(arrows)* is also observed around blood vessels *(BVs)*. (B, C) Scanning electron micrographs of the interface between epithelium and connective tissue in the palate. (B) The underside of oral epithelium and the circular orifices into which the cone-shaped papillae of connective tissue that are illustrated in (C). (A, Courtesy A. Kauzman; B, C, from Klein Szanto AJP, Schroeder HE: Architecture and density of the connective tissue papillae of the human oral mucosa, *J Anat* 123:93–109, 1977.)

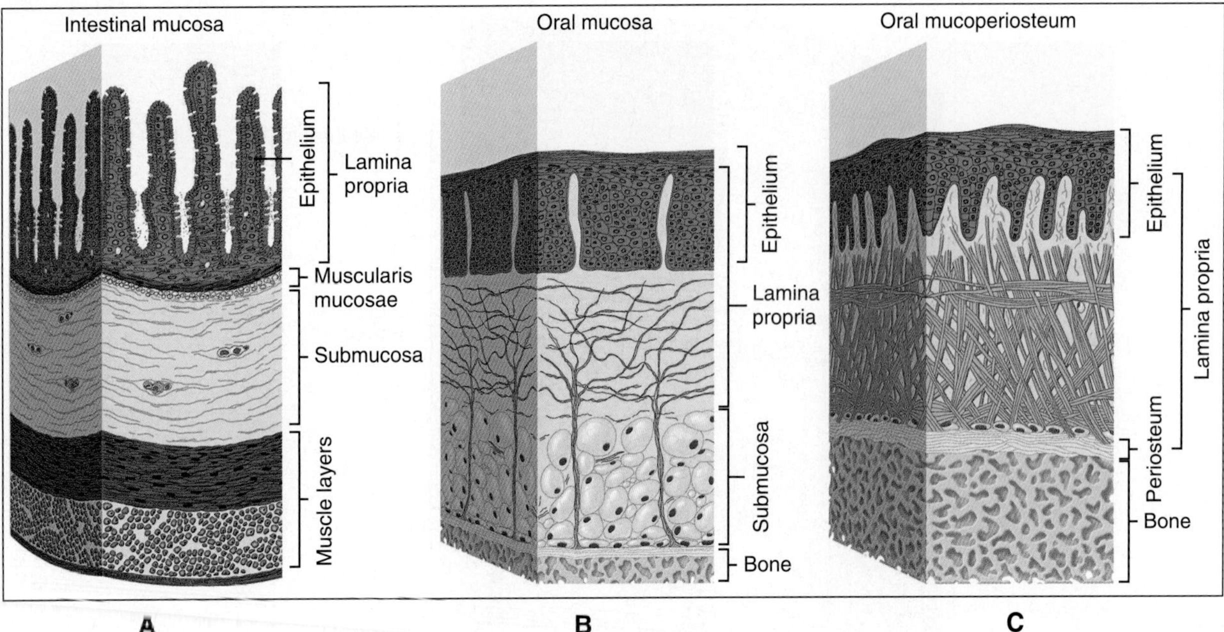

Fig. 12.6 Arrangement of tissue components. (A) Intestinal mucosa. (B) Oral mucosa. (C) Oral mucoperiosteum.

as *Waldeyer ring.* Small lymphoid nodules also may occur sometimes in mucosa of the soft palate, ventral surface of the tongue, and floor of the mouth.

ORAL EPITHELIUM

The oral epithelium at the surface of the oral mucosa constitutes the primary barrier between the oral environment and deeper tissues. The oral epithelium is a stratified squamous epithelium consisting of cells tightly attached to each other and arranged in several distinct layers (strata). Like other epithelia, the oral epithelium maintains its structural integrity by a process of continuous renewal in which cells produced by mitotic divisions in the deepest layers mature and undergo terminal differentiation as they migrate passively toward the surface to replace those that are shed. The end phase of this pathway is indeed regarded as a unique form of programmed cell death (see Chapter 7). The cells of the epithelium thus can be considered to consist of two functional populations: a progenitor population (the function of which is to divide and provide new cells) and a maturing population (which continually differentiate or mature to form a protective surface layer).

Maturing cells in stratified squamous epithelia assemble at the surface a specialized protective layer called the cornified cell envelope, which consists essentially of keratins embedded in an insoluble amalgam of proteins surrounded by lipids (Fig. 12.7). The process begins with the synthesis of an immature envelope on the cytoplasmic face of the plasma membrane. The cells produce keratohyalin granules (discussed later), which release the precursor of the intermediate filament protein filaggrin. This protein aggregates keratin filaments, promoting the collapse and flattening of keratinocytes, which are thereafter referred to as *corneocytes.* Concurrently, several other proteins, including involucrin, loricrin, trichohyalin, and small proline-rich proteins, are synthesized. These proteins are cross-linked by transglutaminases in relation to the aggregated keratin filaments just below the plasma membrane. This cornified cell envelope eventually replaces the plasma membrane of corneocytes and becomes coated with lipid consisting mainly of ceramides, cholesterol, and free fatty acids and acts as an essential water barrier. Corneocytes are tightly attached to each other by modified desmosomes that undergo proteolytic degradation to permit cells to desquamate.

Epithelial Proliferation

The progenitor cells are situated in the basal layer in thin epithelia (e.g., the floor of the mouth) and in the lower two to three cell layers in thicker epithelia (cheeks and palate). Dividing cells tend to occur in clusters that are more abundant at the bottom of epithelial ridges than at the top. Studies on the epidermis and the oral epithelium indicate that the progenitor compartment is not homogeneous but consists of two functionally distinct subpopulations of cells. A small population of progenitor cells cycle slowly and are considered to represent stem cells, the function of which is to produce basal cells and retain the proliferative potential of the tissue. The larger portion of the progenitor compartment is composed of amplifying cells, the function of which is to increase the number of cells available for subsequent maturation. Despite their functional differences, these proliferative cells cannot be distinguished by appearance. Regardless of whether the cells are of the stem or amplifying type, cell division is a cyclic activity. After cell division, each daughter cell recycles in the progenitor population or enters the maturing compartment. Apart from measuring the number of cells in division, estimating the time necessary to replace all the cells in the epithelium is also possible. This is known as turnover time of the epithelium and is derived from knowledge of the time taken for a cell to divide and pass through the entire epithelium. The turnover time has been estimated at 52 to 75 days in the skin, 4 to 14 days in the gut, 41 to 57 days in the gingiva, and 25 days in the cheek. Regional differences in the patterns of epithelial maturation appear to be associated with different turnover rates (e.g., nonkeratinized buccal epithelium turns over faster than keratinized gingival epithelium).

Scientific views on the mechanisms that control the proliferation and differentiation of oral mucosa, skin, and many other tissues have been clarified by the identification of various cytokines that may influence epithelial proliferation. Examples include epidermal growth factor, keratinocyte growth factor, interleukin-1 (IL1), and transforming growth factors α and β.

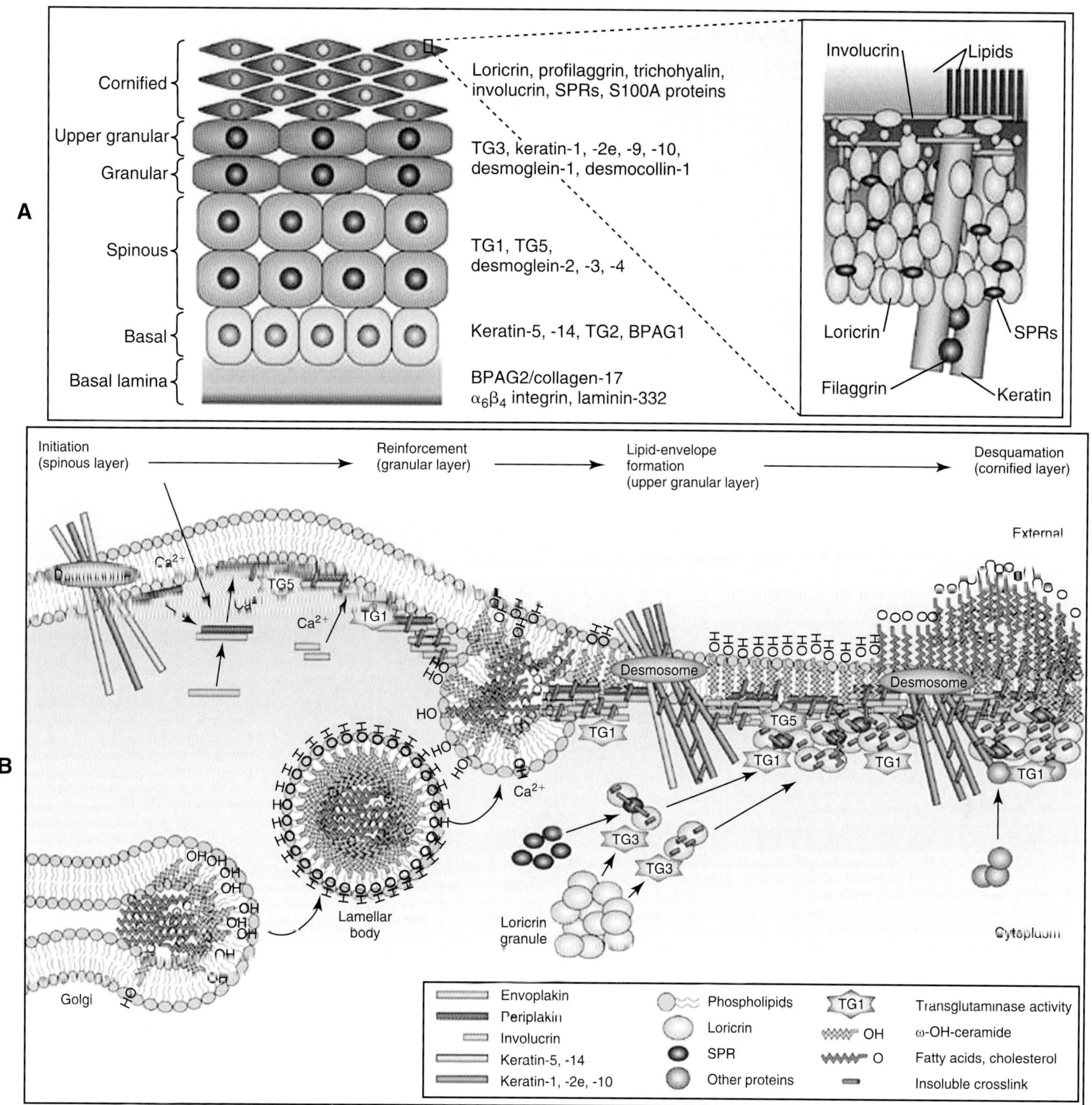

Fig. 12.7 (A) Representation of the organization and various layers of the cornified epithelium. (B) Molecular changes during epithelial maturation.

Because cancer chemotherapeutic drugs block mitotic division, a significant number of patients taking them develop oral ulcers (breakdown of the oral squamous epithelium) and thus experience pain and difficulty in eating, drinking, and maintaining oral hygiene.

Epithelial Maturation

Cells arising by division in the basal or parabasal layers of the epithelium undergo a process of maturation as they are passively displaced toward the surface. In general, maturation in the oral cavity follows two main patterns: keratinization and nonkeratinization (Table 12.1).

Keratinization

The epithelial surface of the masticatory mucosa (e.g., that of the hard palate and gingiva and in some regions of specialized mucosa on the dorsum of the tongue) is inflexible, tough, resistant to abrasion, and tightly bound to the lamina propria. It is covered by a layer of keratinized cells, and the process of maturation leading to its formation is called keratinization or cornification. In routine histologic sections, a keratinized epithelium shows several distinct layers or strata (Fig. 12.8A). The basal layer (stratum basale) consists of cuboidal or columnar cells adjacent to the basal lamina. Above the basal layer are several rows of larger elliptic or spheric cells known as the *prickle cell layer* (stratum spinosum). This term arises from the appearance of the cells in histologic preparation; they typically shrink away from each other, remaining in contact only at points known as *intercellular bridges* (desmosomes) (Fig. 12.9). This alignment gives the cells a spiny or pricklelike profile.

The basal and prickle cell layers together constitute between one-half and two-thirds of the thickness of the epithelium. The next layer

TABLE 12.1 Major Features of Maturation in Keratinized and Nonkeratinized Epithelia

KERATINIZED EPITHELIUM		NONKERATINIZED EPITHELIUM	
Features	**Cell Layer**	**Features**	**Cell Layer**
Cuboidal or columnar cells containing bundles of tonofibrils and other cell organelles; site of most cell divisions	Basal	Cuboidal or columnar cells containing separate tonofilaments and other cell organelles; site of most cell divisions	Basal
Larger ovoid cells containing conspicuous tonofibril bundles; membrane-coating granules appear in upper part of this layer	Prickle/spinosum	Larger ovoid cells containing dispersed tonofilaments; membrane-coating granules appear in upper part of layer; filaments become numerous	Prickle/spinosum
Flattened cells containing conspicuous keratohyalin granules associated with tonofibrils; membrane-coating granules fuse with cell membrane in upper part; internal membrane thickening also occurs	Granular	Slightly flattened cells containing many dispersed tonofilaments and glycogen	Intermediate
Extremely flattened and dehydrated cells in which all organelles have been lost; cells filled only with packed fibrillar material; when pyknotic nuclei are retained, parakeratinization occurs	Keratinized	Slightly flattened cells with dispersed filaments and glycogen; fewer organelles are present, but nuclei persist	Superficial

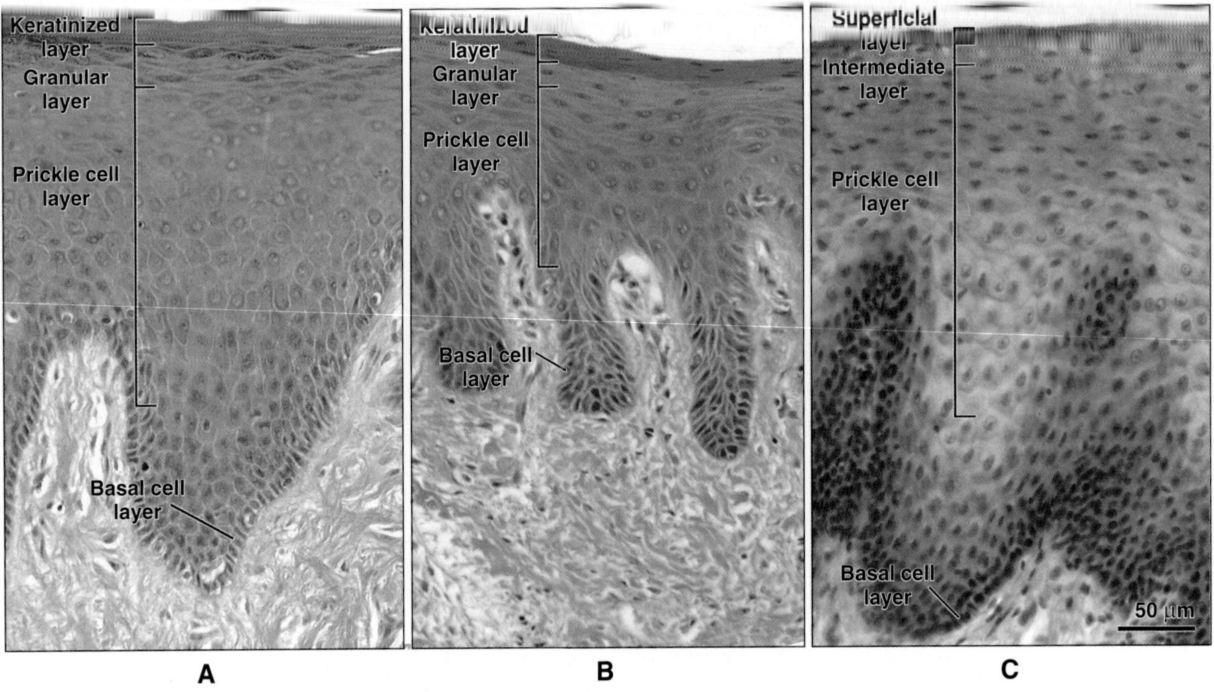

Fig. 12.8 Histologic sections of the main types of maturation in oral epithelium (at the same magnification). (A) Orthokeratinization in human gingiva. Nuclei are lost in the keratinized surface layer. Keratohyalin granules are visible in the granular layer. (B) Parakeratinization in human gingiva. The keratin squames retain their pyknotic nuclei. (C) Nonkeratinization in primate buccal epithelium. No clear division of strata exists, and nuclei are apparent in the surface layer. The differences in thickness and epithelial ridge pattern, as well as in the patterns of maturation, are apparent.

consists of larger flattened cells containing small granules that stain intensely with acid dyes such as hematoxylin (i.e., they are basophilic). This layer is the granular layer (stratum granulosum), and the granules are called keratohyalin granules (see Fig. 12.9A). The surface layer is composed of flat (squamous) cells (squames) that stain bright pink with the histologic dye eosin (i.e., they appear eosinophilic) and do not contain nuclei. This layer is the keratinized layer (stratum corneum or cornified layer). The pattern of maturation of these cells often is termed *orthokeratinization*.

The masticatory mucosa, parts of the hard palate and much of the gingiva, can show a variation of keratinization, known as *parakeratinization*. In parakeratinized epithelium (see Fig. 12.8B), the surface layer stains for keratin, as described previously, but shrunken (or pyknotic) nuclei are retained in many or all of the squames. Keratohyalin granules may be present in the underlying granular layer, although usually fewer than in orthokeratinized areas, so this layer is difficult to recognize in histologic preparations. Parakeratinization is a normal event in oral epithelium and does not imply disease; this is not true for

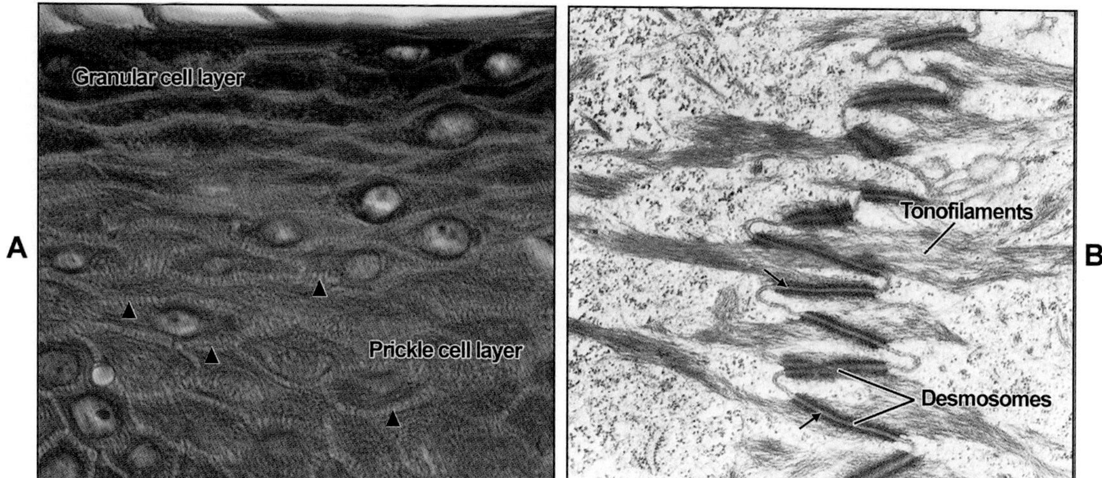

Fig. 12.9 Intercellular junctions. (A) Light micrograph showing the granular cell layer whose cells contain keratohyalin granules (punctate dark staining) and the prickle cell layer in keratinized oral epithelium the intercellular bridges (prickles, *arrowheads*) between adjacent cells. (B) Electron micrograph; in this oral epithelium preparation, minimal shrinkage has occurred so that cells are closely apposed, and the numerous desmosomes holding the cells together are clearly seen. A clear specialized intercellular zone *(arrows)* can be seen between the attachment plaques into which tonofilaments insert.

epidermis, where parakeratinization may be associated with diseases such as psoriasis.

Nonkeratinization

The lining mucosa of the oral cavity, which is present on the lips, buccal mucosa, alveolar mucosa, soft palate, underside of the tongue, and floor of the mouth, has an epithelium that is usually nonkeratinized (see Fig. 12.8C). In some regions, such as the lips and buccal mucosa, the lining mucosa is thicker than keratinized epithelium and shows a different ridge pattern at the connective tissue interface. The basal and prickle cell layers of nonkeratinized oral epithelium generally resemble those described for keratinized epithelium, although the cells of nonkeratinized epithelium are slightly larger, and the intercellular bridges or prickles are less conspicuous. For this reason, some prefer not to use the term *prickle cell layer* for nonkeratinized epithelium. No sudden changes in the appearance of cells above the prickle cell layer occur in nonkeratinized epithelium, and the outer half of the tissue is divided rather arbitrarily into two zones: intermediate (stratum intermedium) and superficial (stratum superficiale). A granular layer is not present, and the cells of the superficial layer contain nuclei that are often plump. This layer does not stain distinctively, as does the surface of keratinized or parakeratinized epithelium.

From the histologic appearance of oral epithelium it is apparent that the tissue shows a well-ordered pattern of maturation and successive layers that contain cells of increasing age (i.e., progressive stages of maturation). Furthermore, the pattern of maturation differs in different regions of the oral mucosa so that two main types can be recognized: keratinization and nonkeratinization. The next section describes the fine structure of the epithelial cell and the main events that take place at the cellular level during maturation of these two types of epithelia (Table 12.2; see also Table 12.1).

Ultrastructure of the Epithelial Cell

Cells of the basal layer are the least differentiated oral epithelial cells. They contain typical organelles present in the cells of other tissues as well as certain characteristic structures that identify them as epithelial cells and distinguish them from other cell types. These structures are the filamentous strands called *tonofilaments* and the intercellular bridges or desmosomes (see Chapter 4; also see Fig. 12.9B). One name often given to an epithelial cell because of its content of keratin filaments is keratinocyte. This serves to distinguish these epithelial cells from the nonkeratinocytes that are described later.

Keratins represent a large family of proteins of differing molecular weights; those with the lowest molecular weight (40 kDa) are found in glandular and simple epithelia; those of intermediate molecular weight, in stratified epithelia; and those with the highest molecular weight (~67 kDa), in keratinized stratified epithelia. A catalog of keratins has been drawn up to represent the different types. Thus all stratified oral epithelia possess keratins 5 and 14, but differences emerge between keratinized oral epithelium (which contains keratins 1, 6, 10, and 16) and nonkeratinized epithelium (which contains keratins 4, 13, and 19). An important property of any epithelium is its ability to function as a barrier, which depends to a great extent on the close contact or cohesiveness of the epithelial cells. Modifications of the adjacent membranes of cells, the most common of which is the desmosome (macula adherens) (see Fig. 12.9B), into which bundles of intermediate filaments (tonofilaments) insert (see Chapter 4), provide cohesion between cells. Adhesion between the epithelium and connective tissue is provided by hemidesmosomes, which attach the cell to the basal lamina (see later). Like desmosomes, hemidesmosomes also possess intracellular attachment plaques with tonofilaments inserted into them. Tonofilaments, hemidesmosomes, and basal lamina together represent a mechanical linkage that distributes and dissipates localized forces applied to the epithelial surface over a wide area. As discussed in Chapter 4, disease such as pemphigus can lead to the breakdown of this linkage and cause splitting of the epithelial layers.

Two other types of connection are seen between cells of the oral epithelium: gap junctions and tight junctions. As shown in Chapter 4, the gap junction is a region where membranes of adjacent cells run closely together, separated by only a small gap. Small interconnections are apparent between the membranes across these gaps. Such junctions may allow electrical or chemical communication between the cells and are sometimes called communicating junctions; they are seen only occasionally in oral epithelium. Even rarer in oral epithelium is the tight (occluding) junction where adjacent cell membranes are so tightly apposed as to exclude intercellular space.

TABLE 12.2 Characteristics of Nonkeratinocytes in Oral Epithelium

Cell Type	Level in Epithelium	Specific Staining Reactions	Ultrastructural Features	Function
Melanocyte	Basal	Dopa oxidase–tyrosinase; silver stains	Dendritic; no desmosomes or tonofilaments; premelanosomes and melanosomes present	Synthesis of melanin pigment granules (melanosomes) and transfer to surrounding keratinocytes
Langerhans cell	Predominantly suprabasal	CD1a; cell surface antigen markers	Dendritic; no desmosomes or tonofilaments; characteristic Langerhans granule	Antigen trapping and processing
Merkel's cell	Basal	Probably periodic acid–Schiff positive	Nondendritic; sparse desmosomes and tonofilaments; characteristic electron-dense vesicles and associated nerve axon	Tactile sensory cell
Lymphocyte	Variable	Cell surface antigen markers (CD3—T cells; CD20—B cells)	Large circular nucleus; scant cytoplasm with few organelles; no desmosomes or tonofilaments	Associated with the inflammatory response in oral mucosa

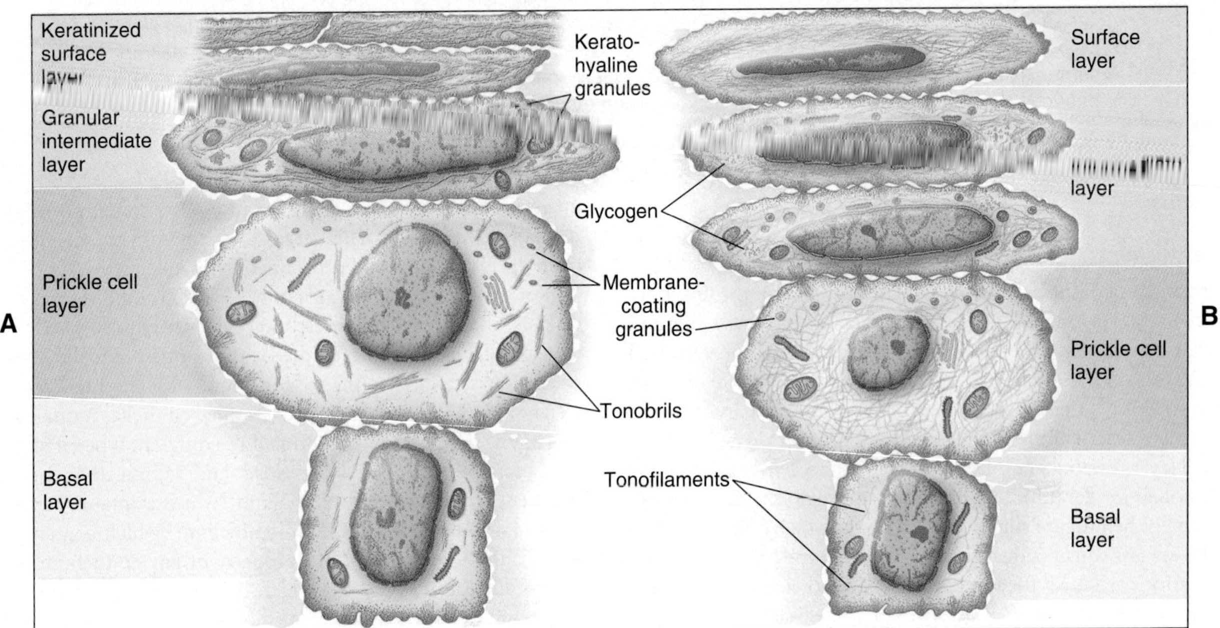

Fig. 12.10 Principal structural features of epithelial cells in successive layers. (A) Orthokeratinized oral epithelium. (B) Nonkeratinized oral epithelium. Note that cells are not drawn to scale. (From Squier CA, et al.: *Human oral mucosa: development, structure, and function,* Oxford, UK, 1976, Blackwell Scientific.)

Cellular Events in Maturation

The major changes involved in cell maturation in keratinized and nonkeratinized oral epithelia are presented in Fig. 12.10 (also see Table 12.1). In both types of epithelia, the changes in cell size and shape are accompanied by a synthesis of more structural protein in the form of tonofilaments, the appearance of new organelles, and the production of additional intercellular material. Some changes, however, are not common to both epithelia and serve as distinguishing features. The cells of both epithelia increase in size as they migrate from the basal to the prickle cell layer, but this increase is greater in nonkeratinized epithelium. A corresponding synthesis of tonofilaments occurs in both epithelia, but whereas the tonofilaments in keratinized epithelium are aggregated into bundles to form tonofibrils, those in nonkeratinized epithelium remain dispersed and so appear less conspicuous (Fig. 12.11). The chemical structure of keratin filaments also is known to differ between layers so that various patterns of maturation can be identified by the keratins that are present.

In the upper part of the prickle cell layer a new organelle appears, called the *membrane-coating* or *lamellate granule.* These granules are small membrane-bound structures containing glycolipid. In keratinized epithelium the granules are elongated and exhibit a series of parallel lamellae. In nonkeratinized epithelium, by contrast, the granules appear to be circular with an amorphous core (Fig. 12.12). As the cells move toward the surface, these granules accumulate close to the cell membrane where they release lipids that participate in establishing a permeability barrier.

The next layer, called the granular layer in keratinized epithelium and the intermediate layer in nonkeratinized epithelium, contains cells that have a greater volume but are more flattened than those of the prickle cell layer. In the upper part of this layer, in both keratinized and nonkeratinized epithelia, the membrane-coating granules appear to fuse with the superficial cell membrane and to discharge their contents into the intercellular space. In keratinized oral epithelium and epidermis, the discharge of granule contents is associated with the formation

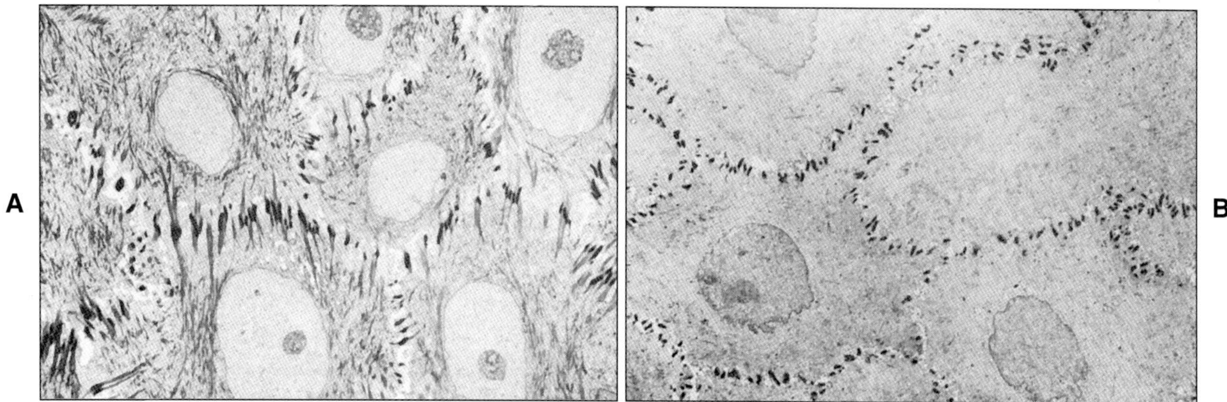

Fig. 12.11 Low-magnification electron micrographs of prickle cells from (A) keratinized gingival epithelium and (B) nonkeratinized buccal epithelium. Filaments are assembled into distinct bundles (tonofibrils) in the keratinized tissue but are inconspicuously dispersed in the nonkeratinized epithelium.

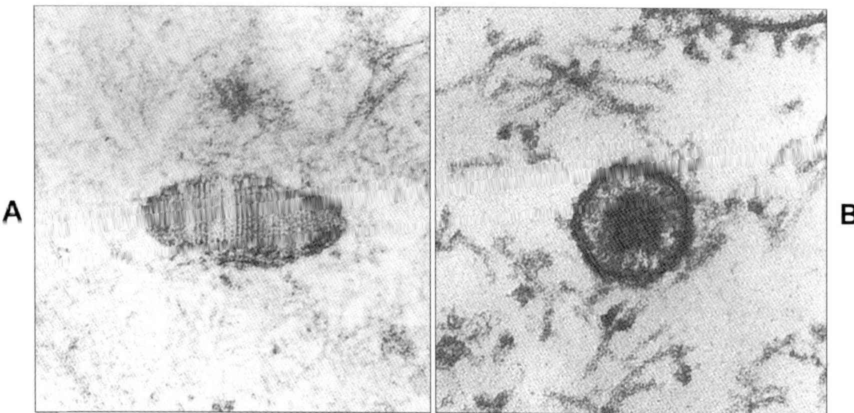

Fig. 12.12 Electron micrographs of membrane-coating granules in oral epithelium. (A) Elongated lamellate type seen in keratinized epithelium. (B) Circular type with a dense core found in nonkeratinized epithelium.

of a lipid-rich permeability barrier that limits the movement of aqueous substances through the intercellular spaces of the keratinized layer. The granules seen in nonkeratinized epithelium probably have a similar function, but the contents have a different lipid composition and do not form as effective a barrier as that in keratinized epithelia.

Cells in the more superficial part of the granular layer develop a cornified cell envelope on the inner (intracellular) aspect of their membrane that contributes to the considerable resistance of the keratinized layer to chemical solvents (see Fig. 12.7). One of the major constituents of this thickening is a protein known as *involucrin.* A similar but less obvious thickening often is seen in the surface cells of nonkeratinized epithelia. The remaining events during epithelial maturation are greatly different in keratinized and nonkeratinized epithelia and so are described separately.

Keratinized Epithelium

The most characteristic feature of the granular layer of keratinized epithelium is the keratohyalin granules, which appear as irregular-shaped basophilic granules under light microscope and as electron-dense structures in the electron microscope (Fig. 12.13). Keratohyalin granules also are associated intimately with tonofibrils, and they are thought to facilitate the aggregation and formation of cross-links between the cytokeratin filaments of the keratinized layer. For this reason, the protein making up the bulk of these granules has been named filaggrin, although they may also comprise a sulfur-rich component called loricrin. As the cells of the granular layer reach the junction with the keratinized layer, a sudden change in their appearance occurs (Fig. 12.14A). All the organelles, including the nuclei and keratohyalin granules, disappear. The cells of the keratinized layer become packed with filaments cross linked by disulfide bonds, which facilitates their dense packing. As part of the process, the cells modify their desmosomes into corneodesmosomes.

The cells of the keratinized layer become dehydrated and flattened and assume the form of hexagonal disks (squames) (see Fig. 12.14C). Squames are lost (by the process of desquamation) and are replaced by cells from the underlying layers. Shedding of squames occurs in a matter of hours. The mechanism of desquamation is an active process resulting from the progressive enzymatic breakdown of proteins (desmoglein I, desmocollin, desmoplakin, and corneodesmosin) comprising corneodesmosomes. Rapid clearance of the surface layer is probably important in limiting the colonization and invasion of epithelial surfaces by pathogenic microorganisms, including the common oral fungus *Candida albicans.*

The keratinized layer in the oral cavity may be composed of up to 20 layers of squames and is thicker than that in most regions of the skin except the soles and palms. The tight packing of cytokeratins within an insoluble and tough envelope makes this layer resistant to mechanical and chemical damage.

In parakeratinization (see Fig. 12.8B), incomplete removal of organelles from the cells of the granular layer occurs; the nuclei remain as shrunken pyknotic structures, and remnants of other organelles may be present in the keratinized layer.

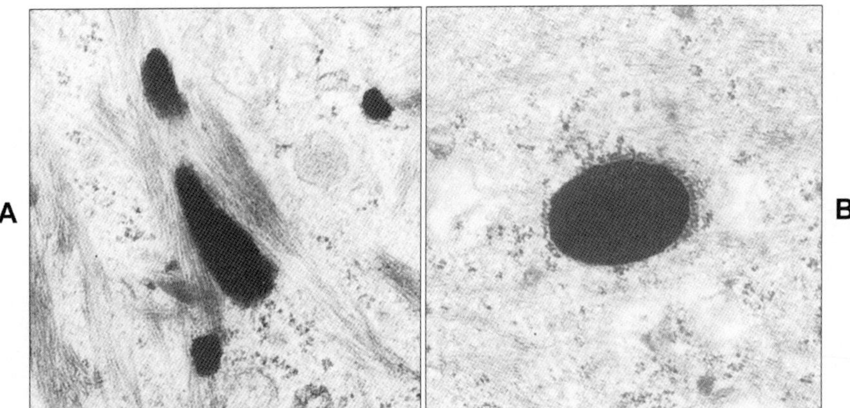

Fig. 12.13 Electron micrographs of keratohyalin granules in oral epithelium. (A) From the granular layer, irregularly shaped granules are associated intimately with tonofilaments. (B) A granule of the type occasionally seen in nonkeratinized oral epithelium is regular in shape but is not associated with tonofilaments.

Nonkeratinized Epithelium

In nonkeratinized oral epithelium, the events taking place in the upper cell layers are far less dramatic than those in keratinized epithelium (see Fig. 12.14A and B). A slight increase in cell size occurs in the intermediate cell layer, as well as an accumulation of glycogen in cells of the surface layer. On rare occasions, keratohyalin granules can be seen at this level, but they differ from the granules in keratinized epithelium and appear as regular spheric structures not associated with tonofilaments (see Fig. 12.13B). Keratohyalin granules often remain, even in the surface cells, where they may be evident in surface cytologic preparations.

In the superficial layer the cells appear more flattened than in the preceding layers and contain dispersed tonofilaments and nuclei, the number of other cell organelles having diminished (see Fig. 12.14B). The surface layer of nonkeratinized epithelium thus consists of cells filled with loosely arranged filaments that are not dehydrated. Thus they can form a surface that is flexible and tolerant of compression and distention.

Although the distribution of keratinized and nonkeratinized epithelia in different anatomic locations is determined during embryologic development, often some variation of this basic pattern occurs in adults (e.g., when the normally nonkeratinized buccal mucosa develops a thin keratin layer [linea alba] along the occlusal line). Similarly, the normal keratin layer of the palate may become thick in smokers because of the irritant effects of tobacco smoke, but such hyperkeratotic epithelium in other ways appears normal. In general, hyperkeratosis of oral epithelium that normally is keratinized represents a physiologic response of the epithelium to chronic irritation, similar to that occurring in callous formation on the palms and soles. Hyperkeratosis of nonkeratinized oral epithelium may be physiologic but also can be associated with abnormal cellular changes that eventually lead to cancer of the squamous epithelium. Squamous cell carcinoma accounts for over 90% of all malignancies in the oral cavity and are characterised by cell and tissue changes. The occurrence, clinical appearance, and histopathologic changes of oral squamous cell carcinomas are discussed in Box 12.1.

Finally, the presence of inflammation in regions such as the gingiva can reduce the degree of keratinization so that it appears parakeratinized or even nonkeratinized.

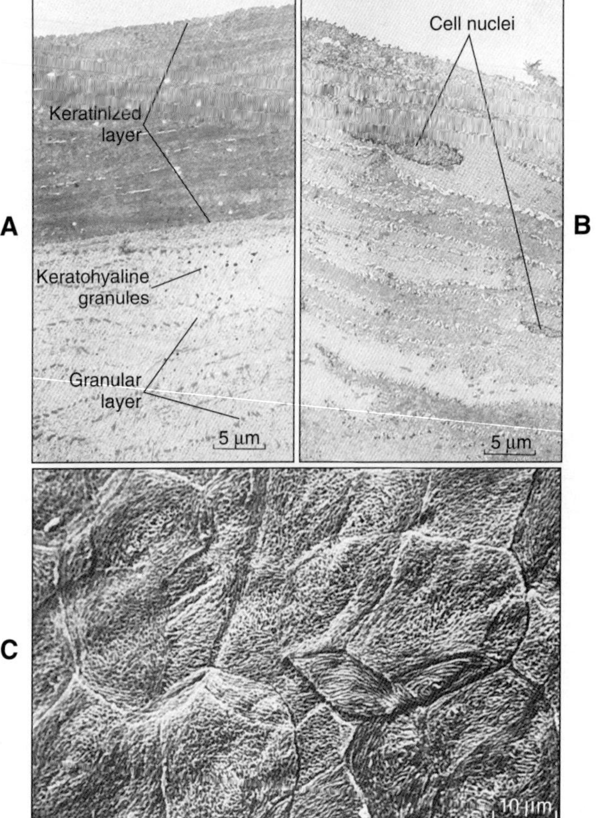

Fig. 12.14 Surface layer of keratinized and nonkeratinized oral epithelium. (A, B) Transmission electron micrographs. (A) The granular and keratinized layers in gingival epithelium. Small keratohyalin granules are visible in the granular layer; the cells (squames) of the keratinized layer are flattened and appear uniformly dense. (B) The corresponding region of nonkeratinized buccal epithelium. The cells undergo only slight changes as they move to the surface. All the cells appear flattened, and organelles (including cell nuclei) can be seen even in the superficial layers. (C) Scanning electron micrograph of the surface cells (squames) of keratinized oral epithelium. The squames are flat disks with a polygonal outline, and their surface shows a reticulate pattern of fine ridges. (C, Courtesy J. Howlett.)

BOX 12.1 Oral Squamous Cell Carcinoma

Oral cancer represents the 16th most common malignancy globally. A 5-year overall relative survival rate of 65% reflects the challenge in treating this disease. In the oral cavity, squamous cell carcinoma (SCC) accounts for over 90% of all malignancies. Oral squamous cell carcinoma (OSCC) arises from the oral mucosal lining epithelium. It is often preceded by a preexistent, clinically evident, oral potentially malignant disorder (e.g., leukoplakia, erythroplakia, oral submucous fibrosis). These precursor lesions can show variable degrees of epithelial dysplasia histologically (Box 12.1 Fig. 1).

Well-documented risk factors include tobacco smoking, alcohol (particularly in combination with smoking), immunosuppression (e.g., acquired immunodeficiency syndrome, iatrogenic immunosuppression in transplant recipients), and betel quid use. Although human papillomavirus (HPV) is the most common cause of oropharyngeal cancer, it is estimated that only approximately 5% of OSCC cases are caused by HPV. At the exception of rare inherited syndromes such as Fanconi anemia and Li-Fraumeni syndrome, the role of inherited genetic predispositions remains elusive. Most OSCCs are genetically heterogeneous and are characterized by numerous somatic genetic variations and epigenetic alterations affecting keratinocytes. The most altered genes in OSCC include tumor suppressor genes *TP53, CDKN2A, FAT1, NOTCH1,* and *PIK3CA* (an oncogene involved in regulation of cell proliferation and invasion).

OSCC cases are most common in middle-age to older adults with a male predominance. The most frequently affected sites include the floor of the mouth, the lateral and ventral surfaces of the tongue, the gingiva, and the buccal mucosa. The clinical appearance of OSCC is variable. It may present as a white, red, or mixed red and white plaque, which may be ulcerated. Some lesions may appear more endophytic and present as deep, necrotic ulcerations with rolled borders. OSCC may also present as an exophytic, red or red and white mass with a papillary, granular, or verruciform surface. Gingival and palatal lesions over time may erode bone, imparting an irregular, ragged radiolucent appearance on radiographic examination. OSCC may be indurated on palpation, reflecting one or more of the following: invasion of cancer cells, fibrosis in the tumor microenvironment, and significant inflammation. Early lesions are often asymptomatic, which may lead to a delay in seeking care.

Histopathologically, most OSCC are conventional, variably keratinizing SCCs. They are characterized by invasive, irregular nests and cords of squamous cells with an eosinophilic cytoplasm and distinct intercellular bridges. Squamous pearls composed of concentric layers of keratin may be identified within these islands. Some tumors may show more extensive nuclear and cellular pleomorphism, nuclear hyperchromatism, and increased mitotic activity, including atypical mitoses. A host inflammatory response to the tumor is often observed. Perineural and lymphovascular invasion may be identified, particularly in high-grade tumors, and are independent negative prognostic factors. Epithelial dysplasia at tumor margins can also increase the risk of recurrence

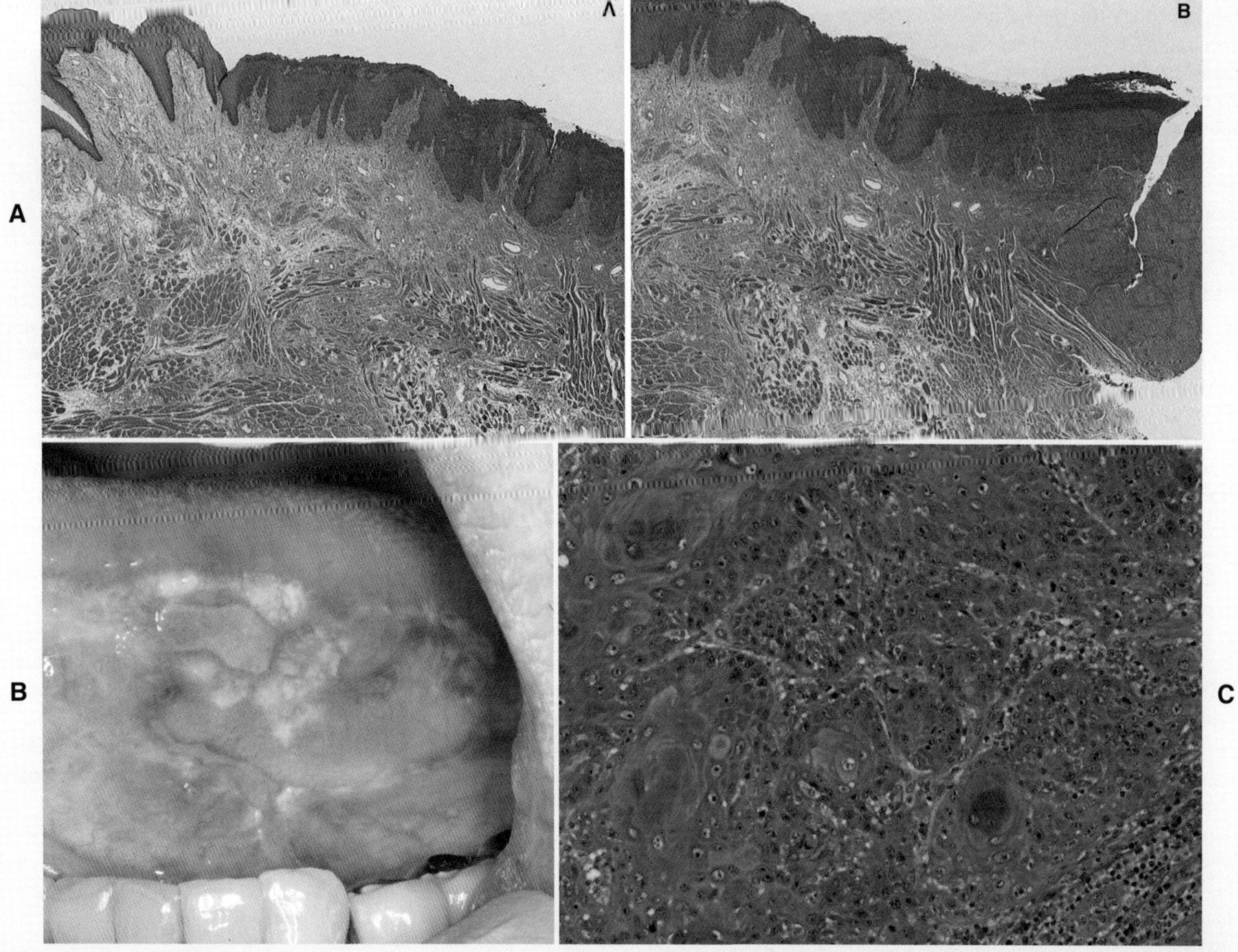

Box 12.1 Fig. 1 (A) Biopsy of the lateral tongue showing a transition from normal epithelium *(A, far left)* to dysplastic epithelium *(A, middle to far right; B, far left to right)* to oral squamous cell carcinoma (OSCC) *(B, far right)*. (B) OSCC of the left lateral tongue presenting as an ulcerated and eroded, mixed erythematous and white plaque. (C) Invasive nests of squamous epithelial cells exhibiting cellular and nuclear pleomorphism, prominent nucleoli, and areas of keratinization. Apoptotic cells and mitoses are abundant.

Continued

BOX 12.1 Oral Squamous Cell Carcinoma—Cont'd

Treatment of OSCC usually requires surgery and in numerous cases induction chemotherapy followed by radiation therapy. Immunotherapy has been approved for nonoperable, recurrent or metastatic OSCC. Despite these aggressive protocols, 35% of patients will die from the disease or its recurrence. In addition, the associated morbidity reduces drastically the quality of life of affected individuals. Patients frequently suffer from complications, which can affect mastication, speech, deglutition, airway management, and integrity of the mucosal surfaces. Diagnosis of OSCC at an early stage of the disease reduces treatment complications and drastically improves the prognosis, thus ensuring the most favorable outcome for patients.

Caroline Bissonnette, DMD
Adel Kauzman, BDS, DMD, MSc, FRCD(C)
Department of Stomatology
Faculty of Dental Medicine
Université de Montréal
Montreal, Quebec, Canada

References

Leemans C, et al.: The molecular landscape of head and neck cancer, *Nat Rev Cancer* 18:269–282, 2018.

Lingen MW, et al.: Low etiologic fraction for high-risk human papillomavirus in oral cavity squamous cell carcinomas, *Oral Oncol* 49(1):1–8, 2013.

Warnakulasuriya S, et al.: Oral potentially malignant disorders: a consensus report from an international seminar on nomenclature and classification, convened by the WHO Collaborating Centre for Oral Cancer, *Oral Dis* 8(27):1862–1880, 2020.

World Health Organization: Classification of head and neck tumours. In El-Naggar AK, et al., editors: *WHO/IARC classification of tumours*, ed 4, Geneva, Switzerland, 2017, WHO, vol. 9.

World Health Organization: *Lip, oral cavity factsheet. Globocan*, 2020. https://gco.iarc.fr/today/data/factsheets/cancers/1-Lip-oral-cavity-fact-sheet.pdf. Accessed April 8, 2023.

Permeability and Absorption

One function of the oral epithelium is forming an impermeable barrier; unlike the intestinal lining, the oral epithelium does not have an absorptive capacity. This permeability barrier consists of lipids derived from the membrane-coating granules that become aligned in a precise pattern after they are released in the intercellular spaces.

Differences in permeability exist between regions depending on the thickness of the epithelium and the pattern of maturation. Thus one of the thinnest epithelial regions, the floor of the mouth, is more permeable; certain drugs (e.g., nitroglycerin administered to relieve the pain of angina pectoris) are absorbed successfully when held under the tongue. Nevertheless, the oral mucosa clearly can limit the penetration of toxins and antigens produced by microorganisms present in the oral cavity, except in the specialized region of the dentogingival junction.

Nonkeratinocytes in the Oral Epithelium

Many histologic sections of oral epithelium contain a distinct cell type (clear cells) that differs in appearance from other epithelial cells because of a clear halo around the nuclei (Fig. 12.15). These nonkeratinocytes include pigment-producing cells (melanocytes), Langerhans cells, Merkel's cells, and inflammatory cells (e.g., lymphocytes); they make up as much as 10% of the cell population in the oral epithelium. All (except Merkel's cells) lack desmosomal attachments to adjacent cells so that during histologic processing the cytoplasm shrinks around the nucleus to produce the clear halo. None of these cells contain the large numbers of tonofilaments seen in epithelial keratinocytes, and none participate in the process of maturation seen in oral epithelia Table 12.2 summarizes their structure and function.

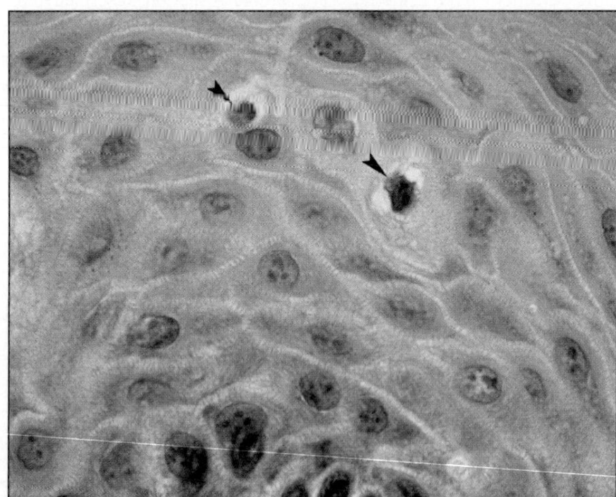

Fig. 12.15 Photomicrograph of the prickle cell layer of gingival epithelium. The clear cells *(arrowheads)* have dark nuclei surrounded by a light halo.

Melanocytes and Oral Pigmentation

The color of the oral mucosa is the net result of a number of factors, one of which is pigmentation. The pigments that most commonly contribute to the color of the oral mucosa are melanin and hemoglobin. Melanin is produced by specialized pigment cells (melanocytes) situated in the basal layer of the oral epithelium. Melanocytes arise embryologically from the neural crest ectoderm (see Chapter 2). In the epithelium they divide and maintain themselves as a self-reproducing population. Melanocytes possess long dendritic (branching) processes that extend between the keratinocytes, often passing through several layers of cells. Melanin is synthesized as small structures called melanosomes (Fig. 12.16), which are transferred into the cytoplasm of adjacent keratinocytes by the dendritic processes of melanocytes. Groups of melanosomes often can be identified under the light microscope in sections of heavily pigmented tissue stained with hematoxylin and eosin. These groups are referred to as *melanin granules*. In lightly pigmented tissues the presence of melanin can be demonstrated only by specific histologic and histochemical stains.

Lightly and darkly pigmented individuals have the same number of melanocytes in any given region of skin or oral mucosa; color differences result from the relative activity of the melanocytes in producing melanin and from the rate at which melanosomes are broken down in the keratinocytes. In persons with heavy melanin pigmentation, cells containing melanin originating from the uptake of melanosomes produced by melanocytes in the epithelium may be seen in the connective tissue. The regions of the oral mucosa where melanin pigmentation is seen most commonly clinically are the gingiva (Fig. 12.17), buccal mucosa, hard palate, and tongue. Despite considerable individual variation, a direct relationship tends to be seen between the degrees of pigmentation in the skin and in the oral mucosa. Light-skinned persons rarely show any oral melanin pigmentation.

Langerhans Cells

Another dendritic cell sometimes seen above the basal layers of epidermis and oral epithelium is the Langerhans cell. The Langerhans cell is

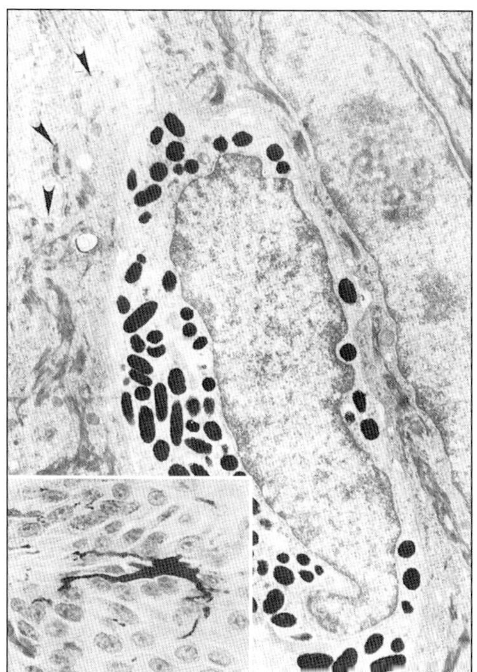

Fig. 12.16 Electron micrograph of a melanocyte in the basal layer of pigmented oral epithelium. The dense melanosomes are abundant. Arrowheads indicate the basal lamina. (Inset) Photomicrograph of a histologic section showing a dendritic melanocyte. The cell appears dark because it has been stained histochemically to reveal the presence of melanin.

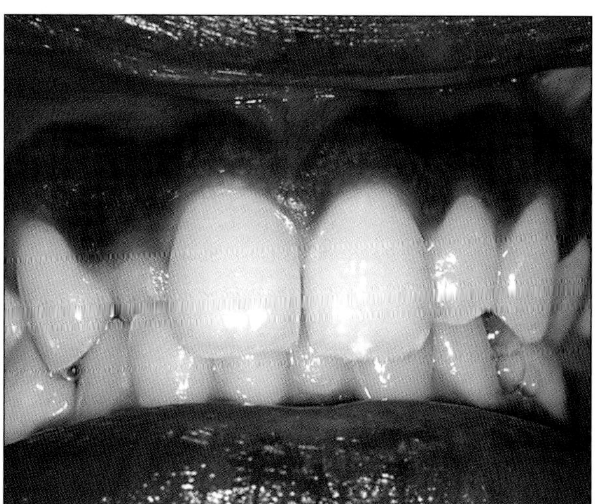

Fig. 12.17 Melanin pigmentation of the attached gingiva in a dark-skinned individual. (Courtesy A. Kauzman.)

characterized ultrastructurally by a small rod- or flask-shaped granule (Birbeck granule, after the person who first described it) (Fig. 12.18). The Langerhans cell usually is demonstrated by specific immunochemical reactions that stain cell-surface antigens.

Langerhans cells appear in the epithelium at the same time as, or just before, the melanocytes, and they may be capable of limited division within the epithelium. Unlike melanocytes, they move in and out of the epithelium, and their source is the bone marrow. Langerhans cells have an immunologic function, recognizing and processing antigenic material that enters the epithelium from the external environment and presenting it to T lymphocytes. Langerhans cells may migrate from epithelium to regional lymph nodes.

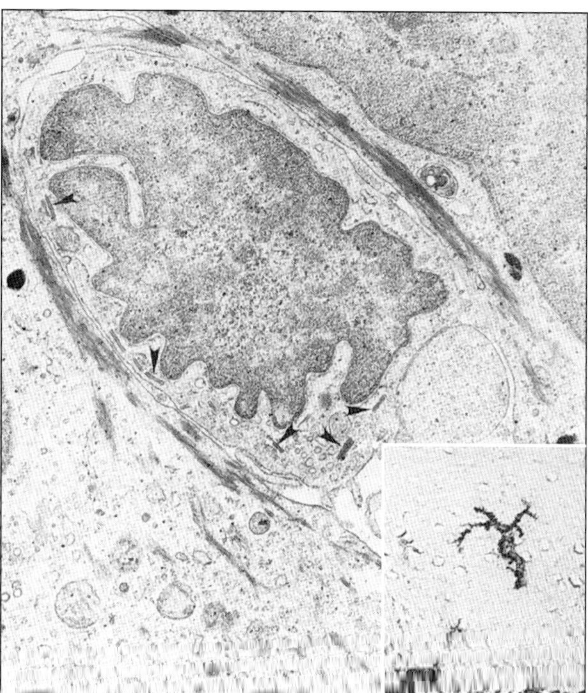

Fig. 12.18 Electron micrograph of a Langerhans cell from the oral epithelium. The cell has a convoluted nucleus and lacks tonofilaments and desmosome attachments to adjacent cells but contains a number of characteristic rodlike granules *(arrowheads)*. (Inset) A dendritic Langerhans cell in a light microscope preparation. Revealed by adenosine triphosphatase staining, the cell is visible in its characteristic suprabasal location. (Inset, Courtesy I.C. Mackenzie.)

Merkel's Cells

Merkel's cell is situated in the basal layer of the oral epithelium and epidermis. Unlike the melanocyte and Langerhans cell, Merkel's cell is not dendritic and possesses keratin tonofilaments and occasional desmosomes linking it to adjacent cells. The characteristic feature of Merkel's cells is the small membrane-bound vesicles in the cytoplasm, sometimes situated adjacent to a nerve fiber associated with the cell (Fig. 12.19). These granules may liberate a transmitter substance across the synapselike junction between Merkel's cell and the nerve fiber and thus trigger an impulse. This arrangement is in accord with neurophysiologic evidence suggesting that Merkel's cells are sensory and respond to touch. Merkel's cells arise from the differentiation of an epidermal progenitor during embryonic development.

Inflammatory Cells

When sections of epithelium taken from clinically normal areas of mucosa are examined microscopically, a number of inflammatory cells often can be seen in the nucleated cell layers. These cells are transient and do not reproduce themselves in the epithelium as the other nonkeratinocytes do. The most common cell type is the lymphocyte, although the presence of polymorphonuclear leukocytes and mast cells is not uncommon. Lymphocytes often are associated with Langerhans cells, which can activate them. A few inflammatory cells are commonplace in the oral epithelium and can be regarded as a normal component of the nonkeratinocyte population.

Clearly, the association between nonkeratinocytes and keratinocytes in skin and oral mucosa represents a subtle and finely balanced interrelationship in which cytokines are the controlling factors. Thus keratinocytes produce cytokines that modulate the function of Langerhans cells. In turn, the Langerhans cells produce cytokines such

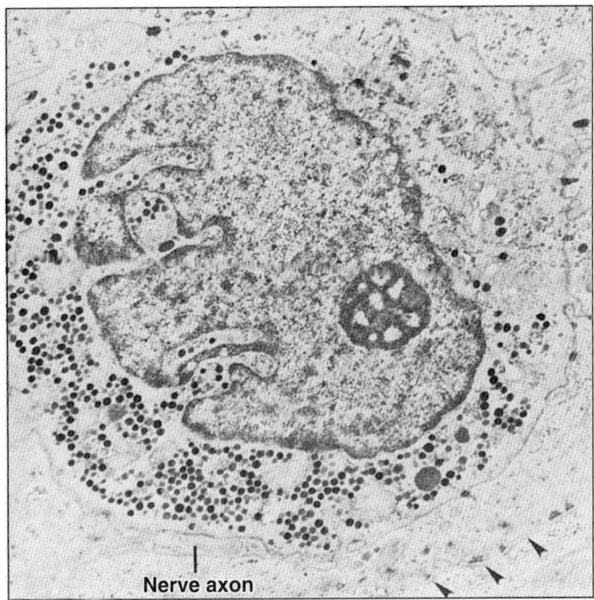

Fig. 12.19 Electron micrograph of Merkel's cell in the basal layer of oral epithelium. The cytoplasm of this cell is filled with small, dense vesicles situated close to an adjacent unmyelinated nerve axon. Arrowheads point to the site of the basal lamina. (Courtesy S.Y. Chen.)

as IL1, which can activate T lymphocytes so that they are capable of responding to antigenic challenge. IL1 also increases the number of receptors to melanocyte-stimulating hormone in melanocytes and so can affect pigmentation. The influence of keratinocytes extends to the adjacent connective tissue, where cytokines produced in the epithelium can influence the activity of fibroblasts.

JUNCTION OF THE EPITHELIUM AND LAMINA PROPRIA

The region where connective tissue of the lamina propria meets the overlying oral epithelium is an undulating interface at which papillae of the connective tissue interdigitate with the epithelial ridges. The connective tissue at the interface consists of ridges, conical papillae, or both, projecting into the epithelium (see Fig. 12.5). This arrangement makes the surface area of the interface larger than a simple flat junction providing better attachment and enabling forces applied at the surface of the epithelium to be dispersed over a greater area of connective tissue. In this respect, masticatory mucosa interestingly has the greatest number of papillae per unit area of mucosa; in lining mucosa, the papillae are fewer and shorter. The junction also represents a major interface for metabolic exchange between the epithelium and connective tissue because the epithelium has no blood vessels.

Basal laminae cannot be visualized directly by light microscopy. In histologic sections of oral mucosa stained by the periodic acid–Schiff reaction, the basal lamina appears as a bright, structureless band at the interface between the epithelium and subjacent connective tissue (see Fig. 12.5A). The basal lamina runs parallel to the basal cell membrane of the epithelial cells; at the ultrastructural level it consists of three zones: lamina lucida, lamina densa, and lamina fibroreticularis. The lamina densa appears as a homogeneous, finely fibrillar planar assembly of extracellular matrix molecules separated from the adjacent cell by the lamina lucida. The latter appears as a clear zone but is not always evident (Fig. 12.20C). The lamina densa consists essentially of a supramolecular network of type IV collagen and laminins. Additional proteins such as heparan sulfate proteoglycan (perlecan), nidogen, and fibulin reinforce this network (see Fig. 12.20C). The lamina lucida essentially contains two membrane-spanning components (i.e., integrin $\alpha_6\beta_4$ and collagen XVII [also known as the *bullous pemphigoid antigen BPAG2*]). Integrin $\alpha_6\beta_4$ acts as a receptor for laminin-332 found in the basal lamina and is thus not part of the hemidesmosome. Collagen type VII anchoring fibrils found in the lamina densa anchor the basal lamina and subjacent connective tissue. Most of the basal lamina components are synthesized by the epithelium (some components of the lamina fibroreticularis are produced by connective tissue cells such as fibroblasts).

Several genetic defects and autoimmune diseases cause defects in the basal lamina. When the mucosa blisters, as in the lesions of pemphigoid, separation of the epithelium from connective tissue occurs at the level of the lamina lucida. This separation is believed to result when individuals produce antibodies that attack the basal lamina BPAG2 (collagen type VII). Mutations in integrin and laminin-332 genes also can cause blistering, the later at the basal lamina connective tissue interface.

LAMINA PROPRIA

The connective tissue supporting the oral epithelium is termed *lamina propria* and consists of cells, blood vessels, neural elements, and fibers embedded in an amorphous ground substance (Fig. 12.21B). For descriptive purposes it can be divided into two layers: the superficial papillary layer (associated with the epithelial ridges) and the deeper reticular layer (which lies between the papillary layer and the underlying structures). The term *reticular* in this case means "net-like" and refers to the arrangement of the collagen fibers. The difference between these two layers reflects the relative concentration and arrangement of the collagen fibers. In the papillary layer, collagen fibers are thin and loosely arranged, and many capillary loops are present. By contrast, the reticular layer has collagen fibers arranged in thick bundles that tend to lie parallel to the surface plane (see Fig. 12.21B).

Like the overlying oral epithelium, the lamina propria shows regional variation in the proportions of its constituent elements, particularly in the concentration and organization of fibers.

Cells

The lamina propria contains several different cells, including fibroblasts, macrophages, mast cells, and lymphocytes. As in other parts of the body, the type of inflammatory cell depends on the nature and duration of the injury. In acute conditions, polymorphonuclear leukocytes are the dominant cell type, whereas more chronic conditions (e.g., periodontal disease) are associated with lymphocytes, plasma cells, monocytes, and macrophages. Table 12.3 lists the major cells of the lamina propria.

Fibroblasts

The principal cell in the lamina propria of oral mucosa is the fibroblast, which is responsible for the elaboration and turnover of fiber and ground substance (Fig. 12.22). The fibroblast thus plays a key role in maintaining tissue connective integrity (see Chapter 4). Fibroblasts have a low rate of proliferation in adult oral mucosa except during wound healing, when their numbers increase because of fibroblast division in the adjacent uninjured tissues. Fibroblasts can become contractile and participate in wound contraction, in which case their actin content increases. In certain disease states (e.g., the gingival overgrowth sometimes seen with phenytoin; calcium channel blockers such as nifedipine; and cyclosporine A, an immunosuppressant drug used

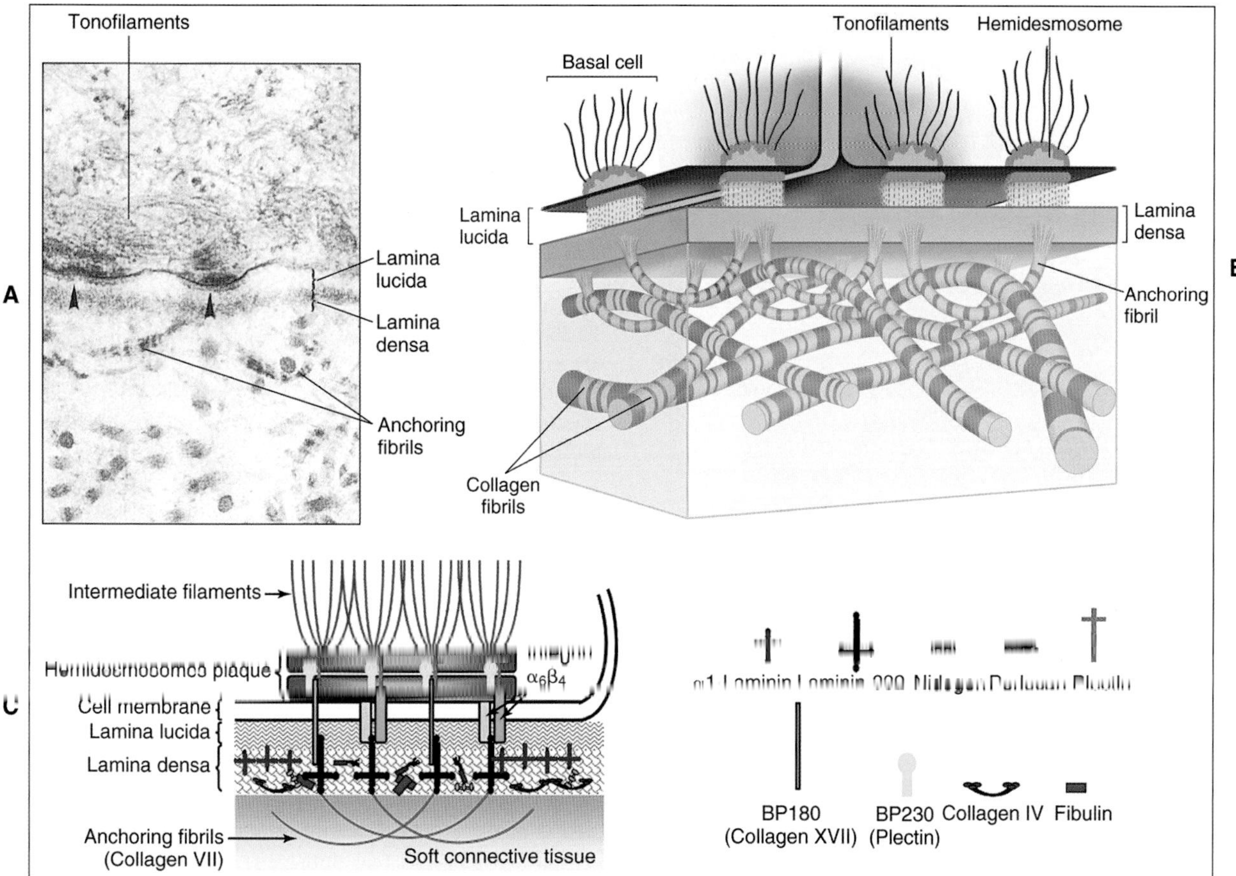

Fig. 12.20 Ultrastructure of basal lamina. (A) High-magnification electron micrograph of the complex in oral mucosa. Hemidesmosomes *(arrowheads)* at the plasma membrane of epithelial basal cells receive bundles of intermediate filaments (tonofilaments). Adjacent to the membrane are the lamina lucida and lamina densa. Several striated anchoring fibrils loop into the lamina densa, and some contain within their loops cross sections of collagen fibrils. (B) Schematic representation of the junction between epithelium and connective tissue. (C) The location of principal molecular constituents of the junction.

in organ transplants), fibroblasts may be activated and secrete more ground substance than normal.

Macrophages

Under light microscope the macrophage is difficult to distinguish from fibroblasts unless it has phagocyted extracellular debris. Ultrastructurally, macrophages have smaller and denser nuclei and less-developed protein synthetic organelles (Fig. 12.23). The macrophage has a number of functions, the principal one being to ingest damaged tissue or foreign material in phagocytic vacuoles that fuse intracytoplasmically with lysosomes and initiate breakdown of these materials. The processing of ingested material by the macrophage may be important in increasing its antigenicity before it is presented to cells of the lymphoid series for subsequent immunologic response. Another important function is the stimulation of fibroblast proliferation necessary for repair.

In the lamina propria of the oral mucosa, two special types of macrophages can be identified specifically: the melanophage and the siderophage. The melanophage, which is common in pigmented oral mucosa, is a cell that has ingested melanin granules extruded from melanocytes within the epithelium. The siderophage is a cell that contains hemosiderin derived from red blood cells that have been extravasated into the tissues as a result of mechanical injury. This material can persist within the siderophage for some time, and the resultant brownish color appears clinically as a bruise.

Mast Cells

The mast cell is a large spheric or elliptic mononuclear cell (Fig. 12.24). The nucleus of the mast cell is small relative to the size of the cell and in histologic preparations commonly is obscured by the large number of intensely staining granules that occupy mast cell cytoplasm. In humans the principal contents of the granules are histamine and heparin.

This immune response cell produces a plethora of molecules implicated in protection against pathogens and in the inflammatory response. Among these, histamine is known to be important in initiating the vascular phase of an inflammatory process.

Lymphocytes

Histologically, the lymphocyte and plasma cell (B-lymphocyte–secreting antibodies) may be observed in small numbers scattered throughout the lamina propria, but apart from specialized regions such as the lingual tonsil, other inflammatory cells are found in significant numbers only in connective tissue, after an injury (e.g., a surgical incision), or as part of a disease process. When inflammatory cells are present in significant numbers, they influence the behavior of the overlying epithelium by releasing cytokines.

Fibers and Ground Substance

The intercellular matrix of the lamina propria consists of two major types of fibers, collagen and elastin, that together with fibronectin

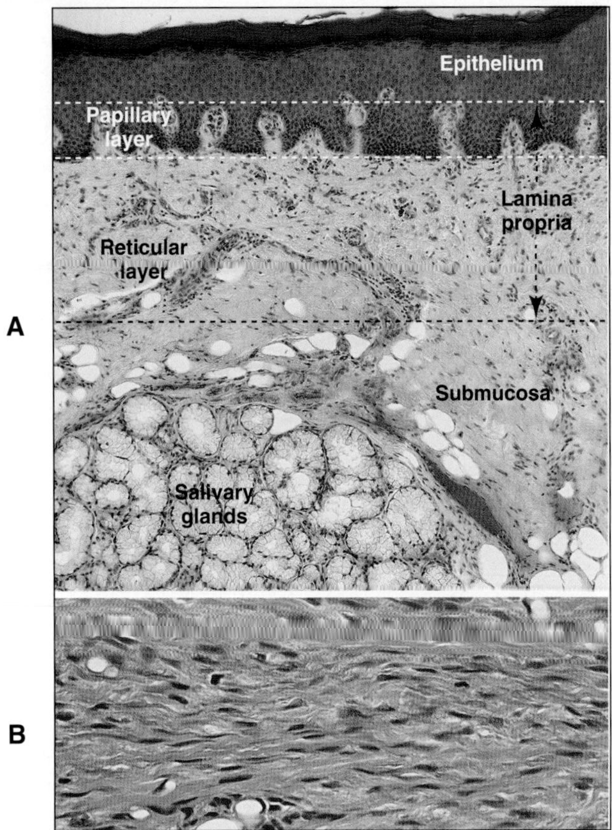

Fig. 12.21 (A) Photomicrograph of palatal mucosa showing the approximate boundaries of the papillary and reticular layers. The group of minor salivary glands in the submucosa is apparent. (B) Higher magnification in the region of the reticular layer showing cells, mostly fibroblasts, and densely packed collagen bundles.

embed in a ground substance composed of glycosaminoglycans and serum-derived proteins, all of which are highly hydrated.

Collagen

Collagen in the lamina propria is primarily types I and III, with types IV and VII occurring as part of the basal lamina. Type V may be present in inflamed tissue. (A full account of the biology of collagen is given in Chapter 4.)

Elastic Fibers

When stained using specific methods, some elastic fibers (see Fig. 12.23) can be seen in most regions of the oral mucosa, but they are more abundant in the flexible lining mucosa, where they function to restore tissue form after stretching. Unlike collagen fibers, elastic fibers branch, anastomose, and run singly rather than in bundles.

Ground Substance

Although the ground substance of the lamina propria appears by light and electron microscopy to be amorphous at the molecular level, it consists of heterogeneous molecular complexes permeated by tissue fluid. Chemically these complexes can be subdivided into two distinct groups: proteoglycans and glycoproteins.

The proteoglycans consist of a polypeptide core to which glycosaminoglycans (consisting of hexose and hexuronic acid residues) are attached. In the oral mucosa the proteoglycans are represented by hyaluronan, heparan sulfate, versican, decorin, biglycan, and syndecan. Proteoglycans in the matrix are different from those associated with the cell surface, and interaction between them and with cell surface molecules (e.g., integrins) is probably important in modulating the behavior and function of the cell. The glycoproteins, by contrast, have a polypeptide chain to which only a few simple hexoses are attached.

TABLE 12.3 Cell Types in the Lamina Propria of Oral Mucosa

Cell Type	Morphologic Characteristics	Function	Distribution
Fibroblast	Stellate or elongated with abundant rough endoplasmic reticulum	Secretion of fibers and ground substance	Throughout lamina propria
Histiocyte	Spindle-shaped or stellate; often dark-staining nucleus; many lysosomal vesicles	Resident precursor of functional macrophage	Throughout lamina propria
Macrophage	Round with pale-staining nucleus; contains lysosomes and phagocytic vesicles	Phagocytosis, including antigen processing	Areas of chronic inflammation
Mast cell	Round or oval with basophilic granules staining metachromatically	Secretion of certain inflammatory mediators and vasoactive agents (histamine, heparin, serotonin)	Throughout lamina propria; often subepithelial
Polymorphonuclear leukocyte (neutrophil)	Round with characteristic lobed nucleus; contains lysosomes and specific granules	Phagocytosis and cell killing	Areas of acute inflammation within lamina propria; may be present in epithelium
Lymphocyte	Round with dark-staining nucleus and scant cytoplasm with some mitochondria	Some lymphocytes participate in humoral or cell-mediated immune response	Areas of acute and chronic inflammation
Plasma cell	Cartwheel nucleus; intensely basophilic cytoplasm with abundant rough endoplasmic reticula	Synthesis of immunoglobulins	Areas of chronic inflammation, often perivascularly
Endothelial cell	Normally associated with a basal lamina; contains numerous pinocytotic vesicles	Lining of blood and lymphatic channels	Lining vascular channels throughout lamina propria

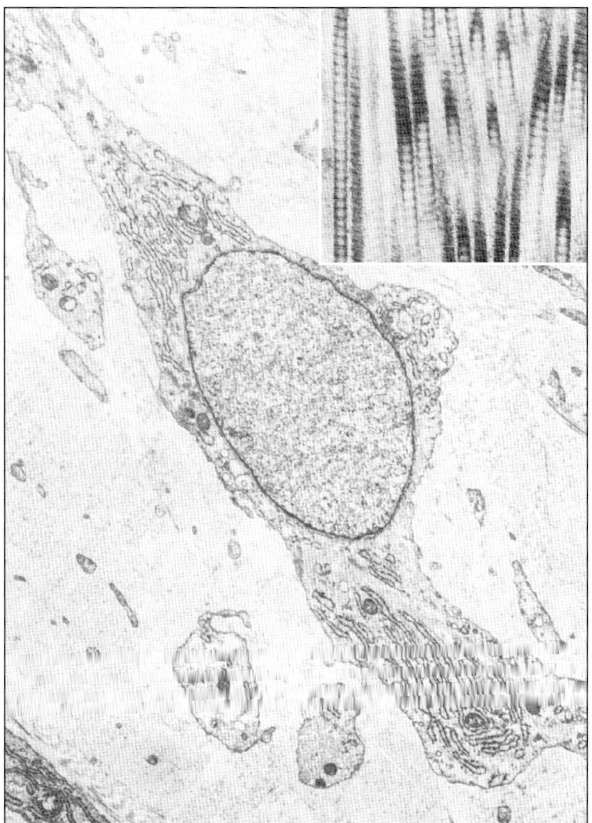

Fig. 12.22 Electron micrograph of a fibroblast in the lamina propria. (Inset) Collagen type I fibrils. The typical cross-banding pattern is apparent.

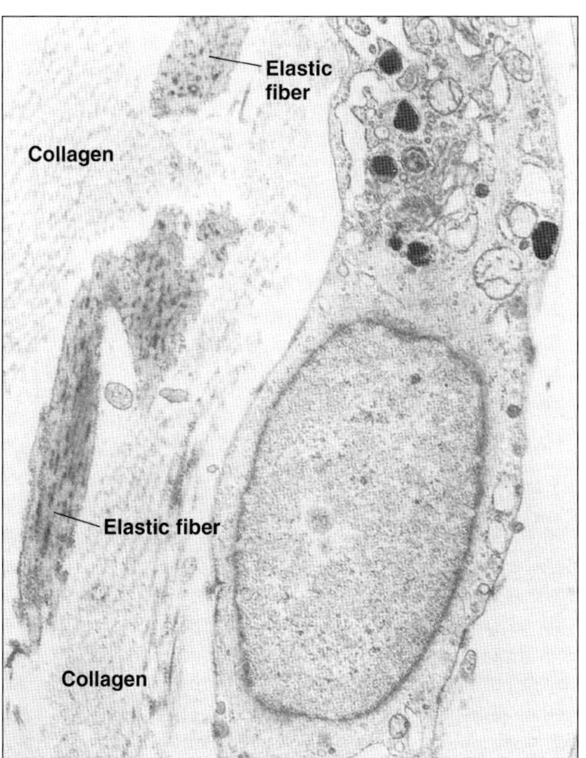

Fig. 12.23 Electron micrograph of a macrophage in the lamina propria. The cell has a number of phagosomes containing dense material. Adjacent to the cell are elastic fibers composed of filaments embedded in a less dense matrix; they appear distinctly different from the adjacent collagen.

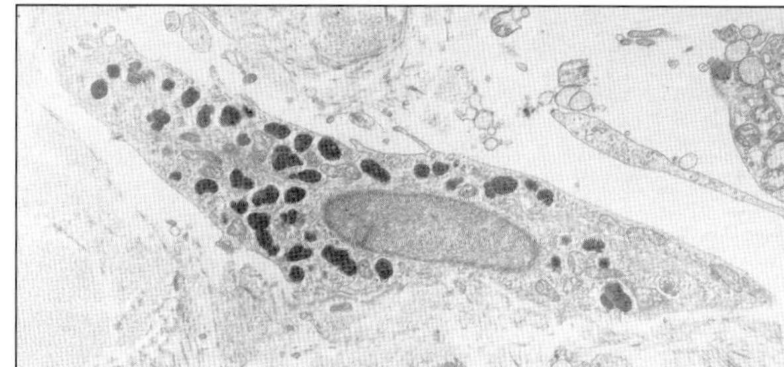

Fig. 12.24 Electron micrograph of a mast cell from the lamina propria. The dense granules in the cytoplasm, characteristic of this cell type in human beings, are apparent.

BLOOD SUPPLY

The blood supply of the oral mucosa (Table 12.4) is rich and is derived from arteries that run parallel to the surface in the submucosa or, when the mucosa is tightly bound to underlying periosteum and a submucosa is absent, in the deep part of the reticular layer. These vessels give off progressively smaller branches that anastomose with adjacent vessels in the reticular layer before forming an extensive capillary network in the papillary layer immediately subjacent to the basal epithelial cells. From this network, capillary loops pass into the connective tissue papillae and come to lie close to the basal layer of the epithelium (Fig. 12.25). The arrangement in oral mucosa is much more profuse than in skin, where capillary loops are found only in association with hair follicles (which may explain the deeper color of oral mucosa).

Regional modifications occur in this basic pattern. In tissues such as the cheek, where the connective tissues may undergo extensive deformation, the arterioles follow a tortuous path and show more extensive branching.

Blood flow through the oral mucosa is greatest in the gingiva, but in all regions of the oral mucosa blood flow is greater than in the skin at normal temperatures. To what extent inflammation of the gingiva (gingivitis), which is almost inevitably present, may be responsible for this greater flow is uncertain. Unlike the skin, which plays a role in temperature regulation, human oral mucosa lacks arteriovenous shunts but has rich anastomoses of arterioles and capillaries, which undoubtedly contribute to its ability to heal more rapidly than skin after injury.

NERVE SUPPLY

Because the mouth is the gateway to the alimentary and respiratory tracts, the oral mucous membrane is innervated densely so that it can monitor all substances entering. A rich innervation also serves to initiate and maintain a variety of voluntary and reflexive activities involved in mastication, salivation, swallowing, gagging, and speaking. The nerve supply to the oral mucous membrane is therefore overwhelmingly sensory (Table 12.5).

The efferent supply is autonomic, supplies the blood vessels and minor salivary glands, and may modulate the activity of some sensory receptors. The nerves arise mainly from the second and third divisions of the trigeminal nerve, but afferent fibers of the facial (VII), glossopharyngeal (IX), and vagus (X) nerves also are involved. The sensory nerves lose their myelin sheaths and form a network in the reticular layer of the lamina propria that terminates in a subepithelial plexus.

The sensory nerves terminate in free and organized nerve endings. Free nerve endings are found in the lamina propria and within the epithelium, where they commonly are associated with Merkel's cells. Apart from the nerves associated with Merkel's cells, intraepithelial nerve endings have a sensory function. Such nerves are not surrounded

TABLE 12.4 Arterial Blood Supply to the Oral Mucosa

Oral Region	Subterminal Branches
Upper lip	Superior labial artery (anastomoses with buccal artery)
Upper gingiva	
Anterior	Anterior superior alveolar artery
Lingual	Major palatine artery
Buccal	Buccal artery
Posterior	Posterior superior alveolar artery
Hard palate	Major palatine artery
	Nasopalatine artery
	Sphenopalatine artery
Soft palate	Minor palatine artery
Cheek	Buccal artery
	Some terminal branches of facial artery
	Posterior alveolar artery
	Infraorbital artery
Lower lip	Inferior labial artery (anastomoses with buccal artery)
	Mental artery
	Branch of inferior alveolar artery
Lower gingiva	
Anterior buccal	Mental artery
Anterior lingual	Incisive artery and sublingual artery
Posterior lingual	Inferior alveolar artery and sublingual artery
Posterior buccal	Inferior alveolar artery and buccal artery
Floor of mouth	Sublingual artery
	Branch of lingual artery
Tongue (dorsal and ventral surfaces)	
Anterior two-thirds	Deep lingual artery
Posterior one-third	Dorsal lingual artery to base of tongue about posterior third

From Stablein MJ, Meyer J: The vascular system and blood supply. In Meyer J, et al., editors: *The structure and function of oral mucosa,* New York, NY, 1984, Pergamon Press.

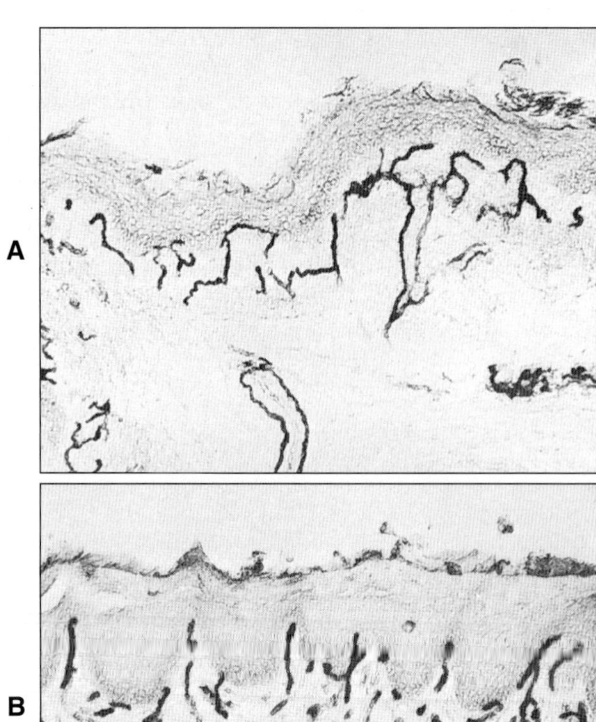

Fig. 12.25 Micrographs showing the relationships between capillaries in the lamina propria and overlying epithelium. Mucosal epithelium is from the floor of the mouth (A) and the cheek (B). The sections were prepared to demonstrate histochemically the distribution of alkaline phosphatase. In (B), staining of the muscle also occurred. (Courtesy G. Zoot.)

by Schwann cells as in connective tissue but run between the keratinocytes (which may ensheath the nerves and so form a mesaxon). These nerves terminate as simple endings in the middle (or upper) layers of the epithelium (Fig. 12.26).

Within the lamina propria, organized nerve endings usually are found in the papillary region. They consist of groups of coiled fibers surrounded by a connective tissue capsule. These specialized endings have been grouped according to their morphology as Meissner or Ruffini corpuscles, Krause bulbs, and the mucocutaneous end-organs. The density of sensory receptors is greater in the anterior part of the mouth than in the posterior region, with the greatest density where the connective tissue papillae are most prominent.

The primary sensations perceived in the oral cavity are warmth, cold, touch, pain, and taste. Although specialized nerve endings are differentially sensitive to particular modalities (e.g., Krause bulbs appear to be most sensitive to cold stimuli and Meissner corpuscles to touch), no evidence indicates that any one receptor is responsible for detecting only one type of stimulus. Possibly, however, each modality is served by specific fibers associated with each termination.

Sensory nerve networks are more developed in the oral mucosa lining the anterior than in the posterior regions of the mouth, and this pattern is paralleled by the greater sensitivity of this region to a number of modalities. For example, touch sensation is most acute in the anterior part of the tongue and hard palate. By comparison, the sensitivity of the fingertips falls between those of the tongue and the palate. Touch receptors in the soft palate and oropharynx are important in the initiation of swallowing, gagging, and retching. Similarly, temperature reception is more acute in the vermilion border of the lip, at the tip of the tongue, and on the anterior hard palate than in more posterior regions of the oral cavity. The detection of pain is understood poorly. The sensation of pain appears to be initiated by noxious stimuli causing tissue damage and thereby activating polypeptides in the interstitial fluid, which in turn act on free nerve endings of slow-conducting unmyelinated and thin myelinated nerves.

A specialized receptor that occurs only in the oral cavity and pharynx is the taste bud. Although some taste buds lie within the epithelium of the soft palate and pharynx, most are found in the fungiform, foliate, and circumvallate papillae of the tongue (Figs. 12.27 and 12.28).

Histologically, the taste bud is a barrel-shaped structure composed of 30 to 80 spindle-shaped cells (see Fig. 12.28C). At their bases, the cells are separated from underlying connective tissue by the basal lamina, whereas their apical ends terminate just below the epithelial surface in a taste pit that communicates with the surface through a small

TABLE 12.5 Principal Sensory Nerve Fibers Supplying the Oral Mucosa

Oral Region	Innervation
Upper lip and vestibule	Twigs from infraorbital branch of maxillary nerve
Upper gingivae	Anterior, posterior, and (when present) middle superior alveolar branches of maxillary nerve
Hard palate	Greater, lesser, and sphenopalatine branches of maxillary nerve
Soft palate	Lesser palatine branch of maxillary nerve, tonsillar branch of glossopharyngeal nerve, and nerve of pterygoid canal (taste; originating from facial nerve)
Cheek	Twigs from infraorbital branch of maxillary nerve, superior alveolar branch of maxillary nerve, buccal branch of mandibular nerve, and possibly some terminal branches of facial nerve
Lower lip and vestibule	Mental branch of inferior alveolar nerve and buccal branch of mandibular nerve
Lower gingivae: buccal	Inferior alveolar branch of mandibular nerve, buccal branch of mandibular nerve, and sublingual branch lingual of lingual nerve
Anterior two-thirds of tongue	Lingual branch of mandibular nerve (taste provided by fibers carried in lingual nerve but originating in facial nerve and passing by way of chorda tympani to the lingual nerve)
Posterior one-third of tongue, facial, and tonsillar	Glossopharyngeal nerve (taste and general sensation)

From Holland GR: Innervation of oral mucosa and sensory perception. In Meyer J, et al., editors: *The structure and function of oral mucosa*, New York, NY, 1984, Pergamon Press.

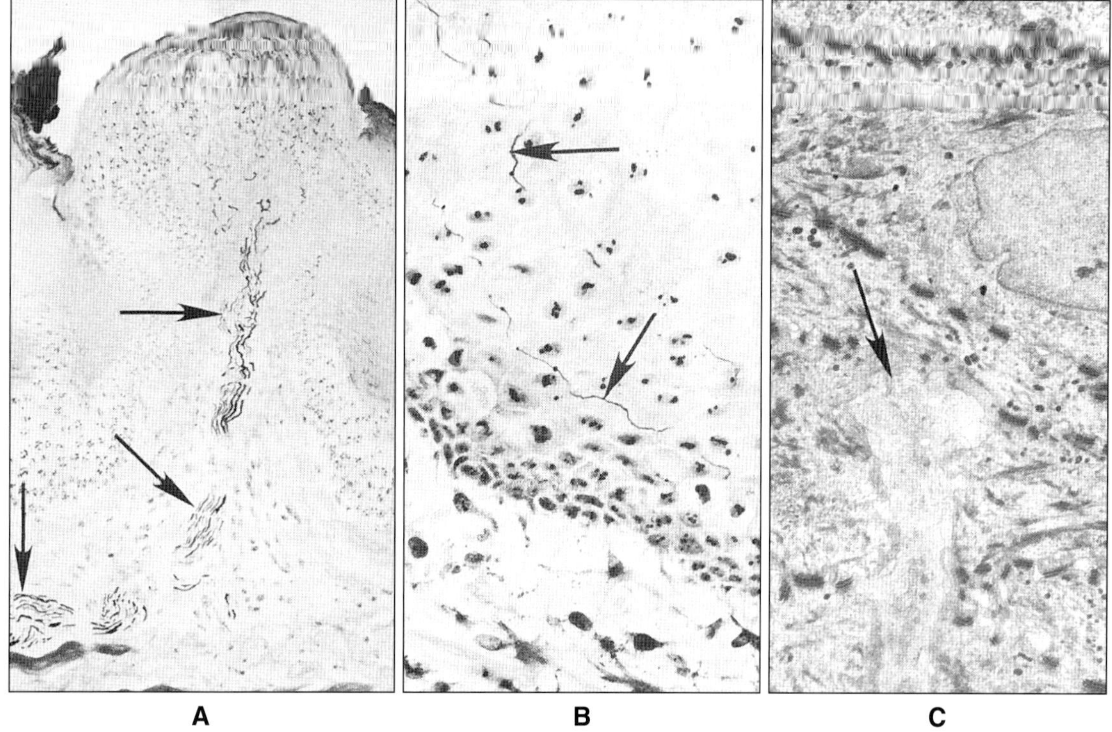

Fig. 12.26 Nerves in the oral mucosa. (A) A nerve bundle *(arrows)* running into the epithelium of a fungiform papilla on the dorsum of the tongue. (B) The appearance of intraepithelial nerves *(arrows)* running between cells of the buccal epithelium. (C) An electron micrograph of a free nerve ending *(arrow)* between the upper prickle cells in human gingiva. (A, B, Courtesy J. Linder.)

opening (taste pore). The cells of the taste bud have been divided into three types: dark (type I), light (type II), and intermediate (type III). Type I (dark) cells are the most common, representing about half of all cells in the taste bud and are generally considered to be support cells that resemble glial cells in the nervous system. These dark cells show an electron-dense cytoplasm and elongated nuclei. Type II cells are more spindle-shaped cells than type I cells. They are also called receptor cells and contain G protein–coupled receptors for bitter, sweet, and umami taste stimuli. Type II cells express voltage-gated sodium and potassium channels essential for producing action potentials. They are replaced continually, and their existence depends on a functional gustatory nerve. Type III (presynaptic) cells are the most neuronlike cells. They exhibit well-defined synapses onto afferent nerve fiber and release the neurotransmitters serotonin and gamma-aminobutyric acid in response to sour taste stimuli. The apical ends of these cells are joined tightly together by junctional complexes, somewhat like those in intestinal mucosa, so that the initial events stimulating sensation of taste appear to involve the amorphous material within the taste pits and the microvilli of constituent cells that project into those pits. Taste stimuli probably are generated by the adsorption of molecules onto membrane receptors on the surface of the taste bud cells, which activates a signaling cascade mediated by membrane-associated proteins, such as transducin and gustducin. The change in membrane polarization that follows stimulates release of transmitter substances, which

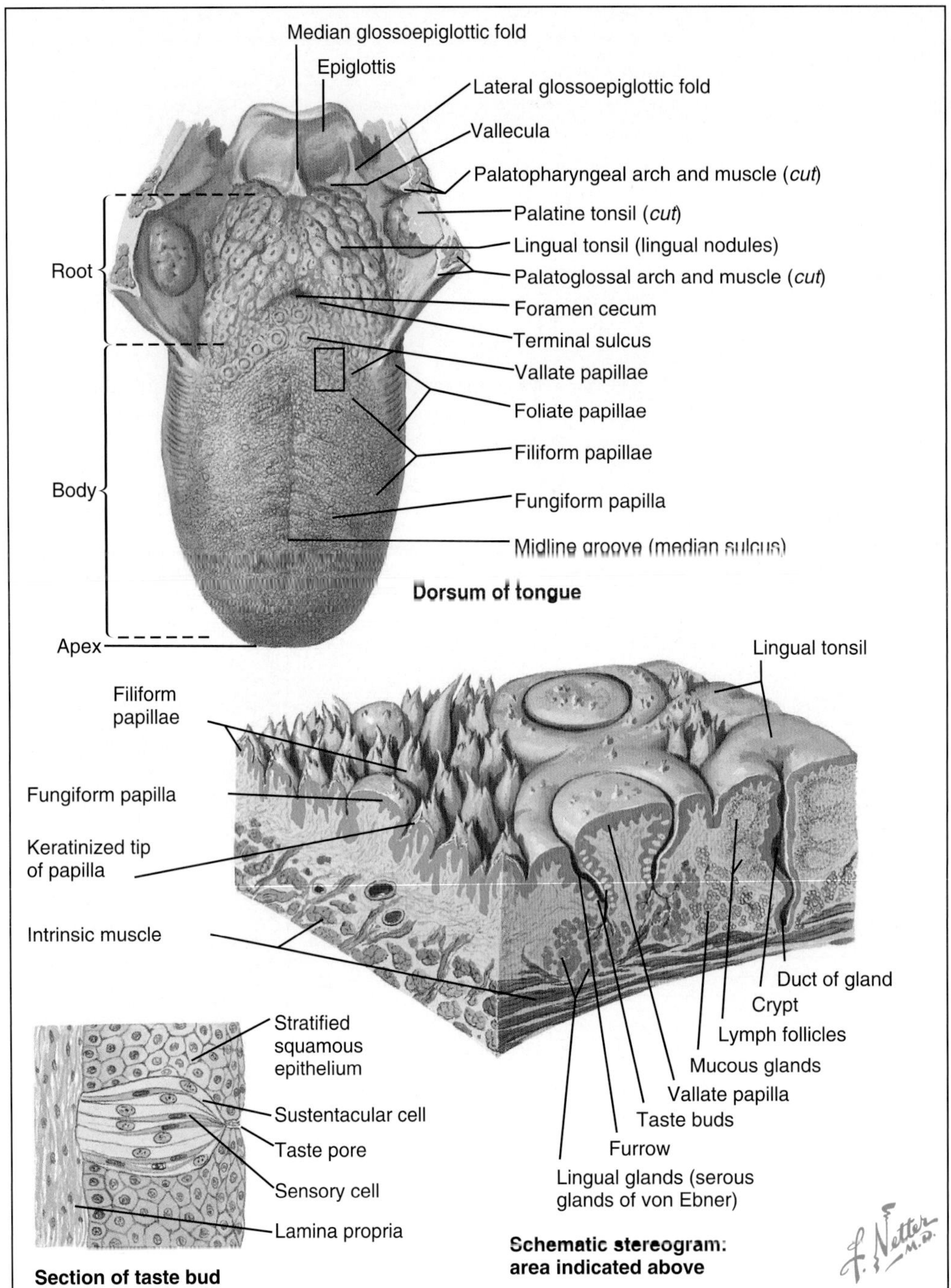

Fig. 12.27 Schematic representation of the distribution and types of lingual papillae on its dorsal surface. (Netter illustration from www.netterimages.com. © Elsevier, Inc. All rights reserved.)

in turn stimulate unmyelinated afferent fibers of the glossopharyngeal nerve (IX) that surround the lower half of the taste cells. Taste bud cells, with Merkel's cells, are the only truly specialized sensory cells in the oral mucosa.

Although the sensitivity of taste buds to sweet, salty, sour, and bitter substances shows regional variation (sweet at the tip, salty and sour on the lateral aspects, and bitter and sour in the posterior region of the tongue), no distinct structural differences have been observed among taste buds in these regions. The identification of different substances likely depends on binding different membrane receptors.

STRUCTURAL VARIATIONS

By now it should be apparent that the human oral mucosa shows considerable variation in structure not only in the composition of the lamina propria, form of the interface between epithelium and connective tissue, and type of surface epithelium but also in the nature of the submucosa and how the mucosa is attached to underlying structures. Fortunately, the organization of component tissues shows similar patterns in many regions. The oral mucosa can be divided into three main types: masticatory, lining, and specialized. The areas occupied by each type are illustrated in Fig. 12.1. In the following

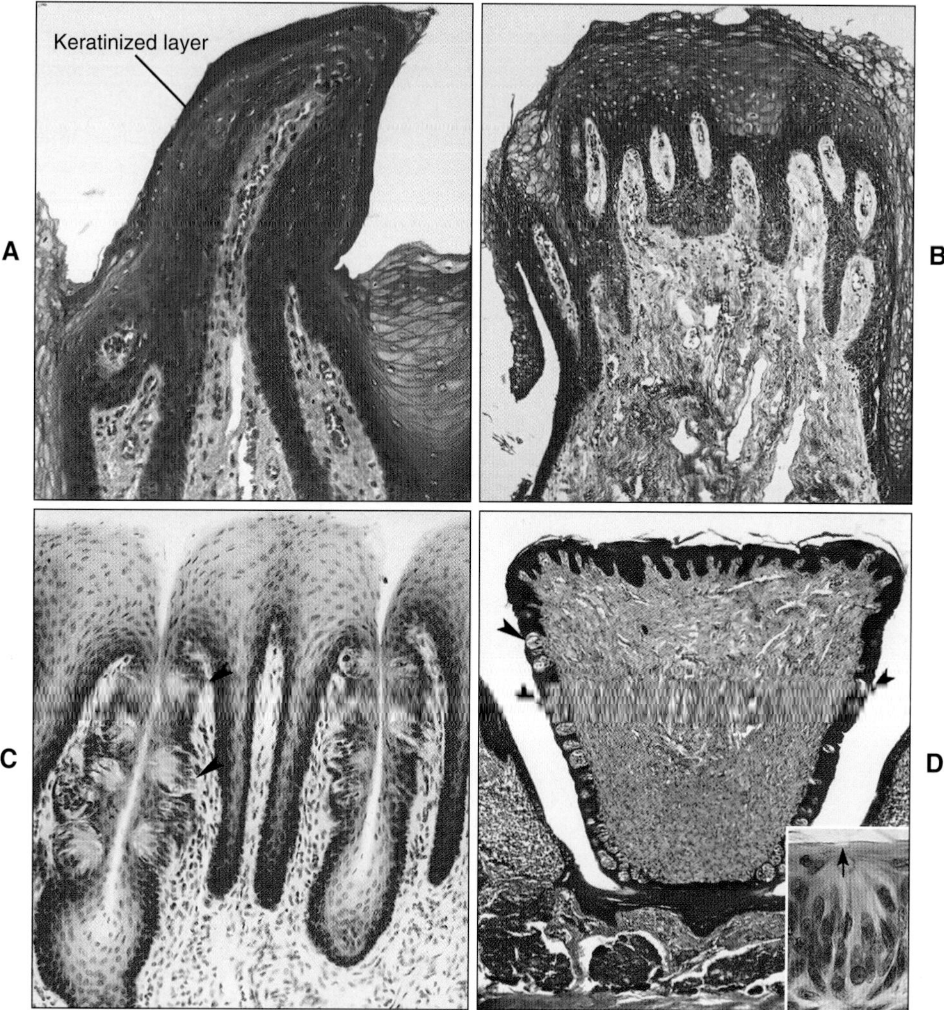

Fig. 12.28 Histologic sections of four types of lingual papillae. (A) Filiform papilla and (B) a fungiform papilla from the anterior part of the tongue. The epithelium of the filiform papillae is keratinized; that of the fungiform papilla is keratinized thinly or nonkeratinized. (C) Section through foliate papillae. The nonkeratinized epithelium covering the papillae contains numerous taste buds *(arrowheads)* situated laterally. (D) Histologic section through a circumvallate papilla from the dorsum of the tongue. A deep groove runs around the papilla, and the glands of Ebner empty into it. The arrowheads indicate the numerous taste buds on the lateral walls of the papilla. (Inset) Enlarged view of a taste bud with its barrel-like appearance and apical pore *(arrow)*. (Courtesy B. Kablar.)

sections, each type of mucosa is described. A summary of the structures within the various anatomic regions occupied by each appears in Table 12.6. Finally, a brief account is given of several junctions between different types of mucosa that are of morphologic interest and clinical importance.

Masticatory Mucosa

Masticatory mucosa covers those areas of the oral cavity such as the hard palate (Fig. 12.29) and gingiva (Fig. 12.30) that are exposed to compressive and shear forces and to abrasion during the mastication of food. The dorsum of the tongue has the same functional role as other masticatory mucosa, but because of its specialized structure it is considered separately.

The epithelium of masticatory mucosa is moderately thick and commonly orthokeratinized, although normally parakeratinized areas of the gingiva and occasionally of the palate occur. Both types of epithelial surface are inextensible and well adapted to withstanding abrasion. The junction between epithelium and underlying lamina propria is convoluted, and the numerous elongated papillae probably provide good mechanical attachment and prevent the epithelium from being stripped off under shear force. The lamina propria is thick, containing a dense network of collagen fibers in the form of large, closely packed bundles. They follow a direct course between anchoring points so that the tissue has little slack and does not yield on impact, enabling the mucosa to resist heavy loading.

Masticatory mucosa covers immobile structures (e.g., the palate and alveolar processes) and is bound firmly to them directly by the attachment of lamina propria to the periosteum of underlying bone, such as in mucoperiosteum, or indirectly by a fibrous submucosa. In the lateral regions of the palate, this fibrous submucosa is interspersed with areas of fat and glandular tissue that cushion the mucosa against mechanical loads and protect the underlying nerves and blood vessels of the palate.

Lining Mucosa

The oral mucosa that covers the underside of the tongue (Fig. 12.31), inside of the lips (Fig. 12.32), cheeks, floor of the mouth, and alveolar processes as far as the gingiva (see Fig. 12.30) is subject to movement.

TABLE 12.6 Structure of the Mucosa in Different Regions of the Oral Cavity

Region	Covering Epithelium	Lamina Propria	Submucosa
Lining Mucosa			
Soft palate	Thin, nonkeratinized stratified squamous epithelium; taste buds present	Thick with numerous short papillae; elastic fibers forming on elastic lamina; highly vascular with well-defined capillary network	Diffuse tissue containing numerous minor salivary glands
Ventral surface of tongue	Thin, nonkeratinized, stratified squamous epithelium	Thin with numerous short papillae and some elastic fibers; a few minor salivary glands; capillary network in subpapillary layer; reticular layer relatively avascular	Thin and irregular; may contain fat and small vessels; where absent, mucosa is bound to connective tissue surrounding tongue musculature
Floor of mouth	Very thin, nonkeratinized, stratified squamous epithelium	Short papillae; some elastic fibers; extensive vascular supply with short anastomosing capillary loops	Loose fibrous connective tissue containing fat and minor salivary glands
Alveolar mucosa	Thin, nonkeratinized, stratified squamous epithelium	Short papillae, connective tissue containing many elastic fibers; capillary loops close to the surface supplied by vessels running superficially to the periosteum	Loose connective tissue containing thick elastic fibers attaching it to periosteum of alveolar process; minor salivary glands
Labial and buccal mucosa	Very thick, nonkeratinized, stratified squamous epithelium	Long, slender papillae; dense fibrous connective tissue containing collagen and some elastic fibers; rich vascular supply giving off anastomosing capillary loops into papillae	Mucosa firmly attached to underlying muscle by collagen and elastin; dense collagenous connective tissue with fat, minor salivary glands, and sometimes sebaceous glands
Lips: vermilion zone	Thin, orthokeratinized, stratified squamous epithelium	Numerous narrow papillae; capillary loops close to surface in papillary layer	Mucosa firmly attached to underlying muscle; some sebaceous glands in vermilion border, minor salivary gland and fat in intermediate zone
Lips: intermediate zone	Thin, parakeratinized, stratified squamous epithelium	Long, irregular papillae; elastic and collagen fibers in connective tissue	–
Masticatory Mucosa			
Gingiva	Thick, orthokeratinized or parakeratinized, stratified squamous epithelium often showing stippled surface	Long, narrow papillae; dense collagenous connective tissue; not highly vascular but has long capillary loops with numerous anastomoses	No distinct layer; mucosa firmly attached by collagen fibers to cementum and periosteum of alveolar process (mucoperiosteum)
Hard palate	Thick, orthokeratinized (often parakeratinized in parts), stratified squamous epithelium thrown into transverse palatine ridges (rugae)	Long papillae; thick, dense collagenous tissue, especially under rugae; moderate vascular supply with short capillary loops	Dense collagenous connective tissue attaching mucosa to periosteum (mucoperiosteum); fat and minor salivary glands are packed into connective tissue in regions where mucosa overlies lateral palatine neurovascular bundles
Specialized Mucosa			
Dorsal surface of tongue	Thick, keratinized and nonkeratinized, stratified squamous epithelium forming three types of lingual papillae, some bearing taste buds	Long papillae; minor salivary glands in posterior portion; rich innervation especially near taste buds; capillary plexus in papillary layer; large vessels lying deeper	No distinct layer; mucosa is bound to connective tissue surrounding musculature of tongue

These regions, together with the soft palate, are classified as lining mucosa.

The epithelium of lining mucosa is nonkeratinized and generally thin. The surface is thus flexible and able to withstand stretching. The interface with connective tissue is smooth, although slender connective tissue papillae often penetrate into the epithelium.

The lamina propria is generally thicker than in masticatory mucosa and contains fewer collagen fibers, which follow a more irregular course between anchoring points. Thus the mucosa can be stretched to a certain extent before these fibers become taut and limit further distention. Associated with the collagen fibers are elastic fibers that tend to control the extensibility of the mucosa. Where lining mucosa covers muscle, the mucosa is attached by a mixture of collagen and elastic fibers. As the mucosa becomes slack during masticatory movements, the elastic fibers retract the mucosa toward the muscle and so prevent it from bulging between the teeth and being bitten.

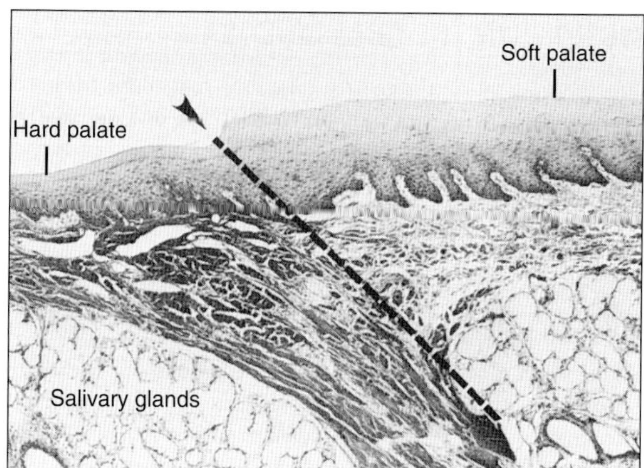

Fig. 12.29 Photomicrograph of the junction *(dashed line)* between mucosa covering the hard and the soft palate. The difference in thickness and the ridge pattern between keratinized epithelium of the hard palate and nonkeratinized epithelium of the soft palate is apparent. The section has been stained by the van Gieson method to demonstrate collagen; the lamina propria of the hard palate contains thick dense bundles, whereas collagen forms thinner fibers in the soft palate. Minor salivary glands occur beneath the mucosa.

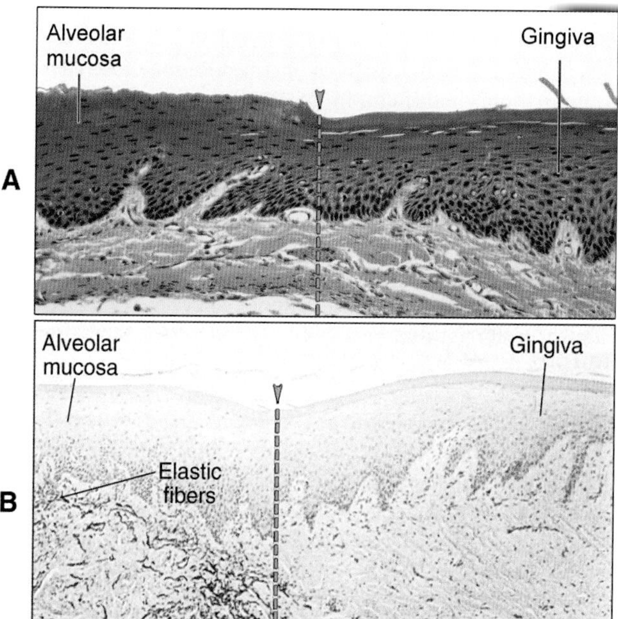

Fig. 12.30 Sections through the mucogingival junction *(dashed line)*. In (A) the differences in thickness, ridge pattern, and keratinization between epithelium of the gingiva and alveolar mucosa are seen. The preparation was stained by the Papanicolaou method, which reveals variations in keratinization. The junction in (B) was stained by the Hart method to demonstrate elastic fibers in the connective tissue. Although little change in the epithelium occurs in this specimen, a striking difference appears in the concentration of elastic fibers in the lamina propria between masticatory mucosa of the gingiva and lining mucosa of the alveoli. (From Squier CA, et al.: *Human oral mucosa: development, structure, and function*, Oxford, UK, 1976, Blackwell Scientific.)

The alveolar mucosa and mucosa covering the floor of the mouth are attached loosely to the underlying structures by a thick submucosa. Elastic fibers in the lamina propria of these regions tend to restore the mucosa to its resting position after distention. By contrast, mucosa of the underside of the tongue is bound firmly to the underlying muscle.

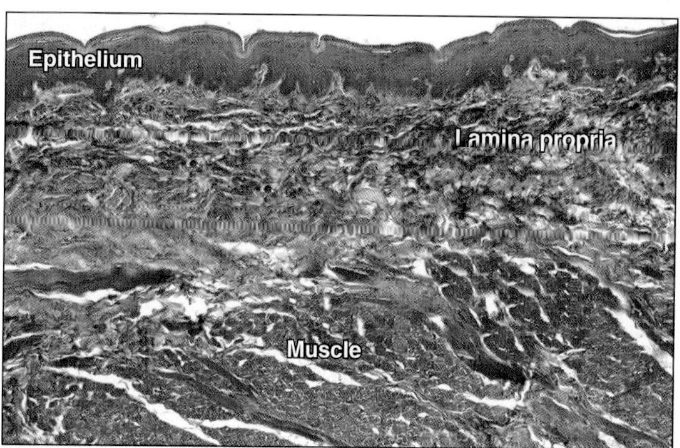

Fig. 12.31 Photomicrograph of lining mucosa from the underside of the tongue. The nonkeratinized epithelium is thin with only a slight ridge pattern and is bound to the underlying muscle by a narrow lamina propria.

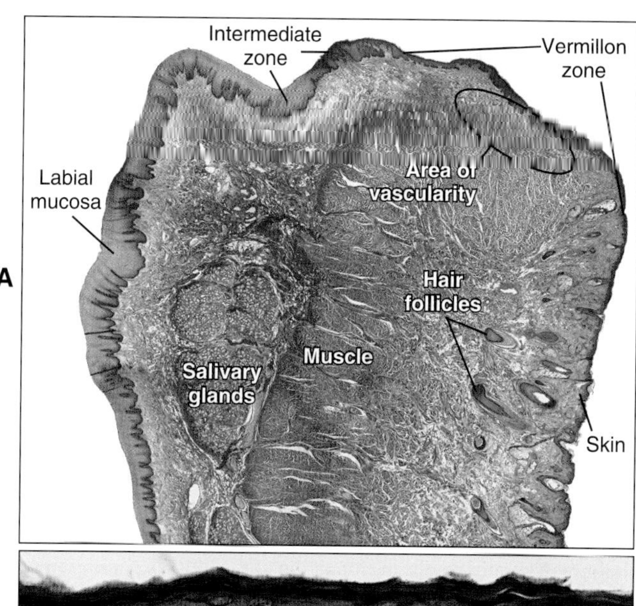

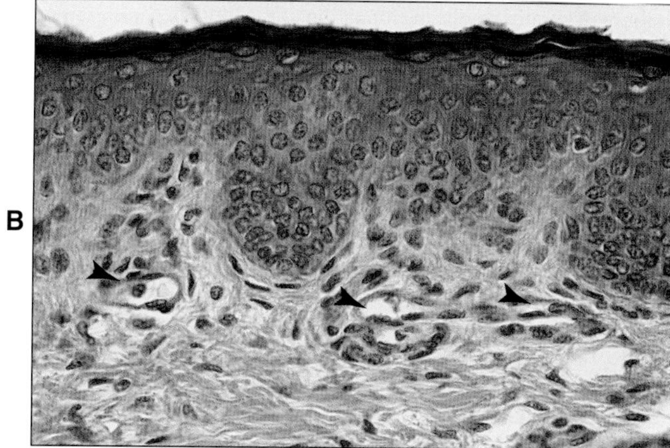

Fig. 12.32 Sagittal section through the lip. (A) The skin covering the external aspect has a thin epidermis and contains hair follicles. Continuous with this is the vermilion zone, which has a thin epithelium overlying an area of extensive vascularity. Between the vermilion zone and the labial mucosa of the oral cavity is the intermediate zone. Minor salivary glands occur beneath the labial mucosa, and the extensive muscular tissue represents part of the orbicularis oris. (B) Higher magnification of the area of vascularity in the vermilion border showing multiple capillary loops *(arrowheads)* in the connective tissue, close to the surface.

The soft palate is flexible but not highly mobile, and its mucosa is separated from the loose and highly glandular submucosa by a layer of elastic fibers.

Specialized Mucosa

The mucosa of the dorsal surface of the tongue is unlike that anywhere else in the oral cavity because, although covered by what is functionally a masticatory mucosa, it is also a highly extensible lining and in addition has different types of lingual papillae. Some of them possess a mechanical function, whereas others bear taste buds and therefore have a sensory function.

The mucous membrane of the tongue (see Fig. 12.27) is composed of two parts with different embryologic origins (see Chapter 3) and is divided by a V-shaped groove, the sulcus terminalis (terminal groove). The anterior two-thirds of the tongue, where the mucosa is derived from the first pharyngeal arch, often is called the body, and the posterior third, where the mucosa is derived from the third pharyngeal arch, is the base. The mucosa covering the base of the tongue contains extensive nodules of lymphoid tissue (lingual tonsils).

Fungiform Papillae

The anterior portion of the tongue bears the fungiform (funguslike) and filiform (hairlike) papillae (see Fig. 12.28A). Single fungiform papillae are scattered between the numerous filiform papillae at the tip of the tongue. The fungiform papillae are smooth, round structures that appear red because of their highly vascular connective tissue core, visible through a thin, nonkeratinized covering epithelium. Taste buds normally are present in the epithelium on the superior surface.

Filiform Papillae

Filiform papillae cover the entire anterior part of the tongue and consist of cone-shaped structures, each with a core of connective tissue covered by a thick keratinized epithelium (see Fig. 12.28A). Together they form a tough, abrasive surface that is involved in compressing and breaking food when the tongue is apposed onto the hard palate. Thus the dorsal mucosa of the tongue functions as a masticatory mucosa. Buildup of keratin results in elongation of the filiform papillae in some patients. The dorsum of the tongue then has a hairy appearance called hairy tongue.

The tongue is highly extensible, with changes in its shape accommodated by the regions of nonkeratinized, flexible epithelium between the filiform papillae.

Foliate Papillae

Foliate (leaflike) papillae sometimes are present on the lateral margins of the posterior part of the tongue, although they are more common in mammals other than human beings. These pink papillae consist of parallel ridges that alternate with deep grooves in the mucosa, and a few taste buds are present in the epithelium of the lateral walls of the ridges (see Fig. 12.28B).

Circumvallate Papillae

Adjacent and anterior to the sulcus terminalis are 8 to 12 circumvallate (walled) papillae, large structures each surrounded by a deep, circular groove into which open the ducts of minor salivary glands (the glands of Ebner) (see Figs. 12.27 and 12.28C). These papillae have a connective tissue core that is covered on the superior surface by a keratinized epithelium. The epithelium covering the lateral walls is nonkeratinized and contains taste buds.

JUNCTIONS IN THE ORAL MUCOSA

Within the oral mucosa are three junctions that merit further discussion: the mucocutaneous (between the skin and mucosa), the mucogingival (between the gingiva and alveolar mucosa), and the dentogingival (interface between the gingiva and the tooth). The junction between the epithelium and the enamel is the principal seal between the oral cavity and the underlying tissues, and hence represents a first line of defense against periodontal disease.

Mucocutaneous Junction

The skin, which contains hair follicles and sebaceous and sweat glands, is continuous with the oral mucosa at the lips (see Fig. 12.32). At the mucocutaneous junction is a transitional region where appendages are absent except for a few sebaceous glands (situated mainly at the angles of the mouth). The epithelium of this region is keratinized but thin, with long connective tissue papillae containing capillary loops. This arrangement brings the blood close to the surface and accounts for the strong red coloration in this region, called the red (vermilion) zone of the lip. The line separating the vermilion zone from the hair-bearing skin of the lip is called the vermilion border. In young people, this border is demarcated sharply, but as a person is exposed to ultraviolet radiation the border becomes diffuse and poorly defined.

Because the vermilion zone lacks salivary glands and contains only a few sebaceous glands, it tends to dry out, often becoming cracked and sore in cold weather. Between the vermilion zone and the thicker, nonkeratinized labial mucosa is an intermediate zone covered by parakeratinized oral epithelium. In infants this region is thickened and appears more opalescent, which represents an adaptation to suckling called the suckling pad.

Mucogingival Junction

Although masticatory mucosa meets lining mucosa at several sites, none is more abrupt than the junction between attached gingiva and alveolar mucosa. This junction is identified clinically by a slight indentation called the mucogingival groove and by the change from the bright pink of the alveolar mucosa to the paler pink of the gingiva (see Fig. 12.2B).

Histologically, a change occurs at this junction, not only in the type of epithelium but also in the composition of the lamina propria (see Fig. 12.30). The epithelium of the attached gingiva is keratinized or parakeratinized, and the lamina propria contains numerous coarse collagen bundles attaching the tissue to periosteum. The stippling seen clinically at the surface of healthy attached gingiva probably reflects the presence of this collagen attachment, the surface of the free gingiva being smooth. The structure of mucosa changes at the mucogingival junction, where the alveolar mucosa has a thicker, nonkeratinized epithelium overlying a loose lamina propria with numerous elastic fibers extending into the thick submucosa. These elastic fibers return the alveolar mucosa to its original position after distention by the labial muscles during mastication and speech.

Coronal to the mucogingival junction is another clinically visible depression in the gingiva, the free gingival groove, the level of which corresponds approximately to that of the bottom of the gingival sulcus. This demarcates the free and attached gingivae, although unlike the mucogingival junction, no significant change in the structure of the mucosa occurs at the free gingival groove.

Dentogingival Junction

The region where the oral mucosa meets the surface of the tooth is a unique junction of considerable importance because it represents

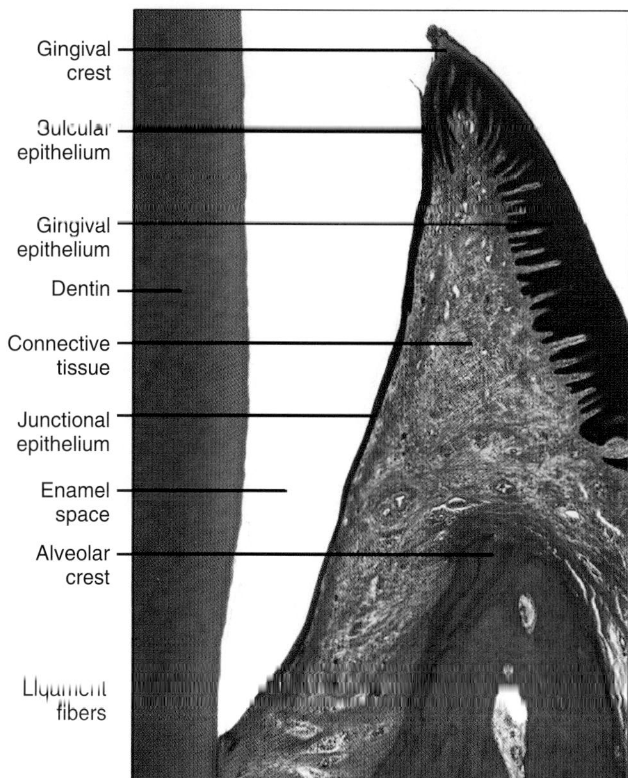

Fig. 12.33 The dentogingival junction. Together, the sulcular and junctional epithelium constitute the dentogingival junction. The junctional epithelium attaches to the tooth surface. Decalcification of the specimen has removed the tooth enamel, leaving an enamel space. The sulcular epithelium is short in this preparation because the tooth is not fully erupted.

a potential weakness in the otherwise continuous epithelial lining of the oral cavity. The dentogingival junction consists of a sulcular epithelium which extends cervically to become the junctional epithelium that attaches to the tooth surface. The sulcular epithelium is separated from the tooth by a space referred to as the *sulcus.* When the tooth first becomes functional, the bottom of the sulcus usually is found on the cervical half of the anatomic crown; with age a gradual migration of the sulcus bottom occurs that eventually may pass onto the cementum surface. The walls of the sulcus are lined by epithelium derived from and continuous with that of the rest of the oral mucosa. This has been designated oral sulcular epithelium and has the same basic structure as nonkeratinized oral epithelium elsewhere in the oral cavity. The orthokeratinized or parakeratinized surface of the free gingiva (or oral epithelium) is continuous with the oral sulcular epithelium at the level of the gingival crest (Fig. 12.33).

The sulcus contains fluid that has passed through the junctional epithelium and a mixture of desquamated epithelial cells from the junctional and sulcular epithelia and inflammatory cells. Indeed, cells of the inflammatory series, particularly polymorphonuclear leukocytes, continually migrate into the junctional epithelium and pass between the epithelial cells to appear in the gingival sulcus and eventually in the oral fluid.

The bacteria that are inevitably present on the tooth surface continually produce substances capable of eliciting inflammation and damage if they enter the mucosal tissues. In the average human mouth, in which mild gingival inflammation is invariably present, the gingival sulcus (see Fig. 12.33) has a depth of 0.5 to 3 mm, with an average of 1.8 mm. Any depth greater than 3 mm generally can be considered pathologic; a sulcus this deep is known as a *periodontal pocket.*

The presence of various molecular constituents from different origins in the sulcular fluid holds the promise for the diagnostic progression of periodontal disease.

Junctional epithelium is derived from the reduced enamel epithelium of the tooth germ (see Chapter 7). As the tooth erupts and the crown passes through the overlying oral epithelium, a fusion occurs between the reduced enamel epithelium and the oral epithelium so that epithelial continuity is never lost. The junctional epithelium is basically a stratified squamous nonkeratinizing epithelium, the cells of which derive from basal cells situated away from the tooth surface. The basal cells rest on a typical basal lamina that interfaces with the subjacent dermal connective tissue (Fig. 12.34A). This so-called outer basal lamina is similar to that which attaches epithelium to connective tissue elsewhere in the oral mucosa. Suprabasal cells have a similar appearance; they are largely flattened cells oriented parallel to the tooth surface and tapering from 3 to 4 layers in thickness apically to 15 to 30 layers coronally. Remarkably, these cells maintain some ability to undergo cell division and turn over rapidly, at least in some species. The most superficial cell layer provides the actual attachment of gingiva to the tooth surface (enamel or sometimes cementum) by means of a structural complex called the epithelial attachment. This complex consists of a specialized inner basal lamina (formed and maintained by the flattened superficial cells), which adheres to the tooth surface and to which the cells are attached by hemidesmosomes (see Fig. 12.34B). Thus the junctional epithelium cells do not "directly" attach to the tooth surface. This basal lamina is unique because it binds to calcified surfaces rather than connective tissue. For many years, the only information about its composition was that it is enriched in glycoconjugates. It is now known that basal laminae applied to tooth surfaces (and the basal lamina associated with maturation-stage ameloblasts; see Chapter 7) contain laminin-332, whereas components such as gamma-1 chain–containing laminins and type IV and VII collagens are not present, setting them apart functionally and compositionally. It has now been demonstrated that the inner basal lamina of the junctional epithelium, which is a specialized basal lamina, contains amelotin (AMTN), odontogenic ameloblast–associated (ODAM) protein, and secretory calcium-binding phosphoprotein proline-glutamine rich 1 (SCPPPQ1) (Fig. 12.35), three secreted proteins that as shown in Chapter 7 are also expressed by maturation-stage ameloblasts. ODAM is particularly interesting because it is also present among cells of the junctional epithelium; hence it could potentially have multiple functions. As such, it has been proposed to behave as a matricellular protein with both cellular and matrix functions that are contextual. The functions of AMTN, ODAM, and SCPPPQ1 remain to be fully-determined, but as part of the inner basal lamina it is likely that they may play a role in its supramolecular organization and participate, directly or indirectly, in mediating its adhesion to the tooth surface. Consistent with this hypothesis, a mouse model in which *Odam* expression has been inactivated shows junctional epithelium changes that mimic those observed in mild periodontal disease in humans and slows its regeneration. It has also been reported that the presence of ODAM increases in the crevicular fluid of patients with periodontitis.

Genetic basal lamina defects are known to cause debilitating epidermal detachments and clearly would be problematic at the level of the junctional epithelium, which must withstand severe physical and chemical forces. Like epidermal bullosa, mutations in components of the junctional epithelium attachment apparatus may explain the etiology of elusive refractory forms of periodontal disease that are not directly associated with bacterial attack and cause premature loss of teeth. In this context, early onset of periodontal disease has been noted

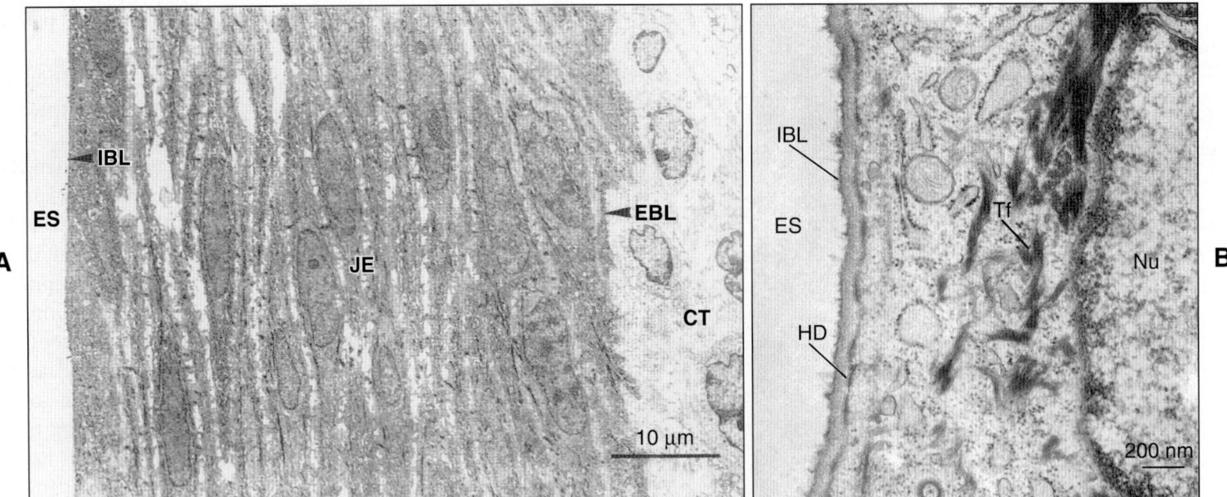

Fig. 12.34 (A) An electron micrograph of junctional epithelium *(JE)* showing the attachment to the enamel surface at the internal basal lamina *(IBL)* and to the connective tissue *(CT)* by the external basal lamina *(EBL)*. The lack of differentiation of the epithelium and the wide intercellular spaces are notable. (B) An electron micrograph showing the fine structure of the attachment of a junctional epithelial cell to the enamel surface via the internal basal lamina. Hemidesmosomes *(HDs)* are evident at the surface of the cell. *ES*, Enamel space; *Nu*, nucleus; *Tf*, tonofilament. (A, From Schroeder HE, Listgarten MA: *Fine structure of the developing attachment of human teeth*, Basel, Switzerland, 1977, S Karger.)

in patients with Weary-Kindler syndrome, and their junctional epithelium is believed to be abnormal.

The junctional epithelium is not simply an area of nonkeratinized oral epithelium but a unique, incompletely differentiated epithelium that shows a controlled level of inflammation from the moment it first forms. The ultrastructural characteristics of junctional epithelial cells are relatively constant throughout the epithelium and differ considerably from those of other oral epithelial cells. Junctional epithelial cells contain fewer tonofilaments and desmosomal junctions, and the cytokeratins present represent those seen in basal epithelial cells (K5, K14, and K19) and in simple epithelia (K8 and K18). Although the cells of the junctional epithelium divide and migrate to the surface, they show no sign of differentiation to form a keratinized surface epithelium. These features, as well as the common presence of infiltrating neutrophil leukocytes and mononuclear cells, may contribute to the permeability of the tissue.

As in all epithelia, the deeper cells adjacent to the connective tissue undergo cell division to replenish those lost at the surface. The rate of cell division is high, and those cells produced move to within two or three cell layers of the tooth surface (where the cells are attached to the tooth surface) and then join a main migratory route in a coronal direction, paralleling the tooth surface, to be desquamated into the gingival sulcus.

Recent cell-lineage tracing studies in rodents have shown that single and/or multiple stem cell populations maintain the junctional epithelium and that a wingless-related integration site (Wnt)-responsive stem cell niche is implicated. One of the remarkable properties of the junctional epithelium is that it readily regenerates if it is damaged or surgically excised. Interestingly, studies in rodents have shown that ODAM and SCPPPQ1 appear early during the process. The new junctional epithelium has all the characteristics of the original tissue, including the same types of cytokeratins and an attachment to the tooth that is indistinguishable from the original one. This raises interesting questions as to the nature of the signals responsible for inducing the formation of a junctional epithelium. Contact with a mineralized surface and a connective tissue influence may be implicated. A comprehensive understanding of the junctional epithelium formation, maintenance and reformation, and the molecular mediators implicated has potential clinical implications for prevention and treatment of periodontal disease, and formation of a periimplant epithelium.

Connective Tissue Component

Examination of the connective tissue supporting the epithelium of the dentogingival junction shows that it is structurally different than supporting the gingival epithelium and contains, even in clinically normal gingiva, a physiologic inflammatory infiltrate believed to be initiated at the time of tooth eruption.

Experimental evidence indicates that the connective tissue supporting junctional epithelium is also functionally different from that supporting the rest of the oral epithelium, and such a difference has important connotations for the pathogenesis of periodontal disease and regeneration of the dentogingival junction after periodontal surgery.

Tissue recombination experiments have shown that connective tissue plays a key role in determining epithelial expression. Subepithelial connective tissue of the lamina propria supports normal maturation of a stratified squamous epithelium. However, when epithelium is combined with deeper connective tissue, it does not mature and assumes a state resembling that of junctional epithelium. At the dentogingival junction, presumably the sulcular epithelium is in contact with superficial connective tissue that supports its differentiation along a keratinization pathway. Instead, the junctional epithelium is exposed to deeper connective tissue that maintains an undifferentiated status.

The inflammation of the connective tissue associated with the dentogingival junction also influences epithelial expression. Thus the oral sulcular epithelium, in distinction to the gingival epithelium, is nonkeratinized, yet both are supported by gingival lamina propria. This difference in epithelial expression may be a direct consequence of the inflammatory process.

The junctional epithelium also is influenced by inflammation. Epithelia maintained experimentally in association with deep connective tissue show little capacity to proliferate but can be induced to

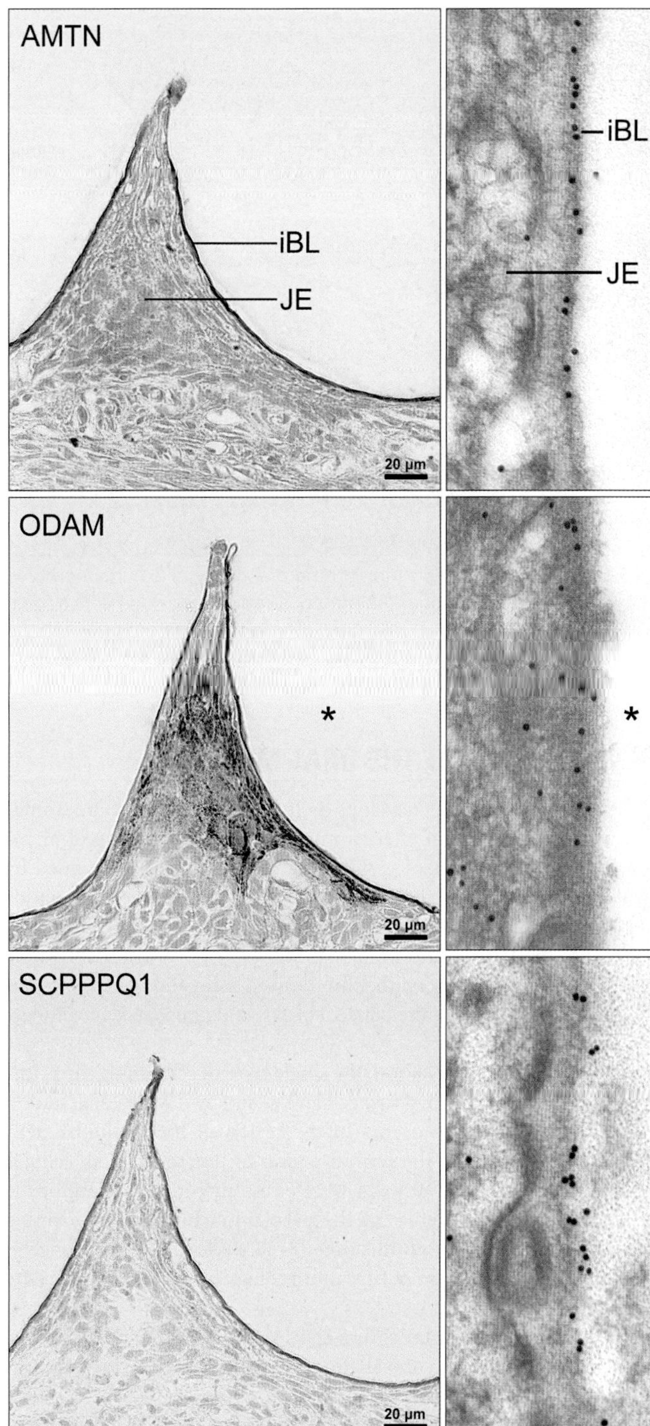

Fig. 12.35 Immunoperoxidase *(left panels)* and corresponding immunogold *(right panels)* preparations for amelotin *(AMTN)*, odontogenic ameloblast-associated *(ODAM)*, and secretory calcium-binding phosphoprotein proline-glutamine rich 1 *(SCPPPQ1)*. Labeling for AMTN and SCPPPQ1 is restricted to the inner basal lamina *(iBL)* at the interface between the junctional epithelium *(JE)* and the enamel (here seen as a space *[*]* in these decalcified preparations). ODAM is likewise found in the basal lamina but is also distinctively present among the cells of the junctional epithelium. (Courtesy K. Ponce [preparations] and A. Fouillen [images].)

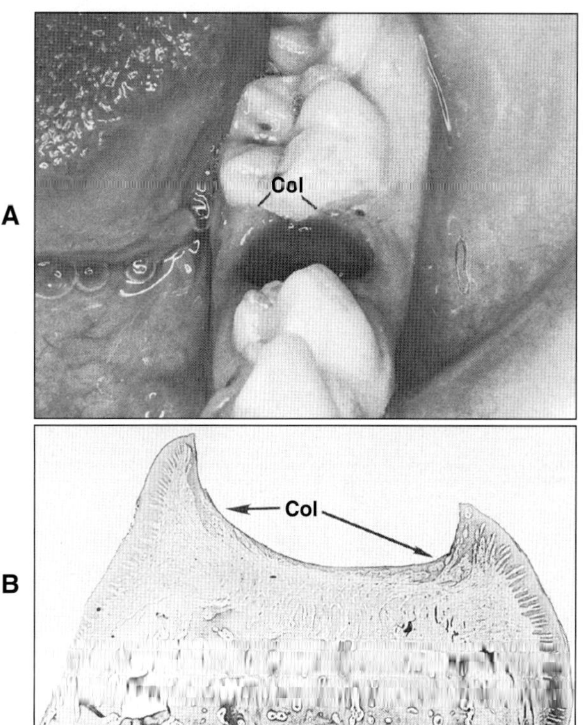

Fig. 12.36 Dental col. (A) Clinical appearance. (B) Histologic section. The distinction between the keratinized gingival epithelium and the epithelium of the col is evident.

do so by mediators of inflammation. Clinically, when inflammation increases, active proliferation and migration of the junctional epithelium occur, resulting in a periodontal pocket and apical movement of attachment level.

A similar set of biologic events occurs in relation to the proliferation of epithelial cell rests of Malassez. Cell rests are supported by the deep connective tissue of the periodontal ligament and proliferate only in the presence of inflammation within that connective tissue.

Although it remains to be demonstrated, a number of observations suggest that ODAM may be implicated in epithelial cell status. It is not found in keratinized epithelia but is expressed by the incompletely differentiated cells of the junctional epithelium. As epithelial cells become neoplastic and gradually acquire an undifferentiated phenotype, they now express ODAM in high amounts. Cells of the rests of Malassez do not normally produce ODAM, yet when periodontal integrity is disrupted, they produce the protein (see Chapter 9).

Col

The previous description of the dentogingival junction applies to all surfaces of the tooth, even though interdentally the gingiva seems to be different. Interdental gingiva appears to have the outline of a col (depression), with buccal and lingual peaks guarding it (Fig. 12.36). Col epithelium is identical to junctional epithelium, has the same origin (from enamel epithelium), and is replaced gradually by continuing cell division. No evidence indicates that the structural elements of the col increase vulnerability to periodontal disease. Rather, the incidence of gingivitis interdentally is greater than in other areas because the contours between the teeth allow bacteria, food debris, and plaque to accumulate in this location.

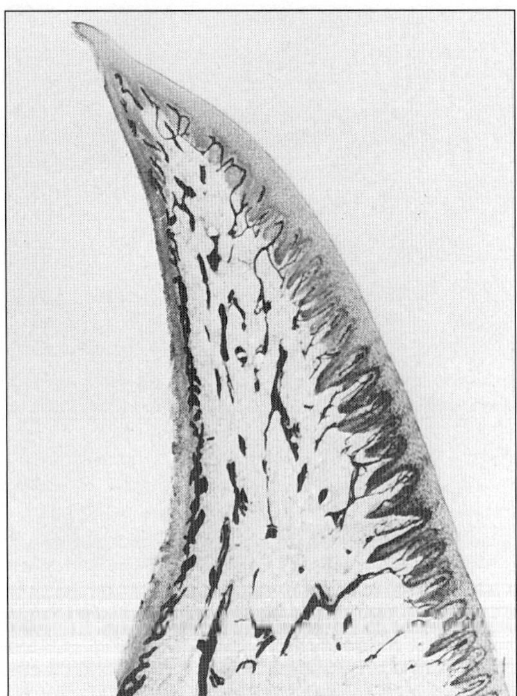

Fig. 12.37 Photomicrograph of the blood supply to the dentogingival junction. The differences in the shape of vessels related to the gingiva and the dentogingival junction are apparent. (From Egelberg J: The blood vessels of the dento-gingival junction, *J Periodontal Res* 1:163–179, 1966.)

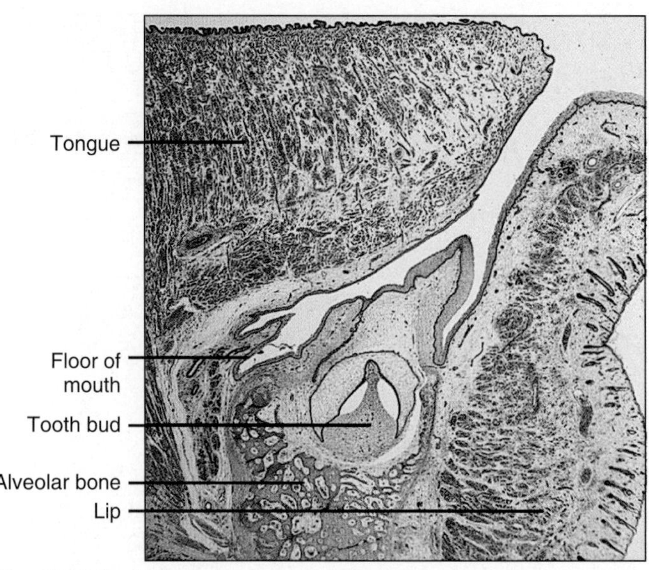

Fig. 12.38 Sagittal section through the oral cavity of a human embryo showing the tongue, floor of the mouth, alveolar bone ridge with a tooth bud, and lip. Differences in thickness are already apparent between the epithelia of the labial mucosa, alveolar ridge, floor of the mouth, and tongue; however, keratinization has not yet begun.

Blood Supply

The blood supply to the gingiva is derived from vessels in the periosteum of the alveolar process. Branches from these vessels are perpendicular to the surface and form loops within the connective tissue papillae of the gingiva. Vessels supplying the dentogingival junction are derived from the continuation of interalveolar arteries as they pierce the alveolar crest. These vessels are parallel to the sulcular epithelium and form a rich network just below the basal lamina (Fig. 12.37).

For descriptive purposes, the blood supply to the periodontium can be divided into three zones: to the periodontal ligament, to the gingiva facing the oral cavity, and to the gingiva facing the tooth. Interconnections among the three zones permit collateral circulation.

Nerve Supply

The gingival component of the periodontium is innervated by terminal branches of periodontal nerve fibers and by branches of the infraorbital and palatine, or lingual, mental, and buccal nerves. In the attached gingiva, most nerves terminate within the lamina propria, and only a few endings occur between epithelial cells. In the dentogingival junction of rat molars, a rich innervation of the junctional epithelium has been demonstrated, with free nerve endings between epithelial cells at the connective tissue and the tooth surface of the epithelium. Vesicular structures and neuropeptides have been demonstrated in these nerve endings.

Why the junctional apparatus should have such an extensive blood and nerve supply is an interesting question. As has been pointed out, when the tooth erupts, inflammation occurs in the connective tissue related to the junction, and this inflammation persists as an almost normal feature of the dentogingival junction. A relationship exists among vascular elements, immunocompetent cells, and secreted neuropeptides, and the described vascular and neural supply may reflect this relationship and function.

DEVELOPMENT OF THE ORAL MUCOSA

The primitive oral cavity develops by fusion of the embryonic stomatodeum with the foregut after rupture of the buccopharyngeal membrane, at about 26 days of gestation, and thus comes to be lined by epithelium derived from ectoderm and endoderm. The precise boundary between these two embryonic tissues is defined poorly, but structures that develop in the branchial arches (e.g., tongue, epiglottis, pharynx) are covered by epithelium derived from endoderm, whereas the epithelium covering the palate, cheeks, and gingivae is of ectodermal origin.

By 5 to 6 weeks of gestation, the single layer of cells lining the primitive oral cavity has formed two cell layers, and by 8 weeks of gestation a significant thickening occurs in the region of the vestibular dental lamina complex. In the central region of this thickening, cellular degeneration occurs at 10 to 14 weeks, resulting in separation of the cells covering the cheek area and the alveolar mucosa and thus forming the oral vestibule. At about this time (8–11 weeks), the palatal shelves elevate and close, and the future morphology of the adult oral cavity is apparent.

The lingual epithelium shows specialization at about 7 weeks of gestation when the circumvallate and foliate papillae first appear, followed by the fungiform papillae. Within these papillae, taste buds soon develop. The filiform papillae that cover most of the anterior two-thirds of the tongue become apparent at about 10 weeks. By 10 to 12 weeks of gestation, the future lining and masticatory mucosa show some stratification of the epithelium and a different morphology.

Those areas destined to become keratinized (e.g., hard palate and alveolar ridge of gingiva) have darkly staining, columnar basal cells that are separated from the underlying connective tissue by a prominent basal lamina. Low connective tissue papillae also are evident. By contrast, the epithelium that will form areas of lining mucosa retains cuboidal basal cells, and the epithelium–connective tissue interface remains flat. Between 13 and 20 weeks of gestation, all the oral epithelia thicken (Fig. 12.38), and with the appearance of sparse keratohyalin granules, a distinction between the prickle cell and granular layer can be made. Differences are evident between the cytokeratins of epithelia of the developing masticatory and lining regions. During this period, melanocytes and Langerhans cells appear in the epithelium. The surface layers of the epithelium show parakeratosis; orthokeratinization of the masticatory mucosa does not occur until after the teeth erupt during the postnatal period.

While these changes are occurring in the oral epithelium, the underlying ectomesenchyme shows progressive changes. Initially the ectomesenchyme consists of widely spaced stellate cells in an amorphous matrix, but by 6 to 8 weeks of gestation extracellular reticular fibers begin to accumulate. As in the epithelium, regional differences can be seen in the ectomesenchyme. The connective tissue of lining mucosa contains fewer cells and fibers than that of the future masticatory mucosa. Between 8 and 12 weeks of gestation, capillary buds and collagen fibers can be detected; although the collagen initially shows no orientation, as the fibers increase in number they tend to form bundles. Immediately subjacent to the epithelium, these bundles are perpendicular to the basal lamina. Elastic fibers become prominent only in the connective tissue of lining mucosa between 17 and 20 weeks of gestation.

AGE CHANGES

Clinically, the oral mucosa of an elderly person often has a smoother and drier surface than that of a younger individual and may be described as atrophic or friable, but these changes likely represent the cumulative effects of systemic disease, medication use, or both, rather than an intrinsic biologic aging process of the mucosa.

Histologically, the epithelium appears thinner, and a smoothing of the epithelium–connective tissue interface results from the flattening of epithelial ridges. The dorsum of the tongue may show a reduction in the number of filiform papillae and a smooth or glossy appearance, such changes being exacerbated by any nutritional deficiency of iron or B complex vitamins. The reduced number of filiform papillae may make the fungiform papillae more prominent, and patients erroneously may consider it to be a disease state.

Aging is associated with decreased rates of metabolic activity, but studies on epithelial proliferation and rate of tissue turnover in healthy tissue are inconclusive. Langerhans cells become fewer with age, which may contribute to a decline in cell-mediated immunity.

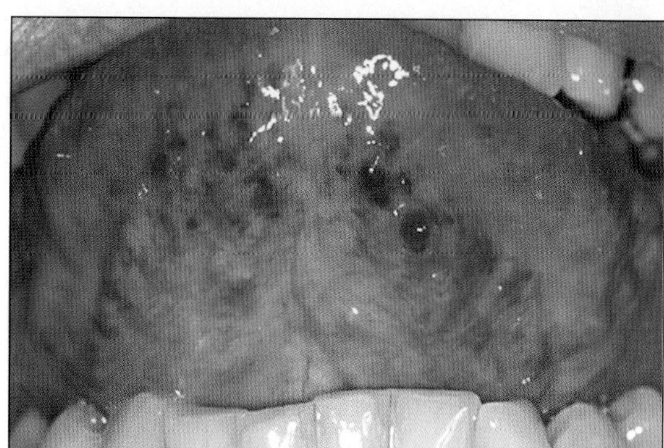

Fig. 12.39 Ventral surface of the tongue in an elderly patient showing varicosities. (Courtesy A. Kauzman.)

Vascular changes may be prominent, with the development of varicosities. A striking and common feature in elderly persons is nodular varicose veins on the undersurface of the tongue (sometimes called caviar tongue) (Fig. 12.39). Although such changes appear to be unrelated to the cardiovascular status of the patient, they are more common in patients with varicose veins of the legs. In the lamina propria a decreased cellularity occurs with an increased amount of collagen, which is reported to become more highly cross-linked. Sebaceous glands (Fordyce spots) of the lips and cheeks also increase with age, and the minor salivary glands show considerable atrophy with fibrous replacement.

Elderly patients, particularly postmenopausal women, may have symptoms such as dryness of the mouth, burning sensations, and abnormal taste. Whether such symptoms reflect systemic disturbances or local tissue changes is not clear.

RECOMMENDED READING

Presland RB, Dale BA: Epithelial structural proteins of the skin and oral cavity: function in health and disease, *Crit Rev Oral Biol Med* 11:383–408, 2000.

Schroeder HE: *Differentiation of human oral stratified epithelia*, Basel, Switzerland, 1981, S Karger.

Squier C, Brogden K: *Human oral mucosa, development, structure & function*, Oxford, UK, 2011, Wiley-Blackwell.

13

The Mastication Apparatus

Antonio Nanci and Barry Sessle

OUTLINE

Mastication, or chewing as it is often termed, is a fundamental function necessary for the breakup of foodstuffs and their mixing with saliva so that they are in a suitable form that is safe to swallow. Mastication is a highly complex biomechanical function involving the coordinated activity of numerous muscles in the craniofacial region. While it also uses a skeletal substrate of bones, teeth, and joints to allow for muscle-produced jaw movements to receive and manipulate foodstuffs and to pierce, crush, and grind the foodstuffs, it is driven and regulated by motor outputs from the brain. Furthermore, its underlying pattern of muscle activities may be modified by sensory inputs into the brain from the craniofacial region, and the brain uses these sensory inputs to regulate the motor outputs to the muscles. Thus mastication can be viewed as the expression of a system involving the brain as well as bones, muscles, teeth, the temporomandibular joint (TMJ), and other craniofacial tissues. And mastication is a function closely allied to Dentistry since a major goal of many areas of Dentistry and allied fields is to ensure that patients maintain a high level of masticatory performance as part of their oral health. The following outlines the various components of this biomechanical system.

The bones involved in the articulation of the lower jaw with the cranium and upper facial skeleton are the mandible and the temporal bone, and the joint, therefore, is designated the TMJ. The joint is unique to mammals. In other vertebrates the lower jaw is compound, consisting of several bones including the bone-bearing teeth (dentary) and the articular bone (formed from the posterior part of Meckel's cartilage) and articulates with the quadrate bone of the skull (Fig. 13.1). As mammals evolved, the compound lower jaw was reduced to a single bone (the mandible), bearing teeth that articulate with the newly developed articulating surface on the temporal bone. Thus in phylogenetic terms, the TMJ is a secondary joint. The primary vertebrate jaw joint is still present in human anatomy (as the incudomalleolar articulation), with the bones involved (incus and malleus) now positioned in the middle ear (Fig. 13.2).

CLASSIFICATION OF JOINTS

Fig. 13.3 shows a common, simple classification of joints.

Fibrous Joints

In a fibrous joint, two bones are connected by three types of fibrous tissue joints. The first is the suture, a joint that permits little or no movement. The histology of the suture clearly indicates that its function is to permit growth because its articulating surfaces are covered by an osteogenic layer responsible for new bone formation to maintain the suture as the skull bones are separated by the expanding brain. The second type of fibrous joint is the gomphosis, the socketed attachment of tooth to bone by the fibrous periodontal ligament. Functional movement is restricted to intrusion and recovery in response to biting forces (long-term movement of teeth in response to environmental pressures or orthodontic treatment represents remodeling of the joint rather than functional movement). The third type of fibrous joint is the syndesmosis, examples of which are the joints between the fibula and tibia and between the radius and ulna. The two bony components are some distance apart but are joined by an interosseous ligament that permits limited movement.

Cartilaginous Joints

In a primary cartilaginous joint, bone and cartilage are in direct apposition (e.g., the costochondral junction). In a secondary cartilaginous joint, the tissues of the articulation occur in the sequence as bone–cartilage–fibrous tissue–cartilage–bone (e.g., the pubic symphysis). Cartilaginous joints and fibrous joints permit little if any movement between the involved bones.

Synovial Joints

In a synovial joint, which generally permits significant movement, two bones (each with an articular surface covered by hyaline cartilage) are united and surrounded by a capsule that thereby creates a joint cavity. This cavity is filled with synovial fluid formed by a synovial membrane that lines the nonarticular surfaces. The cavity in some joints may be divided by an articular disk. Various ligaments are associated with synovial joints to strengthen the articulation and check excess movement.

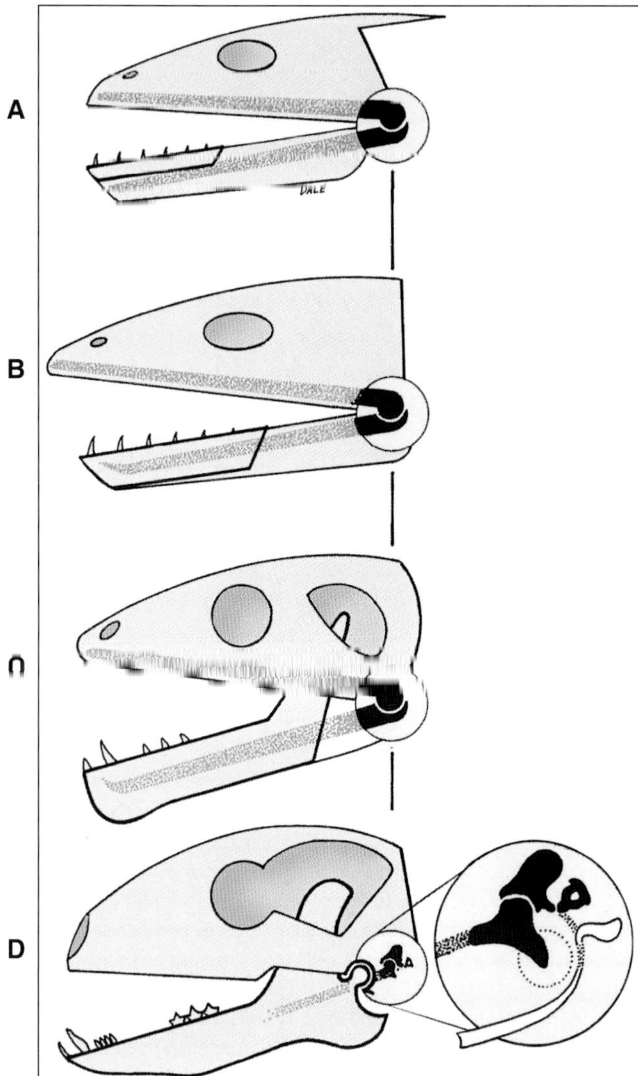

Fig. 13.1 Evolution of the mammalian jaw joint. (A) Amphibian skull. The teeth are confined to the dentary bone. The articulation is between the terminal portion of Meckel's cartilage (the articular) and the palatoquadrate bar. (B) Reptile skull. The jaw joint is still between the articular and the palatoquadrate bar, but the dentary bone is of increased size. (C) The skull of a fossil mammal-like reptile. The dentary bone is enlarged greatly and has a coronoid process. The jaw articulation, however, is still between the articular and palatoquadrate bar. (D) In mammals the dentary bone has formed an articulation with the temporal bone. The original joint now constitutes part of the inner ear. (From DeBrul EL: Origin and adaptations of the hominid jaw joint. In Sarnat BG, Laskin DM, editors: *The temporomandibular joint: a biological basis for clinical practice*, ed 4, Philadelphia, PA, 1992, WB Saunders.)

Synovial joints are classified further by the number of axes in which the bones involved can move (uniaxial, biaxial, or multiaxial) and by the shapes of the articulating surfaces (planar, ginglymoid [hinged], pivot, condyloid, saddle, and ball and socket).

TYPE OF JOINT

The temporomandibular articulation is a synovial joint. The anatomy of the TMJ varies considerably among mammals, depending on masticatory requirements, so a single, all-embracing descriptive classification is not possible. In carnivores, for example, movement is restricted to a simple hinge motion by the presence of well-developed anterior and posterior bony flanges that clasp the mandibular condyle. The badger provides an extreme example of this—the flanges clasp and envelop the condyle to such an extent that it is not possible to dislocate the mandible from the skull. In human beings a different situation exists; the masticatory process demands that the mandible be capable not only of opening and closing movements but also of protrusive, retrusive, and lateral movements and combinations thereof. To achieve them, the condyle undertakes translatory and rotary movements; therefore the human TMJ is described as a synovial sliding–ginglymoid joint (Fig. 13.4).

DEVELOPMENT OF THE JOINT

At 3 months of gestation, the secondary jaw joint (TMJ) begins to form. The first evidence of TMJ development is the appearance of two distinct regions of mesenchymal condensation, the temporal and condylar blastemata. The temporal blastema appears before the condylar, and initially both are positioned some distance from each other. The condylar blastema grows rapidly in a dorsolateral direction to close the gap. Ossification begins first in the temporal blastema (Fig. 13.5A). While the condylar blastema is still condensed mesenchyme, a cleft appears immediately above it that becomes the inferior joint cavity (see Fig. 13.5B). The condylar blastema differentiates into cartilage (condylar cartilage), and then a second cleft appears in relation to the temporal ossification that becomes the upper joint cavity (see Fig. 13.5C). With the appearance of this cleft, the primitive articular disk is formed.

BONES OF THE JOINT

The bones of the temporomandibular articulation are the glenoid fossa (on the undersurface of the squamous part of the temporal bone) and the condyle (supported by the condylar process of the mandible). The glenoid fossa is limited posteriorly by the squamotympanic and petrotympanic fissures. The glenoid fossa is limited medially by the spine of the sphenoid and laterally by the root of the zygomatic process of the temporal bone. Anteriorly, the glenoid fossa is bounded by a ridge of bone described as the articular eminence, which also is involved in the articulation (Fig. 13.6). The middle part is a thin plate of bone, the upper surface of which forms the middle cranial fossa (housing the temporal lobe of the brain). The condyle is the articulating surface of the mandible. In the sagittal plane, the glenoid fossa is 15 to 20 mm long (from medial to lateral extreme) and 8 to 12 mm thick. The articular surface of the condyle is strongly convex in the anteroposterior direction and slightly convex mediolaterally. The medial and lateral ends are termed *poles.* The medial pole extends farther beyond the condylar neck than the lateral pole does and is positioned more posteriorly so that the long axis of the condyle deviates posteriorly and meets a similar axis drawn from the opposite condyle at the anterior border of the foramen magnum. Variations in the shape of the condyle are common, and often the condylar surface is divided by a sagittal crest into medial and lateral slopes.

Unlike most synovial joints, the articular surfaces of which are covered with hyaline cartilage, the temporomandibular articulation is covered by a layer of fibrous tissue (Fig. 13.7). This histologic distinction has been used to argue that the TMJ is not a weightbearing joint, but the reality for this distinction can be found in the developmental history of the joint. The only other synovial joints with articular surfaces covered by fibrous tissue are the acromioclavicular and sternoclavicular joints, linking the clavicle to the appendicular skeleton. The mandible and the clavicle are bones formed directly from an intramembranous ossification center and are not preformed in cartilage, cartilage that persists in the long bones to cover articular surfaces following the appearance of ossification centers.

The glenoid fossa always is covered by a thin fibrous layer that directly overlies the bone, much as periosteum does (Fig. 13.8), but this layer becomes appreciably thicker where it covers the slope of the articular eminence (Fig. 13.9).

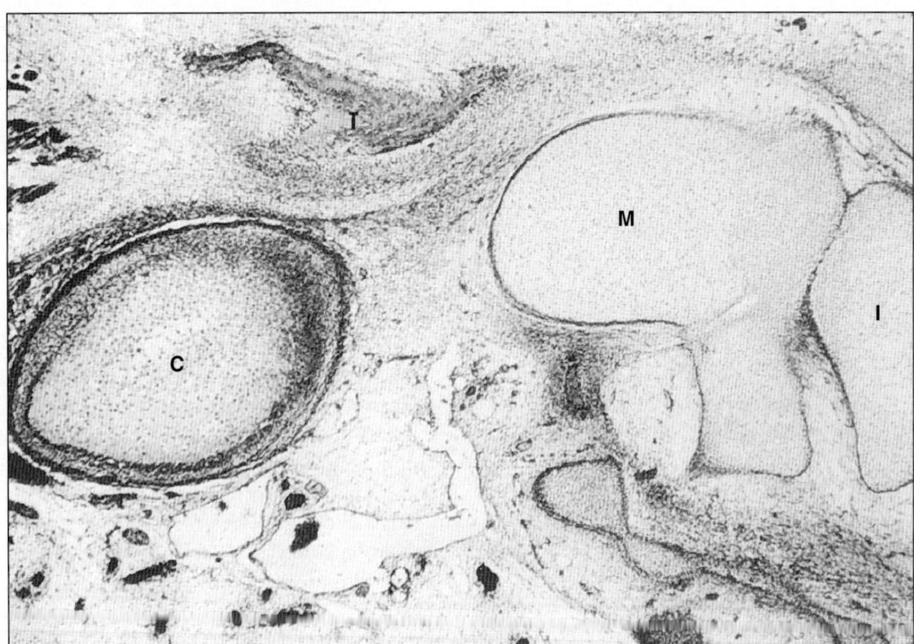

Fig. 13.2 Sagittal section through a 67-mm fetus showing the primary and secondary jaw joints. The developing temporal bone *(T)* and condylar blastema *(C)*, together, form the secondary joint. The malleus *(M)* and incus *(I)* represent the primary joint. (From Perry HT, et al.: The embryology of the temporomandibular joint, *Cranio* 3:125–132, 1985.)

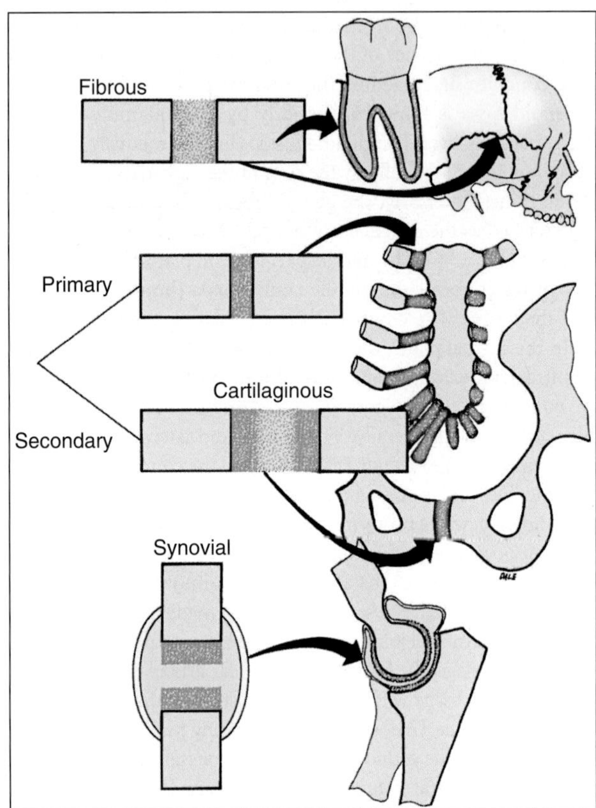

Fig. 13.3 Classification of joints.

CARTILAGE ASSOCIATED WITH THE JOINT

Earlier accounts of TMJ histology indicated that the surface coverings of the joint consist of fibrocartilage rather than fibrous tissue. Although with age the fibrous covering layer might contain some cartilage cells, no evidence indicates that this is normal. However, firm evidence indicates that fibrocartilage is associated with the articulation deep to the fibrous layer in the condyle and on the articular eminence (Fig. 13.10). The occurrence of such cartilage has a developmental explanation: A secondary growth cartilage associated with the developing TMJ forms within the blastema, the condylar cartilage, and is in some ways akin to the epiphyseal cartilage of a developing long bone. The condylar cartilage consists essentially of a proliferative layer of replicating cells that function as progenitor cells for the growth of cartilage (Fig. 13.11). These cells become chondroblasts and elaborate proteoglycans and type II collagen to form the extracellular matrix of cartilage in which they become entrapped as chondrocytes. At the same time, an increase in the size of the chondrocytes occurs (hypertrophy). After the production of this cartilage, endochondral ossification occurs, which involves mineralization of the cartilage, vascular invasion, loss of chondrocytes, and differentiation of osteoblasts to produce bone on the mineralized cartilaginous framework (Fig. 13.12; see also Fig. 13.11). The only difference in this process between condylar and epiphyseal cartilages in long bones is the absence of ordered columns of cartilaginous cells (which characterize the epiphyseal growth cartilage and result from chondroblast cell division). The absence of well-defined, elongated columns of chondroblast daughter cells in condylar cartilage has key significance. A typical long bone epiphyseal plate characterized by well-defined columns is committed to an essentially unidirectional mode of growth; that is, the proliferation of cells by mitotic division is such that the whole bone necessarily elongates in a manner determined by the columns of dividing cells. The mandibular condyle, by contrast, has a multidirectional growth capacity, and its cartilage can proliferate in any combination of superior and posterior directions as needed to provide for the best anatomic placement of the mandibular arch.

The classic model of endochondral ossification holds that chondrocytes undergo a cellular cascade leading to hypertrophy and programmed cell death (apoptosis). Bone forms on calcified cartilage by invading osteoprogenitor cells brought to the site by vascular invasion (see Chapter 6). There is now growing evidence that at least a subset of chondrocytes evades apoptosis and transdifferentiates into osteoblasts in the growth plate and during bone healing and regeneration. Data from cell lineage tracing work in rodents further support the direct transformation of chondrocytes into bone-forming cells during mandibular condyle ramus formation, and

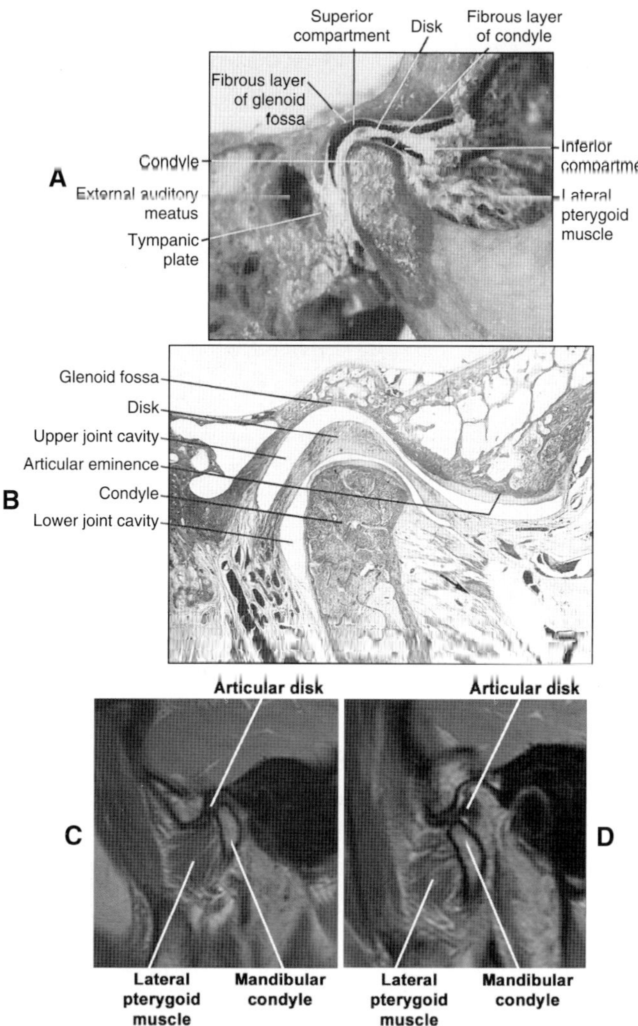

Fig. 13.4 The temporomandibular joint. (A) The macroscopic appearance of the joint. (B) Histologic section through the joint. (C, D) Sagittal T1-weighted magnetic resonance scans of a normal temporomandibular joint in a closed (C) and open (D) mouth. Note the synchronous displacement of the mandibular condyle and articular disk during movement. (A, From Liebgott WB: *The anatomical basis of dentistry*, St. Louis, MO, 1986, Mosby; 1986; B, from Griffin CJ, et al.: Anatomy and histology of the human temporomandibular joint, *Monogr Oral Sci* 4:1–26, 1975; C, D, courtesy Maria Grazia Piancino.)

the mandible would essentially be formed by a mosaic of chondrocyte-derived bone cells (neck and ramus center) and intramembranous bone cells (body) (Fig. 13.13).

A transient growth cartilage also has been found in association with development of the articular eminence. No eminence exists at birth; its development starts with a slender strip of growth cartilage (involving the same layers as already described for the condyle) situated along the slope of the eminence. Whereas the lifespan of these cartilages differs—the condylar cartilage existing until the end of the second decade, the eminence cartilage lasting a much shorter time—the subsequent history is the same for both. The proliferative activity of cells in the proliferative layer ceases, but the cells persist (Fig. 13.14; see also Fig. 13.9). The cartilage immediately below converts to fibrocartilage and, in the mandible, eventually mineralizes to a degree even greater than that of the mineralized bone (Fig. 13.15). Thus fibrocartilage is found in the mandible and on the slope of the articular eminence. Certainly in both instances, cells of the proliferative layer can resume their proliferative activity if the occasion demands. Thus remodeling of the articular surfaces can occur in response to functional changes throughout life and in response to orthodontic treatment. Additions to the joint surfaces may occur, increasing the vertical dimension of the face. Regressive remodeling creates a loss of the vertical dimension, and peripheral remodeling adds tissue to the margins of the articulation (often an arthritic change). Remodeling also compensates for the changing relationships of the jaws brought about by tooth wear and loss.

In summary, although fibrocartilage is associated with the temporomandibular articulation, it does not form part of the articulation and has no formal functional role to play in the everyday movements occurring between the two bones of the joint.

CAPSULE, LIGAMENTS, AND DISK OF THE JOINT

The capsule of a synovial joint consists of dense collagenous membrane that seals the joint space and provides passive stability that is enhanced by increased local thickenings in its walls to form anatomically recognizable ligaments, as well as active stability from proprioceptive nerve endings in the capsule. Furthermore, extensions of the fibrous capsule into the joint cavity in some joints, including the TMJ, form disks that function as articular surfaces and divide the joint into two compartments (Fig. 13.16; see also Figs. 13.10 and 13.11). The disk consists of coarse collagen fibers with numerous interspersed fibroblastic cells (see Fig. 13.16A). In some regions the collagen fibers appear wavy, which is believed to relate to their ability to accommodate tensional forces (see Fig. 13.16B).

Recognizing the disk as an extension of the capsule, the capsule of the TMJ can be described as a fibrous, nonelastic membrane surrounding the joint, which is attached above to the squamotympanic fissure posteriorly, the margins of the glenoid fossa laterally, and the articular eminence anteriorly. Inferiorly, the capsule is attached to the neck of the condyle. Above the disk the capsule is fairly lax, whereas below it is attached tightly to the condyle. The lateral aspect of the capsule is thickened to form a fan-shaped ligament known as the *temporomandibular ligament,* which runs obliquely backward and downward from the lateral aspect of the articular eminence to the posterior aspect of the condylar neck. The ligament consists of two parts: (1) an outer oblique portion arising from the outer surface of the articular eminence and extending backward and downward to insert into the outer surface of the condylar neck, and (2) an inner horizontal portion with the same origin but inserting into the lateral pole of the condyle (Fig. 13.17). The capsule and its lateral thickening form the ligament of the joint. This ligament restricts joint movements by limiting the distance that the bones forming the articulation can be separated from each other without causing tissue damage. The temporomandibular ligament restricts displacement of the mandible in three different planes. First, the ligament functions in a way similar to collateral ligaments of other joints because of the bilateral nature of the articulation. By preventing lateral dislocation of one joint, it prevents medial dislocation of the other. Second, its oblique component limits the amount of inferior displacement; third, its horizontal component prevents or limits posterior displacement. This anatomic configuration means that, if dislocation occurs, it is forward with the head of the condyle slipping in front of the articular eminence. Two other ligaments are included in conventional descriptions of the joint, although neither has a functional role. The first is the sphenomandibular ligament, running from the lingula and shielding the opening of the interior alveolar canal to the spine of the sphenoid. This ligament represents the residual perichondrium of Meckel's cartilage. The second is the stylomandibular ligament, running from the styloid process to the angle of the mandible. This ligament represents the free border of the deep cervical fascia.

An inward circumferential extension of the capsule forms a tough, fibrous disk that divides the joint into upper and lower compartments; provides an articular surface for the head of the condyle; and, because

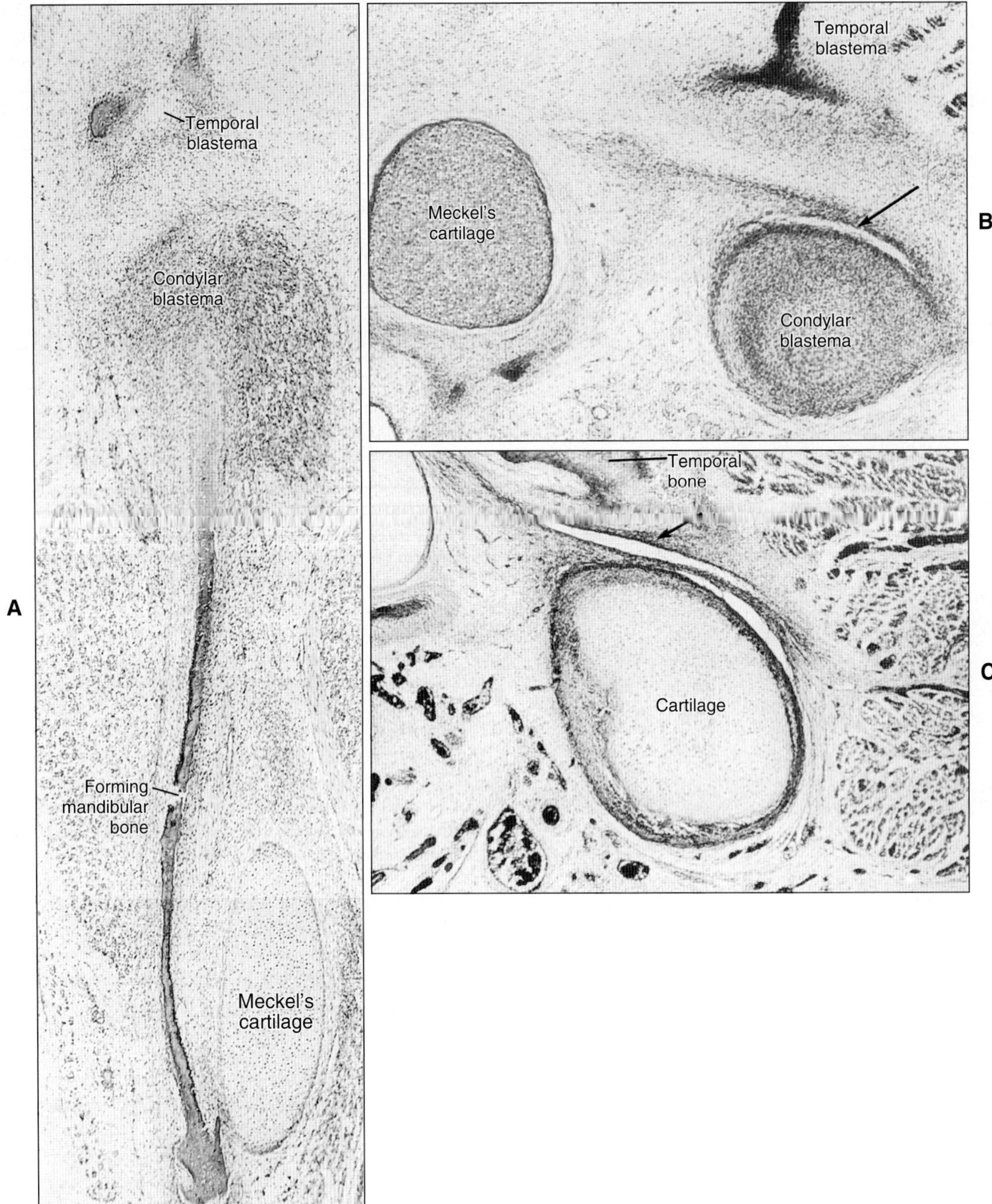

Fig. 13.5 Developing temporomandibular articulation. (A) Coronal section through a 12-week-old (61-mm crown-to-rump) fetus. Bone formation has begun in the temporal blastema. The condylar blastema is still undifferentiated. The membranous bone forming the body of the mandible on the lateral aspect of Meckel's cartilage is apparent. (B) Sagittal section of the temporomandibular joint (TMJ) in a fetus (67 mm crown-to-rump) showing the developing inferior joint cavity *(arrow)*. Bone formation has begun in the temporal blastema, but the condylar blastema still consists of undifferentiated cells. Meckel's cartilage is to the left of the developing joint. (C) Sagittal section of the TMJ of a fetus (70 mm crown-to-rump) showing the developing superior joint cavity *(arrow)*. Cartilage has formed in the condylar blastema, and the developing temporal bone is indicated. (A, From Chi JG, et al.: *Sequential atlas of human development,* Seoul, 1997, Medical Publishing; B, C, from Perry HT, et al.: The embryology of the temporomandibular joint, *Cranio* 3:125–132, 1985.)

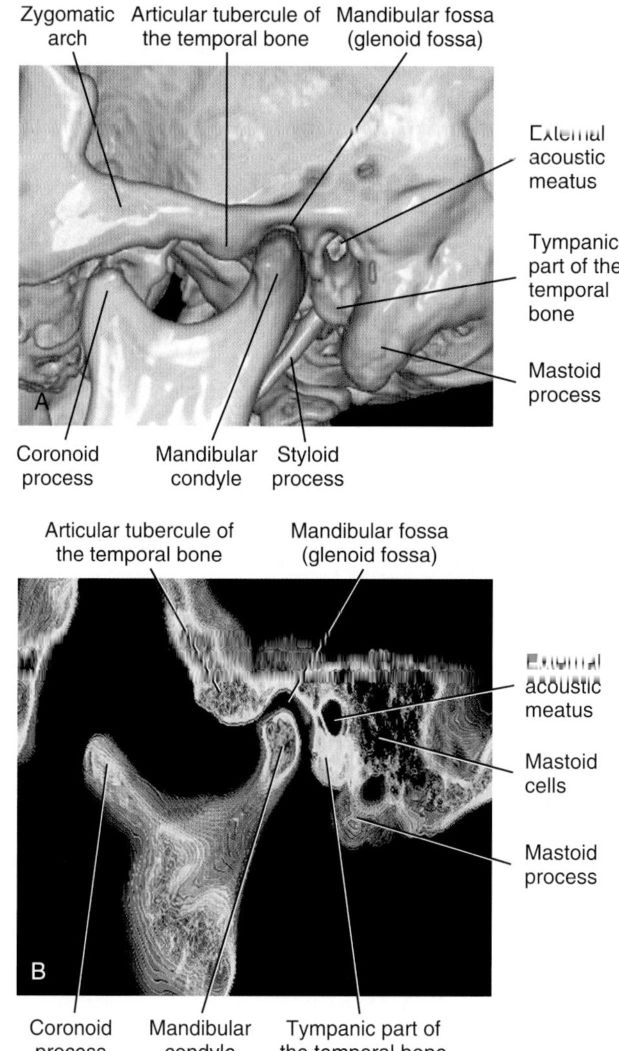

Fig. 13.6 Skeletal components of the temporomandibular articulation. (A) Three-dimensional computed tomography (CT) reconstruction of the skull (lateral view). (B) Sagittal CT slice through the temporomandibular articulation. (Courtesy M. Schmittbuhl.)

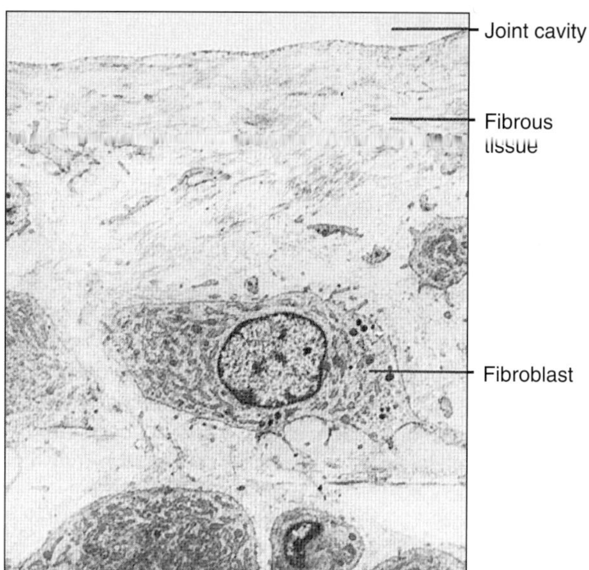

Fig. 13.7 Transmission electron micrograph showing the fibrous articular tissue covering the mandibular condyle. (From Goose DH, Appleton JI: *Human dentofacial growth*, New York, NY, 1982, Pergamon Press.)

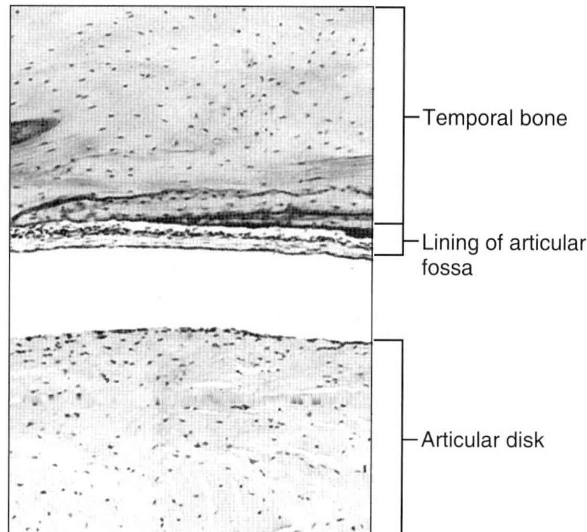

Fig. 13.8 Section through the temporal bone showing the thin lining of the articular surface of the glenoid fossa. (From Blackwood HJJ: The mandibular joint: development, structure and function. In Cohen B, Kramer IRH, editors: *Scientific foundations of dentistry*, London, 1976, William Heinemann Medical Books.)

the lower half of the capsule is tightly bound to the condyle, moves with the condyle during translation. The disk consists of dense fibrous tissue (see Fig. 13.4), and its shape conforms to that of the apposed articular surfaces. Thus the lower surface of the disk is concave and generally matches the convex contour of the condyle. The upper surface of the disk also presents a concave surface because its posterior and anterior components are considerably thickened, delimiting a central thinner component. At rest, this central thinner component of the disk separates the anterior slope of the condyle from the slope of the articular eminence. The thickened posterior portion occupies the gap between the condyle and the floor of the glenoid fossa, and the anterior portion lies slightly anterior to the condyle. The type I collagen bundles that constitute the disk generally are arranged loosely and are oriented randomly, except in the central region where they are more tightly bound in organized bundles. Coronal sections of the disk show it to be thicker medially.

The anterior portion of the disk fuses with the anterior wall of the capsule. Above the point of fusion, the capsule runs forward to blend with the periosteum of the anterior slope of the articular eminence. Below, the capsule merges with the periosteum of the front of the neck of the condyle. As explained previously, this appearance in section creates the impression that the anterior portion of the disk splits into two lamellae. Posteriorly, the disk also appears to divide into two lamellae, but, again, these lamellae represent the posterior wall of the capsule. The upper part of the capsule, or lamella, consists of fibrous and elastic tissue (the only part of the capsule where elastic fibers are found) and inserts into the squamotympanic fissure. The lower part of the capsule, consisting of collagen only, is nonelastic and blends with the periosteum of the condylar neck.

Between these two lamellae a space is created that is filled with a loose, highly vascular connective tissue. The disk is well supplied with vascular and neural elements at its periphery but is avascular and not innervated in its central region (Fig. 13.18). During function, the disk makes only short movements in a passive manner to fit best with the changing relationships of the condylar head, the glenoid fossa, and the articular eminence. Such adaptation is permitted by the shape of the disk and the slippery environment of the joint cavity, although some influence also is exerted by superior fibers of the lateral pterygoid and the tight relationship created by taut capsular fibers running from the margins of the disk to the condyle.

SYNOVIAL MEMBRANE

The capsule is lined on its inner surface by a synovial membrane (Fig. 13.19). Generally, the synovial membrane is considered to line the entire capsule, with folds or villi of the membrane protruding into the joint cavity, especially in its fornixes and its upper posterior aspect. These folds increase in number with age and are more prominent in joints affected by a pathologic process. The synovial membrane does not cover the articular surfaces of the joint or the disk, except for its bilaminar posterior region. Essentially, any synovial membrane consists of two layers: a cellular intima resting on a vascular subintima (Fig. 13.20) and the fibrous tissue of the capsule into which the subintima blends. The subintima is a loose connective tissue containing vascular elements together with scattered fibroblasts, macrophages, mast cells, fat cells, and some elastic fibers, which prevent folding of the membrane. The intima varies in structure, having one to four layers of synovial cells embedded in an amorphous, fiber-free intercellular matrix. Often cellular deficiencies exist, and the subintimal connective tissue directly borders the joint cavity. These cells are not connected by junctional complexes and do not rest on a basal lamina. The joint cavity therefore is not lined by epithelium. The cells forming this discontinuous layer are of two types: a predominant type A (macrophage-like) cell and a type B (fibroblast-like) cell. Type A cells have surface filopodia, many plasma membrane invaginations, and associated pinocytotic vesicles. Their cytoplasm contains numerous mitochondria and lysosomal elements and a prominent Golgi complex. Profiles of rough endoplasmic reticulum are few. Type B cells, by contrast, contain many profiles of rough endoplasmic reticulum. Type A cells exhibit significant phagocytotic properties, and type B cells synthesize the hyaluronate found in synovial fluid.

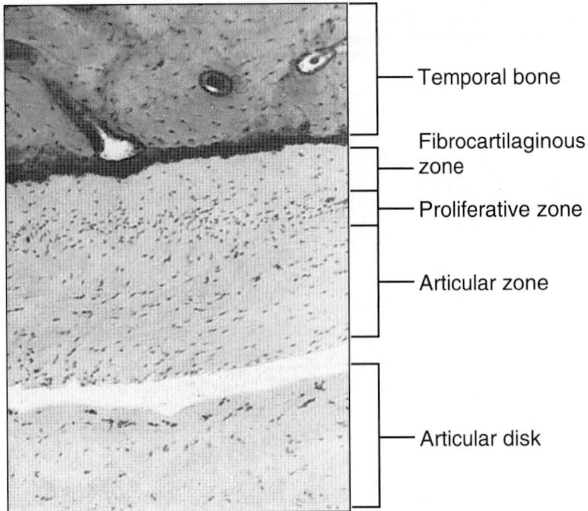

Fig. 13.9 Section through the articular eminence in an adult mandibular joint showing the thick articular covering of this area of the joint. (From Blackwood HJJ: The mandibular joint: development, structure and function. In Cohen B, Kramer IRH, editors: *Scientific foundations of dentistry*, London, 1976, William Heinemann Medical Books.)

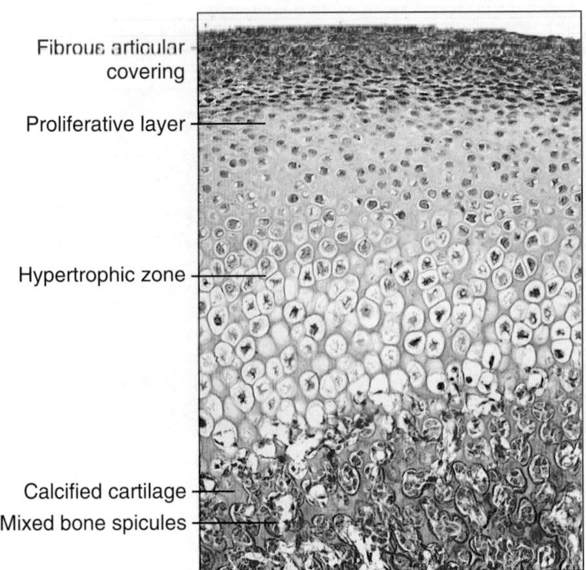

Fig. 13.11 Section through the growth cartilage of the condyle illustrating endochondral transformation into bone.

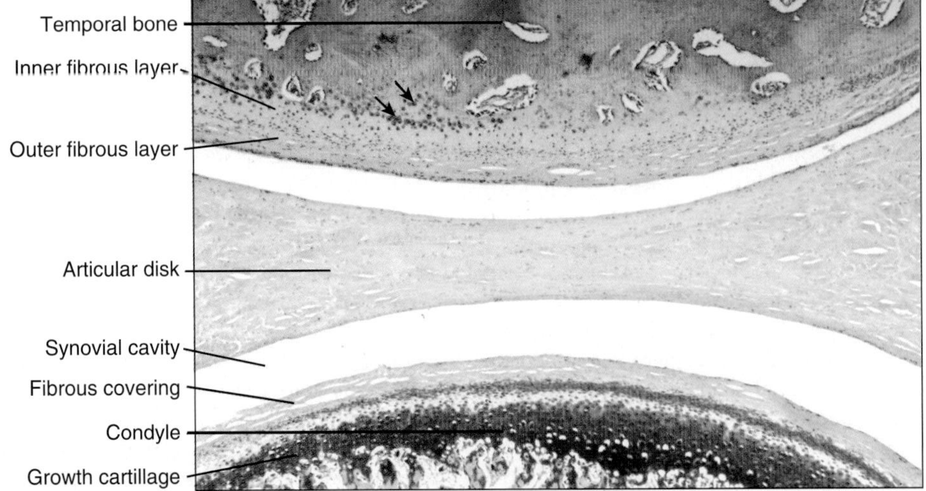

Fig. 13.10 Histologic section through the temporomandibular joint illustrating the relationship between the temporal bone, articular disk, and head of the condyle. Occasionally, chondrocytes are found in the inner fibrous layer of the temporal bone covering *(arrows)*.

The chemical composition of synovial fluid indicates that it is a dialysate of plasma supplemented with proteins and proteoglycans. The synovial membrane is responsible for controlling the passage of plasma components and producing the additional components. Synovial fluid also may contain a small population of varying cell types such as monocytes, lymphocytes, free synovial cells, and occasionally polymorphonuclear leukocytes. Synovial fluid is characterized by well-defined physical properties of viscosity, elasticity, and plasticity. The function of this fluid is to provide (1) a liquid environment for the joint surfaces, and (2) lubrication to increase efficiency and reduce erosion. Synovial fluid also is believed to act as a nutrient fluid for the avascular tissues covering the articular surfaces and for the disk.

MUSCLE CONTRACTION

Muscle cells (fibers) that make up the bundles (fasciculi) are long and narrow. A fiber can be several centimeters long and up to 0.1 mm in diameter. In any given muscle, the fibers tend to be of uniform length. The cell membrane of the fiber is called the *sarcolemma*, immediately beneath which the nucleus of the cell is found. Within each cell, the sarcoplasm is packed with myofibrils, arranged in such a way that their close packing creates the pattern of striations seen under light microscopy. Another feature of the muscle fiber is its sarcoplasmic reticulum, a branching endoplasmic network that surrounds each myofibril. Muscle contraction depends on the availability of calcium ions, which

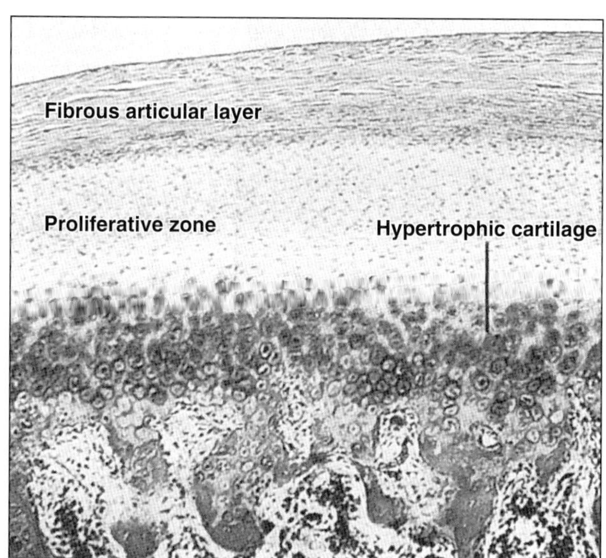

Fig. 13.12 Section through the growing condylar cartilage of a 13-year-old child. (From Goose DH, Appleton J: *Human dentofacial growth*, New York, NY, 1982, Pergamon Press.)

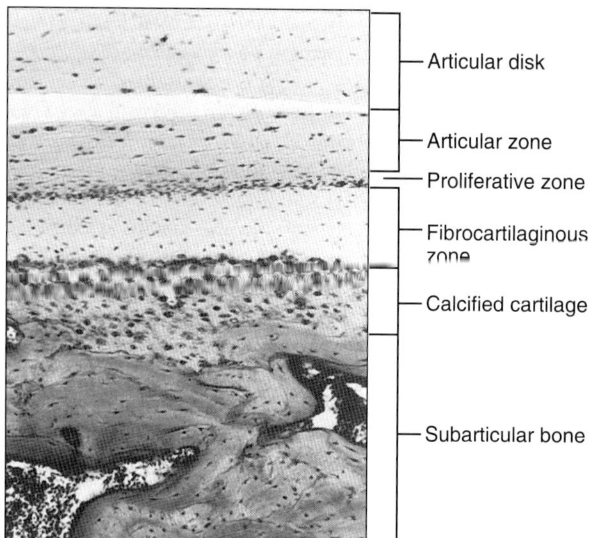

Fig. 13.14 Section through the articular covering of an adult mandibular condyle. (From Blackwood HJJ: The mandibular joint: development, structure and function. In Cohen B, Kramer IRH, editors: *Scientific foundations of dentistry*, London, 1976, William Heinemann Medical Books.)

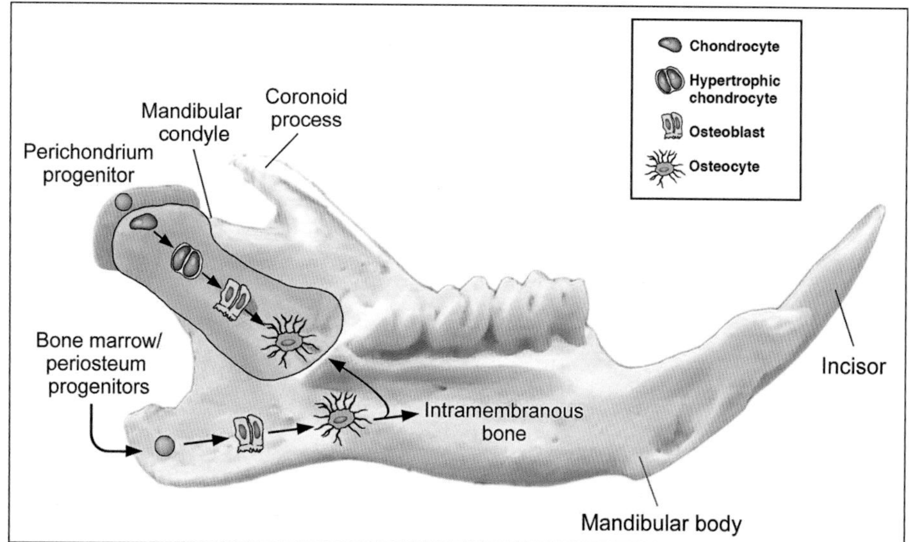

Fig. 13.13 Schematic illustration of the contribution of chondrocyte to the mandible. New findings using the cell lineage approach in rodents support the concept that chondrocytes directly transform into bone-forming cells during the formation of the condylar neck and ramus of the mandible. (Adapted from Hinton RJ, et al.: Roles in chondrocytes in endochondral bone formation and fracture repair, *J Dent Res* 96:23–30, 2017.)

are transferred back and forth from the sarcoplasmic reticulum. Finally, the sarcoplasm contains variable numbers of mitochondria, glycogen, and myoglobin (the last acts as an oxygen-storing pigment).

There are slow- and fast-twitch fibers, and histochemical studies have revealed the presence of an intermediate category. This distinction is mirrored in the histology and histochemistry of the individual muscle fiber; the slow-twitch fiber is generally narrower than the fast-twitch fiber, has poorly defined myofibrils, contains slow myosin, possesses many mitochondria, and exhibits high oxidative-enzyme and low phosphorylase activity. This last trait reflects the fact that slow fibers also have a well-developed aerobic metabolism. As a result, they resist fatigue. By contrast, the type II or fast-twitch fibers have fewer mitochondria, possess an extensive sarcoplasmic reticulum, contain fast myosin, and show a lower oxidative enzyme activity (which is balanced by increased phosphorylase activity). Fast-twitch fibers thus rely more on anaerobic (glycolytic) activity and fatigue more easily.

With this distinction understood, it is important to recognize that most, if not, all muscles contain a mixture of fast and slow fibers in varying proportions, reflecting the function of that muscle (Fig. 13.21). Also important is recognition that individual muscle fibers can be transformed (e.g., as a result of training) and that the innervation of the fibril determines its characteristics. In experiments in which nerves to red and white muscle fibers are cut, crossed, and reconnected, the fibers change their morphology and physiology accordingly.

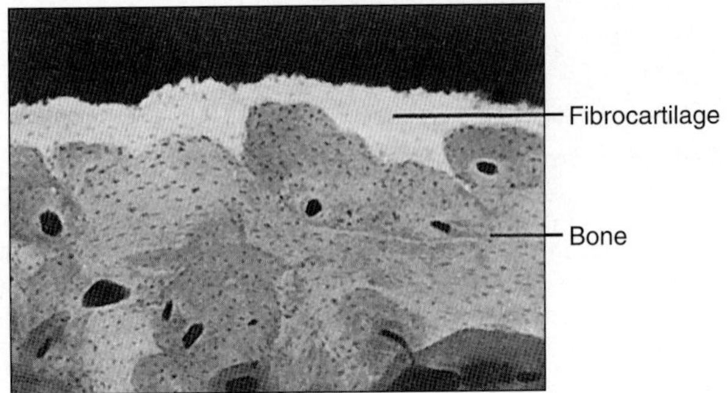

Fig. 13.15 Microradiograph showing the subarticular bone and mineralization of the adjacent fibrocartilaginous layer. (From Blackwood HJ: Cellular remodeling in articular tissue, *J Dent Res* 45:480–489, 1966.)

MOTOR UNIT

Voluntary skeletal muscle obviously requires innervation for contraction to take place. A single nerve may innervate a single muscle fiber (fine control) or, by branching, supply as many as 160 fibers. No matter the pattern, the complex is known as a *motor unit* (Fig. 13.22), and innervation is achieved through a structure known as the *motor end plate.* At the site of innervation, the nerve loses its myelin sheath but not the covering of Schwann cells and forms a terminal dilation that comes to occupy a corresponding dimple in the muscle cell surface. Between the nerve termination and the sarcolemma is a gap (the synaptic cleft) where the sarcolemmal surface is thrown into a series of junctional folds. A motor unit supplies fibers of a single type.

Two other neuronal structures need to be described in relation to muscle contraction: the muscle spindle and the Golgi tendon organ.

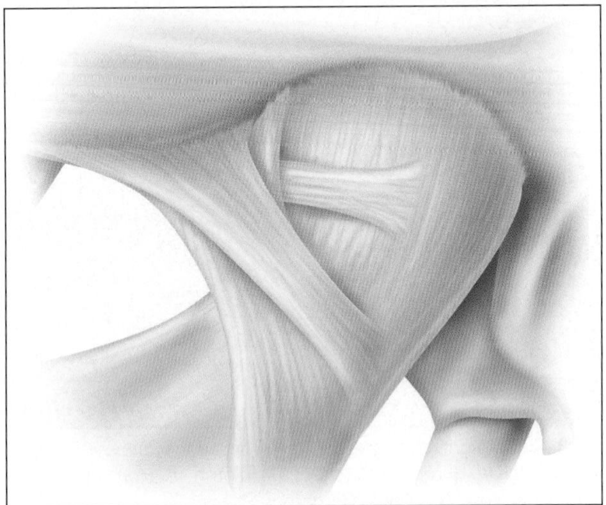

Fig. 13.17 The lateral (or temporomandibular) ligament. This diagram emphasizes two functional components of the capsular ligament preventing posterior and inferior displacement. The total ligament also prevents lateral and medial displacement (of the opposite joint).

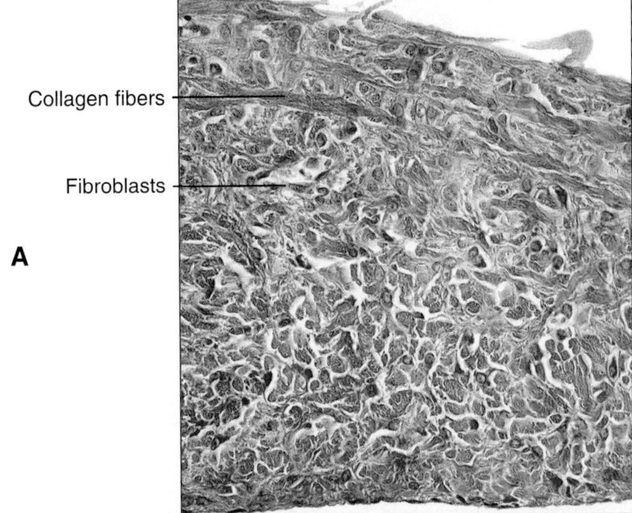

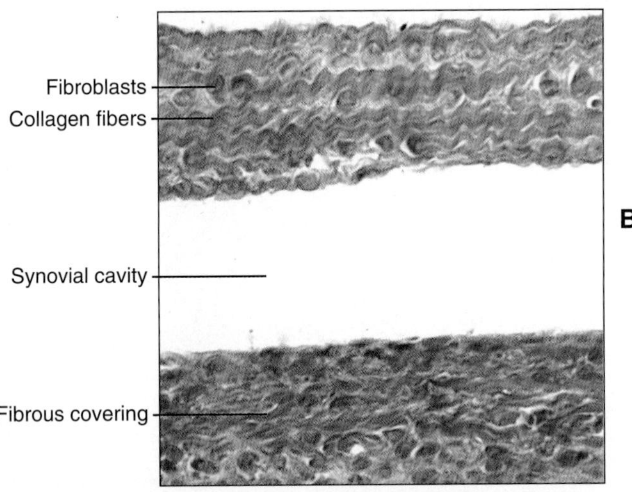

Fig. 13.16 Light microscope images of the articular disk showing (A) the coarse collagen fiber network constituting it and interposed fibroblastic cells and (B) the wavy appearance of the fibers in some regions that contributes to the biomechanical properties.

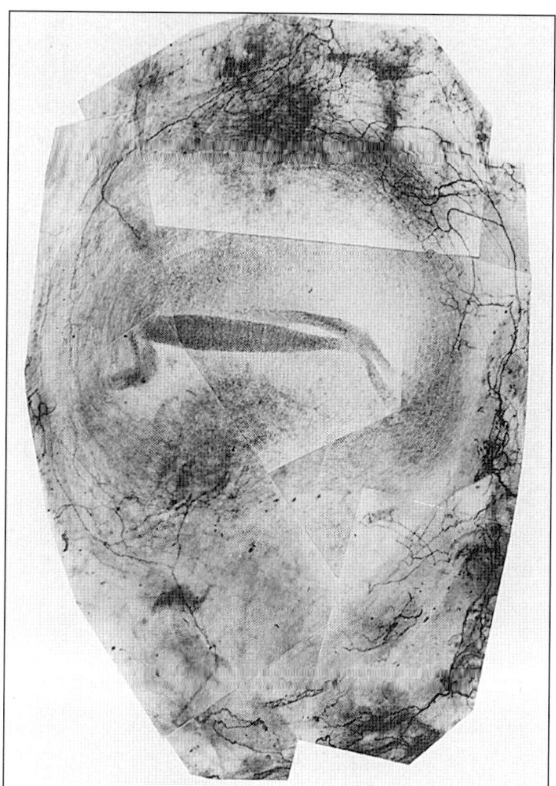

Fig. 13.18 Nerve distribution shown in a whole mount preparation of a rat disk. The absence of nerves from the central portion of the disk is notable. (From Shimizu S, et al.: Postnatal development of protein gene product 9.5- and calcitonin gene-related peptide-like immunoreactive nerve fibers in the rat temporomandibular joint, *Anat Rec* 245:568–576, 1996.)

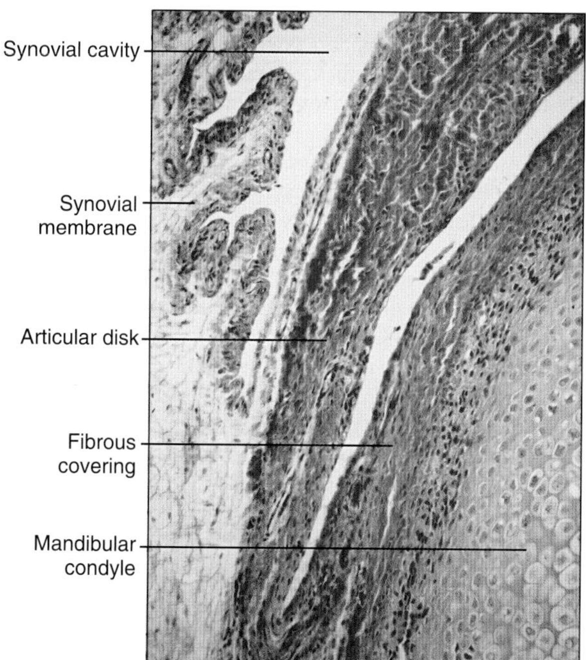

Fig. 13.19 Histologic section through the temporomandibular joint showing the synovial membrane, articular disk, and articular surface of the condyle. The synovial membrane is a bilayered structure with folds or villi that regulate formation of the synovial fluid that fills the joint cavities and lubricates articular surfaces.

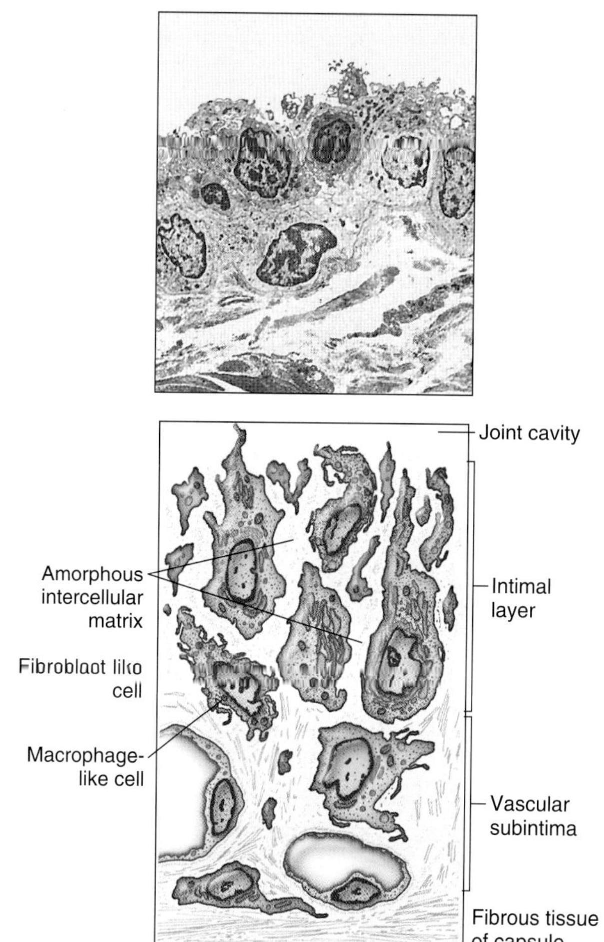

Fig. 13.20 Synovial membrane. *(Top)* Electron micrograph. *(Bottom)* Diagrammatic representation. (Micrograph courtesy W. Feagens.)

Muscle Spindle

The muscle spindle is an encapsulated proprioceptor that detects changes in length. In the craniofacial region, only jaw-closing and tongue muscles have spindles. These consist of a connective tissue sac 5 mm long and 0.2 mm in diameter containing 2 to 12 specially adapted muscle fibers (intrafusal fibers). Intrafusal fibers are narrower than extrafusal fibers and assume two forms. The first is described as a nuclear bag fiber because of the concentration of many nuclei in its centrally expanded portion, and the second as a nuclear chain fiber because its nuclei are aligned in a single row. The nuclear bag fiber is innervated by a nerve that spirals around the bag (the primary afferent). The nuclear chain fiber is innervated from a primary terminal supplying the central region of the chain and a secondary terminal on either side of the primary (Fig. 13.23). These afferents are responsible for the jaw stretch reflex. The primary terminal is believed to be involved with responses to the degree and rate of stretch, and the secondary terminal is believed to be involved with responses involved only with the degree of stretch. Muscle spindle intrafusal fibers retain their efferent supply.

Golgi Tendon Organ

Golgi tendon organs are found at the junctions between muscles and the tendons (aponeuroses) on which they pull. Golgi tendon organs are approximately half the size of a muscle spindle and consist of a capsule surrounding a group of collagen fibrils. The afferent nerve breaks up within the capsule, and the terminal fibers ramify between the collagen bundles. The nerves are stimulated by compression between the bundles when the tendon is under compression.

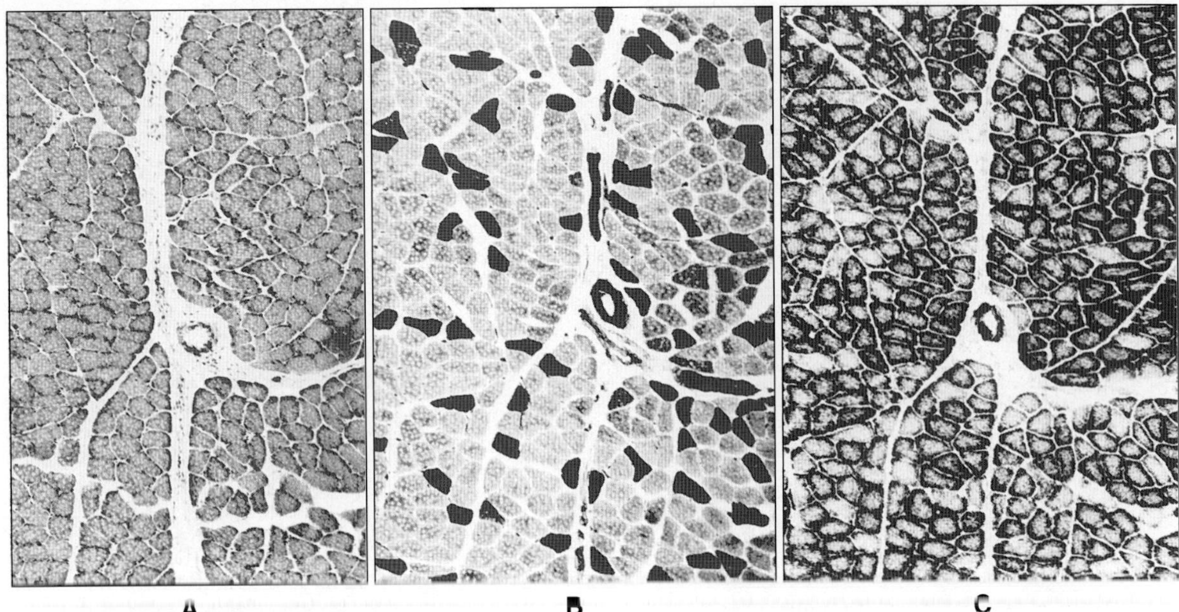

Fig. 13.21 Three successive sections of the lateral pterygoid muscle. (A) The muscle has been stained with hematoxylin and eosin, and all the fibers appear the same. (B) The muscle has been stained to demonstrate adenosinetriphosphatase activity, and this treatment clearly distinguishes two types of fiber—the slow oxidative (unstained) and the fast glycolytic. (C) The same muscle is stained to demonstrate reduced nicotinamide adenine dinucleotide. The majority of fibers that stained strongly with adenosinetriphosphatase now are not stained, but some indicate a fast oxidative fiber.

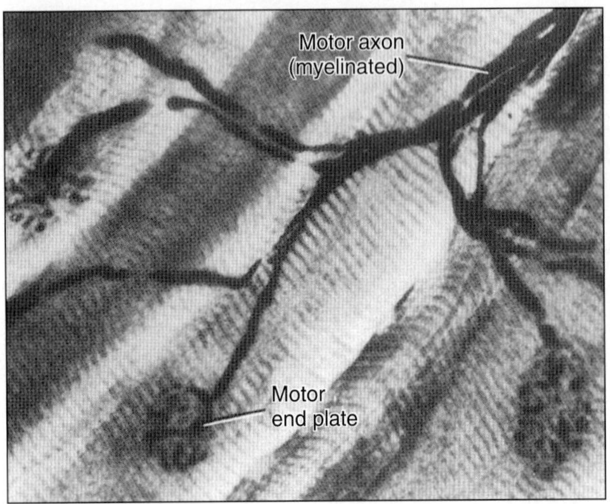

Fig. 13.22 Motor end plates on skeletal muscle fibers (stained with gold chloride). (From Cormack DH: *Introduction to histology*, Philadelphia, PA, 1984, Williams & Wilkins.)

From this abbreviated account of muscle, its heterogeneity can be appreciated as providing the tremendous adaptation of structure necessary to function, which is especially evident in the muscles of mastication.

MUSCLES OF MASTICATION

Classically, the muscles of mastication are the masseter, the medial (inferior) pterygoid, the lateral (superior) pterygoid, and the temporalis (Fig. 13.24). In functional terms, other muscle groups are involved in mastication, such as the postcervical group, which stabilizes the cranial base, the infrahyoid group, which stabilizes the hyoid bone and permits the mylohyoid muscle and anterior belly of the digastric muscle to influence mandibular position and the tongue and facial muscles, which aid chewing by helping to position foodstuff between the teeth.

The masseter and medial pterygoid muscles together have a sling-like configuration, clasping the angle of the mandible, and are the principal elevators of the jaw. Both muscles are multipennate and quadrate, and each has two heads.

The variety of coordinated and precise muscle activities and movement patterns that characterize mastication reflect, in part, the neuromuscular compartmentalization of the masticatory muscles. This is especially evident in the masseter, which comprises different portions, each with a different function. This compartmentalization is further denoted by the fact that each compartment is supplied by its own unique set of motor unit axons and biomechanical properties (see later).

The masseter consists of a superficial portion and a deep portion (or head), which, although originating separately, have a common insertion and blend together at the anterior border of the muscle. The superficial head has a tendinous portion, originating from the zygomatic process of the maxilla, and a fleshy portion, arising from the inferior border of the anterior two-thirds of the zygomatic arch. The fibers of the superficial head run inferoposteriorly to insert into the angle and lower border of the mandibular ramus. They cover the fibers of the deep portion of the muscle, which arise from the inner aspect and inferior border of the posterior third of the zygomatic arch and run almost vertically downward to insert into the upper border and lateral aspect of the ramus. Although anatomically this muscle has two components, the components can be distinguished readily and can be seen in functional terms to consist of four components: deep anterior, deep posterior, superficial anterior, and superficial posterior.

The medial pterygoid also has two portions, or heads. The bulk of the muscle originates from the medial aspect of the lateral pterygoid plate, with a slip of fibers originating from the maxillary tuberosity.

Analysis of fiber composition of these two powerful, elevator muscles confirms regional differences. Both muscles exhibit a preponderance of slow-twitch fibers, indicating a muscle that (in conjunction with the multipennate structure) is adapted to resisting fatigue at low

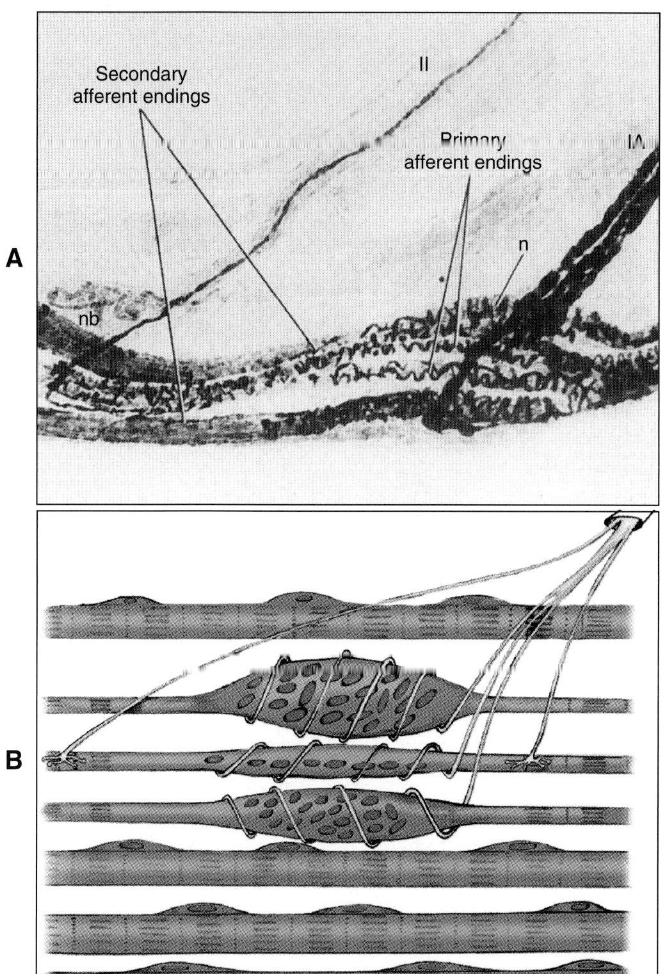

Fig. 13.23 (A) Photomicrograph of the structure and innervation of a muscle spindle (cat; stained with gold chloride) showing primary annulospiral afferent endings and secondary flower spray endings. (B) The spindle. (For clarity the capsule has been omitted.) Primary annulospiral fibers envelop the nuclear bag and the nuclear chain intrafusal fibers. The flower spray secondary endings are associated with the nuclear chain fiber. *nb,* Nuclear bag; *n,* nuclear chain fibers. (A, From Boyd IA: The structure and innervation of the nuclear bag muscle fiber system and the nuclear chain muscle fiber system in mammalian muscle spindles, *Philos Trans R Soc Lond B Biol Sci* 245:81–136, 1962.)

force levels. The posterior portions of both muscles, however, are characterized by possessing a high concentration of fast-twitch, rapidly contracting motor units and are sensitive to fatigue; they can generate large forces intermittently in the molar region of the mandible.

The temporalis is a fan-shaped muscle arising from the side of the skull that inserts into the coronoid process and the anteromedial border of the mandibular ramus. The muscle is covered by a strong sheet of fascia attached (above) to the superior temporal line and (below) to the medial and lateral aspects of the zygomatic arch, the undersurface of which also provides origin for fleshy muscle fibers. The temporalis is bipennate. An inner layer of fibers converges vertically down the lateral wall of the cranium to form a central tendon that inserts into the coronoid process and the anterior edge of the ascending ramus. The outer layer fibers (arising from the temporal fascia) descend in a more medial direction.

Functionally, the temporalis acts as two muscles: its anterior fibers as an elevator and its posterior horizontally disposed fibers as a retractor of the mandible. The muscle also shows variation in its fiber composition. The bipennate superficial portion has 50% fast-twitch fibers, indicating a capacity for acceleration coupled with an ability to develop tension. The posterior portion, however, contains a preponderance of slow-twitch fibers and many muscle spindles, indicating adaptation to a postural function. Thus, in general, the masseter and the medial pterygoid are power producers, and the temporalis is concerned more with moving and stabilizing the mandible.

The lateral pterygoid muscle has two heads, superior and inferior, arising from the roof of the infratemporal fossa and the lateral pterygoid plate, respectively. No debate exists over the insertion of fibers of the lower head; they run posteriorly, inferiorly, and slightly laterally to insert into the pterygoid fovea on the anterior surface of the condylar neck and, on contraction, bring about downward-forward and medial movement of the condyle. The insertion of the fibers of the superior head has been the subject of debate. No doubt exists that most of the fibers of this head insert into the pterygoid fovea on the condyle, but the question resides on whether some of the superior fibers insert into the disk. The upper fibers of the muscle may (1) gain insertion into the condyle by merging with the central tendon of the muscle, (2) insert directly into the pterygoid fovea, or (3) insert directly into the disk at its most medial aspect. Because the bulk of the muscle inserts into the condyle logically, however, its main activity is to move the condyle. Electromyographic studies indicate a reciprocal activation of the two heads of the muscle, with the inferior head involved in opening the jaw and the superior head involved in closure (by seating the condylar head against the posterior slope of the articular eminence). The attachment of the upper fibers to the disk directly or indirectly is believed to stabilize the disk at closure. Again, these functional differences are reflected in fiber composition, with the slow-twitch fiber predominating, indicating a capacity for endurance during continuous work at low force levels.

Finally, the intrafusal fibers of muscle spindles in the masseter not only have a different enzyme profile from that in the extrafusal fibers but also are different from the intrafusal fibers in the limbs and trunk. This suggests special functional characteristics for this masticatory muscle.

NEURAL BASIS OF MASTICATION

Mastication, or chewing as it is more commonly called, is a highly coordinated sensorimotor function in humans that has evolved from the primitive feeding behavior of lower invertebrates. While most of the structural components in muscles and the brain that are required for chewing are present at birth, chewing is not fully expressed in all its sophistication in the newborn. This complex function typically displays a rhythmic series of vertical movements of jaw opening and jaw closing produced by the contraction of the jaw-closing muscles (e.g., masseter, temporalis) and jaw-opening muscles (e.g., anterior digastric). However, it often may include less rigidly patterned horizontal jaw movements (protrusive, lateral) as well as movements of the tongue and lips or cheeks (e.g., to ensure the appropriate placement of a food bolus between the teeth during chewing). Thus in the full sense of the word (mastication), when we refer to the masticatory muscles, this term needs to encompass muscles of facial expression and tongue as well as jaw muscles. Furthermore, it needs to be appreciated that humans, like other mammals, are not born as chewing animals, but rather at birth have an inherent ability to suckle. There is a considerable and variable postnatal learning period before the sophisticated sensorimotor patterns comprising mastication develop, which are built on some of the sensorimotor patterns characteristic of suckling and triggered in part by the eruption of teeth. Thus mastication can be viewed, at least in part, as a learned sensorimotor behavior that is

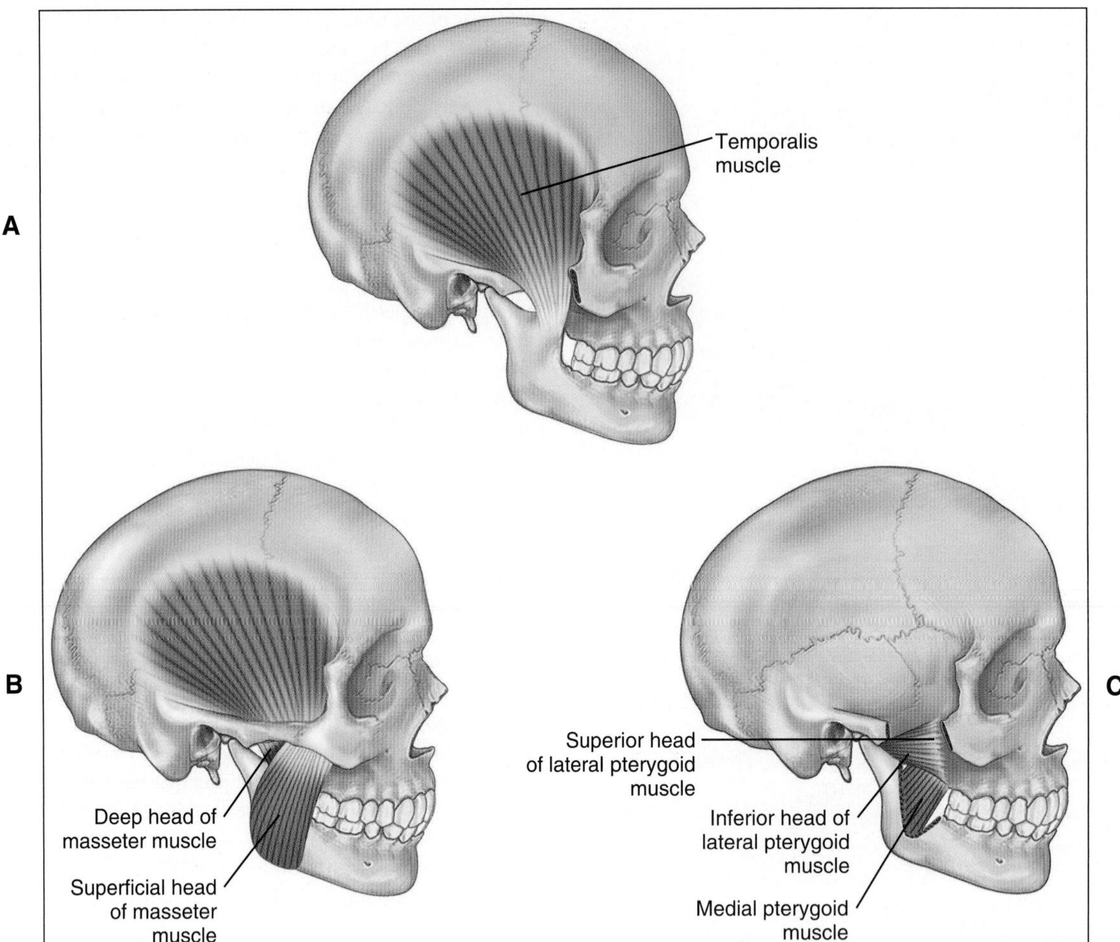

Fig. 13.24 Jaw-closing muscles involved in mastication. (A) Temporalis. (B) Masseter. (C) Lateral and medial pterygoids.

dependent on circuits in the central nervous system (CNS) that underlie the processes associated with learning (see later).

The complex arrangement of the masticatory muscles reflects the multiplicity of motor behaviors in which the muscle may participate. Thus some parts of a muscle may or may not be active depending on the motor behavior, and, for example, two parts of the muscle may be active at the same time for some movements but at different times for other movements. Consequently, the muscle as a whole can participate in producing a wide range of movements.

Clearly, such a complex array of muscle activities requires a neural substrate that comprises sophisticated and adaptive neural circuits providing for the initiation and control of the masticatory muscles during masticatory behaviors and for the integration of their activities with associated sensorimotor behaviors such as swallowing, speech, and respiration. The neural substrate for mastication also involves sensory receptors in orofacial tissues and their primary afferent inputs into the CNS, as well as the muscles to produce movements associated with mastication. The structural and functional features of the muscles are outlined earlier in this chapter, including the contractile and histochemical profiles of their muscle fibers as well as some of the sensory receptors found in muscle (e.g., muscle spindle, Golgi tendon organ). It is interesting that, whereas muscle spindles and Golgi tendon organs are abundant in muscles supplied by spinal nerves, these receptors in primates are limited to the jaw-closing and tongue muscles, and in subprimates they occur only in jaw-closing muscles. In contrast to the jaw-closing and other skeletal muscles, facial and jaw-opening muscles have few or no muscle spindles and Golgi tendon organs. Nonetheless, the limited sensory information that the CNS receives from the facial and jaw-opening muscles may be compensated for by the rich sensory input to the CNS derived from primary afferent nerve fibers that supply receptors in facial skin, oral mucosa, periodontium, TMJs, and other orofacial tissues. The vast majority of these primary afferents have their cell bodies in the trigeminal ganglion, although in the case of jaw muscle spindles and some periodontal mechanoreceptors, their cell bodies are located in the trigeminal mesencephalic nucleus; this is the only instance in the whole body where primary afferent cell bodies are found within the CNS.

These various afferent inputs into the CNS provide orofacial sensory information that is relayed in ascending sensory pathways through the brainstem to higher brain levels (e.g., thalamus, cerebral cortex) and that is used for perceptual, motivational, and affective functions. However, this sensory information also may be used at each of these levels as feedforward and feedback information important for sensorimotor integration and control. In addition, these afferent inputs into the CNS may contribute to brainstem circuits underlying reflexes (e.g., jaw-opening, gagging) evoked in the masticatory muscles by orofacial stimuli activating receptors that signal pain, touch, joint position, muscle stretch, tension, etc. These brainstem circuits include brainstem sensory and motor nuclei and adjacent brainstem interneuronal sites as well as integrative centers (e.g., chewing center, swallow center) that are central pattern generators (CPGs) that play important roles in the elaboration of the motor output patterning that characterize chewing and swallowing.

The sensory nuclei and motor nuclei are arranged into distinct neuronal pools in the brainstem and receive the afferent inputs from orofacial tissues mentioned earlier, as well as inputs from other brainstem sites and from areas at higher levels of the CNS that regulate the activity of the neuronal pools. The motor nuclei contain the brainstem motoneurons that provide the motor output to the masticatory muscles; these include (1) the motoneurons of the trigeminal motor nucleus, which, through their motor axons (alpha efferents), provide the motor innervation of most jaw muscles; (2) the motoneurons of the facial motor nucleus, which innervate the muscles of facial expression; and (3) the motoneurons of the hypoglossal nucleus, which innervate the intrinsic and extrinsic muscles of the tongue. The major sensory nuclei involved in mastication are the trigeminal brainstem sensory nuclear complex and the solitary tract nucleus. These sensory nuclei are the major relays of the orofacial sensory information that (as noted earlier) is relayed in ascending sensory pathways to higher brain levels involved in perceptual, motivational, and affective functions and sensorimotor integration and control. They also serve as major interneuronal sites contributing to the neural circuits underlying mastication because they relay the afferent inputs that they receive from the orofacial tissues or from higher brain areas to the motoneurons. There are other important brainstem interneuronal sites involved in mastication, and they include the intertrigeminal and supratrigeminal nuclei, as well as components of the reticular formation that lie immediately adjacent to the trigeminal brainstem complex and the solitary tract nucleus. Thus these various interneuronal regions provide a neural substrate that allows for the initiation or modulation of the brainstem reflexes mentioned earlier, which can be evoked by stimuli applied to various orofacial tissues. Some of these regions also provide part of the neural circuitry and processes constituting the CPGs that are so crucial in the initiation and control of mastication and swallowing. Fig. 13.25 gives an overview of some orofacial afferent inputs and CNS pathways involved in the initiation or modulation of the activities of the brainstem motoneurons and CPGs.

In the case of the CPG for mastication (the chewing center), this is a network of neurons in the brainstem between the rostral poles of the trigeminal motor nucleus and facial motor nucleus that generates or modulates chewing movements through their excitatory and inhibitory projections to the motoneurons in the trigeminal, facial, and hypoglossal motor nuclei. The CPG utilizes its orofacial afferent inputs, especially those from periodontal mechanoreceptors and jaw muscle spindles, together with inputs that it receives from higher brain areas (e.g., sensorimotor cortex) to provide guidance and modification of the movements. The left and right sides of the CPG are connected by axons of neurons in the CPG that cross the midline at several levels of the brainstem. Some of the neurons that form the core of the CPG reside in the medial reticular formation, but most of the neurons forming the core of the CPG are located within the principal nucleus (NVsnpr) of the trigeminal brainstem sensory nuclear complex. Neurons of the dorsal part of NVsnpr have intrinsic properties, enabling them to have a rhythmic pattern of activity, and they are thought to form the rhythmogenic core of the CPG. They have two distinct types of patterns of activity: one that is reflected in a sustained and regular firing of action potentials (i.e., tonic) and one consisting of bursts of action potentials recurring at regular intervals (i.e., rhythmic). These two modes of activity enable the neurons to participate in two quite different functions. As illustrated in Fig. 13.26, neuronal firing in the tonic mode allows them to relay the sensory information that they receive to other nearby brainstem neurons and to higher CNS areas, whereas in the rhythmic bursting mode they generate a rhythmic motor command that is conveyed to the motoneurons producing the rhythmic movements that characterize mastication. The rhythmic

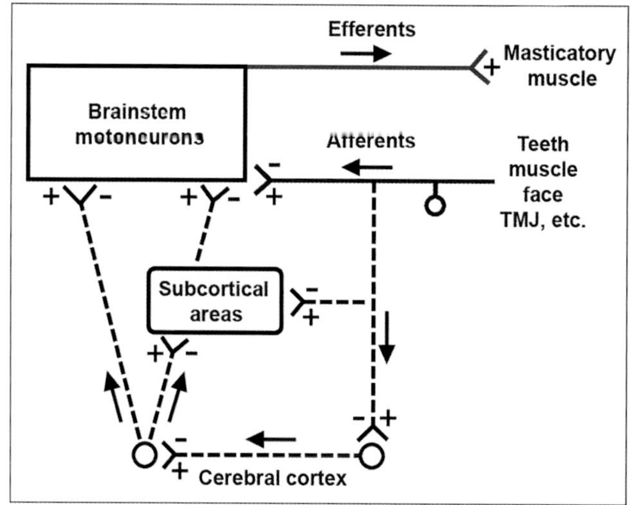

Fig. 13.25 Overview of orofacial sensory inputs and central nervous system (CNS) pathways involved in regulating motoneurons in brainstem motor nuclei (e.g., trigeminal, facial, hypoglossal). The activity of the motoneurons can be influenced (excited, +; inhibited, -) by inputs from sensory receptors in teeth, muscle, face, temporomandibular joint (TMJ), and other orofacial tissues as well as by inputs from other cerebral cortical areas (e.g., sensorimotor) and subcortical areas (e.g., basal ganglia, cerebellum, reticular formation, central pattern generators [CPG]). The projections from the cerebral cortex can influence the motoneurons through relatively direct effects or through indirect effects via its connections with the subcortical areas. The orofacial sensory inputs can also relatively directly influence the brainstem motoneurons, but, in addition, they can indirectly influence the motoneurons via their projections through ascending pathways to many of the subcortical areas (e.g., CPG) and higher CNS areas (e.g., sensorimotor area).

mode of activity depends on a sodium-persistent current that is voltage dependent and is regulated by the extracellular concentration of Ca^{2+}. It is notable that recent research has also documented that the nonneuronal cells called *glia* (in particular, astrocytes) (see Chapter 4) play an important role in the functioning of the CPG through their interactions with some of the neuronal elements of the CPG (see Fig. 13.26). Inactivation of astrocytes or blockade of S100β completely impedes the cell's ability to switch from a tonic to a rhythmic firing pattern, indicating that astrocytes and endogenous release of S100β are absolutely required for this process to occur. This is compelling evidence that astrocytes are much more than housekeepers and play an important role in neural processing.

Thus the stereotyped rhythmic opening and closing jaw movements typical of chewing are patterned by the CPG, although they can also be varied and programmed to function in an integrated manner with other movements, such as those of the tongue and cheeks to allow for repositioning of a food bolus and for changes in masticatory force and jaw velocity and displacement as the bolus is crushed and manipulated. These processes explain why factors such as food composition and hardness, bite force, and number of teeth can influence the masticatory process and allow the bolus to be reduced to a size suitable for swallowing. The CPG can also modulate the intraoral sensory inputs that it receives from the teeth, tongue, cheeks, etc. to provide a form of central control that, on one hand, may inhibit afferent inputs to the motoneurons that would otherwise produce undesirable perturbations and reflexes that could disrupt the ongoing masticatory process. On the other hand, however, it may not inhibit nociceptive afferent inputs but allow them to access the masticatory motoneurons and thereby provide protection of the masticatory apparatus during mastication.

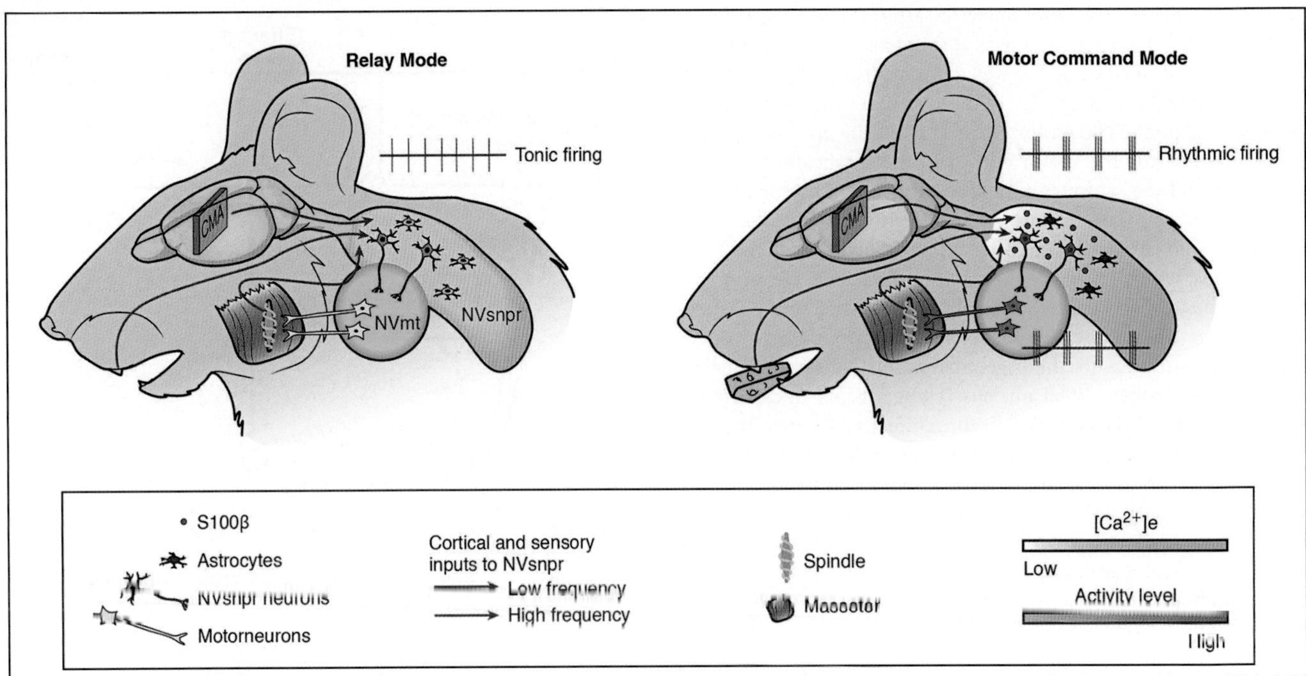

Fig. 13.26 Jaw muscles executing masticatory movements are controlled by trigeminal motoneurons that receive a rhythmic motor command from a central pattern generator (CPG) located in the brainstem. Neurons forming the core of the CPG produce this rhythmic motor command under conditions in which mastication needs to be triggered (i.e., under voluntary control from the cortex) or when there is a sustained stimulation of the sensory fibers innervating the jaw muscles, the teeth, or the interior of the oral cavity. The neurons most likely to form the core of the CPG are in the dorsal part of the trigeminal nucleus (NVsnpr). These neurons fulfill a dual function. Most of the time they faithfully transmit to higher brain areas sensory information that they receive with a tonic firing mode. Under conditions in which mastication needs to be triggered, the level of inputs arriving from the cortex and/or sensory fibers increases importantly. This in turn activates astrocytes in NVsnpr and leads to release of S100β (a calcium-binding protein found in astrocytes) and subsequent decrease of the extracellular concentration of Ca^{2+} ($[Ca^{2+}]e$). This drop of $[Ca^{2+}]e$ then potentiates INaP and causes NVsnpr neurons to fire rhythmically. Because of the voltage dependency of INaP, this would occur only within a defined membrane potential range, between approximately −60 and −50 mV in our cells. This would provide the cells with a means to have graded activity in function of the incoming inputs and to trigger bursting in motor neurons of the trigeminal motor nucleus (NVmt) and, thereafter, chewing when this input reaches a certain level. If the level of sensory inputs decreases, then the process slowly stops. (Courtesy A. Kolta.)

The jaw-opening reflex mentioned earlier is a common example of this central control in operation. In this case, the CPG may not inhibit nociceptive afferent inputs during mastication but indeed allow for the interruption of mastication and for the jaw-opening reflex to be elicited by a noxious stimulus. An example is that of a fish bone piercing the oral mucosa when an individual is eating a fish meal. In such an instance, it is important for chewing to be halted and for the jaw to open reflexively to prevent further damage to the mucosal tissues.

Returning to the influences of higher brain areas that were only briefly mentioned earlier, these descending modulatory influences arise from many different areas of the CNS (Fig. 13.27). These include the limbic system, lateral hypothalamus, basal ganglia, cerebellum, and the sensorimotor area and cortical masticatory area, both of which are in the cerebral cortex. Each of these CNS areas plays an important role in modulating mastication in relation to one or more functions in which each may be involved (e.g., emotion, stress, fine sensorimotor control) and can affect mastication. Take, for instance, the two cerebral cortical areas: the sensorimotor area and cortical masticatory area, which are especially important in orofacial sensorimotor functions, including mastication. They play an integral role in the sensorimotor control of masticatory and other orofacial sensorimotor functions through their descending projections, which exert regulatory influences on the orofacial sensory and motor circuits in the brainstem and other parts of the CNS. A clinical example of the importance of these cortical areas is the loss of sensorimotor control of orofacial movements needed for speech, chewing, or swallowing that can follow a stroke affecting the cortical masticatory area or that part of the sensorimotor area normally controlling orofacial motor functioning. It should also be noted that the sensorimotor area of the cerebral cortex may also contribute to the learning of new motor skills such as that associated with learning to play a musical instrument or a skilled sport or in the case of a dental clinician or student learning to manually control a new dental restorative technique. The sensorimotor area is also involved in the learning of mastication by the infant and in the relearning of masticatory skills after a stroke affecting this part of the brain. The brain's remarkable capacity for neuroplasticity, even in the elderly, underpins these abilities. The process of neuroplasticity of these parts of the brain involved in the initiation and modulation of orofacial sensorimotor functions allows for the acquisition or modification of sensorimotor skills that are manifested as mastication. Neuroplasticity of these parts of the brain have also been shown to occur with the loss of teeth or other alterations to the dental occlusion (e.g., dental implants, orthodontically induced tooth movement) or other intraoral tissues (e.g., pain).

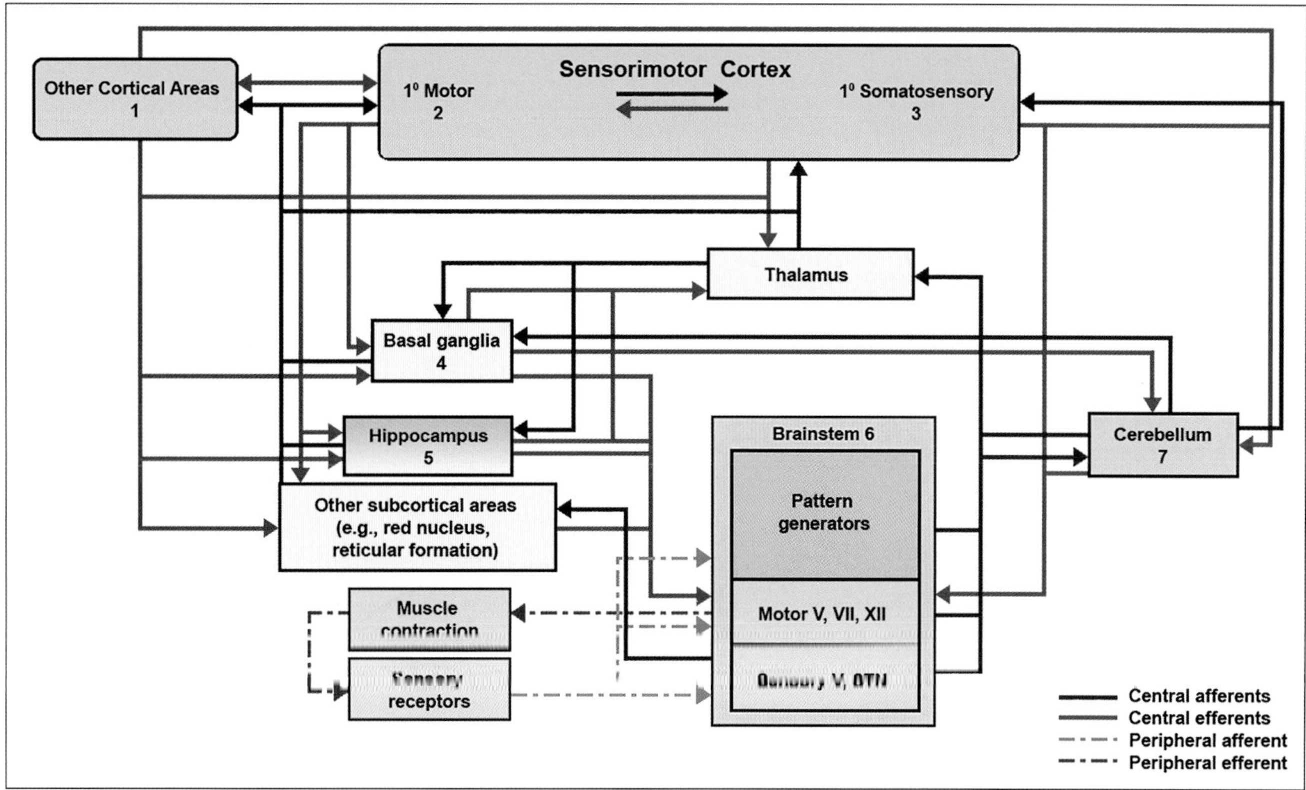

Fig. 13.27 Major afferent projections from orofacial tissues to the brain and efferent projections from the brain to jaw muscles. This complex circuitry is crucial for optimal coordination of the bilateral orofacial movements. Central nervous system areas play an important role in modulating mastication in relation to one or more of the following functions: *1,* motivation, emotion, cognition, attention, memory, and motor planning; *2,* sensorimotor integration, execution, control, and learning; *3,* multisensory processing and integration; *4,* sensorimotor control and learning; *5,* memory and spatial coding; 6, initiation and modulation of sensorimotor functions; and *7,* sensorimotor integration, control, timing, and learning. (Cortices and cerebellum, *green;* thalamus and subcortical areas, *yellow;* peripheral activity and nerves, *blue;* hippocampus regions, *green-yellow;* pattern generators, *orange.*) *STN,* Solitary tract nucleus. (From Avivi-Arber L, Sessle BJ: Jaw sensorimotor control in healthy adults and effects of ageing, *J Oral Rehab* 45:50–80, 2018.)

Such neuroplasticity is necessary for the person's ability to adapt (or not) to the altered intraoral environment and modify accordingly the masticatory function or other orofacial sensorimotor behaviors.

BIOMECHANICS OF THE JOINT

The muscles act on the TMJ to achieve opening and closing, protrusion and retrusion, and alternate lateral movements of the jaw and to provide stability. Because these movements rarely occur in isolation, most involve complex combinations of muscle activity. The role of the muscles in providing stability should not be overlooked, for during mastication, the forces applied to the joint not only are great but also are changing constantly; when this is considered with the destabilizing effects of translatory movement, the functional role of muscle becomes more obvious. An example is biting, which demands that the disk be stabilized in a slightly forward position. This stabilization is achieved by the upper fibers of the lateral pterygoid muscle.

Based on the anatomic configuration of the muscles and remembering that most movements of the joint involve rotatory and translatory movement, muscle function now can be grouped as follows (Fig. 13.28):

1. The masseter, medial pterygoid, anterior part of the temporalis, and upper head of the lateral pterygoid combine to close the jaw.
2. The inferior head of the lateral pterygoid, the anterior belly of the digastric, and the mylohyoid (the latter two not strictly muscles of mastication as defined) are responsible for opening movements.
3. The inferior head of the lateral pterygoid and the elevator group bring about protrusive movement, and the posterior fibers of the temporalis and the elevator group retrude the mandible.
4. Lateral movement is achieved by combined action of the elevator muscles, the posterior part of the temporalis (retrusion on the working side), and the lateral pterygoid (protrusion on the non-working side).

Because movements at the joint involve rotation and translation, the functional significance of the disk becomes more apparent (Fig. 13.29, see also Fig. 13.4C and D). The disk is not comparable to the meniscus in some other joints but is a unique feature of the temporomandibular articulation in that it enables a complexity of movement to be performed that cannot be done in any other joint. As has been pointed out already, the disk moves passively according to and dictated by its shape and the changing relationships of the bones involved in the temporomandibular articulation. The description is simplistic, however, because the direct and indirect relationships of the superior head of the lateral pterygoid to the disk clearly play a part in its function.

INNERVATION OF THE JOINT

The innervation of any joint (the TMJ included) involves four types of nerve endings: the first (type I) are Ruffini corpuscles; the second (type II), Pacini corpuscles; the third (type III), Golgi tendon organs; and the fourth (type IV), free nerve endings. The first three types are

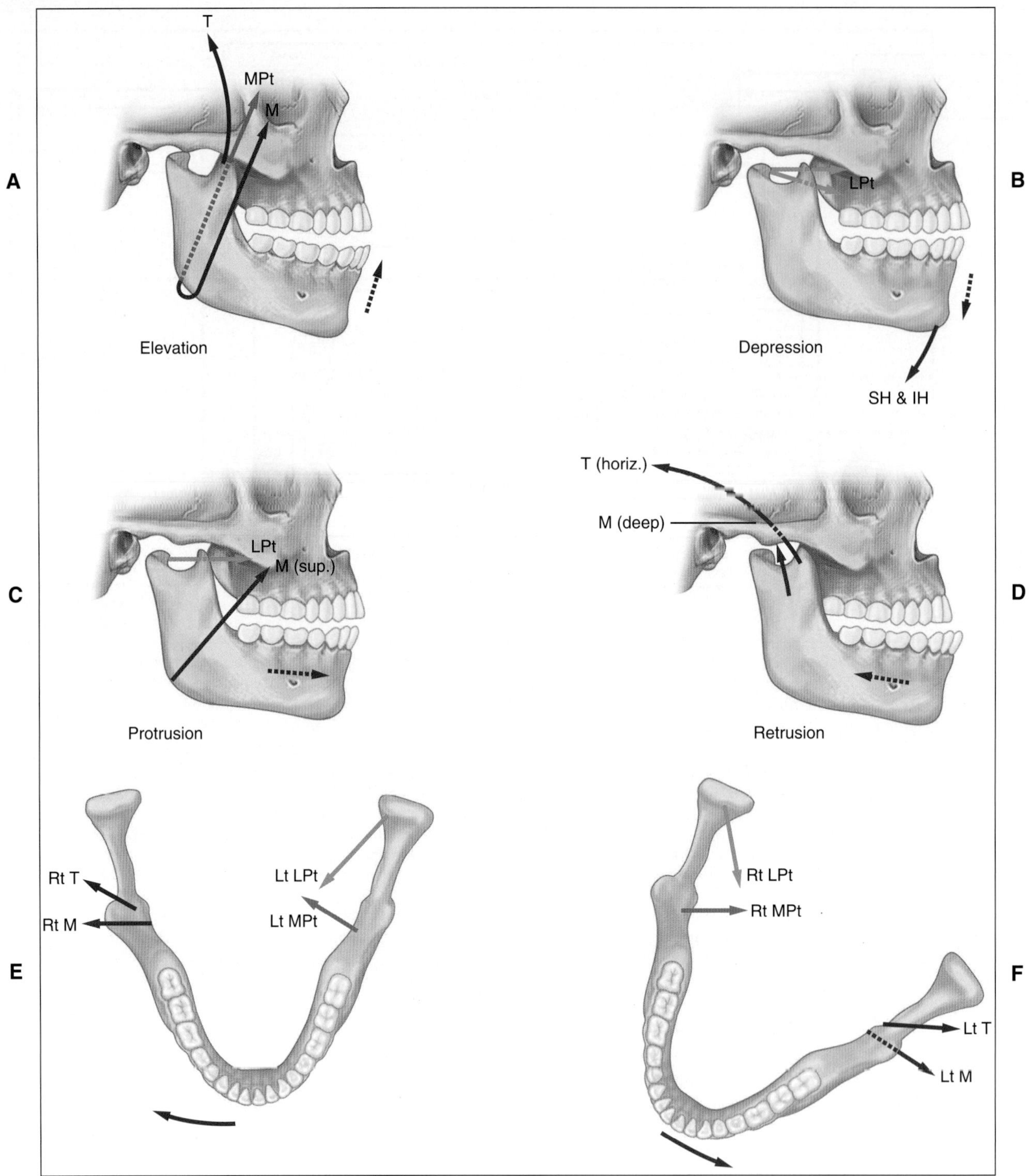

Fig. 13.28 Actions of the muscles of mastication. (A) Elevation. (B) Depression. (C) Protrusion. (D) Retrusion. (E) Right lateral excursion of the mandible. (F) Left lateral excursion of the mandible. *IH,* Infrahyoid; *LPt,* lateral pterygoid; *Lt LPt,* left lateral pterygoid; *Lt M,* left masseter; *Lt MPt,* left medial pterygoid; *Lt T,* left temporalis; *M,* masseter; *M (deep),* masseter, deep fibers; *M (sup.),* masseter, superficial fibers; *MPt,* medial pterygoid; *Rt LPt,* right lateral pterygoid; *Rt MPt,* right medial pterygoid; *Rt M,* right masseter; *Rt T,* right temporalis; *SH,* suprahyoid; *T,* temporalis; *T (horiz.),* temporalis, horizontal fibers.

encapsulated, with the first two (Ruffini and Pacini corpuscles) limited to the capsule of a joint and the third (Golgi tendon organs) confined to the ligaments associated with the joint. Free nerve endings have a wider distribution. Ruffini corpuscles show a striking resemblance to Golgi tendon organs (already described), so making a distinction between them, other than to point out that Golgi tendon organs are located specifically in tendons or ligaments, is difficult to justify. The Pacini corpuscle has a characteristic microanatomy. The corpuscle is an ovoid encapsulated structure, 1 to 2 mm long and 0.5 to 1 mm in diameter. Within the capsule, concentric layers of modified elongated Schwann cells wrap around a central axon much like the successive layers of an onion, with the inner layers compacted and the outer ones

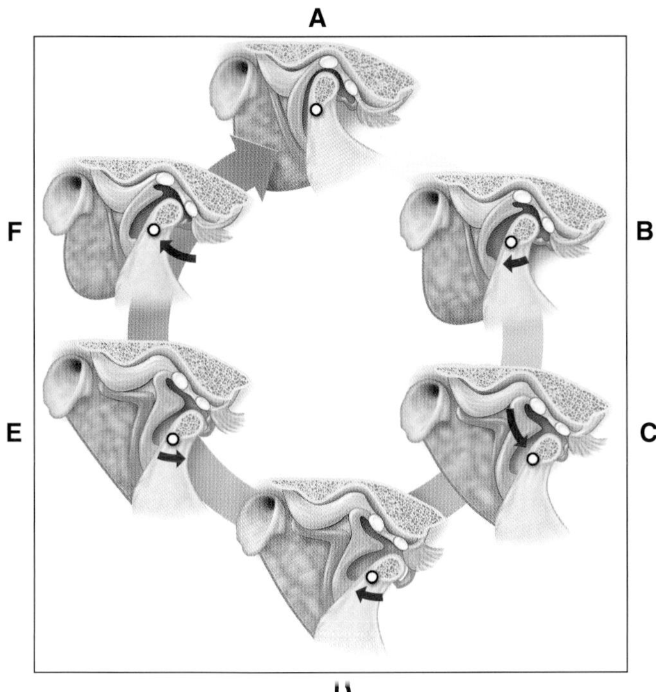

Fig. 13.29 Changing position of the mandible during opening and closing. (A–D) During opening. (E, F) During closing.

having wider connective tissue spaces between the cells. The corpuscle is adapted to register changes in pressure and vibration.

The TMJ is no different from other joints with respect to its innervation. Free nerve endings are the most abundant, with Ruffini, Golgi, and Pacini endings following in descending order. Generally, the anatomic and functional designations for each type of nerve ending, with its reflex role, are as listed in Table 13.1. However, neurophysiologic studies are limited in their ability to attribute single nerve discharges to specific endings. In particular, the role of free nerve endings is confusing because elsewhere in the body such endings are sensitive to thermal, mechanical, and noxious stimuli.

Regardless, a common pattern for innervation of the TMJ can be summarized as follows: Ruffini endings exist in clusters in the superficial layers of the joint capsule and are believed always to be active in every position of the joint (even when the joint is immobile) so that they signal static joint position, changes in intraarticular pressure, and the direction, amplitude, and velocity of joint movements. Pacini corpuscles are rapidly acting mechanoreceptors with a low threshold found mainly in the deeper layers of the capsule that signal joint acceleration and deceleration. Golgi tendon organs, limited as they are to the ligaments and sparsely distributed in the superficial layers of the lateral ligament, remain completely inactive in immobile joints, becoming active only when the joint is at the extremes of its range of movement. The distribution and significance of free nerve endings in joints usually are considered secondary to the roles of the other specialized receptors, yet they are the most commonly occurring terminal in a joint, are generally believed to be associated with nociception, and are distributed widely. Some debate has occurred as to whether free nerve endings occur in the disk of the TMJ and the synovial membrane. Immunocytochemical studies have shown that nerves do indeed occupy the periphery of the disk (see Fig. 13.18) and the synovial membrane.

Branches of the mandibular division of the fifth cranial nerve (i.e., the auriculotemporal, deep temporal, and masseteric) supply the afferent innervation to the joint.

TABLE 13.1 Anatomic and Functional Designations for Nerve Endings

Anatomic Designation	Functional Designation
Ruffini corpuscle	Posture (proprioception)—dynamic and static balance
Pacini corpuscle	Dynamic mechanoreception—movement accelerator
Golgi tendon organ	Static mechanoreception—protection (ligament)
Free nerve ending	Pain (nociception)—protection (joint)

BLOOD SUPPLY TO THE JOINT

The vascular supply to the TMJ comes from branches of the superficial temporal, deep auricular, anterior tympanic, and ascending pharyngeal arteries, all of which are branches of the external carotid artery.

RECOMMENDED READING

Dellow PG, Lund JP: Evidence for central timing of rhythmical mastication, *J Physiol (London)* 215:1–13, 1971.

Kolta A, et al.: Trigeminal motor system. In *Neuroscience and biobehavioral psychology*, Oxford, UK, 2017, Elsevier.

Morquette P, et al.: An astrocyte dependent mechanism for neuronal rhythmogenesis, *Nat Neurosci* 18:844–854, 2015.

Nozawa-Inoue K, et al.: Synovial membrane in the temporomandibular joint—its morphology, function and development, *Arch Histol Cytol* 66:289–306, 2003.

Schmolke C: The relationship between the temporomandibular joint capsule, articular disc and jaw muscles, *J Anat* 184:335–345, 1994.

Sessle BJ: Mechanisms of oral somatosensory and motor functions and their clinical correlates, *J Oral Rehab* 33:243–261, 2006.

14

Facial Growth and Development

Clarice Nishio, James K. Hartsfield Jr., and Antonio Nanci

OUTLINE

Growth of the face is a gradual and differential maturational process that takes many years and requires a succession of changes in regional proportions and relationships of various parts (Fig. 14.1). An understanding of the mechanisms of growth and development of the face is pertinent to dentistry in general and essential for the practice of dentistry. The objective of this chapter is to present an overall view of events occurring during craniofacial growth and development.

BASIC CONCEPTS OF FACIAL GROWTH

Two common but incorrect assumptions must be discarded before an understanding of facial growth is possible. The first is that various individual bones (e.g., mandible, maxilla, ethmoid, and sphenoid) enlarge simply by a symmetric expansion of the outer contours (Fig. 14.2). The second is that a bone grows by a combination of periosteal deposition on its outer surface and endosteal resorption on its inner surface. Beginning students often assume (incorrectly) that the bone of growing cortex must necessarily be produced by the periosteum. Actually, half or more of the compact bone tissue of the face and cranium is laid down by endosteum, the inner membrane lining the medullary cavity, and about half the periosteal surfaces of most bones in the face and neurocranium are resorptive (with about half depository) (Fig. 14.3). The reason is that remodeling is required to increase the size of any given bone. Here the term *remodeling* is intended in the dental context (see Enlow and Hans in Recommended Reading) as opposed to its use in bone biology (see Chapter 6; also see Roberts et al. in Recommended Reading).

Three essential processes bring about the growth and development of various cranial and facial bones: size increase, remodeling, and displacement. The first two are closely related and are produced simultaneously by a combination of bony resorption and deposition. The third (displacement) is a movement of all the bones away from each other at their articular junctions as each undergoes size increases. In clinical procedures, to control properly and thereby make use of the complex processes of growth, the following concepts must be fully and thoroughly understood.

Size Increases and Remodeling

As a bone enlarges and remodels, there is addition of new bone on one side and old bone resorption from the opposite side, leading to an overall repositioning of the bone in the direction of deposition. The composite of repositioning changes throughout the bone brings about its overall enlargement.

The term *growth center* is an area in which the tissue has an intrinsic tissue separating capacity and ability to grow in a primary fashion by itself (e.g., a synchondrosis). In contrast, a growth site is used to designate some area or part that responds to changes in growth/displacement of adjacent tissues (e.g., mandibular condyle and sutures).

All parts and areas of a bone and their covering membranes, however, participate directly in the growth sequence, regardless of whether they are specially designated. A mosaic of remodeling fields blankets all outside and inside surfaces of all individual bones (see Fig. 14.3), and these growth fields produce the enlargement of each bone. Although some changes in a given bone shape may be involved, the essential function of remodeling is to move the various parts of a bone to successively new locations (relocation) so that the whole bone can then enlarge (Figs. 14.4 and 14.5). Remodeling fields represent the morphogenetic activity of the enclosing periosteum, endosteum, and other soft tissues. Thus the entire bone is involved in the growth process, not just certain restricted growth sites or growth centers.

Displacement Process

As all the various muscles, epithelia, connective tissues, and other soft tissues of the head grow and expand, a separation effect occurs at the articular joints among the different bones, which are physically carried away from each other by masses of enlarging soft tissue. This process is termed *displacement,* and the bone's osteogenic membranes and cartilages are immediately triggered to respond by producing overall bone enlargement and remodeling. The displacement movements of the bones, in effect, create the space into which bones grow. Spaces as such never develop, of course, because displacement and subsequent bone growth are virtually simultaneous. When a functional and biomechanical equilibrium is attained between the soft tissues and the bones, the stimulus for skeletal growth ceases.

Thus, as stated, the mandible is continuously displaced in an anteroinferior direction but enlarges by equal amounts posteriorly and superiorly (Fig. 14.6). All the various bones of the nasomaxillary complex also become separated from each other at their various sutural junctions by displacement, and the sutural membranes (comparable

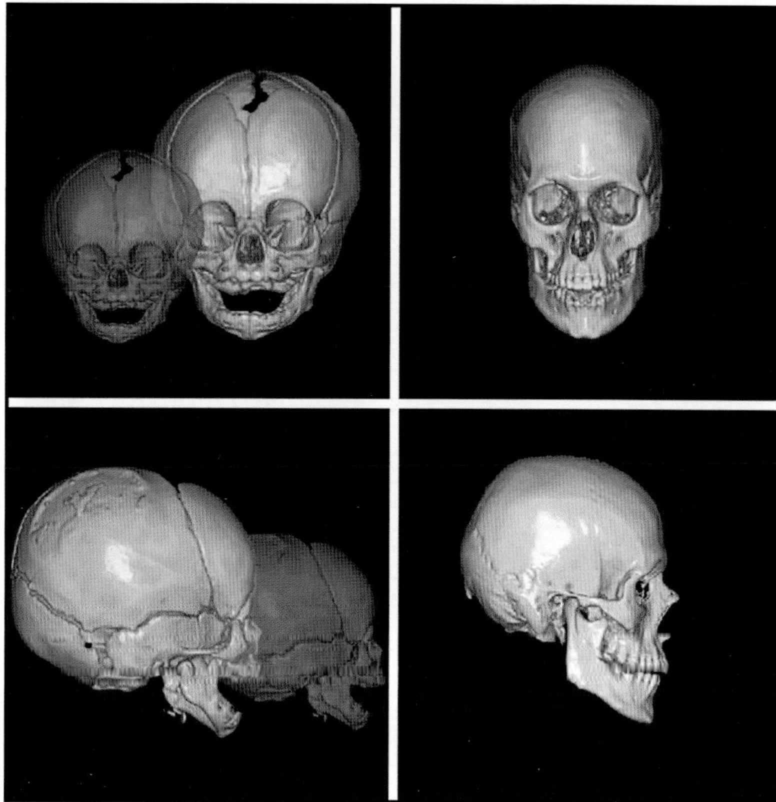

Fig. 14.1 Changes in craniofacial proportions between an infant (2 months; *left panels*) and an adult *(right panels)*. The skull at about birth has been enlarged to match the adult skull to illustrate the differences in form and proportions of craniofacial complex components. Note that the neurocranium in the infant is prominent, whereas the face predominates in the adult and represents a large part of the whole skull.

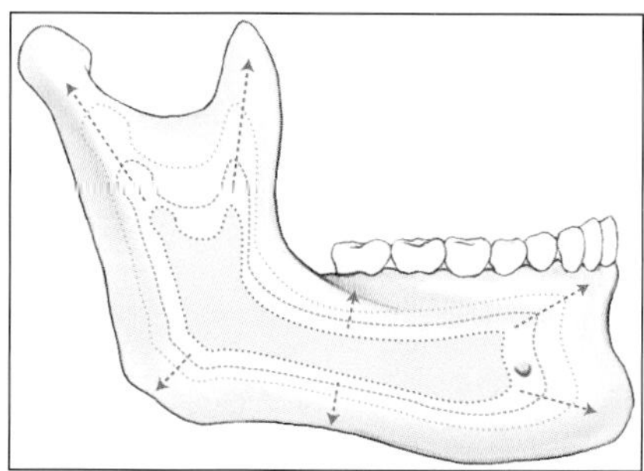

Fig. 14.2 Erroneous schema of bone growth. Bone does not simply grow by symmetric expansion. Rather, it undergoes a complex remodeling process throughout all its regions and parts. Compare with Fig. 14.3.

to periosteal membranes) deposit bone in an amount equal to that lost by the displacement separation.

MANDIBULAR CONDYLE AND GROWTH

In Chapter 13 the condylar cartilage was described as having, along with the remainder of the ramus, a special developmental role to accomplish: an adaptive function involved in the continued placement of the mandibular arch in juxtaposition with the maxillary arch and cranial base as they all grow to become an interrelated whole. Because the mandible articulates with the cranial base at one end (at the temporomandibular joints) and with the maxilla through tooth contact in the occlusal plane, its growth must be adaptable to the wide range of dimensional, anatomic, rotational, and developmental variations that occur in the nasomaxillary complex, dentition, and neurocranium. The ramus and its condyle have the capacity to provide for this developmental adaptability, within normal latitude, by varying the amount and direction of their growth to accommodate whatever nasomaxillary and dental height, length, and width exist during the changing course of growth. Similar variations occurring in the cranium are also accommodated.

The mandibular growth process involves a feedback mechanism. Continuously changing growth circumstances (e.g., physiologic changes, soft tissue increases, biomechanical forces, bioelectric alterations, neurologic changes, hormones, and possibly other factors) trigger the ramus and condyle to grow or stop growing in more or less upward and backward directions. This is an exceedingly important and fundamental growth function carried out by the condyle and the ramus as a whole.

A summary of the facial growth changes that have been discussed in this chapter appears in Fig. 14.7, which depicts the face and skull from 3 to 18 years of age.

FACIAL TYPES

There are three general head types: The dolichocephalic head is relatively narrow and long, the brachycephalic head is wider and rounder, and the mesocephalic head is the type between the dolichocephalic and brachycephalic with intermediate length and width dimensions (Fig. 14.8). Each type gives rise to corresponding general facial types. These facial types are the long and narrow (leptoprosopic), the round and broad (euryprosopic), and the intermediate (mesoprosopic).

Although many intermediate types of head forms and facial patterns exist in any general population, the dolichofacial and the brachyfacial skull configurations (see Fig. 14.8A and C) tend to be associated with

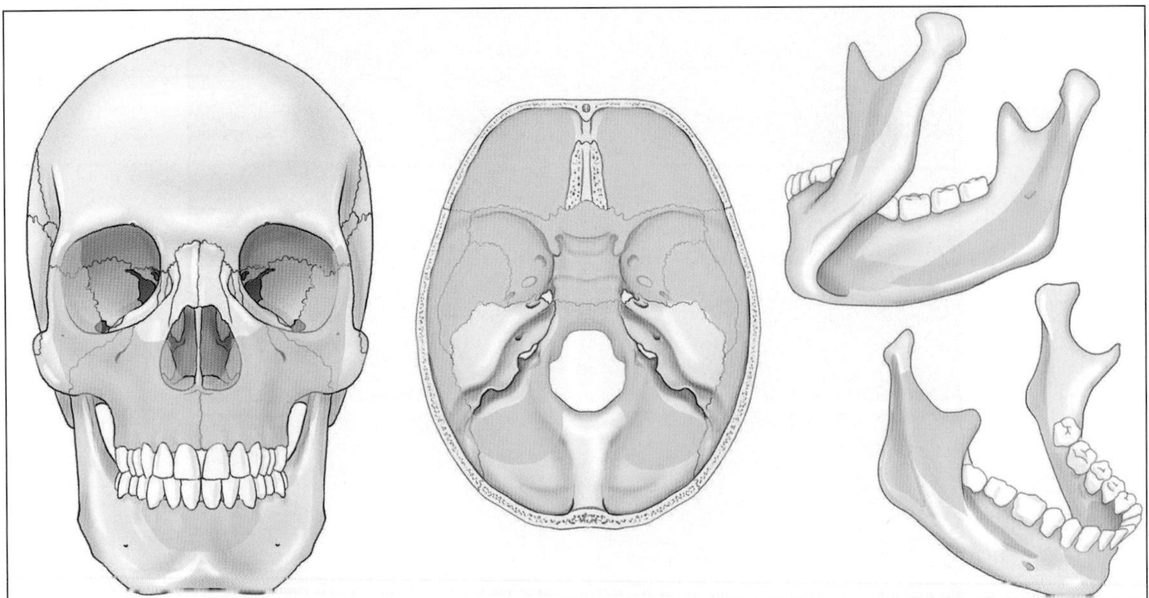

Fig. 14.3 Growth and remodeling fields. The entire facial and neurocranial skeleton is covered, inside and out, by a characteristic spread of regional growth and remodeling fields. Resorptive fields are shaded. Depository fields are free of shading.

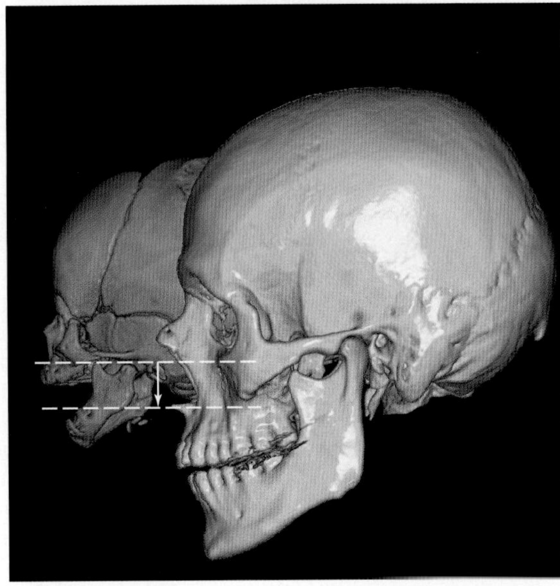

Fig. 14.4 Growth of the hard palate, illustrating the process of relocation and remodeling. In the infant (2 months old), the level of the hard palate is just slightly inferior to the level of the inferior orbital rim *(left)*. As the nasal cavities expand, the bony palate becomes relocated downward.

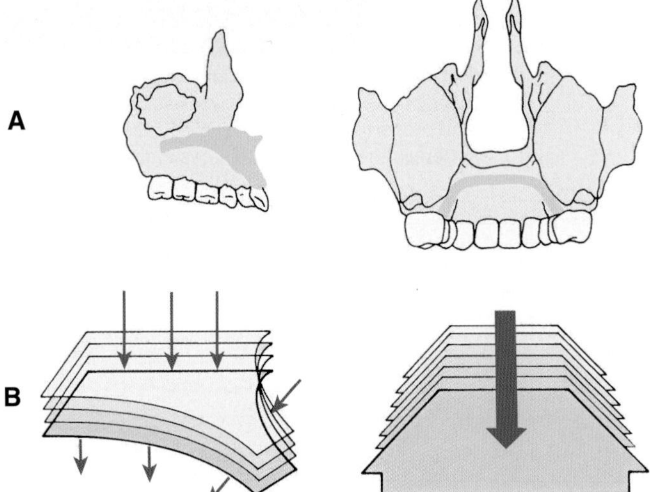

Fig. 14.5 Downward remodeling of the palate. (A) This is produced by deposition on the inferior-facing (oral) side and resorption from the superior-facing (nasal) side, thus bringing about a progressive and continuous inferior relocation of the whole palate and maxillary arch. (B) The maxillary teeth are moved downward at the same time by a process of vertical drift associated with remodeling (resorption and deposition) of alveolar bone. (From Proffit WR: *Contemporary orthodontics*, ed 4, St. Louis, MO, 2007, Mosby.)

characteristic facial features. The narrow facial type tends to have a convex profile with a prognathic maxilla and a retrognathic mandible. The forehead slopes because the forward growth of the upper part of the face carries the outer table of the frontal bone with it. A larger frontal sinus is characteristic of this facial type because of the greater separation of inner and outer bony tables of the forehead, whereas the inner table remains fixed to the dura of the frontal lobe of the cerebrum. The glabella and supraorbital rims are prominent, and the nasal bridge is high. There is a tendency toward an aquiline or Roman nose because the more prominent upper part of the nasal region induces a bending or curving of the nasal profile. Because the face is relatively narrow, the eyes appear close set, and the nose is correspondingly thin. The nose is also typically prominent and quite long, and its point has a tendency to tip downward. The lower lip and mandible are often set in a somewhat recessive position because the long dimension of the nasal chambers leads to a downward and backward rotational placement of the lower jaw (the dolichocephalic head type also has a more open cranial base flexure, which adds to the downward mandibular rotation). These factors contribute to a downward inclination of the occlusal plane and a marked curve of occlusion.

The round and broad facial type is characterized by a more upright and bulbous forehead, with the upper nasal part of the face less prominent than in the dolichocephalic face. The nasal chambers are horizontally shorter but wider, in contrast to the narrow but more prominent

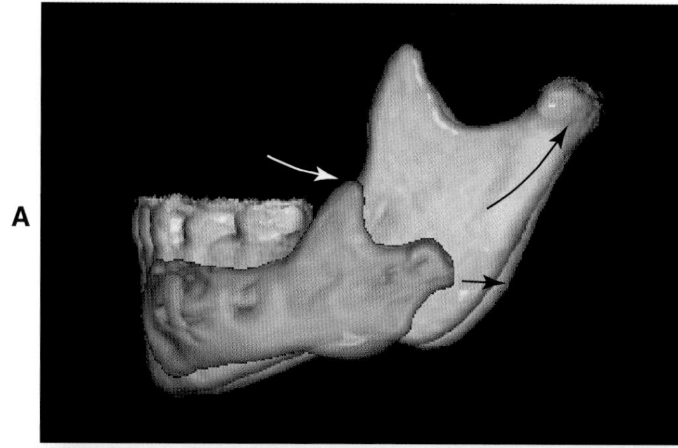

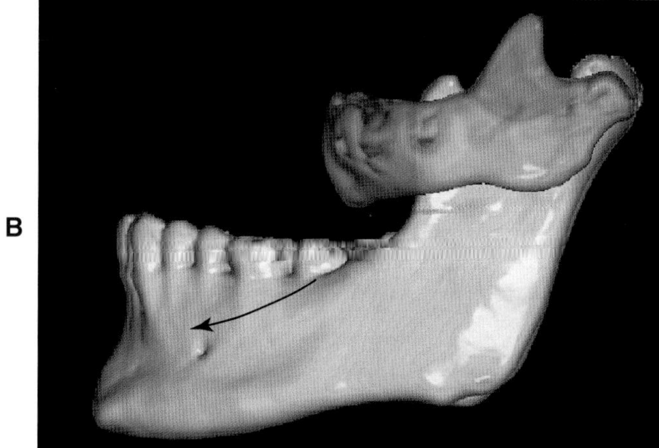

Fig. 14.6 Superimposed growth stages of the mandible from a child (5 years old) compared with that of an adult. (A) Remodeling of the infant mandible occurs by local combinations of resorption and deposition. This process relocates the ramus in posterior and superior directions and provides for a lengthening of the corpus. (B) During growth, the whole mandible undergoes an anterior and inferior displacement.

nasal region characterizing the dolichocephalic head form. The net capacity of the airway in both instances is thus equivalent. There is less protrusion by the supraorbital ridges, the glabella is less prominent, and the frontal sinus is smaller. The nose is shorter vertically as well as horizontally. The nasal bridge is lower, the nasal sides are broader, and the end of the nose often tips upward. The eyes appear widely set, and the zygomatic bones seem prominent because the nose and forehead are less prominent. The face appears quite flat and broad, in contrast to the more angular, narrower, deeper, and topographically bold appearance of the dolichocephalic face. The cranial base angle of the brachycephalic skull tends to be more closed, and there is a greater tendency toward an orthognathic (straight-jawed) profile.

FACIAL PROFILES

There are three basic types of facial profiles (Fig. 14.9): (A, in figure) the orthognathic profile or straight-jawed type; (B and C) the retrognathic profile or convex type, which has a retruding chin and is the most common one among white populations; and (D) the prognathic profile or concave type, which is characterized by a prominent lower jaw and chin.

To identify a person's profile type, imagine a line projecting horizontally from the orbit. Drop a perpendicular line from this, just brushing the surface of the upper lip. If the chin touches this vertical line, the profile is orthognathic; if it falls behind or ahead, the profile is retrognathic or prognathic. For a female face, the vertical line generally passes through the nose at a point about halfway along its upper slope. In male faces that are longer and narrower than females, however, the more marked extent of the upper nasal prominence is such that more of the nose sometimes lies forward of the vertical line.

People with a dolichocephalic head form (a characteristic feature of some white populations in northernmost and southernmost Europe, North Africa, and the Middle East) tend to have a retrognathic face. Those with a brachycephalic head form (a characteristic feature of Middle Europe and East Asia) have a greater tendency toward prognathism. Also, Asians commonly have a maxillary and mandibular dentoalveolar protrusion characterized by labial tipping of the maxillary incisors, resulting from a protrusive mandibular

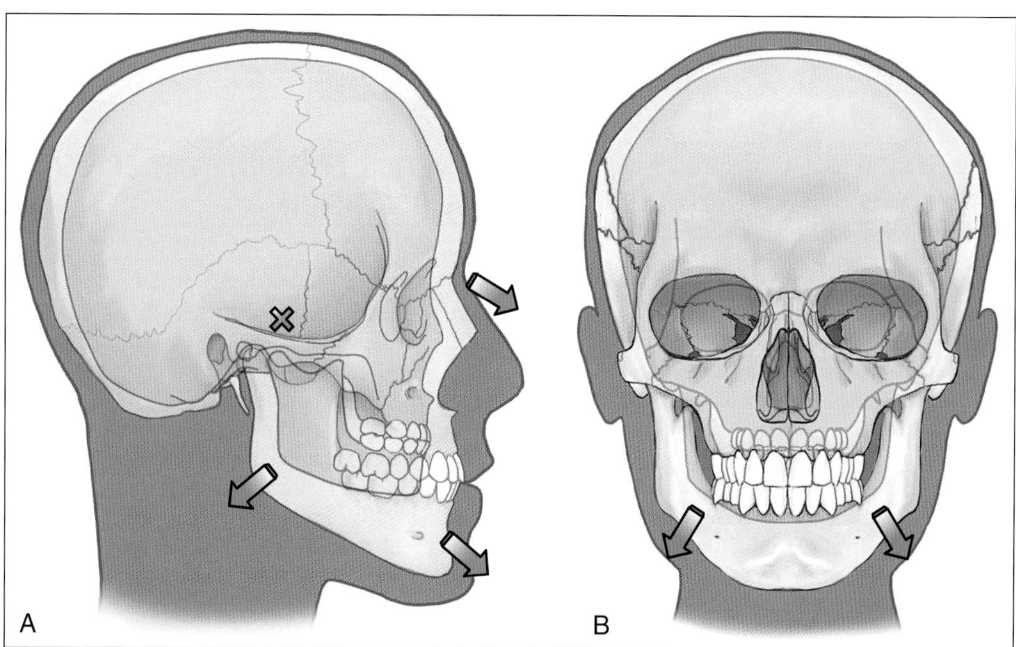

Fig. 14.7 Summary of postnatal growth and development from 3 to 18 years of age. (A) Lateral view. The location of the sella turcica is denoted by x. (B) Frontal view.

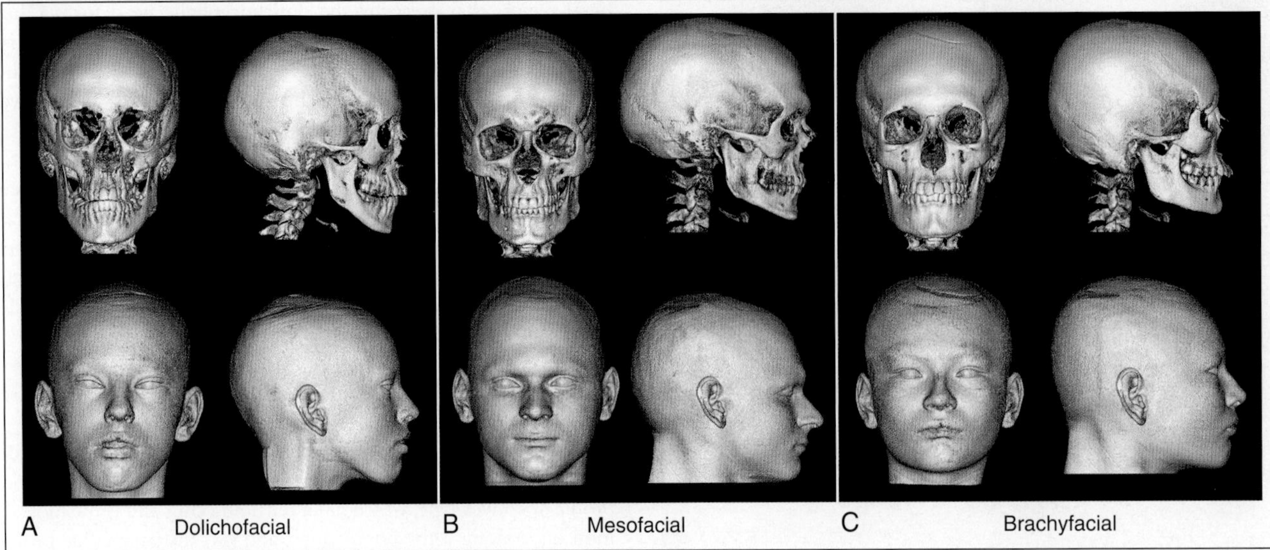

Fig. 14.8 Skeletal head types and the corresponding general facial patterns. (A) Dolichocephalic head gives rise to a narrow and long facial type. (B) Mesocephalic head presents a relatively proportional width and vertical facial pattern. (C) Brachycephalic head is associated with a more round and wider facial feature. (Courtesy D. Turgeon.)

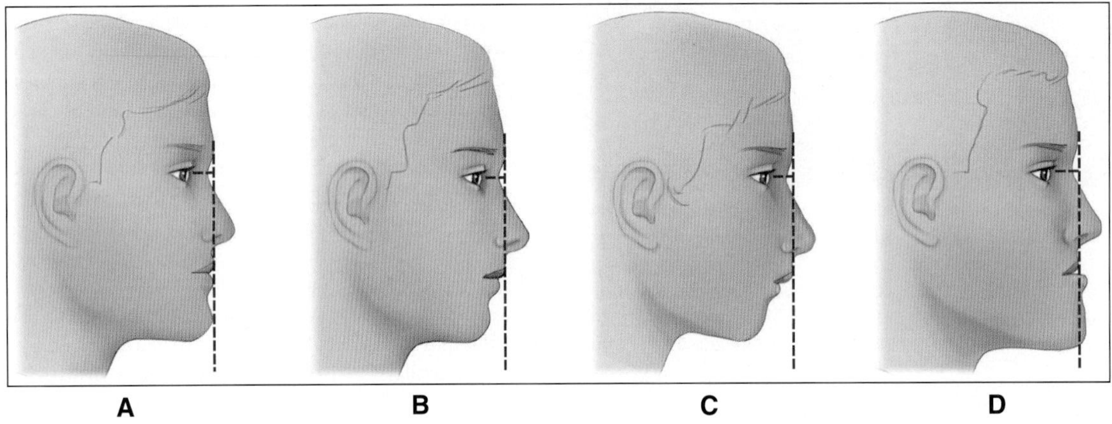

Fig. 14.9 (A) An orthognathic profile; the chin touches a vertical line along the upper lip perpendicular to the neutral orbital axis. (B) A slightly retrognathic profile; the chin tip falls several millimeters behind this line. (C) A severely retrognathic face; the chin is well behind the vertical line. The lower lip also is much less prominent. (D) A prognathic profile; the chin tip lies well forward of this vertical line.

dentition. Thus there are more malocclusions involving protruding maxillary teeth in some white populations and more malocclusions involving protruding mandibular teeth with dentoalveolar protrusion in Asian populations.

An important intrinsic developmental process of compensation functions to offset and reduce the anatomic effects of built-in tendencies toward malocclusions. A genetically predisposed retrognathic mandibular placement caused, for example, by some rotational factor in the cranial base can be compensated by the development of a broader mandibular ramus. Thus the whole mandible becomes longer and reduces the amount of retrognathism. Because latitude exists for compensatory adjustments, only a relatively slight degree of retrognathism, or some other anatomic imbalance, occurs in most persons (Fig. 14.10). For narrow-faced individuals, 3 to 4 mm of mandibular retrognathism (a mild malocclusion with some crowding of the incisors) is typical. A perfect occlusion is hardly to be considered normal because relatively minor dental arch or facial skeleton irregularities are almost universal. Only when the compensatory process fails do severe malocclusions occur.

GENETICS, ENVIRONMENT, EPIGENETICS, AND MALOCCLUSION

The exploration of how faces grow has changed over the years. While the initial facial growth theory placed an emphasis on genetics determining growth, the modern growth theory also explores how specific environmental and epigenetic factors interact with our DNA to affect growth and development (Fig. 14.11). The clinical importance of understanding how facial growth and development occur has long been founded on the belief that treatment should be based upon the etiology of the variation in growth and development, which gave rise to a malocclusion. However, it is now well appreciated that variations in how individuals respond to treatment are frequently based on a combination of genetic, environmental, and/or epigenetic factors. In this discussion we will refer to what we can see or measure about an individual as a phenotype (e.g., the presence of a diastema or the amount of facial convexity, respectively). In contrast, a specific genetic factor is termed a *genotype*, and the collective sum of all genotypes that make up an individual is called the *genome*.

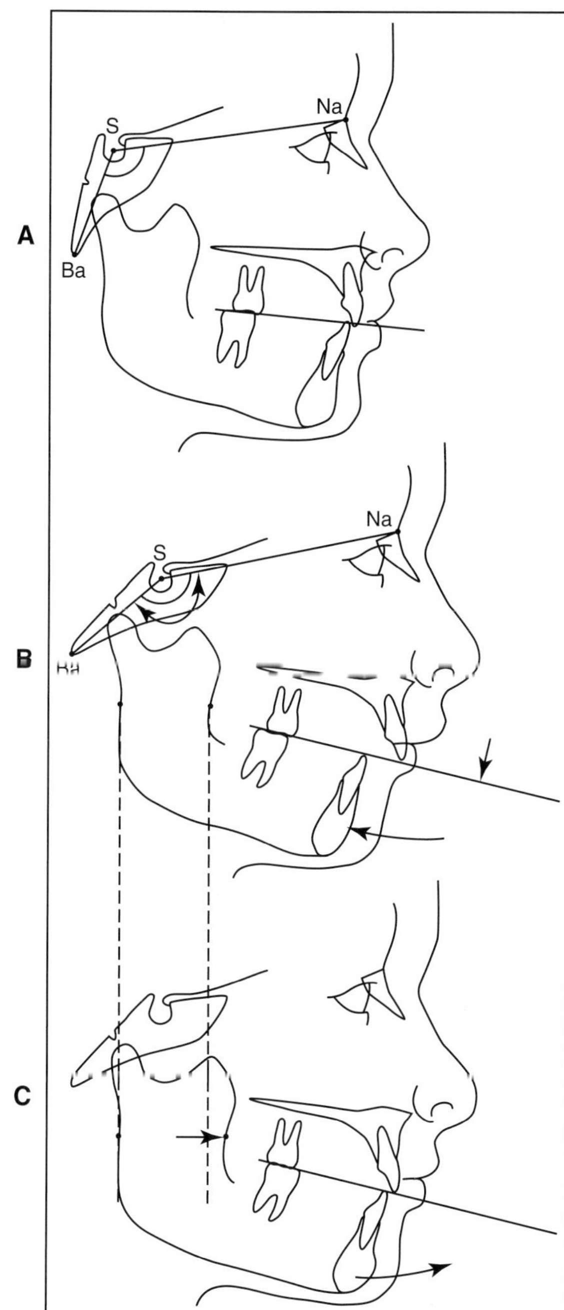

Fig. 14.10 Mandibular compensation (A) represents the normal mandible; the cranial base is open angled *(BaSNa)* and (B) has the anatomic effect of placing the mandible in a retrognathic position. Because the whole mandible is in a backward and downward position, the occlusal plane has a slight downward inclination. The retruding tendency of the mandible is often compensated during facial growth by the development of a wider ramus (C), thus placing the mandibular arch in a more forward position.

Although most of our somatic cells contain an identical copy of our genome, they differentiate into a wide variety of different cell types throughout the body, each with unique and highly specialized functions. This occurs due to the differentially regulated patterns of gene expression within individual cells or groups of cells. Specialized proteins (e.g., transcription factors) along with enzymes that can add or remove methyl groups on cytosine within the DNA backbone (e.g., DNA methylases and demethylases, respectively) and enzymes that add or remove methyl, acetyl, and/or other regulatory molecules on

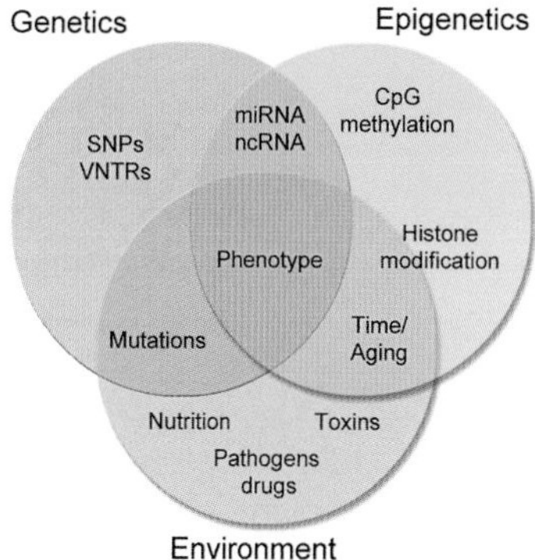

Fig. 14.11 Genetics, environment, and epigenetics. The DNA genetic sequence (including single nucleotide polymorphisms *[SNPs]* and variable number of tandem repeats *[VNTRs]),* environmental factors that can directly affect the DNA sequence (mutations) and epigenetic factors that can be affected by environmental factors over time and can then affect the use of the DNA sequence for gene expression ultimately into proteins are all components of growth and development. (Courtesy L.A. Morford, from Dwivedi RS, et al.: Beyond genetics: epigenetic code in chronic kidney disease, *Kidney Int* 79(1):23–32, 2011.)

the histone proteins, which help package the DNA (e.g., histone methyltransferases, histone acetyltransferases, histone demethylases, and histone deacetylases), work in a coordinated manner to modulate gene expression at the transcriptional level.

These forms of gene regulation impact the type, amount, location, and timing of gene transcription (i.e., the production of messenger RNA [mRNA]) and the corresponding protein production within each cell (Fig. 14.12). The overall impact on protein production may be programmed within the genome itself and can reflect changes caused by environmental influences (e.g., diet, stress, smoking). These changes may be transient or may be of a more permanent nature such that they could be inherited. RNA moieties (such as microRNA and long noncoding RNA) may also regulate gene expression at the posttranscriptional level by targeting the destruction of specific mRNA molecules when they are no longer needed (see Fig. 14.12).

The term *epigenetic regulation* is used to describe heritable changes to the chromatin (DNA packaged around histones) that directly influence how and when a gene is turned off or on, as well as the production of regulatory RNAs that posttranscriptionally help determine how long to make the corresponding protein from the mRNA copy of the gene. These types of regulation occur in the absence of any nucleotide changes within the DNA sequence and can be reversible. Hence it is our DNA code that provides the necessary instructions for how to make a protein (i.e., the recipe), and a person's epigenetic landscape helps determine what polypeptides (proteins) will be made, when they will be made, and where they will be made.

A trait is a particular aspect or characteristic of a phenotype. One example of a trait is mandibular prognathism (i.e., a longer than normal mandible), which is one subtype of the Angle Class III malocclusion. The way a trait is inherited is termed its *mode of inheritance.* There are two main types of genetic influence on the way traits are inherited: (1) Mendelian inheritance is monogenic and predominately involves a single gene with the possibility of other influencing genetic and environmental factors; (2) complex inheritance is when many genetic and environmental factors potentially interact though epigenetics. There are multiple mendelian modes of inheritance based on the effect of the variation(s) of a gene (referred to as *alleles*) located at a specific spot on a chromosome called a *locus.* The modes are referred to as *autosomal dominant, autosomal recessive, X-linked recessive,* and *X-linked dominant.* The nonrandom recognized association of more than one

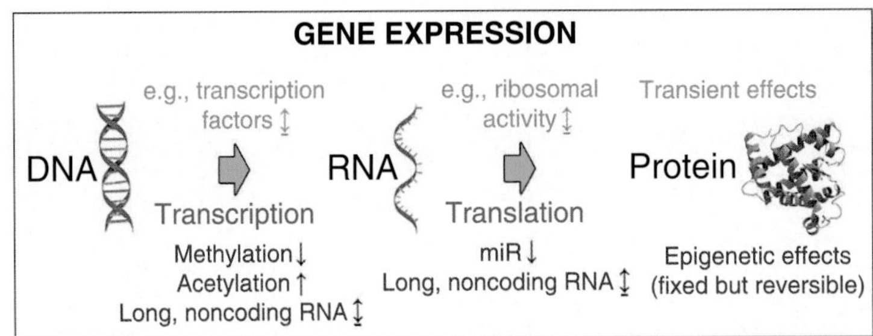

Fig. 14.12 Various factors acting upon gene regulation impact the type, amount, location, and timing of gene transcription (i.e., the production of messenger RNA) and the corresponding protein production within each cell. (Courtesy L.A. Morford.)

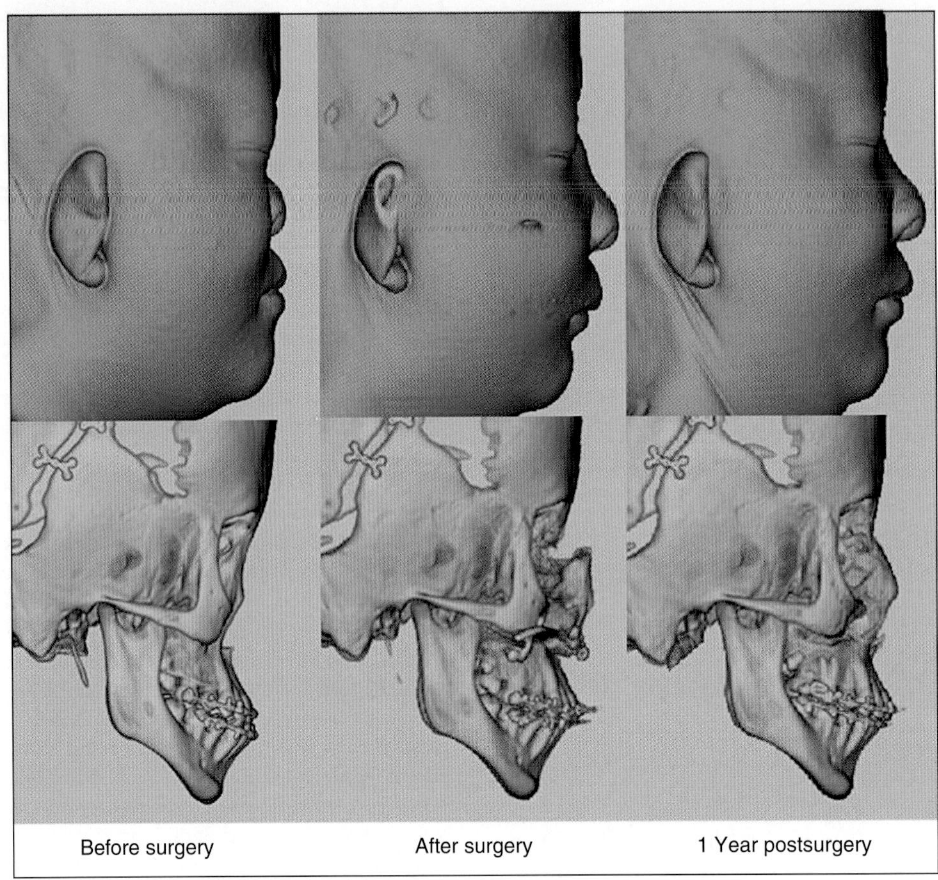

Fig. 14.13 Crouzon syndrome is a craniofacial dysostosis characterized by the early fusion of different cranial sutures. The orthognathic surgeries Le Fort I and II are treatment options to move the maxilla and midface forward to compensate the insufficient growth of the midface. (Courtesy E. Tanaka.)

trait is a syndrome, which may have a mendelian or complex mode of inheritance, or other etiology. Crouzon syndrome, for example, is a craniosynostosis syndrome with an autosomal dominant mode of inheritance (Fig. 14.13). Mandibular prognathism that is not part of a syndrome (i.e., nonsyndromic) has been observed in many families as a mendelian trait with an autosomal dominant mode of inheritance.

Even in families in which some members present mandibular prognathism as an autosomal dominant mode of inheritance, there may be a family member who has the same genotype as the affected family members but with no clinical sign of the prognathic mandible. This type of trait occurrence is called *incomplete penetrance.* Likewise, if there is some clinical sign of mandibular prognathism in another family member, it may be of a lesser or greater severity than the other family members, a situation in genetics referred to as *variable expressivity.* This variance in the phenotype even in the presence of the same genotype may be due to the interaction of other proteins during development and influenced by environmental/epigenetic factors.

While a mendelian mode of inheritance may be associated with developmental dental dysplasias, such as the types of amelogenesis imperfecta and with mandibular prognathism, most variation in facial growth is not inherited in a mendelian mode. For many craniofacial traits, the factor that influences facial growth in most people is not a protein generated from a single gene but rather the proteins that come from many genes and/or the environmental factors that influence the production of the proteins (i.e., gene expression). This highlights the principle that growth in general, including facial growth, is the result of the interactions of several genetic and environmental factors. Thus in most patients their facial growth is a complex trait.

Even if a patient's craniofacial growth is influenced heavily by one gene (i.e., monogenic in familial skeletal Angle Class III) as opposed to multiple genetic factors, there is no guarantee that future growth will necessarily or absolutely be predetermined, and therefore it cannot be absolutely predicted. Nor does it mean that growth will proceed on a particular immutable track, although traits with a monogenic influence may be less amenable to environmental (treatment) intervention than traits influenced by multiple genes, unless a specific gene or protein therapy can be applied sufficiently early in growth and development to change the expected outcome.

Sometimes various facial and dental arch traits are said to be highly or largely genetic, implying that their size, shape, and/or relationships are determined by genetic factors and would be difficult to change. This presumption is often based on the inappropriate interpretation of heritability (h^2) estimates. Analyses comparing the variation in a quantitative trait among individuals who are related (e.g., twins or nontwin siblings), to the degree to which the individuals share the same genetic background, are heritability studies. Heritability estimates range from 0 to 1. A trait with a heritability estimate of 1 would be expressed with complete positive correlation to the genes in common (i.e., no correlation with environmental factors), whereas a heritability estimate of 0 would be expressed with no correlation to the proportion of genes in common. Heritability estimates have been used to estimate the relative influence of additive genetic factors versus environmental factors on a quantitative trait. They do not measure the interaction of genetic and environmental/epigenetic factors.

Furthermore, heritability studies can only estimate the proportion of the total phenotypic variation for a quantitative trait that can be attributed to genetic differences between individuals within the specific sample being examined up to the time of the analysis. Heritability estimates reflect clinical variation correlated with the proportion of genes in common and are not a measure of specific genes or proteins themselves. Thus as environmental factors can vary, estimates of heritability may change with time, and they do not necessarily relate to one individual in the sample being studied. Heritability studies do not determine the type of genetic influences or their mode of inheritance (i.e., whether the trait is a single gene [monogenic] trait or a complex trait with the effects of multiple genetic and environmental factors). Therefore they cannot predict how easily a quantitative trait may be changed or the likelihood of the change being permanent.

When growth and development is outside of what is considered the normal range of variation, and treatment is indicated, there may be one or more options that will help most patients. However, the usual treatment protocol(s) are sometimes not as effective in some patients as they are in most. In addition, some patients may have an adverse reaction to medication(s) or other therapies. The concept of personalized medicine (precision medicine) refers to the tailoring of treatment and disease prevention to the individual characteristics of each patient. This tailoring may consider differences in people's lifestyle, environment, genetics, and epigenetics to classify individuals into subpopulations that differ in their susceptibility to a particular disease and/or their response to a specific treatment. Research involving genetic association, family linkage, whole exome sequencing, and whole genome sequencing investigations into the genetic, environmental, and epigenetic factors that interact in facial growth and development, especially where the mode of inheritance appears to be mendelian, is ongoing to determine how these data may contribute to precision treatment in the future in oral and, indeed, general health.

The polygenic systems have the capacity to protect developmental processes against potential hostile environmental influence. However, when a substitution of deleterious genes decreases this protection beyond the level where environmental factors can be counterbalanced, a skeletal developmental defect is developed, such as cleft lip and palate, a facial asymmetry, or syndromes. The developmental disruption between the genetic-environmental interactions may not only cause craniofacial abnormalities but also play an important role in the regulation of maxillary, mandibular, and tooth morphologies.

CURVE OF OCCLUSION

Because of the notably long vertical human face, there is a tendency for the mandible and occlusal plane to have a downward- and backward-rotated position. This rotational alignment would produce an anterior open bite except for a compensatory action on the part of the dentition (Figs. 14.14, 14.15, and 14.16). The mandibular incisors and their

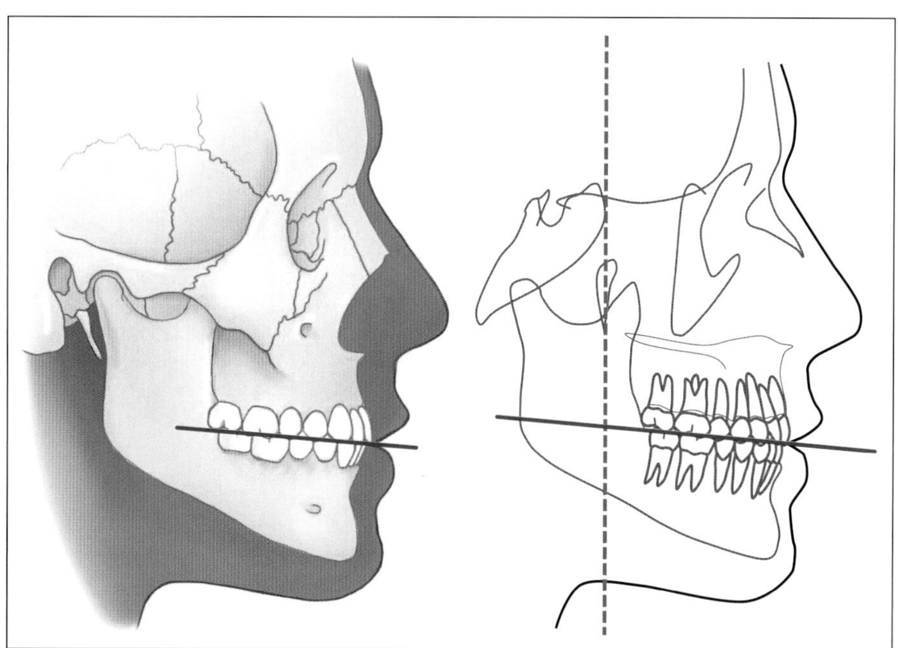

Fig. 14.14 Perfectly balanced craniofacial composite. The occlusal plane is approximately perpendicular to the maxillary tuberosity. It is rotated neither upward nor downward to any marked extent and is approximately parallel to the neutral orbital axis. In most faces, some degree of occlusal plane rotation occurs. (Courtesy E. Tanaka.)

alveolar sockets undergo additional upward drift, which closes the occlusion in the incisor region. The occlusal plane has a characteristic curve as a result that tends to be relatively marked according to the downward rotation of the mandible produced by vertical growth of the nasomaxillary region. As the mandibular anterior teeth undergo this vertical drifting process, their axial inclinations shift to a more upright alignment, which continues until they come into occlusion with the upright-oriented maxillary teeth. Incisor alignment contrasts with alignment of the mandibular posterior teeth, which tend to be inclined slightly anterior because of the downward mandibular rotation.

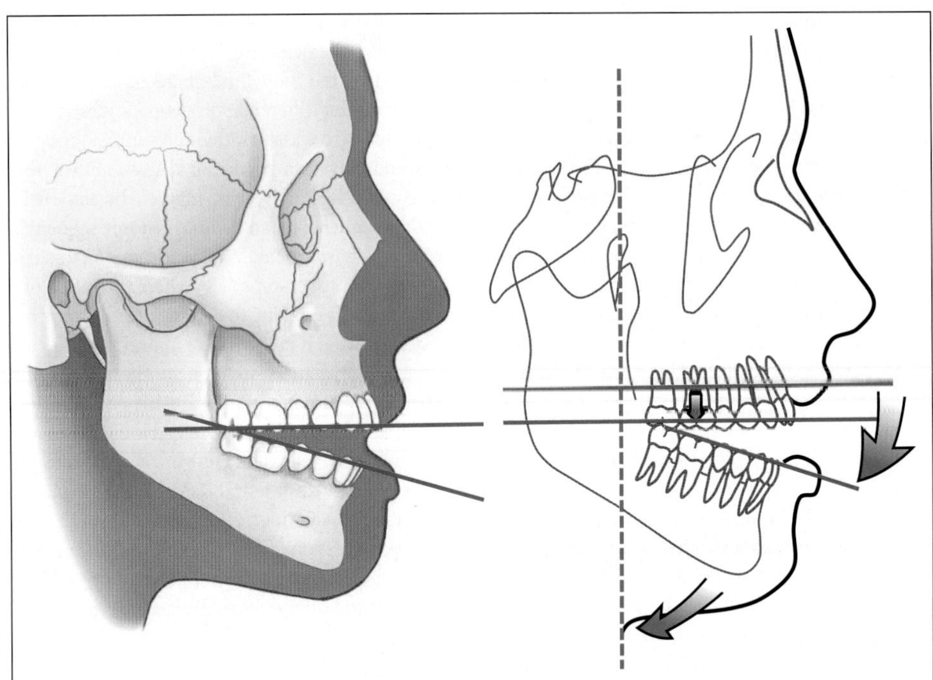

Fig. 14.15 Lowered maxillary arch resulting in a downward and backward alignment of the mandible. Note also the retrusion of the chin and lower incisors. This, in part, is the anatomic basis for a Class II malocclusion among persons having a long, narrow head form. (An open cranial base angle has the same effect and adds to the extent of the mandibular retrognathism.) (Courtesy E. Tanaka.)

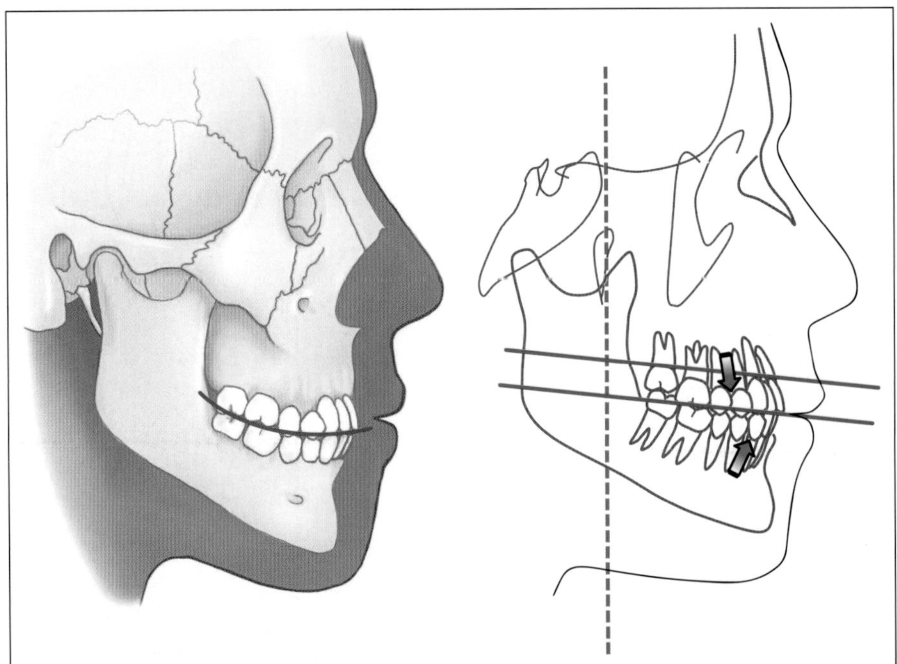

Fig. 14.16 Dental compensations precluding an anterior open bite as a consequence of the mandibular rotation seen in Fig. 14.15. The anterior mandibular teeth drift vertically in a superior direction, the anterior maxillary teeth drift inferiorly, and the result (commonly encountered) is the curve of occlusion. (Courtesy E. Tanaka.)

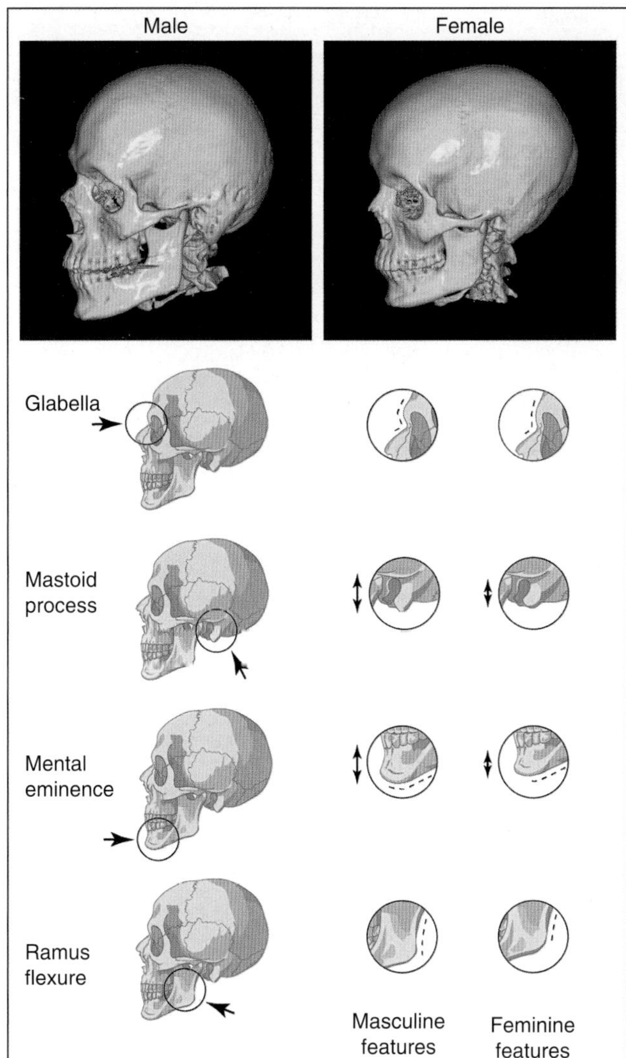

Fig. 14.17 Comparison of male and female craniofacial features. Relative to female crania, male crania are generally characterized by greater robusticity, massive glabellar prominence that forms a rounded and well-developed projection commonly associated with prominent supraorbital ridges and a larger mastoid process that projects downward. The male mandible also generally exhibits a massive mental eminence and a relative flexure of the posterior border of the ramus.

MALE AND FEMALE FACES

Until about 12 years of age, male and female faces are essentially comparable. Shortly after puberty, the female face has attained most of its size and structural maturity, and growth ceases. Growth and development of the male facial complex, however, continue into the early 20s, bringing about noticeable differences between male and female faces (Fig. 14.17).

Male and female faces, irrespective of the narrow or broad type, have a composite of key topographic characteristics. On a scale from extreme masculine to extreme feminine, most individuals usually have intermediate features. In general, however, the male face tends to be noticeably more protuberant and more knobby, bulky, or coarse. Female faces tend to be flatter, more delicate, and less bumpy.

The characteristically larger nose of the male face creates several related facial differences. The whole nasal region is larger because of the requirement for a greater airway capacity. Thus the relatively wide and long male nose contrasts with the thinner and less prominent female nose. The hard palate forms the floor of the nasal cavity and the roof of the oral cavity. When the upper skeletal part of the nasal region becomes markedly prominent, a constraint is imposed on the lower part of the nasal skeleton by the palate and maxillary arch (i.e., the upper part of the nose can become so prominent that the nasal profile necessarily bends to give a resultant aquiline or Roman nose configuration). Alternatively, upper nasal prominence can produce a rotation of the whole nasal profile into a distinctively more vertical alignment. In this classic male Greek nasal configuration, the nasal profile drops nearly straight down from the prominent forehead. There is a great deal of ethnic variation in nasal shapes; in some population groups an aquiline configuration, for example, is as common among females as males. Generally, however, the smaller, thinner female nose tends to have a concave-to-straight profile, whereas the male nose has a tendency toward a straight-to-convex profile.

A major difference exists between the sexes in the forehead. In females the supraorbital ridges lie on or very near the same vertical plane as the inferior orbital rims and cheekbones. There are usually no more than a few millimeters of supraorbital overhang in the female face. The female cheekbones therefore tend to appear more prominent, which is especially noticeable in a 45-degree view of the face (see Fig. 14.17). The entire midfacial region, including the upper jaw, also seems more prominent in female faces. The outer bony plate of the forehead in males, because of the greater nasal prominence, is carried forward. The result is a sloping forehead with large frontal sinuses and a supraorbital and glabellar overhang. Because of the more massive extent of both nasal and supraorbital skeleton in males, the zygomatic bones appear less prominent, as does the whole upper jaw. Despite such basic sex differences in the face, recall that there are similar facial differences between long and broad head form types as well.

AGE-RELATED CHANGES

Fig. 14.18 depicts the age-related changes of the skeletal and soft tissue that the human face goes through with time. An infant's face is relatively round and wide because lateral facial growth occurs earlier and to a greater extent than vertical growth. With increasing age and body size, however, vertical facial enlargement exceeds lateral facial growth as the nasal chambers progressively expand inferiorly to provide an increased airway for the enlarging lungs. A baby's face also appears rather flat because the nose is small relative to the broad but short face. Because forward growth of the face has not yet occurred, the forehead is upright and bulbous. Buccal and labial fat pads give a full appearance to the cheeks. Brachycephalic adults usually have a rather juvenile facial character compared with the relatively angular and topographically bolder adult dolichocephalic face. If an adult round face tends toward obesity, thus presenting a fat-padded face, the youthful parallel is augmented. Subcutaneous adipose tissue also tends to smooth out any age wrinkles, which further adds to the illusion of youth. Any marked loss of facial adiposity exaggerates an aged appearance because of consequent skin wrinkling.

The firm, turgid, velvety skin of youth becomes progressively more open pored, leathery, spotted, crinkled, and flabby with advancing age. Overexposure to the sun greatly hastens some of these changes. In middle age the skin begins to sag and droop noticeably because the hypodermis becomes less firmly anchored to the underlying facial muscles and bone. This sag may be the result of weight loss, but biochemical and physical alterations in the connective tissue of the dermis and hypodermis also exert an effect. There is a diminished flexibility of component fibers with a marked decrease in the content of water-bound proteoglycans. The latter results in widespread subcutaneous dehydration, contributing significantly to shrunken facial volume and consequent skin surplus. These

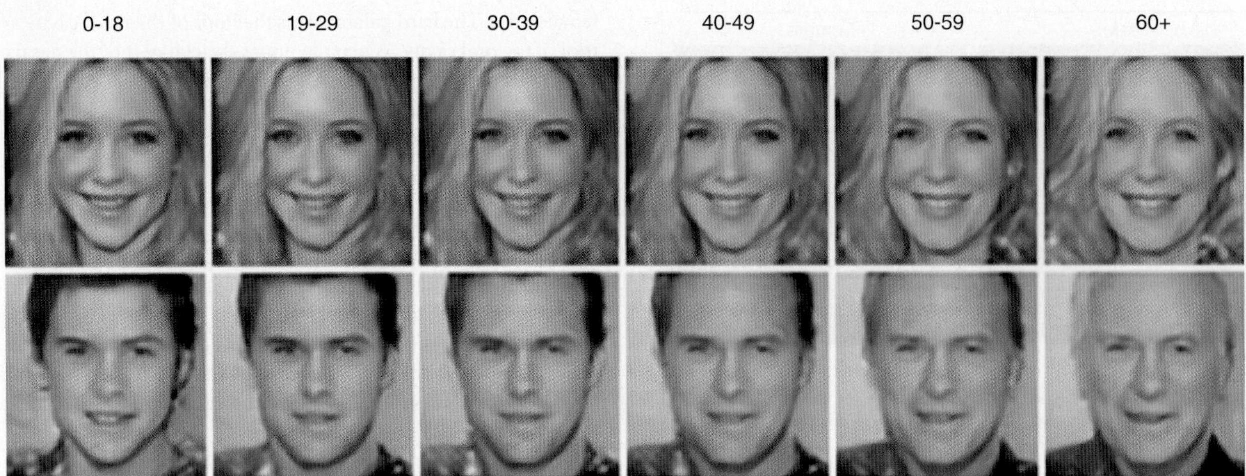

Fig. 14.18 Age-related facial changes. (From Antipov G, et al.: Face aging with conditional generative adversarial networks. In *2017 IEEE international conference on image processing*, Beijing, China, 2017, IEEE, pp 2089–2093.)

factors, in turn, lead to the onset of facial lines and wrinkles, sunken eyes, drooping bags, and suborbital creases.

Facial lines and furrows appear in characteristic locations. One of the first to appear, which is associated with middle age, is the nasolabial furrow (extending down along the sides of the nasal alae lateral to the corners of the mouth) called a *smile line.* This is seen at any age when a face grins, but it becomes a permanent integumental mark during the late 30s or early 40s. In individuals who look younger than their years, the onset of these and other telltale lines may be delayed or are at least less noticeable. Other permanent lines that appear with advancing age include forehead furrows, suborbital creases, crow's feet at the lateral corners of the eyes, vertical corrugations over the glabella and on the upper lip, lines extending down from the corners of the mouth on both sides of the chin, bags below the cheekbones, and jowls along the sides of the mandible. In advanced old age, the face can become an expansive carpet of noble ripples and may be characterized by a decrease in the vertical dimension resulting from loss of teeth.

RECOMMENDED READING

Enlow DH, Hans MG: *Essentials of facial growth*, Philadelphia, PA, 1996, Saunders.

Hartsfield Jr JK, et al.: Precision orthodontics, limitations and possibilities in practice. In *Biological mechanisms of tooth movement*, ed 3, Hoboken, NJ, 2021, John Wiley & Sons Ltd.

Krishnan V, et al.: *Biological mechanisms of tooth movement*, ed 3, Hoboken, NJ, 2021, John Wiley & Sons Ltd, pp 189–198.

Richmond S, et al.: Facial genetics: a brief overview, *Front Genet* 9:462, 2018.

Roberts WE, et al.: Remodeling of mineralized tissues, part II: control and pathophysiology, *Semin Orthod* 12:238–253, 2006.

Roberts WE, et al.: Remodeling of mineralized tissues, part I: the Frost legacy, *Semin Orthod* 12:216–237, 2006.

INDEX

Page numbers followed by "*f*" indicate figures, "*t*" indicate tables, and "*b*" indicate boxes.